Van Mildert College

from the 1st author.

Dec. 1992

D1826736

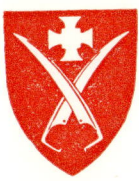

Work-Related Lung Disorders

To J. C. Gilson

Work-Related Lung Disorders

J. E. COTES

DM, FRCP, FFOM
*Reader, University Department
of Occupational Health and Hygiene
External scientific staff of
Medical Research Council
Honorary Consultant Physician
Newcastle upon Tyne*

J. STEEL

PhD, Dip.Occ.Hyg., FIOH, FFOM
*Senior Lecturer in Occupational Hygiene
University of Newcastle upon Tyne*

in collaboration with

G. L. LEATHART

MD, FRCP, DIH, FFOM
*formerly Senior Lecturer
in Occupational Health and
Honorary Consultant Physician
Newcastle upon Tyne*

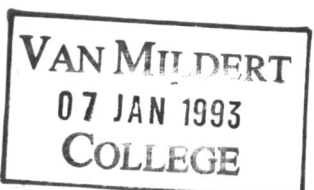
OXFORD

Blackwell Scientific Publications

LONDON EDINBURGH BOSTON

MELBOURNE PARIS BERLIN VIENNA

© 1987 by
Blackwell Scientific Publications
Editorial Offices:
Osney Mead, Oxford OX2 0EL
25 John Street, London WC1N 2BL
23 Ainslie Place, Edinburgh EH3 6AJ
3 Cambridge Center, Suite 208
    Cambridge, Massachusetts 02142, USA
54 University Street, Carlton
    Victoria 3053, Australia

First published 1987
Reprinted 1990

Set by Katerprint Typesetting Services
Printed in Great Britain by
William Clowes Ltd, Beccles, Suffolk

DISTRIBUTORS
Marston Book Services Ltd
PO Box 87
Oxford OX2 0DT
(*Orders*: Tel: 0865 791155
          Fax: 0865 791927
          Telex: 837515)
USA
Year Book Medical Publishers
35 East Wacker Drive
Chicago, Illinois 60601
(*Orders*: Tel: (312) 726-9733)
Canada
The C.V. Mosby Company
5240 Finch Avenue East
Scarborough, Ontario
(*Orders*: Tel: (416) 298-1588)
Australia
Blackwell Scientific Publications
(Australia) Pty Ltd
54 University Street
Carlton, Victoria 3053
(*Orders*: Tel: (03) 347-0300)

British Library
Cataloguing in Publication Data

Cotes, J.E.
    Work-related lung disorders.
    1. Lungs—Diseases 2. Lungs—Dust
    diseases 3. Occupational diseases
    I. Title II. Steel, J. III. Leathart, G.L.
    616.2′4   RC756

    ISBN 0 632 01511 X

Contents

Preface

The lung is a robust organ. Each day it is expanded at least twenty thousand times and humidifies, cleans and exchanges gas with $10\ m^3$ to $30\ m^3$ of air. Despite this exposure the lung usually continues to function efficiently into old age. The risk of it not doing so is greatest for cigarette smokers and those whose work brings them in contact with polluted atmospheres. Where pollution is a problem the practice of occupational hygiene should reduce the exposure to a level at which the body's defences can cope or where the risk to the exposed person is not unacceptable. The pollutant may be a particulate of mineral or biological origin, a vapour, a gas or a mixture of all three. In addition the lung may be harmed by an inclement physical environment.

As a result of exposure the lung is the organ most vulnerable to occupational disorders; these can be prevented but seldom cured. The prime responsibility for prevention lies with the occupational physician, the hygienist and the safety engineer. If symptoms develop the patient's first contact is usually with the general practitioner and chest physician who will often make the diagnosis, conduct the clinical management including rehabilitation and give advice on eligibility for compensation. This book provides a guide for all these persons, and for others, including postgraduate students, epidemiologists and research workers needing an overall view of occupational lung disorders.

Here are descriptions of the techniques of environmental monitoring and control and of chest radiology, lung physiology, epidemiology and the other components of occupational respiratory surveys. All the occupational respiratory disorders are described including those associated with high altitude and hyperbaric conditions. Prevention, clinical management and aspects of compensation are reviewed and the whole is set in the context of historical evolution of the subject: this is reflected in the occupational health and safety legislation of the U.K. and the U.S.A.

Publication comes at a time when occupational respiratory medicine is in transition. Pneumoconiosis of coal workers is becoming a rare disease, asbestosis is on the decline, and whilst mesothelioma is now affecting many previously exposed persons the recent epidemic of asbestos-related diseases is past its peak. Measures to control beryllium disease, farmers' lung and some other occupational respiratory diseases also show evidence of success. By contrast the occupational components of asthma, chronic bronchitis, emphysema, alveolitis and lung cancer persist and are incompletely understood; some research is proceeding but in the U.K. the Medical Research Council is reducing its support and there has not been a compensating increase in funding from employers' organizations, trades unions or other bodies such as the Department of Employment or the European Economic Community. Sadly, in all instances, the excuse is short-term expediency but the need for prevention, good clinical management and understanding basic mechanisms requires that research should proceed. This book provides some of the tools and contains suggestions as to where they should be applied. The book also looks to the past to describe conditions which fortunately are now rare and to learn from earlier mistakes. To this end there are full accounts of diseases in decline with illustrative cases which have been chosen for their completeness. The cases are of particular value because due to passage of time and associated decay the material evidence is now scarce. A little of what is left is preserved in these pages.

These considerations justify a new book which in many respects complements Parkes' *Occupational Lung Disorders*. Here is a new theoretical text and practical handbook for persons concerned with lung disorders of occupations. The contributors will have succeeded in their task if the book proves to be a useful guide.

Acknowledgements

The stimulus for this book came from the first author's experience at the MRC Pneumoconiosis Unit (now sadly closed), from preparing commissioned posters for a European Symposium on occupational lung disorders and from moving, without premeditation, from a research unit to a university department. Here, Dr. John Steel wrote the chapter on environmental monitoring. All chapters went out to referees; most were also read by Dr. J.C. Gilson and by Dr. G.L. Leathart who subjected them to detailed scrutiny. The illustrative cases included many from Dr. J.E.M. Hutchinson. These supplemented cases seen in the course of medical practice. Additional cases came via Dr. T. Ashcroft, Dr. A.E. Cockcroft, Dr. G.L. Leathart, Dr. K. McConnochie, Dr. S.J. Pearce and others whose help is indicated in the captions. Drs. A. Bundgaard (Copenhagen), D.J. Hendrick (Newcastle), A.W. Jones (Manchester) and K.B. Robinson (Durham) also contributed material. Access to chest radiographs was by courtesy of MRC Pneumoconiosis Unit, Pneumoconiosis Medical Panels in Newcastle (Dr. J.E.M. Hutchinson) and Cardiff (Dr. D.J. Jones) and National Health Service. The pathological specimens were prepared for the Pneumoconiosis Medical Panels or came from the collections of Dr. T. Ashcroft, Dr. R.M.E. Seal and Dr. J.C. Wagner. The authors of diagrams are acknowledged in the captions which also indicate the source. The ownerships of copyrights are brought together opposite. Mr. R.T. Harris, formerly of MRC Pneumoconiosis Unit, undertook the photography and Mr. F.M. Clay prepared the line illustrations. References were scrutinized by Mrs. J. Thompson and M. Brown. The text was prepared by Mrs. M.E. Hyam who also read the proofs. Many of the latter were also scrutinized by Dr. G.L. Leathart, Dr. J. Steel and Dr. S.J. Pearce. The printing was overseen by Messrs J.L. Robson and E. Wates, and the publication by Mr. Per Saugman, of Blackwell Scientific Publications. The indexes were prepared by Mrs. E. Passe and Mrs. K. Ollerenshaw.

The book is a collaborative venture to which many persons have contributed. To all of them I am grateful, as I am to the individuals and publishing companies who kindly allowed the reproduction of material for which they hold the copyright. In this respect as in the preparation of the text a strenuous attempt has been made to achieve accuracy and completeness. However, some lapses are inevitable and for all of these I both accept responsibility and ask indulgence. A letter pointing out any error or omission would be welcomed.

J.E. Cotes

Chapter Referees

Place names are of universities; numbers refer to chapters; other referees are named in the text.
Dr. T. Ashcroft, *Newcastle* (10)
Mr. G. Berry, *Sydney* (6)
Dr. G. Bird, *Newcastle* (15)
Professor P.G. Blain, *Newcastle* (13)
Dr. P.S. Burge, *Birmingham* (16)
Dr. A.E. Cockcroft, *London* (5 and 9)
Dr. K.J. Collins, *London* (7)
Dr. M.R. Cross, *Newcastle* (7)
Dr. F.M. El-Gamal, *Alexandria* (6 and 8)
Dr. E.M. Gillanders, *Employment Medical Advisory Service* (1)
Mr. T.G.E. Gillanders, *British Shipbuilders* (2 and 3)
Professor A. Harris, *Newcastle* (12)
Dr. R.M. Harrison, *Newcastle* (12)
Jr. J.E.M. Hutchinson, *Pneumoconiosis Medical Panel* (1)
Dr. S. Kagamimori, *Toyama* (1)

Professor G. Kazantzis, *London* (12)
Professor W.R. Lee, *Manchester* (14)
Professor R.I. McCallum, *Newcastle* (7)
Miss V. J. Male, *Northern Regional Health Authority* (6)
Dr. P.D. Oldham, *MRC Pneumoconiosis Unit* (6)
Dr. S.J. Pearce, *Dryburn Hospital, Durham* (19)
Mr. G.H. Pigott, *I.C.I.* (4)
Dr. F.S. Preston, *British Airways* (7)
Dr. J.W. Reed, *Newcastle* (18)
Professor R.S.F. Schilling, *London* (14)
Professor H. Weill, *New Orleans* (1)
Professor J.G. Widdicombe, *London* (4)
Dr. J.F. Wollaston, *Occupational Health and Safety Service* (1)

Sources of copyright material

Academic Press, New York
Acta Crystallographica (International Union of Crystallography)
American Conference of Governmental Industrial Hygienists, Cincinnati, Ohio
Annals of Occupational Hygiene (Pergamon Press)
Annals of the Academy of Medicine of Singapore
Blackwell Scientific Publications
British Journal of Industrial Medicine (British Medical Association)
British Medical Journal
Bulletin Européen de Physiopathologie Respiratoire (Societas Europaea Physiologiae Clinicae Respiratoriae)
Chapman and Hall
Churchill Livingstone
Clinical Allergy (Blackwell Scientific Publications)
Clinical Science (Medical Research and Biochemical Societies)
Grune and Stratton (*Seminars in Oncology*)
Health Physics Society
Her Majesty's Stationery Office, London
International Labour Organization, Geneva
Journal of Applied Physiology (American Physiological Society)
Journal of Occupational Medicine (American Occupational Medical Association and American Academy of Occupational Medicine)
Journal of the Society of Occupational Medicine (John Wright & Sons)
Les Bronches (*Il Pensiero Scientifico*)
Marcel Dekker Inc.
National Coal Board
Taylor & Francis
Thorax (British Medical Association and Thoracic Society)
World Health Organization, Geneva

Chapter 1
The Protection of
Health at Work

How the subject developed
The legislative framework
Effect of health and safety legislation
  on occupational medicine
Safe conditions at work
Moral and ethical dilemmas

How the subject developed

Since the dawn of history, mining has been associated with lethal damage to the lungs; this is apparent in specimens from ancient Egypt, Bolivia and other countries (16). Man's initial reaction was to compel slaves, prisoners of war or convicts to do the most dangerous work. Public awareness of the risks developed slowly, starting early in the 16th century with the observations of Paracelsus (1493–1541) and of Agricola, also known as Georg Bauer (1494–1555), whose *De Re Metallica* was published in Bohemia in 1556. This book included advice on improving the conditions in which miners worked. Nearly 150 years later in 1700 Ramazzini (1633–1714) published in Padua the first systematic account of diseases of occupations *De Morbis Artificum Diatriba*.

The second half of the 18th century saw the development in the U.K. of water-powered machinery for spinning and weaving cotton. The manual work could then be done by children (mostly orphans or paupers). The awful conditions in rural textile mills recorded by Sir Thomas Percival and others led to the first Factory Act; this was introduced by Sir Robert Peel (senior) in 1802. With the advent of steam power the textile industry moved into the towns. Here overcrowding, occupational and environmental pollution, long working hours and poor sanitation caused severe damage to health, morality and the structure of society. The damage is recorded in Thackrah's book *The effects of the principal arts, trades and professions and of civil states and habits of living on health and longevity*. The book was published

in 1832, a year before Thackrah's death from tuberculosis at the age of 38 years. The evidence he provided contributed to the passing of the Factory Act of 1833; this was introduced into Parliament by Sadler. The Act improved on the conditions in mills and factories stipulated by earlier acts and was the first to establish a factory inspectorate with rights of access and limited powers of enforcement. It was a turning point in factory legislation. Nine years later under the guidance of Cooper, 7th Earl of Shaftesbury, women and children were banned from working in mines and in 1843 the first Inspectors of Mines were appointed. Subsequent acts extended the scope of the regulations to industries other than textiles, improved working conditions and strengthened the powers of the inspectorates. The first Medical Inspector of Factories, Sir Thomas Legge, was appointed in 1898. Meanwhile the regulations for factories and workshops employing less than 50 persons had been brought together in the Factory and Workshop Act of 1878. Two years later saw the passage of the Employers Liability Act and in 1897 the first Workmen's Compensation Act; this led to the appointment by some large firms of industrial medical officers. In 1900 legislative action was taken to reduce accidents amongst railway employees. Further legislation followed but the next major step forward came during the First World War with the setting up of a Health of Munition Workers' committee; this reviewed working practices and conditions with a view to increasing productivity and introduced improvements in first-aid and industrial medical and nursing services. Some firms established hospitals for their employees as a result of the committee's work. Public funding of medical research was introduced by Lloyd George's Medical Insurance Act of 1911; the Medical Research Committee was formed in 1913 and it became the Medical Research Council in 1920. The horizons for occupational research were expanded during the Second World War by the needs of the armed forces for environmental physiology, ergonomics and safety equipment. Associated developments in respiratory physiology by Fenn, Comroe, Gaensler, Mead and others were subsequently applied to occupational diseases. In 1945 the MRC Pneumoconiosis Unit was founded and created many of the tools now taken for granted by the occupational respiratory physician (pages 165 and 220).

In the U.S.A. the initial legislation came later than in the U.K. but the subject developed more rapidly. The Bureau of Labour was founded in 1884, the Bureau of Mines in 1910 and the Public Health Service Office of Industrial Hygiene in 1914. These measures created a body of occupational hygienists, including Dr. Theodore Hatch who subsequently led the world in environmental monitoring and control of the working environment. Some of the conditions encountered were described by Dr. Alice Hamilton who was joined by Dr. Harriet Hardy, (page 232) in the second edition of her book *Industrial Toxicology*. Hygiene legislation moved from being a State to a Federal responsibility only in 1970.

In Italy the lead given by Ramazzini was maintained by the foundation in 1904 of the first Institute of Occupational Health in Milano. For many years, directed by Vigliani, the Clinica del Lavoro was in the forefront of occupational medicine and contributed massively to the development of the International Labour Office in Geneva (see below). Vigliani was for a long time president of the Permanent Commission and International Association on Occupational Health (PCIAOH). In South Africa the first of many contributions to knowledge of the mineral pneumoconioses was made in 1906. In the U.S.S.R. following the revolution the resources allocated to health were used primarily for the prevention of disease. An extensive training programme for industrial

hygiene was introduced and in 1923 a Research Institute of Occupational Health and Safety was founded in Moscow. Subsequently Institutes of Occupational Health were set up in other countries; the number has increased since the end of World War II due partly to the help and inspiration provided by Sven Forssman of Sweden. The recent epidemic of asbestos-related diseases has led to research effort on a world scale commensurate with the wide distribution of mineral and other resources and the equally extensive but different distribution of their utilization. International collaborative studies have also been set up by the aluminium industry. These developments have been assisted by 'the great international agencies which are described below.

The legislative framework

International

International Labour Office. The ILO in Geneva, the oldest international government-supported occupational health agency, is funded by quotas from most countries. It undertakes surveillance of occupational health and safety on a world scale and provides extensive guidance on how this should be done. It works through representatives of government, employers and trades unions and makes use of ad hoc expert committees on specific topics. By this means the ILO International Classification of Pneumoconiosis in Chest Radiographs was developed and is now regularly revised. Much of the surveillance is by analysis of national statistics of occupational health and safety but the ILO also undertakes its own surveys. It supports research into methods, procedures and health standards, arranges international conferences, produces recommendations, and commissions reports by independent experts on all aspects of occupational health including the pneumoconioses. Support is given to training programmes for developing countries. The ILO does not legislate but its recommendations may be incorporated in national legislation. The advice available to ILO is summarized in the Encyclopaedia of Occupational Health and Safety (17).

World Health Organization. The occupational health programme of WHO is integrated with those for environmental health, communicable diseases, nutrition and other medical programmes and is, therefore, directed to the comprehensive health-care of working populations. WHO provides guidance to governments in establishing occupational health services and institutes, helps in the development of research programmes, contributes to training and education at all levels and to the development of guidelines for sound practices (including occupational health standards, 29). It is not itself concerned with legislation. The world programme is supplemented by regional programmes based on WHO regional offices. The European office (EURO) is responsible for promoting international co-operation in environmental health: in this capacity, jointly with the industry, EURO has co-ordinated research on the effects of man-made mineral fibres and of welding fumes.

Union Internationale Contre Cancre. The UICC was established on the initiative of President De Gaulle of France. It has been the vehicle for much international collaborative research into the asbestos-related cancers. The extension of the ILO x-ray classification to all types of pneumoconioses (page 86) and the establishment of standard samples of the different types of asbestos are amongst its achievements.

International Agency for Research into Cancer. The IARC in Lyon is an independent agency under WHO. It undertakes research into problems of cancer on a world scale including cancer of occupational origin, the latter's responsibility having been transferred from ILO. The Agency has also taken over part of the work formerly done by UICC including the geographical pathology of cancer, now directed by Higginson. IARC reports and monographs are of the highest quality: those on chemical carcinogenesis are referred to extensively in chapter 12 (Occupational Lung Cancer).

Regional

The European Economic Community (EEC) incorporates the European Coal and Steel Community (ECSC) which, since its inception, has energetically promoted the health and safety of men in these industries. An extensive research programme has been financed by a levy on production, and progress has been made towards providing European standards for the working environment, work practices including ergonomics, medical surveillance, lung function testing, treatment and rehabilitation. The ECSC recommendations and others by EEC will soon have legal backing within the Community.

National

United Kingdom legislation was overhauled in the Health and Safety at Work etc. Act of 1974 (15); this became law on January 1st 1975. The Act arose from the distinguished report of a committee chaired by Lord Robens on Safety and Health at Work (20) and led to the repeal of a plethora of Acts of Parliament and government regulations extending back to 1802. The Act established a Health and Safety Commission (HSC) with the duty to ensure, so far as it is reasonably practicable, the health, safety and welfare of all persons in employment, both at the place of work and in the adjacent community. To this end the Commission is empowered to draft Regulations for authorization by the relevant Secretary of State, and on its own authority, to issue Codes of Practice and Guidance Notes, and make arrangements for research and training.

Regulations have the force of law despite their not being voted on individually by Parliament. They enable the Commission to replace progressively existing regulations and if necessary to create new ones. Codes of Practice explain the regulations and what they require, including the currently accepted hygiene and safety standards. Guidance notes suggest ways in which the requirements may be met. However, whilst the standards are legally enforceable the methods whereby they are achieved are not; the employer is free to meet the standard by any effective means. The Codes of Practice may be drafted by the Commission and other bodies including the Department of Employment, the British Standards Institution, a trade association or an individual company. Not all Codes of Practice are approved by the Commission. The information they contain is technical and often linked closely to a particular process or type of equipment: it is intended to be readily comprehensible and amenable to rapid change to meet new circumstances. Further improvement of working conditions is likely to follow from the enforcement of the Control of Substances Hazardous to Health regulations which are currently in preparation (13). The regulations are likely to require that medical surveillance records are kept for 30 years from the date of the last entry and the results of environmental monitoring for 5 years. Substances for which surveillance can be indicated are listed in table 1.1.

The Health and Safety Commission is appointed by the Secretary of State for Employment. It has a chairman and 9 representatives, 3 for employers, 3 for trades unions, 2 for local government authorities and 1 independent person. Thus it is a quasi-political body which depends for technical information on a scientific secretariat and on evidence from independent authorities and expert committees including the Advisory Committee on Toxic Substances (ACTS) and the Advisory Committee on Dangerous Pathogens (ACDP). It can also be influenced by pressure groups and the news media. Thus the decisions of HSC are inevitably

compromises and are sometimes made with little regard to the scientific evidence (2). Some of the factors which operate are discussed on page 7 below.

The HSC sets the standards of occupational hygiene and safety. The attainment of these standards within the workplace is primarily the responsibility of the employer through a designated person, usually the managing director or director with responsibility for health and safety. In the event of a failure to conform the employer is liable to prosecution which can lead to a fine or imprisonment. Complying with standards is a joint enterprise involving the Works Safety Officers, the Safety Committee and officers of the Health and Safety Executive or local government authority. The last of these has responsibility for dry cleaning establishments, car parks, swimming pools, offices and other service industries. Many industrial concerns have recruited occupational physicians or use the services of Appointed Doctors; these persons are approved by the HSE to implement regulations which entail biological monitoring of the workforce.

The Health and Safety Executive (HSE) is the executive arm of HSC. It comprises the Director General, the Deputy Director General and the Director of Research and Laboratory Services; these three persons are appointed by the Health and Safety Commission and are responsible to the Commission for implementing the Act. The Executive operates via a management board whose members oversee its principal divisions; these are publications, training, the inspectorate, the Employment Medical Advisory Service, the Occupational Hygiene Laboratories at Cricklewood and the former Safety in Mines Research Establishment at Sheffield (now the Research and Laboratories Services Division of HSE). *The Inspectorate* combines the roles of 7 former inspectorates which were concerned respectively with alkalis, clean air, explosives, factories, mines and quarries, nuclear installations and pipelines. These have been replaced by 5 inspectorates, each with a chief inspector, for agriculture, industrial air pollution, mines and quarries, factories, and nuclear installations. The chief inspectors meet as a Board under the chairman-

Table 1.1. Substances to which exposure can be an indication for medical surveillance (13)

Acrylonitrile	Dichlorobenzidine
Arsenic and compounds	Ortho-toluidine
Benzene	Dianisidine
Cadmium and compounds	Carbon disulphide
Mercury and compounds	Platinum salts
Nickel and compounds	Organophosphorus compounds (in regular use only)
Chloroform	
Paradichlorobenzene	MbOCA
Carbon tetrachloride	Beryllium dust or fume
I-Naphthylamine	VCM
Chromic acid	Any substance which can cause methaemoglobin- aemia in life
Sodium or potassium chromate or dichromate	

ship of the Director General who reports annually on its progress. The inspectors, of whom there are over 1000, are enforcement officers though in practice they act mainly in an advisory and fact-finding capacity; they have right of entry to premises, can demand information and can seize or prohibit the use of articles which may be a source of imminent danger to health. The inspectors can issue mandatory improvement and prohibition notices which, if circumstances warrant, may require the closure of a factory or process. They also instigate proceedings in criminal courts.

The *Employment Medical Advisory Service* (*EMAS*) was set up in 1973 to replace the old appointed Factory Doctors. Its foundation preceded the establishment of HSE, of which it is now an integral part. The purpose was to study medical problems relating to employment and to give advice to persons who might request it; some of these are listed in table 1.2. EMAS employs nearly 100 doctors who are specialists in occupational health or are willing to undertake training. Some are part-time. Their principal duty is to advise the HSE inspectors of factories and, like them, the employment medical advisers have right of entry to a workplace though they cannot instigate proceedings in court. They also conduct medical examinations of workers where there is a statutory requirement to do so or where the service or inspectorate consider it is advisable. Such examinations

usually take place at the workplace during working hours in premises provided by the employer. The examination may form part of an occupational survey (e.g. 8, see also Chapter 7). Statutory medical examinations may alternatively be performed by any medical practitioner who has been appointed by EMAS for this purpose; the appointment is for a specific examination at a particular place of work. Appointed diving doctors (page 135) come into this category. EMAS doctors provide advice for persons undergoing training and rehabilitation under the auspices of the Manpower Services Commission or attending Occupational Rehabilitation Centres. They collaborate with Careers Officers in advising disabled or disadvantaged young persons about employment. Amongst the EMAS doctors there are specialists in occupational lung disorders, psychiatry, dermatology and diving medicine. There are also some 25 employment nursing advisers who advise on aspects of occupational nursing; this is undertaken by trained occupational health nurses who carry much day-to-day responsibility in factories.

The *Safety Officer* is appointed by the management either whole-time or as part of a wider remit; this may embrace training, welfare, hygiene, fire-prevention, security or control of damage and losses of materials. On account of this diversity the appointed person may be called the safety manager, health and safety

Table 1.2. Examples of persons who may turn to EMAS for advice on occupational medical problems

Context	Example
Industry	Employers, trades unions, individual workers
Health and Safety Executive	The inspectorates for agriculture, factories, mines, etc. (page 4)
National Health Service	General practitioners and consultants
Rehabilitation	Potential applicants for places at Employment Rehabilitation Centres
Leaving school	Careers officers, school medical officers
Disabled persons	Disablement resettlement officers of Manpower Services Commission, etc.
Local Authority	Environmental Health Officers (for situations where they are the enforcing authority)

officer, manager or controller, safety and security manager, etc. The Safety Officer should advise management on all aspects of safety from the design stage, through the installation of new plant, to the drawing up of safe systems of work. Either he or a deputy in each building or working unit should carry out regular inspections to ensure that the standards are observed. The Safety Officer investigates accidents, takes steps to ensure they do not recur and prepares accident statistics. He does not have access to health records. The job entails contact with other relevant organizations including EMAS, the inspectorate, local authority, fire brigade and ambulance service.

The active participation of the workforce was an essential feature of the Robens proposals. This aspect is covered by the Safety Representatives and Safety Committees Regulations (1977) which enable the appointment of *Safety Representatives* and provide the framework within which they are entitled to operate. Safety Representatives are appointed by the trades unions with members in the workplace in question. They collaborate with the Safety Officer and may operate through a *Safety Committee* which is set up with representatives of management. The latter should include both senior and line managers and representatives of the maintenance staff, foremen and supervisors. The Safety Officer and the Works Medical Officer are usually ex-officio members. The other members each serve for a limited period, usually 3 years; the chairmanship normally rotates between management and union representatives. The Safety Committee provides a forum for discussing all aspects of safety and is entitled to a quick response from management to any problems which are raised. The agenda, minutes and written evidence about problems which are raised may if necessary be discussed with the HSE inspectorate or with EMAS.

The United States has an impressive history of occupational and environmental protection which for historical reasons was based initially on that in the United Kingdom. Originally the responsibility lay with the states but it was taken over by government which passed statutes and set up agencies for their enforcement. The statutes now cover most aspects of environ-

mental health and safety; some of the agencies are listed in table 1.3. The stimulus for action has often been a scandal or disaster which led to mobilization of public opinion, and the statute has usually been in the form of a directive to the agency to regulate and control or eliminate the respective hazard. The directive has usually been in general terms and on scrutiny has often been found to extend beyond the original cause for concern or into territory covered by a previous directive. The required level of safety has varied from what is feasible in the case of occupational hygiene standards to zero risk in the case of potential carcinogens in foods (Delaney's amendment). For other suspected carcinogens an intermediate position may be adopted (18, see also page 244). The direct cost of this federal intervention has been high: thus during the decade 1970–1979 the number of staff in the social regulation agencies increased from 108,000 to 662,000 and the total cost of compliance and enforcement rose to equal that of the federal defence budget (1).

The Occupational Safety and Health Act requires that, so far as is feasible, the employment and the place of employment are free from recognized hazards that are causing or are likely to cause death or serious physical harm to employees. Self-employed persons are not included in the act but activities of the self-employed which might harm others are covered by other acts (table 1.3). Three agencies were created to administer the Act which affects some 65 million persons in over 5 million workplaces.

The Occupational Safety and Health Administration (OSHA) is part of the Department of Labor. It is responsible for establishing safety and hygiene standards and for their enforcement: to this end it helps to set up, monitor and evaluate state programmes and promotes education and training. Its activities are directed to employers, employees and the Compliance Health and Safety Officers (CHSO) who are federal inspectors with the job of enforcing the Act. The huge legal involvement in occupational health in the U.S.A has led to OSHA having on its staff some 600 attorneys; this compares with fewer than 20 lawyers employed by the U.K. Health and Safety Commission.

The National Institute for Occupational

Table 1.3. U.S. enforcement agencies for health, safety and the environment and the topics of some of the acts for which they are responsible

Department of Health and Human Services (HHS)	
Food and Drug Administration (FDA)	Food, drugs and cosmetics
National Institute of Occupational Safety and Health (NIOSH)	Mine safety and occupational safety and health
Department of Interior	
National Mine Health and Safety Academy	Mine safety and health
Department of Labour (DOL)	
Mine Safety and Health Administration (MSHA)	Mine safety and health
Occupational Safety and Health Administration (OSHA)	Occupational safety and health
Department of Transport (DOT)	Hazardous materials transportation, ports and waterways, railroad safety
Environmental Protection Agency (EPA)	Atomic energy, clean air, insecticides, etc., marine protection, noise, control, safe drinking water, toxic substances, uranium mill tailings, water pollution control
Other	
Consumer Product Safety Commission (CPSC)	Child protection, flammable fabrics, lead-based paint, poison packaging
Federal Mine Safety and Health Review Commission	Mine safety and health
Occupational Safety and Health Review Commission	Occupational safety and health

Safety and Health (*NIOSH*) is part of the Department of Health and Human Services. It is a research organization which comes under the Centers for Disease Control (CDC) with headquarters in Atlanta and has facilities in Cincinnati, Ohio and Morgantown, West Virginia. NIOSH undertakes research, provides research grants to universities, collates health statistics, provides evidence for and recommends standards, evaluates health hazards for employers or employees and contributes to health education. The latter is pursued through Educational Resources Centres (ERCs) which provide two-year training programmes in occupational nursing, industrial hygiene and safety and in occupational medicine for graduates in medicine. The Division of Lung Diseases, National Institutes of Health and other research institutes also have a concern for and sponsor research into occupational respiratory diseases (25).

The Occupational Safety and Health Review Commission is a legal body employing judges of administrative law who adjudicate in the event of disagreement between OSHA and employers, employees or other interested parties. The legal process is usually completed at this level but may proceed upwards to the Supreme Court.

The OSH Act obliges employers to maintain the safety and hygiene standards which are laid down. Employees and all other interested parties participate in establishing the standards. These are drafted by OSHA or NIOSH but if they are controversial may be reviewed by an ad hoc advisory committee on which employers and workers are represented. The committee must complete its deliberations within 270 days. The proposals are then published in the Federal Register after which all interested parties have 30 days in which to file evidence and to contest the regulation; the appeal procedure can go up to the Supreme Court in which case there is a long delay before the regulation becomes law. Thereafter failure to meet the standard is an offence though in some circumstances the employer may use as a defence that no harm or injury has resulted from the failure to conform (1).

Conformity with the Act is secured by education of employers and employees who have right of access to all health and environmental records; they may also participate in inspections by OSHA compliance officers.

The Federal Mine Safety and Health Act (MSH Act) established a Mine Safety and Health Administration (MSHA) and a Federal Mine Safety and Health Review Commission. It also led to the incorporation into NIOSH of the Institute for Respiratory Disease Studies located in Morgantown, West Virginia. The act extended the scope of the National Mine Health and Safety Academy which is responsible for training inspectors in health and safety for the mines. Mines are inspected two to four times per annum according to circumstances. Miners receive compulsory training on health and safety on entering the industry and subsequently every 2 years.

Compensation

In the U.K. under the Social Security Act of 1975 any employee who is disabled on account of a

Prescribed Disease due to his employment is entitled to *disablement benefit*; this is in addition to sickness or invalidity benefit if he is incapable of work, or retirement pension if he is over pension age and retired. Temporary incapacity confers an entitlement to industrial injuries benefit; this is on the same scale as sickness benefit. The benefit for pneumoconiosis or related disorder is conditional on the disablement being due to one of the conditions listed in table 1.4 (9). The amount of the benefit is determined mainly by the extent of disablement; this is considered in chapter 18. In some circumstances it may also be affected by other factors including the rate of progression (6) and the resulting limitation to employment (e.g. in a coal mine). In the case of coalworkers' pneumoconiosis the occurrence of chronic bronchitis and emphysema or tuberculosis is also taken into account and compensated accordingly. Where the pneumoconiosis disablement exceeds 49% the emphysema and bronchitis are fully compensated. Where it is under 50% they are regarded as aggravating factors which attract additional compensation up to that for the pneumoconiosis. However, unlike in Germany and some other countries, bronchitis and emphysema are not compensated in the

Table 1.4. Lung diseases for which occupational injuries benefit may be claimed through a Pneumoconiosis Medical Panel

Occupational disease	Aggravating conditions	Page
Asbestos-related disease		197
Diffuse pleural thickening (bilateral)		
Asbestosis	Lung cancer	
Diffuse mesothelioma		
Beryllium disease		232
Byssinosis		309
Cadmium poisoning		247
Carcinoma of lung in arsenic workers and some nickel		246
workers		250
Farmers' lung and other occupational causes of extrinsic		
allergic alveolitis		320
Occupational asthma (table 16.6, page 361)		345
Pneumoconiosis due to coal, silica and other dusts	Chronic bronchitis†	145
	Emphysema†	165
	Tuberculosis‡	279
Poisoning by oxides of nitrogen		285

† % disablement from pneumoconiosis determines maximal additional benefit.

‡ disablement 100% during a period of treatment.

absence of pneumoconiosis. The limitation is based on the view that the illnesses are indistinguishable from those developing in the general population as a result of smoking and other factors. However, in the case of emphysema in coalminers with pneumoconiosis (chapter 9) the situation may change in the light of recent studies. The extent of disablement is considered to vary from 1% in the case of early disease without symptoms or disability, to 100% when the affected person is confined to bed and undergoing treatment at home or hospital; in the case of an acute episode the disablement reverts to the previous level following treatment. For historical reasons the development of active tuberculosis in a coalminer or person with silicosis is rated as 100%, despite the disease now being treatable on an out-patient basis. The disablement benefit may be supplemented by a special hardship allowance if the claimant is unable to work, by a constant attendance allowance if in need of constant care and attention, unemployment supplement or by a hospital treatment allowance. The amounts of pension and disablement are rated in 10% increments so a person whose disablement is 1% nonetheless receives a pension which is 10% of the maximum. The money comes from the National Insurance Fund which receives contributions from employers.

Making a claim. Claims for pneumoconiosis and related occupational diseases are made by the affected person on a form which is obtained from and returned to the local office of the Department of Health and Social Security. The application is first scrutinized by the local office to establish that the claim is in respect of one of the conditions listed in table 1.3 and that the applicant has been an employee in a prescribed occupation within the relevant qualifying period. This is since 1948 for coal workers' pneumoconiosis, and the 10 years preceding the claim in cases of occupational asthma. The claim form goes to the local Pneumoconiosis Medical Panel (now the Medical Boarding Centre, Respiratory Diseases) which is authorized to obtain medical information about the applicant from a G.P., hospital consultant or other source. If the claim is for pneumoconiosis, the applicant (unless bed-ridden) attends the

Panel for a chest radiograph which is then sent for scrutiny. Formerly this was done at another panel but now the applicant's own panel may do so instead. The scrutiny determines if there appears to be a compensatable amount of pneumoconiosis, usually category 2 on the International Classification (page 86). Category 1 is certifiable if the applicant is relatively young (e.g. age 35 years) or the change has developed within 10 years of first exposure. If pneumoconiosis is considered to be present or if the claimant has ever worked with asbestos or slate he is assessed clinically and by measurement of ventilatory capacity at the Panel which he first attended. Compensation is awarded on the findings. The claimant is routinely reassessed at intervals of 6 months to 5 years depending on circumstances but may apply for reassessment at any time if his condition deteriorates. If the claimant is turned down at scrutiny he may apply to be examined by a Pneumoconiosis Medical Board. If pneumoconiosis is deemed to be absent by a board he may apply for re-examination, and if again turned down may apply to a Medical Appeal Tribunal. This has a lawyer as chairman and two medical members who are consultants in thoracic medicine with experience of occupational chest disease. If the diagnosis of pneumoconiosis is upheld by the Appeal Tribunal, compensation will be awarded. If the appeal is rejected the applicant may, but seldom does, immediately re-apply for Boarding. If dissatisfied with the amount of the award there can be no appeal against this for 2 years unless there is medical evidence of unforeseen deterioration, such as development of heart failure or cancer. The tribunal procedure is seldom used which is evidence that the pneumoconiosis panels do their work well. When a case does come up the applicant usually turns out not to have radiographic pneumoconiosis but to be disabled by chronic bronchitis and/or emphysema (cf. page 34).

In addition to industrial injuries benefit under the state scheme the affected person may instigate a civil court action for negligence on the part of the employer (4). To be successful the plaintiff must be able to prove that the employer failed to undertake the safety precautions considered necessary at the time of the employment. In practice this has led to most persons with asbestosis and many older persons with silicosis receiving damages from their former employers. Coalminers are idemnified according to a fixed schedule relating to the radiological extent of disease, from the NCB Compensation Scheme set up by Government in 1974; the scheme replaced the right to common law action against the employer in the coal mining industry. The interrelations between the law of tort and the social security system as they affect compensation for death or personal injury suffered in the course of employment was reviewed by the Pearson Commission (5).

In the U.S.A. occupational injury and to a lesser extent occupational diseases are covered by workers' compensation laws. These are intended to reimburse the costs of medical care and rehabilitation and compensate for loss of wages resulting from workplace injury or illness. The maximal payment is usually two-thirds of previous wages plus medical costs. Employers pay contributions into the scheme for each of their employees; the amount is determined by the size of the firm, with large employers being self-insured, the claim experience of the industry and the experience of the individual firms (3).

The compensation laws are specific for individual States; the laws differ widely in the conditions which they cover and the amount of compensation which is provided. In 1976 a measure of standardization was introduced but the coverage still falls short of what was recommended in 1972 by the National Commission on State Workmen's Compensation Laws.

A claim is made through the state compensation board to whom the worker is required to prove that the injury or illness was caused by the job. It is not necessary to prove negligence, but where the claim is for permanent disablement this may be contested by the insurer. In the absence of negligence the successful claimant foregoes the right to sue the employer for damages. When negligence can be proved the compensation is decided by litigation. This has led to large payments being made by firms for occupational lung diseases when these have not been covered by state compensation law. In the case of suspected asbestos-related disease many employees have initiated civil tort litigation against manufacturers of asbestos products on the grounds that the product was defective or the warning of risk inadequate. These product liability cases are currently more numerous than can be dealt with by the courts. The cases have resulted in the payment of large amounts of compensation; a high proportion of awards have gone to individuals who did not have demonstrable disease and to legal fees (24). The litigation has also led to the declared bankruptcy of the principal asbestos-producing company but legislation by congress will in due course transfer the financial liability to the U.S. Federal Government. Similar financial cover is already provided against litigation initiated by Federal employees, longshoremen, harbour workers and coal miners. The latter are covered by the Federal government 'black lung' programme introduced in 1969 to prevent the coalmining industry from going bankrupt as a result of similar litigation. Subsequent amendments to the Act have led to benefit being payable for illnesses and deaths unrelated to coalmining, for example automobile accidents and diving into an empty swimming pool (26)!

The very large discrepancy between the small payments and limited cover provided by the state compensation laws, the almost unlimited and sometimes undeserved damages which may be obtained in the courts, and the amendments to the Federal Coal Mine Health and Safety Act have caused problems in the practice of occupational medicine which have still to be resolved (24). The subject is considered below.

Comparison of the approaches to occupational health and safety in the U.K. and the U.S.A.

The preceding paragraphs have outlined the position in each country separately: they have been summarized in a recent book (28) and using the example of vinyl chloride (12). The differences are highlighted in table 1.5; however, this should be interpreted cautiously as there are exceptions to most of the generalizations which it contains. In addition the position is changing as a result of legislation, new regulations, and the activities of the courts.

Table 1.5. Comparison of approaches to occupational safety and health in the U.K., U.S.A. and Japan

	U.K.	U.S.A.	Japan
Body which sets standards	Health and Safety Commission (HSC)	Occupational Safety and Health Administration (OSHA), other agencies (Table 1.2) State Authorities	Standards Bureau Ministry of Labour
Body which enforces	Health and Safety Executive	OSHA, other agencies, State authorities	Labour Standards Bureau
Adjudicator	The courts (civil and criminal)	Federal Safety and Health Review Commission	The courts
Research input	Medical Research Council (commissioned research for Department of Employment), Major employers (e.g. National Coal Board), trade associations ECSC	National Institute for Occupational Safety and Health (NIOSH)	National Institutes of Industrial Health and of Safety Association of Industrial Health
Day-to-day surveillance	Statutory requirement for safety officers, representatives and committees	Emphasis on measurement, not personnel	Health and safety supervisor in plants
Responsibility of management	Personal	Corporate	Personal
Place of the unions	Integral: in HSC and safety committees	Mainly casual: in ad hoc committees and Review Commission	Integral: in Central Labour Standards Council
Consultation before standards are changed	Often rather limited; decisions rapid	Extensive changes made with difficulty	Changes are not difficult
Availability of industrial compensation	All employees and most occupational disorders	Some employees and disorders	All employees and most occupational disorders
Scale of benefits	National, probably adequate	State based, often inadequate	National, probably adequate
Litigation	Infrequent: damages moderate	Fairly frequent: damages may be enormous	Infrequent: damages moderate

Effects of health and safety legislation on occupational medicine

In the U.K. the passage of the Health and Safety at Work Act of 1974 placed on all employers heavy obligations and the risk of severe penalties. This led to their taking seriously, occasionally for the first time, a responsibility for the health of their employees. The Act required employers to be well-informed about health problems, to have technical competence, often to make sophisticated measurements and to collaborate with trades unions; further responsibilities were added subsequently. The response included the appointment of Occupational Medical Officers with a knowledge of preventive and occupational medicine. Many such persons were recruited from University Departments of Occupational Health who were thereby denuded of staff. Now industry is having to contribute actively to the training of occupational physicians.

The involvement of trades unions in the practice of health and safety was the other great outcome of the Robens report. The trades unions appointed safety representatives, of whom some rapidly acquired a high level of competence, occasionally exceeding that of management. Others were shop stewards accustomed to wage bargaining and a few used their new position to further this end. At least one union decided to provide for the health of its members through a scheme of private health insurance. Thus the response has been varied. There remains massive scope for trades unions to contribute more to the health and safety education of their members, both directly and by initiating research.

In the U.S.A. the major role of the courts in awarding compensation has led to a deep division between the medical practitioners acting for or employed by trades unions and the corporation medical officers. The generally inadequate state workmen's compensation, the prospect of astronomical damages from litigation and an over-abundance of law graduates (attorneys) have led to many law suits being taken on for a contingency fee whereby the attorney's fee (usually one-third to one-half of the damages) is contingent on the case being successful. The morality of this practice is considered later. Meanwhile in both the U.K. and the U.S.A. there is a need for objective medical evidence in the courts to be accepted in advance by both parties so that disagreement is on interpretation, not on matters of fact.

Safe conditions at work

Acceptable risk

Occupational diseases are prevented by enclosing dangerous processes so that there is no human exposure, or by keeping the concentration of hazardous substances, or the risk from hazardous conditions, below that at which there

is a material effect on health. It is seldom possible to define a dose at which there is absolutely no effect; the effect may increase from virtually nil, when the concentration is so low or exposure is so short that the body's natural defences can eliminate the hazard, to death when the concentration is high. Intermediate levels may cause clinical disease, or there may be subclinical impairment of function which is detectable only by physiological, radiological, psychological, or biochemical tests. Individuals differ in their response to respiratory and other hazards so the effect on a group of individuals can be described by a distribution curve, with the impairment occurring at a lower concentration, or with shorter exposure, in some susceptible members of the group than in others who are relatively resistant. Thus before defining what dose is tolerable a decision should be made on the degree of impairment (whether clinical or subclinical) which must be avoided, and if the standard should apply to everybody, even the most susceptible, or whether the latter ought to be further protected in some other way. Atopic individuals and those with some types of immunological responses might be included in the latter category. Some factors which increase the risk of a person developing an occupational lung disorder are given in table 1.6. If the resulting impairment is minor (e.g. simple pneumoconiosis in coal workers) it may be acceptable to allow a fairly large number of workers to be affected, but if it is severe (e.g. mesothelioma from inhaling asbestos fibre) only a very small number of cases will be tolerated. Ideally, protection should be absolute but this ideal may not be attainable without abandoning the process, either because of technical problems or because the cost of complete protection may make the process uneconomic. In addition there may be a natural background level of effect (disease) which cannot be fully separated from that due to the occupational exposure, for example, lung cancer due to background radiation or 'spontaneous' mesothelioma. If the process is to continue the protection must at least reduce the number of persons affected to below that which is tolerable, taking into account the nature of the harmful effect and other factors. The number may be expressed as a proportion of those who

Table 1.6.   Factors which increase a person's chance of developing an occupational lung disorder

Condition	Circumstance
Asbestosis and asbestos cancer	Smoking
Mesothelioma	Exposure long ago; healthy bronchial tree (?)
Beryllium disease	Pregnancy, patch test, withdrawal from exposure
Byssinosis	Smoking, asthma
Cadmium poisoning (acute)	Continuing to work (?)
Coal workers' pneumoconiosis	Mouth breathing, not wearing respirator, propensity for hard work
Farmers' lung	Non-smoking; ability to form IgG_3 immunoglobulin (?)
Occupational asthma	Atopic status (in some instances)
Silicosis	High susceptibility (? hereditary)

are at risk; this factor in conjunction with the dose–response relationship in turn determines the hygiene standard which must be achieved. The question of what risk is acceptable in different circumstances is considered under ethics on page 16; the dose–response relationship is discussed below.

Dose–response relationship

The effect of an environmental hazard upon those who are exposed to it can be described in part by the dose–response relationship. This relates the proportion of subjects who exhibit a defined abnormality to the dose of noxious agent which is considered to be responsible. Some examples are given in fig. 1.1. The curve is sometimes called a quantal dose–response curve to distinguish it from the curve describing the effect of increasing doses of an agent, for example oxygen on the haemoglobin as in the haemoglobin dissociation curve; the latter is also called a dose–effect curve. The dose–response curve often differs between animal

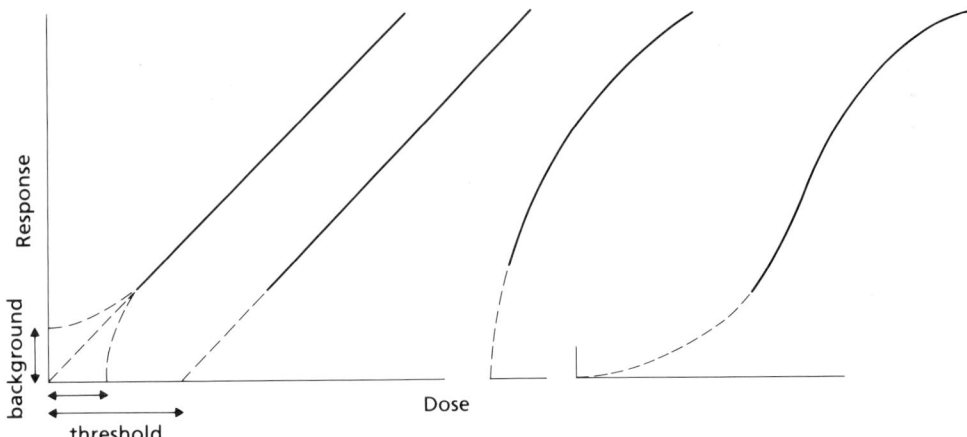

Fig. 1.1. Hypothetical dose-response relationships. The dose reflects the duration and intensity of exposure (e.g. years × fibres/ml). The response could be standardized mortality ratio, x-ray category of pneumoconiosis, prevalence of a respiratory symptom, lung function index, etc. The relationship is usually assumed to be linear but it is as likely to be sigmoid or concave. The origin is seldom defined precisely; there is usually a threshold dose below which there is no response and often a background effect upon which the response is superimposed.

species and from one substance to another so the only reliable estimates are those obtained on man. The dose is related to years of work in different environmental concentrations which may be known or estimated (page 23). The response is one of the attributes given in the caption to fig. 1. The accuracy of the resulting curve is determined by the precision with which the dose and the response can be estimated and by the number of subjects who are exposed to the different doses. The response to a high dose is based on relatively few subjects, those who had the misfortune to be exposed before the danger was realized. The response to a low dose is usually not known precisely because either the dose or the response cannot be estimated with the requisite accuracy. This is the case for lung cancer associated with exposure to asbestos. With high dosage the histology and the high fibre count in the remaining lung provide evidence for aetiology (page 211). With low dosage the rest of the lung is no different from that of other potential lung cancer patients who are usually smokers. Thus an aetiological diagnosis is not possible. At the same time the hypothesis that the prevalence of lung cancer is increased by low dose exposure cannot be tested statistically because the number of subjects required would be too large. The dose–response curve may be extrapolated to low doses from higher ones where it has been measured; usually a linear extrapolation is made because this is safer than assuming a threshold dose below which there is no effect. However, the linear model is implausible in many circumstances (page 244), and does not allow for interactions. Unless the shape of the curve is known on the basis of independent information the extrapolation is only a guess and may be wrong (cf. page 223). Similar considerations apply to estimates of the number of new cases which may occur in the future (22).

The quantal dose–response curve gives the average proportion of workers likely to develop the relevant complication at any level of dose. For any dose the proportion is then the 'risk' run by the average worker, though not by the individual worker for whom the risk may be modified by one of the factors listed in table 1.6. From knowledge of the risk and other factors the acceptable risk and the corresponding dose can be calculated. This determines the hygiene standard for the particular noxious agent. The same agent may have two or more dose–response curves based on different health end-points (19); according to circumstance the appropriate curve should be used for establishing the standard.

The dose–response relationship is obtained by setting up an occupational survey. For lung cancer this is usually a retrospective mortality survey. For other effects of inhaled substances the information is usually obtained initially by a cross-sectional survey. This is followed by a prospective longitudinal study in which both respiratory morbidity and mortality are recorded (chapter 6).

Hygiene standards

The hygiene standard describes the dividing line between what are acceptable and unacceptable environmental conditions 'at work'. Each standard is based on the available medical and environmental information but this is often insufficient to construct a dose–response relationship. In addition the standard is a compromise between what is ethically desirable and what is both financially viable and technically possible at the time. Circumstances change so standards are provisional. Most standards are national ones; very few are agreed internationally. In the U.S.S.R. the standard is nominally the maximal concentration at which, for persons exposed over a working lifetime, there is no disease or deviation from normal health detectable by current methods, either during work or in the long term. The resulting *maximum allowable concentration* (MAC) is an ideal which is seldom attained in practice. In the U.S.A. the standards for most substances were initially set by the American Conference of Governmental Industrial Hygienists (ACGIH, 7). Their standards began as the best guesses which could be made at the date of issue; they were then revised annually to take account of new evidence but only in the case of a few substances did this include reliable information on the effects in man. The ACGIH standard, called the *threshold limit value* (TLV), is the airborne concentration which nearly all workers may be exposed to repeatedly without ill effect. The TLV is not intended to protect the small proportion of individuals who are exceptionally susceptible and might not prevent aggravation in those already affected by, for example, becoming sensitized. The TLV has three categories based on the times needed for an effect to become apparent. For irritants and substances which act instantly (e.g. cyanogen, page 257) there is a *ceiling* which should not be exceeded at any time. For asbestos and other substances which exert a cumulative effect the *time-weighted average* allows for regular work 8h per day. In between, for sensitizing agents and substances which have a short-term cumulative effect the *short-term exposure limit* is for exposures up to 15 min on not more than four separate occasions per day. In 1970 the TLVs were adopted as standards by the U.S. Occupational Safety and Health Administration (OSHA) and they formed the basis for the health standards set by the U.K. Health and Safety Commission (HSC). Subsequently both national organizations modified their standards with a view to more complete protection; in the case of OSHA their *permissible exposure limits* (PEL) where these survived the ratification process (page 7) came to resemble the MAC as defined above whilst the HSC also moved in this direction (14). Meanwhile the ACGIH has also in many instances revised its limits and in the U.S. the National Institute of Occupational Safety and Health (NIOSH) has recommended some additional changes. In Europe the EEC is beginning to promulgate hygiene standards whilst the World Health Organisation has a few internationally agreed standards to its credit. These have been worth the long time taken to achieve them. Some of the conflicting pressures which have had to be overcome are described under ethics below. The hygiene standards currently adopted by HSE for some substances which may affect the lungs are given in table 1.7.

In addition to hygiene standards the control of occupational hazards has led to the introduction of British Standards for the design and performance of equipment, codes of practice for human behaviour and information to employees on the dangers associated with the materials they may handle.

Biological monitoring

The hygiene standards control environmental concentrations; they have been developed in the manner described above from studies using physical systems, bacteria, experimental animals and man. Where no direct information has been available, that on related substances has been used instead. The standards ensure that so far as possible the concentration of substance in the target organ, for example, the lung, is below the level at which there is an unacceptable effect on health. The relationship between this concentration and that in the environment is influenced by a number of factors; they include the nature and action of the substance, the industrial processes of which it forms part, the environmental factors (ventilation, humidity, etc.) which determine the airborne concentration, the characteristics of the equipment for environmental sampling and analysis, the strategy for sampling (chapter 2), the environmental hygiene measures (chapter 3) and the biological factors which determine entry of the material into the lungs, deposition on the respiratory epithelium, clearance by ciliary action or inactivation, by digestion or other processes. The processes vary in their efficiency and have different time constants (chapter 4) so the relationship between the environmental concentration and that in the affected tissue is not a close one.

Where the body burden is of interest the amount of substance in the target organ, body fluid or excreta should be determined directly. This form of monitoring allows for variability in the relationship between exposure and retention and unlike some medical surveillance can be used to identify a risk of undue exposure before the onset of symptoms. Substances which are at least slightly soluble in body fluids, including many chemical substances and the salts of most metals, can be monitored by analysis in blood, urine or saliva. Metabolites of ingested or inhaled substances can be monitored in the same way. Volatile substances and gases which effect an equilibrium across the alveolar capillary membrane can be monitored by analysis of alveolar gas (for example, carbon monoxide and ethanol). Lung concentrations of some insoluble

Table 1.7. Control limits (italics) and recommended exposure limits for respirable substances (diam. <7μm) in workplace air by courtesy of HSE (14), 8h time-weighted average concentrations and factor for 10 min (f_{10})

	mg m^{-3}	ppm	f_{10}		mg m^{-3}	ppm	f_{10}
Acrolein	0.25	0.1	3	Inert dust‡	5		2
Acrylonitrile	4	2		Isocyanates**	0.02		3.5
Aluminium	10*		2	Manganese vapour	1		
Ammonia	18	25	1.5	Man-made mineral			
Antimony	0.5			fibre	5†		
Arsenic (page 247)	0.2			Mercury	0.05		3
Asbestos (page 224)				Nickel (insoluble)	1		3
Barium sulphate	2			(soluble)	0.1		3
Beryllium	0.002			Nickel carbonyl	0.35	0.05	
Bismuth (also Boron)	10			Nitrogen dioxide	5	3	
Cadmium (all forms)	0.05			Oil mist	5		
Carbon black	3.5			Ozone	0.2	0.1	
Carbon dioxide	9 × 10^3	5 × 10^3	3	Paraquat	0.1		
Carbon monoxide	55	50	8	Phosgene	0.4	0.1	
Chlorine	3	1	3	Phthalic anhydride	6	1	4
Chromium(III)	0.5			Platinum (soluble)	0.002		
(VI)	0.05		v	Silica (page 162)			
Coal (page 194)				Starch	10		
Cobalt	0.1			Sulphur dioxide	5	2	2
bis-Chloromethyl				Thallium (soluble)	0.1		
ether	0.005	0.001		Tin (inorganic)	2		
Cyanogen	20	10		Tungsten (soluble)	1		
Ethylenediamine	25	10		Vanadium (dust)	0.5		
Formaldehyde	3	2	1	(fume)	0.05		
Furfuryl alcohol	20	5	3	Vinyl chloride		7	
Hardwood	5						

* Metal and oxide.
** 5 ppb recommended by NIOSH (84, page 371).
† For superfine fibres (diam. <3μm) 1 fibre ml^{-1}.
‡ Iron*, manganese, marble, tungsten, zinc, zirconium.

radio-opaque substances can be monitored by chest radiography (page 82) or x-ray spectro-photometry (e.g. antimony, page 249). Inhaled ferromagnetic dusts (e.g. iron and some salts of nickel, manganese and cobalt) can be assessed by magnetopneumography (page 264). The number and sensitivity of the techniques which can be used are increasing annually and this type of surveillance is now a useful adjunct to environmental monitoring. The maximal acceptable concentrations represent biological standards which complement the environmental standards but do not replace them. Biological monitoring is now a subject in its own right and is at a stage in development at which research input yields a large return.

Moral and ethical dilemmas

Whose standard?

In an ideal world the workplace would present no threat to health and decisions about safety would be solely internal matters for the work force. In practice no job is completely devoid of danger; the danger adds to and interacts with others in the environment and with inherent human frailties. Measures to contain the hazard interact with others and exert a chain reaction throughout industry and society. Conversely almost all activities and substances can be used beneficially in some circumstances (e.g. asbestos which is both a health hazard and protective against fire). The substances can usually be handled safely if enough time, effort, self-discipline and investment are applied.

The community requires from industry the greatest benefit with the least detriment to health, safety and the environment. Within industry the various sub-groups including managers, employees, trades unions, employers' organizations and technical specialists each have their own objectives, both altruistic and selfish. These blend in a continuum which makes it easy to represent a selfish motive as altruistic and vice versa. The difficulty is compounded when, as is often the case, the dose–response relationship is not known precisely, the level of risk which is acceptable is not defined and the benefit is difficult to assess. The risk and the dose–response relationship are considered above. The framework for a cost-benefit analysis is indicated in table 1.8.

The financial burden of occupational injury and disease is made up of the expenditure on safety and hygiene and the costs of ill-health; the former contributes to production costs whilst the latter are shared between the industry (through sick pay schemes, insurance premiums, lost production, litigation, etc.), and the whole community. This is a reason for the community requiring that industry makes a substantial investment in safety and hygiene; the expenditure on prevention and on occupationally induced ill-health are reciprocally related. In addition there is need to achieve the right overall level of expenditure; too much raises costs, reduces competitiveness and leads to loss of jobs. Too little expenditure causes unacceptable hardship to the victim and introduces an unacceptable risk for those who are exposed. The risk is conspicuous when in the form of an occasional disaster; it is much less conspicuous when there is a daily small toll of life or ill health. Some levels of risk which are experienced and in most instances accepted by the community in respect of different hazards are given in tables 1.9 and 1.10.

The difficulty of setting hygiene standards is illustrated by the current controversy on exposure limits for radiation (11) and for asbestos fibres where the problems are very similar. The dose–response relationship for asbestosis and asbestos-related lung cancer is probably better established than that for any other occupational hazard. It points to a safe limit of above 2.0 fibres/ml but with wide confidence limits. However, cases of asbestos lung cancer due to this level of exposure are unlikely to be detectable against the background of lung cancer due to other causes. Meanwhile in all countries new cases continue to occur as a result of previous high exposure and will do so for many years to come. In some countries the media portray the intense suffering which makes emotive television (27). Relatives join with environmentalists and others to campaign for a total ban; the call is taken up by trades unions wishing to show concern for their members, by legislators for whom a sense of responsibility may be blended with a wish for publicity, by lawyers for whom the publicity brings more litigation and increased damages leading to larger contingency fees, by local government officials and by others who may benefit from publicity associated with having the asbestos removed unnecessarily from

Table 1.8. Framework for cost–benefit analysis

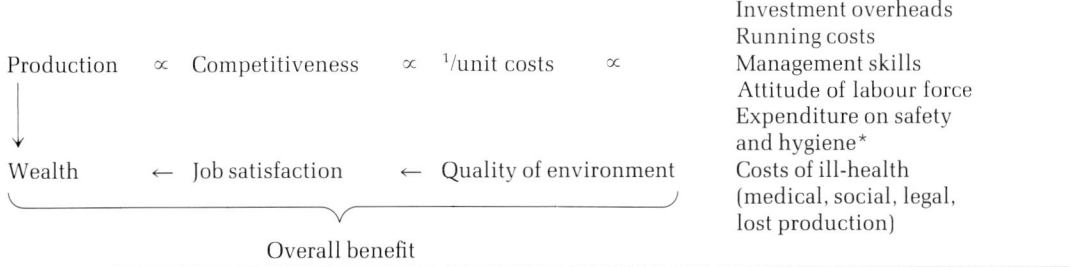

* Independent of benefit this expenditure ought to be cost-effective.

Table 1.9. Loss of life expectancy and risk of premature death from various hazards if exposure is from age 20 years (By courtesy of F. Warner) (23)

Population	Hazard	Starting date (approx.)	Expected av. age at death (yr)	Loss of life expectation (yr)		Proportion of premature deaths
				Affected persons	Average overall	
All women	Complications of pregnancy	1978	77.4	47.4	0.01	0.02%
All men	Motor traffic accidents	1978	72.0	27.1	0.30	1%
Women making service gas masks	Asbestos-related diseases	1942	78.9	21.0	1.51	7%
Underground coal miners	Accidents, pneumoconiosis	1951	68.9	18.2	2.40	13%
Men refining nickel	Respiratory tract cancer	1925	69.3	14.2	3.97	28%
Smoking 15–24 cigs./day	Smoking related diseases	1951	76.3	14.7	5.45	37%

Table 1.10. Risk of death per annum: examples of different categories of risk (23)

Lower limit (per annum)	Assessment of risk	Example
$1:10^2$	Unacceptable	Distilling β-naphthylamine, smoking 20 cigarettes per day, heavy exposure to crocidolite, being President of U.S.A., belonging to 55–59 year age group
$1:10^3$	High	Belonging to 35–39 year age group, accident as deep sea fisherman, oil rig worker, parachutist, hang glider, motor cyclist*
$1:10^4$	Moderate	Accident as car driver*, quarry-man, coal miner, railway worker, shipyard worker
$1:10^5$	Low	Accident as worker in most industries, traveller by rail or air*

* per 16,000km travelled.

intact buildings (10). The list of interested parties is almost endless and the temptation for the regulatory agency to join in by lowering the maximal permitted concentrations is compelling, especially as the cost is indirect. In the case of asbestos less will be used so a few more road vehicles may collide, buildings and installations burn down and ships catch fire, in each case with some loss of life. Buildings including industrial buildings will cost more; some jobs will be lost, there will be more unemployment with its attendant misery and the gross national product will be somewhat reduced. All these misfortunes are acceptable if the measures are on balance beneficial. The analysis needs to take into account both the related costs with their attendant misery and those attributable to the alternative products. For example, the alternatives to asbestos are on average approximately 10% dearer but save on imports by the use of local products (e.g. synthetic fibres for manufacture of reinforced cement products) and this could have a beneficial effect. But some alternative products create new problems or may do so in future.

Meanwhile possibly insufficient attention has been paid to politically less attractive but potentially more effective alternative strategies. In the case of asbestos the main source of unregulated exposure is probably from the demolition of buildings and machinery. More might be done to assist in the recognition of any contained asbestos with a view to its safe disposal. In addition, in the case of amphibole asbestos, a notable reduction in personal risk would be secured by confining any exposure to those over the age of 50 years. The risk of developing asbestosis or asbestos-related lung cancer would similarly be reduced by arranging that only non-smokers worked with asbestos (table 10.4, page 221). The case for these measures deserves a wider hearing.

The different view-points which are brought out by this discussion and example indicate a need for great humility and integrity in deciding what standard to adopt; the outcome of any such debate is likely to be influenced by the value to be placed on human life.

Value of human life

Each human being is unique and within the family or social circle is irreplaceable. On this scale a human life is beyond price. As the bread-winner the employed person provides for all the family. His minimal projected worth is his probable total future earnings. This varies inversely with age and once the person has started on a career is to some extent predictable. Compared with the earnings the value in the family circle has a different relationship to age but both are terminated in the event of natural death when the actual value falls to zero. The endpoint is the average life-expectancy with its standard deviation. Most people might be expected to set it as their target, but very often the preservation of life appears to be given a low priority. The great majority of those who die before the age of 50 years do so as a result of activities for which they are to some extent personally responsible; the activities include smoking, accidents at sport or on the roads, overeating and drinking

heavily. Smoking continues despite dire warnings which might be expected to reduce the 10–50-fold increased mortality from lung cancer of smokers compared with non-smokers (table 10.4, page 221). The practice of these indulgences by nearly 50% of the adult population is evidence that man treats his life relatively lightly, or that he does not fully appreciate the risk. The sum of the indulgences is correlated with social class though whether this is cause or effect is debatable. Either way the propensity to gamble with life has a bearing on what constitutes an acceptable risk; this is apparent in table 1.10 where risks voluntarily undertaken are contrasted with those which might obtain in industry. Some indulgences and some risks are probably essential for man's sanity and overall health but where a man clearly rates his own life lightly, this should perhaps be taken into account when a figure is put on it by others. This is now being done with respect to the use of safety belts by motor vehicle casualties; possibly a similar view should be taken of smoking by persons exposed to asbestos. Persistence despite complete awareness of the risks might influence the amount of damages payable on account of employers' negligence or malpractice which shortens life or leads to illness. The damages should be commensurate with the value which has been lost and not also be used as punishment for the negligent employer. Separate penalties should be awarded for negligence. When this is done the way is open to consider the value of life as assessed by the courts in relation to the amount which might properly be spent prospectively on health and safety measures. One million pounds to prevent one death has been suggested as an upper limit (23) and whilst this figure is hypothetical it is also a starting point for debate.

Moral responsibility

Good health is a precious commodity. It needs to be cultivated by sensible living and enjoyed in exuberance of spirit. Each person is responsible for maintaining his own physical and mental condition as for other aspects of his life. The occupational environment should at best contribute positively and at the worst not exert a stultifying influence. This philosophy underlies the emphasis in the Health and Safety at Work Act on the responsibility of workers individually. It places heavy responsibilities on employers to the same end. The position in the U.K. appears to be improving in consequence, but all concerned could accelerate the process, including all the pressure groups whose involvement is described on page 17 above. The acceptance of personal responsibility for health is encouraged by a promise of fair financial support in the event of personal disablement or catastrophe. However, the prospect of unmerited gain from high damages which are intended to punish the employer as well as recompense the victim encourages the exaggeration of symptoms and may lead to compensation neurosis (page 404). The attendant falsification of or misrepresentation of medical evidence may affect subsequent treatment. Compensation neurosis is promoted by a legal system which allows contingency fees and by emphasis on compensation instead of prevention. The practice in the U.K. of paying a 10% disability pension for a notional 1% disablement also contributes to invalidity by leading the recipient to believe that his condition is more serious than is actually the case. The process of reversing these undesirable practices was assisted by the Robens report but still has far to go; it might usefully include the trades union branch compensation secretaries adopting the title of health secretaries.

Ethical consideration

The occupational physician is in an unusual position. He meets patients in the traditional doctor–patient relationship, as an impartial medical examiner reporting to a third party and sometimes as a research worker into aspects of occupational health (21). In addition the occupational physician gives expert advice and guidance to management, of which he is a part, to employees or their representatives and sometimes to trades unions. The advice may be comparatively unimportant, or crucial to the employee, or to the survival and financial viability of the company, but depending on the state of labour relations and other factors the implications of the medical advice for the company may be anything but obvious. Indeed occasional difficulties are inevitable since the interests and motives of workforce, trades unions and management seldom coincide.

The occupational physician is the leader of a team which includes occupational nurses and the first-aid squad. He has a close working relationship with the safety officer, Union safety representatives and other members of the safety committee and is in contact with the Employment Medical Advisory Service, trade associations and research bodies. He also maintains contact with the patient's personal physician, the trades union medical adviser and other professional colleagues.

In the doctor–patient relationship the occupational physician's primary responsibility is to the patient, including individuals in management whose needs are sometimes overlooked. The responsibility extends to ensuring the confidentiality of the medical records and of information about the patient which might appear to detract from his usefulness to the employer. The patient should be encouraged to disclose information which could be used positively on his behalf, for example information about illness in his family. However, the person's own wishes must be over-ruled where the medical condition requires that he be suspended from work. This is also the case where the patient's condition may result in him being a risk to others, for example on account of alcoholism, tuberculosis or epilepsy.

In the role of medical examiner the physician may have a conflict of interests. Thus in the pre-employment examination of persons for a post where there is a known risk of occupational lung disease those with existing chest disease should be excluded (page 80). If the risk is of occupational asthma there may occasionally be a need to exclude persons who are severely atopic but usually this is not the case (page 80). Smokers and atopic individuals are at increased risk of chronic non-specific lung disease or lung cancer (page 376) so the company's interest might appear to be served by excluding such persons prior to employment. In practice this is seldom true but if it is done the exclusion should be openly stated as company policy and not performed by stealth via the pre-employment examination. Similar considerations apply to a record of truancy from school and other attributes which may mitigate against a responsible attitude to employment. Persons who have lost time from work on account of chest illness are candidates for compulsory redundancy in the event of the company shedding staff. This is similarly a matter for the personnel department. The medical department will be concerned with aspects of disablement and rehabilitation (chapter 19).

The occupational physician's opportunities for research will often be in conjunction with an occupational respiratory survey, of which the features are considered in chapter 6. Whatever he studies he will normally require the explicit agreement of the management, the union, the proposed subjects and the local ethical committee. The latter will require assurances on the appropriateness of the experimental design, the availability of adequate resources for completion and the confidentiality of the personal information which is obtained.

The advisory role of the occupational physician is subject to ethical constraints, but these are unlikely to present problems in medical consultations with employees or managers. However, in connection with new processes or substances, or when hygiene standards are changed or questioned as a result of an incident reported by the media, the occupational physician's role may be very difficult. Excessive caution may raise the cost of hygiene measures or lead to demands for extra wages, as danger money, to a level where the plant may have to close. A too optimistic assessment, possibly based on inadequate information, may lead to company bankruptcy from punitive damages (page 10). Either course may create personal tragedies. The path between these extremes requires of the occupational physician many saintly attributes, an objective analytical approach which sees through the stated views of the several parties to their real interests, and the guile to bring them together. This aspect of occupational medicine is seldom taught but fortunate is the plant where it obtains in practice.

An integrated health service for industry

The occupational physician and associated medical staff are part of a larger team which also includes occupational hygienists and safety engineers. Their overall objective is to provide sufficient professional expertise and functional support to employers and employees to achieve steadily improving standards of occupational health and safety in the workplace.

The occupational hygienist has the responsibility for measuring, assessing and monitoring the environment principally for those substances, materials and physical factors which may pose a risk to health or safety. The measurements can be related to established hygiene standards and used to assess whether an environmental problem exists and if so, what is its extent. The hygienist should then advise on appropriate control and personal protection.

The safety engineer is responsible for those aspects of the plant, machinery or process which affect the safety of the workforce. He is concerned with risk assessment, evaluation of accident statistics and the auditing of safety within the organization. He is also concerned with the development of safe systems of work and shares with the hygiene and medical specialists a responsibility for training of employers and employees.

In a large organization all three specialities should be integrated as a team. At present there are few such organizations and most firms lack this support. It could be provided by the large organizations offering a service to local industry or by the development of non-profit-making occupational health and safety companies. These would provide a professionally independent medical, hygiene and safety service on a contract fee basis. The costs to industry could then be better identified whilst the independent role would be an advantage alike to employer, employee and professional occupational health and safety practitioner.

References

1 Anderson FR. Human welfare and the adminis-tered society: federal regulations in the 1970s to protect health and safety and the environment. In: Rom WN (ed) *Environmental and Occupational Medicine*. Boston: Little, Brown & Co., 1983; 835–64.

2 Anon. Two cheers. Editorial. *J Soc Occup Med* 1983; **33**: 105–6

3 Ashford NA, Andrews RA. Workers compen-sation. In: Rom WN (ed) *Environmental and Occupational Medicine*. Boston: Little, Brown & Co. 1983; 907–12.

4 Britton MG, Hughes DTD, Phillips TJG. A guide to compensation for asbestos-related diseases. *Br Med J* 1981; **282**: 2107–2111.

5 Collinson JM. The Pearson Report—com-promise or step towards effective and just com-pensation for disability? *Br J Industr Med* 1979; **36**: 263–75.

6 Cotes JE. Respiratory disablement: problems and opportunities. *J Soc Occup Med* 1983; **33(1)**: 5–12.

7 Craft BF. Occupational and environmental health standards. In: Rom WN (ed): *Environmental and Occupational Medicine*. Boston: Little, Brown & Co. 1983; 913–24.

8 Davies TAL. Respiratory disease in foundry-men: report of a survey. London: HMSO, 1971.

9 Department of Health and Social Security. The pneumoconiosis, byssinosis and miscellaneous diseases benefit scheme. Leaflets PN1 May 1979 and N1226 December 1979 with subsequent amendments. London: DHSS.

10 Doll R, Peto J. Asbestos, effects on health of exposure to asbestos. London: HMSO, 1985.

11 Dunster J. Are we too frightened of radiation? *New Scientist* 1983; **100**: 70.

12 Hammond EC, Selikoff IJ (eds). Public control of environmental health hazards. Articles by Duncan KP and Cottine BR. *Ann NY Acad Sci* 1979; **329**: 183–200.

13 Health and Safety Commission. Control of sub-stances hazardous to health regulations and approved codes of practice. London: HSE, in preparation.

14 Health and Safety Executive. Substances hazardous to health. Occupational exposure limits 1986. Exposure limits for chemical sub-stances in workplace air. Guidance note EH 40. London: HSE, 1986.

15 Jones WT. *The Health and Safety at Work Act. A practical handbook*. London: Graham and Trotman. 1975

16 Munizaga J, Allison MJ, Gerszten E, Klurfeld DM. Pneumoconiosis in Chilean miners of the 16th century. *Bull NY Acad Med* 1975; **51**: 1281–93.

17 Parmeggiani L (ed). *Encyclopaedia of Occupational Health and Safety*, 3rd ed. Geneva: International Labour Office, 1983.

18 Perera F, Petito C. Formaldehyde. A question of cancer policy. *Science* 1982; **216**: 1285–91.

19 Radford EP. Sensitivity of health endpoints: effect on conclusions of studies. *Environ Hlth Perspect* 1981; **42**: 45–50.

20 Robens, Lord (Chairman). Safety and health at work: Report of the Committee 1970–72. London: HMSO. 1972.

21 Royal College of Physicians: Faculty of Occupational Medicine. *Guidance on Ethics for Occupational Physicians*, 2nd ed. London: FOM, RCP. 1982.

22 Walker AM, Loughlin JE, Friedlander ER, Rothman KJ, Dreyer NA. Projections of asbestos-related disease, 1980–2009. *J Occup Med*, 1983; **25**: 409–25.

23 Warner F. Risk Assessment. Report of a Royal Society group report. London: Royal Society. 1983.

24 Weill H. Asbestos-associated diseases: science, public policy and litigation. *Chest* 1983; **84**: 601–8.

25 Weill H, Turner-Warwick M (eds). Occupational lung diseases: research approaches and methods. In Lenfant C (ed) *Lung Biology in Health and Disease*. Vol 18. New York: Marcel Dekker. 1981.

26 Whitaker PJ. Coalworkers' pneumoconiosis and the compensation dilemma. *J Occup Med* 1981; **23**: 422–6.

27 Willis J. Alice—a fight for life. Yorkshire Television. 1982.

28 Wilson GK. *The Politics of Safety and Health. Occupational Safety and Health in the United States and Britain*. Oxford: Clarendon Press. 1985.

29 World Health Organisation. Technical Report Series No. 647. Recommended health-based limits in occupational exposure to heavy metals. Geneva: WHO. 1980.

Chapter 2
Environmental Monitoring

Sampling for aerosols
Measurement of gases and vapours
Sampling strategy

Measurements of airborne contaminants in the working environment are made primarily to monitor the integrity and performance of hazard control systems or to assess the health risk to the occupants of the workplace. Where the health risk takes the form of an insult to the respiratory tract, contaminant evaluation is essentially a simple process in which a suitable sampling device is used to separate and collect the offending material from a measured volume of the atmosphere. The separated material can be quantified almost instantaneously if the sampling instrument is of the direct reading type or, alternatively, the material may be reserved for analysis at a later stage following the termination of the sampling run. Either procedure then allows the contaminant level in the atmosphere to be established in terms of mass or number concentration for particulates, and mass or volume concentration for gases and vapours.

Regardless of the purpose for which it is required, the accuracy and utility of this information will depend on the proper selection of sampling instrument and sampling strategy. While it may be necessary to take account of factors such as the chemical nature and physiological effects of the contaminant, or the size, portability and power requirements of the measuring instrument, the initial choice of an appropriate sampling system is broadly dictated by the physical form of the airborne material. For this reason, sampling instrument selection is best considered under the main headings of airborne contaminant classification, namely aerosols and gases and vapours.

Sampling for aerosols

Aerosols are solid or liquid particles dispersed in the atmosphere as dusts, fumes, smokes, mists and fogs. In the occupational environment, the aerosols of special interest in connection with respiratory hazards are dusts, particularly those within the respirable size range, and fumes.

Dust particle size

The term 'dust' is used to describe small, solid particles formed by the mechanical attrition or disintegration of larger masses of material. Each of these dust particles is capable of being temporarily suspended in the atmosphere from which it will settle out under the influence of gravitational force at a constant velocity which depends on its size, shape and density. In a dust cloud composed of spherical particles of the same density but differing diameters, each individual particle will attain a terminal velocity which is characteristic of its size. Thus, the size of such a particle may be described in terms of its falling speed.

In the real industrial environment, however, the shape of dust particles may depart markedly from the spherical and variation in density, as well as in size, may also be evident. It is nevertheless still possible to classify these particles on the basis of size by assigning to each a notional diameter which is equivalent to the diameter of a spherical water droplet having the same falling speed as the actual particle. In other words, this aerodynamic equivalent diameter (a.e.d.) is the diameter of a unit density hypothetical sphere having the same terminal settling velocity as the actual airborne particle, irrespective of its geometric size, shape and density.

Inhalable dust measurement

While industrial dusts usually consist of particles of a wide range of sizes, dust measurement is solely concerned with particles that are able to enter the respiratory system by inspiration through the nose or mouth and, within this inspirable or inhalable fraction, those in the respirable category capable of penetrating the pulmonary air spaces.

The International Standards Organization (ISO) has defined the inspirable dust fraction by an inspirability curve (fig. 2.1) which requires an increasing fractional acceptance with decreasing particle size below the somewhat arbitrary acceptance threshold of 185μm a.e.d. (table 2.1). Although there is no dust sampling instrument currently available which complies precisely with the ISO sampling efficiency curve, the sampler specified in the Health and Safety Executive (HSE) method for the measurement of total dust (10) appears to collect a dust fraction which approximates to the ISO inspirable fraction. The HSE sampling head (fig. 2.2) uses a multi-orifice plate located upstream of a 25mm diameter glass fibre filter to achieve an empirical match between the sampling efficiency of the system and the ISO inspirability curve when a smooth airflow of 1 l min⁻¹ is maintained through the filter.

Table 2.1. Values of the inspirable fraction of ambient airborne particles — ISO sampling convention

Aerodynamic equivalent diameter (μm)	Inspirable fraction (%)
0	100
5	83.1
10	73.3
20	60.6
40	44.9
80	26.3
160	4.9
185	0

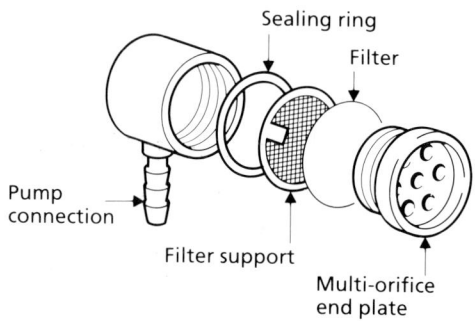

Fig. 2.2. Multi-orifice sampling head.

The measurement of inspirable dust is usually called for when the airborne particles are soluble in tissue fluids or are of an acutely toxic or irritant nature. On the other hand, the measurement of respirable dust is more appropriate where the dust cloud contains relatively

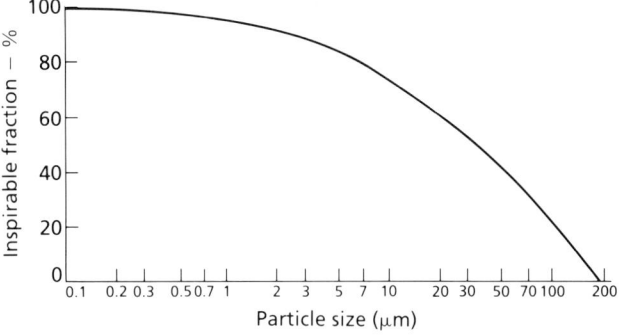

Fig. 2.1. ISO inspirability curve.

insoluble particles which may reach the pulmonary air spaces.

Respirable dust measurement

Insoluble particles deposited in the alveolar region are removed at a very slow rate compared with other regions of the lung which are supplied with more efficient clearance mechanisms, and it is for this reason that the respirable dust fraction is of special concern. The amount of dust deposited in the pulmonary air spaces will largely depend on the distribution of the aerodynamic equivalent diameters of the particles in the inhaled dust. Thus, in order to assess effectively the potential risk of lung damage, it is necessary to make use of a dust monitoring instrument which is able to select and retain that portion of the dust cloud which is capable of entering, and residing for long periods within, the alveolar region. This separation can be brought about in a relatively simple fashion by means of a two-stage respirable dust sampler in which an initial collector simulates the action of the upper respiratory tract by arresting the larger particles in the airborne dust sample while passing the finer, respirable particles for subsequent collection in a second and final collector, usually in the form of a high efficiency filter.

On the basis of limited lung deposition data, the Johannesburg Pneumoconiosis Conference (1959) reiterated an earlier British Medical Research Council proposal that the characterization of respirable dust should be founded on falling speed rather than measurement of linear dimensions of particles, and further recommended that the efficiency of respirable dust measurements should be effectively 100% at 1μm, 50% at 5μm and zero at 7μm, all sizes referring to unit density spherical particles (18). These figures define a curve of removal of particles in the upper respiratory passages and closely approximate the selection characteristics of an elutriator designed to act as the initial separator in the respirable dust sampler proposed by Davies in 1952 (6). Walton (24) has shown that for particles of diameter d in the dust cloud entering such an elutriator, the fraction which will penetrate is given by $1 - (d/D)^2$ where

D is the upper size limit of particles capable of passing through the elutriator. From this relationship it can be seen that an elutriator designed to allow the penetration of 50% of 5μm particles will also pass 98% of 1μm particles, but will prevent the penetration of any particle greater in size than 7.1μm.

An alternative standard for a sampling efficiency curve was established at a conference held in 1961 at Los Alamos by the U.S. Atomic Energy Commission (9), and differed from the BMRC criterion in that it was not based on a particular size-separating device but was derived instead from a model for respirable dust retention which appears to be in good agreement with the experimental data of Brown et al (2) on the retention of particulate matter in the lung. The Los Alamos criterion, slightly modified with respect to the penetration of particles of 2μm diameter and less, was subsequently adopted by the American Conference of Governmental Industrial Hygienists (3) as a practical acceptance curve for size-selective respirable dust samplers.

If the sampling efficiency curves and separation characteristics are compared (fig. 2.3 and table 2.2) it is evident that the ACGIH curve is in better agreement with the pulmonary deposition curve derived by Hatch (9) from the data of Brown et al (2) than is the BMRC curve. A sampling instrument conforming to the latter acceptance curve would, as compared with an instrument following the ACGIH curve, be expected to oversample particles in the 3–6μm range, but in practice it has been observed that for industrial dusts showing a typical size distribution, the performance of a first-stage collector meeting the requirements of the BMRC curve does not differ greatly from that of a collector which obeys the ACGIH criteria.

Most practical respirable dust samplers use as a first-stage separator either a horizontal elutriator or a cyclone collector; these remove the larger particles respectively by sedimentation under the influence of gravity and by centrifugation. Because the Johannesburg convention defines respirable dust as that passing an ideal horizontal elutriator which retains 50% of particles of 5μm a.e.d., it follows that the separation characteristics of a sampling instru-

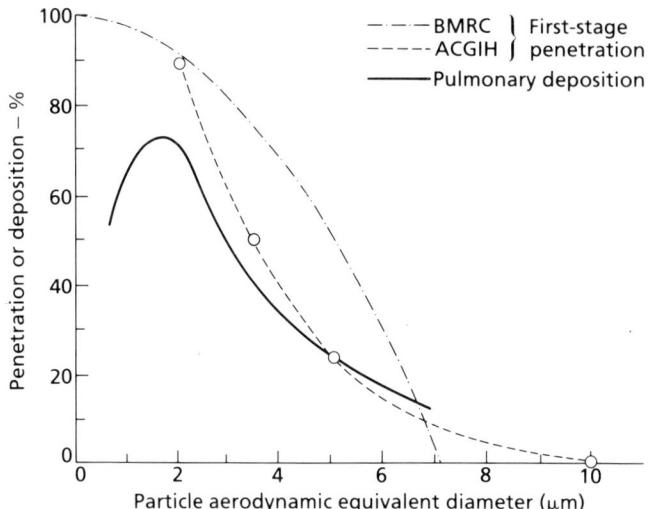

Fig. 2.3. Sampler acceptance curves compared with the pulmonary deposition curve derived by Hatch from the data of Brown *et al.* (Adapted from Hatch & Gross (9), courtesy of Academic Press, Inc.)

ment incorporating such an elutriator as a first-stage collector must, by definition, conform to the BMRC acceptance curve. The cyclone separator, on the other hand, may be empirically designed to match either the ACGIH curve or the BMRC curve.

A system of dust classification by horizontal elutriation makes use of the variation in falling speeds of different sized particles. Under conditions of constant streamline flow through a rectangular duct of length L, width W and height H, the time T taken for air to pass from one end of the channel to the other is given by the relationship

$$T = \frac{LWH}{Q}$$

where Q is the volume flowrate.

Table 2.2. Size-selective performance data of first-stage separators conforming to BMRC or ACGIH respirability criteria

First-stage penetration (%)	Particle size (µm a.e.d.)	
	BMRC	ACGIH
0	7.1	10.0
25	6.1	5.0
50	5.0	3.5
75	3.5	2.5
90	2.2	2.0
100	0	

Dust particles which are transported by the moving air will fall at constant speeds towards the floor of the duct. All particles with falling speeds in excess of some critical terminal velocity, V_c, will settle out on the duct floor within the time taken for the air to pass through the duct; hence

$$V_c = \frac{H}{T} = \frac{Q}{LW}$$

In the case of particles with terminal velocities less than this critical value, some will pass through the duct and some will be captured by deposition on the floor of the duct. The deposited fraction, P, of particles having a terminal velocity, V, where V is less than V_c, will be given by

$$P = \frac{V}{V_c}$$

In order to comply with the BMRC acceptance curve, the value of P must equal 0.5 for 5µm particles (terminal velocity V_m) and

$$V_c = 2 V_m = \frac{Q}{LW}$$

Thus, to satisfy the BMRC criterion for respirable dust sampling, the ratio of volume flow (cm^3 sec^{-1}) to floor area (cm^2) of the elutriator must be numerically equal to twice the terminal velocity (cmsec^{-1}) of a 5μm a.e.d. particle. For air at normal temperature and pressure flowing under streamline conditions, the elutriator volume flow:floor area ratio is 0.145.

The practical application of the horizontal elutriator as a respirable dust selector is demonstrated in the parallel plate size-selecting sampler MRE 113A developed by the Mining Research Establishment (7). This apparatus, originally designed for underground use and now the standard dust monitoring instrument in U.K. and U.S.A. mines, also finds general employment in industry as a static or fixed point respirable dust sampler. The unit uses a battery-powered electric motor to drive a diaphragm pump which draws dust-laden air at a constant flowrate, first through the elutriator and then through a 55mm diameter membrane or glass fibre filter (fig. 2.4). The respirable dust fraction collected on the filter can be assayed by physico-chemical analysis or, after undergoing a suitable equilibration process to bring it to constant weight, weighed directly on a sensitive balance. At the 2.5 l min^{-1} sampling flowrate employed, it can be easily calculated that the elutriator floor area measures close to 285 cm^2. Incorporated into a single duct, this large surface would result in a bulky and unwieldy instrument, and in order to produce a first-stage selector of manageable proportions the area is shared equally between four galleries stacked one above the other. If identical vertical spacings are maintained between the horizontal plates then the air flow will divide equally between the ducts and the required flowrate to floor area ratio will be maintained in each duct as will the separation characteristics under streamline flow conditions. Because separation is independent of duct height, provided the flow rate and floor area are constant, laminar flow through the elutriator may be ensured by making the ducts as thin as practicable.

While the horizontal elutriator will perform consistently in accordance with specifications so long as the air flow is accurately controlled at the design level, it exhibits certain features which render it unsuitable for use as a personal sampling instrument. For example, to make the elutriator sufficiently compact to be mounted on the head, say, of a test subject, the duct floor area would need to be only a small fraction of that used in the static sampling instrument, which in turn would impose on the system a very low flowrate and, hence, an unacceptably protracted sampling period to collect a weighable quantity of respirable dust. Perhaps even more important is the requirement that the elutriator must always be operated in the horizontal position in order to avoid serious errors, a condition almost impossible to fulfil in the case of active subjects.

In contrast, the cyclone functions particularly well as a first-stage separator in a personal size-selective dust sampling instrument. The cyclone separator (fig. 2.5) consists essentially of a conical chamber surmounted by a cylindrical chamber into which dust-laden air is drawn tangentially. As the air rotates in the vortex formed inside the cyclone chamber, the entrained dust particles are subjected to a centrifugal force which drives them towards the relatively still air zone next to the wall from which they slide down to the discharge port at the tip of the cone. Towards the bottom of the cone the descending stream of air reverses direction and, still spinning in the same direction, flows upward through the centre of the vortex to the axial exhaust port.

For a particle of mass m moving in a rotating gas stream in a path of radius R and with a tangential velocity V_t, the radial acceleration is V_t^2/R and the force acting on the particle in a direction away from the centre of the circular

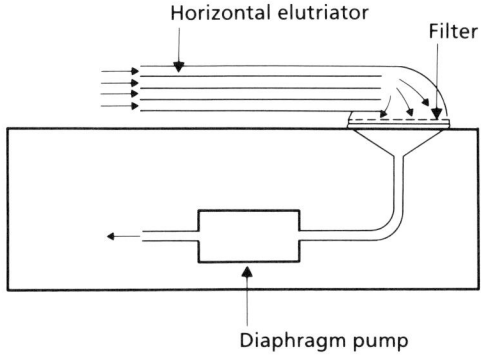

Fig. 2.4. Schematic diagram of MRE 113A size-selective dust sampler.

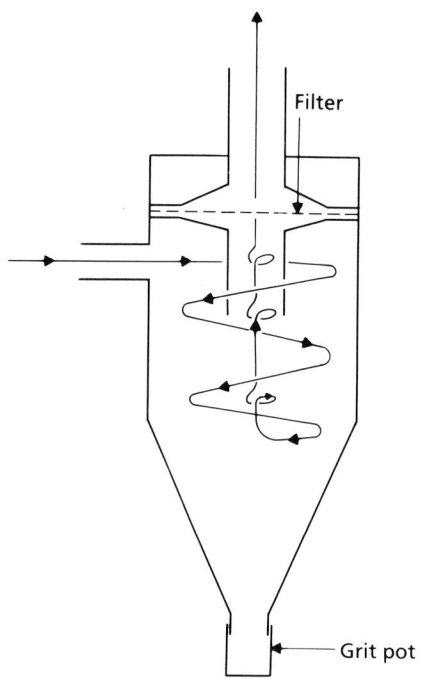

Fig. 2.5. Schematic diagram of cyclone size-selective dust sampler.

path is mV_t^2/R. The force required to overcome the viscous drag on a sphere of radius r moving with a velocity V through a medium of viscosity μ is $6\mu rV\pi$. When the radial movement of a spherical particle in a rotating gas stream reaches the terminal radial settling velocity V_o then

$$6\mu rV_o\pi = \frac{mV_t^2}{R}$$

But

$$6\mu rV_g\pi = mg$$

where V_g = terminal velocity of the particle settling in the same medium under gravitational force.

　Thus

$$V_o/V_g = V_t^2/Rg$$

The separation factor or ratio of the radial settling velocity to the gravitational settling velocity gives a measure of the efficiency of the cyclone as a particle collector and, within the

streamline zone of motion, varies directly with the square of the gas velocity in the apparatus and inversely with the radius of the path of the rotating gas stream. A large separation factor is associated both with a high inlet air velocity, although this must not exceed the level at which turbulence causes re-entrainment of settled particles, and a cyclone chamber of small diameter.

　Dust-laden air must pass through the cyclone at a speed slow enough to permit the removal of particles of the desired minimum size, but because the radial settling velocity may be several hundred times as large as the gravitational settling velocity, the time of passage and internal surface area involved in dust deposition are each required to be only a small fraction of that necessary for comparable efficiency of separation in a horizontal elutriator handling the same volume flow. The resulting compact size of the cyclone and the fact that its performance is not affected by quite large variations in its orientation make it very suitable for use as the primary separator in a personal dust monitoring instrument, although an accurately controlled pulsation-free air flow is essential for the maintenance of design collection efficiency. Cyclone efficiency can be stated in terms of a 'particle cut size' or size of particle that can be separated from the air stream to the extent of 50%. The cut size for any cyclone may be calculated from the physical properties of the dust and gaseous medium, the gas inlet velocity, the cyclone inlet dimensions, and the effective number of turns made by the gas stream in the cyclone (14). The last-mentioned quantity can not be calculated and must be determined experimentally, although its value will be the same for any size of cyclone of the same geometric proportions. By using an empirical approach, it is thus possible to design a cyclone having a cut size corresponding to the 50% retention particle size on either the BMRC or ACGIH criterion and, by making further fine experimental adjustments to flow rate, dimensions and proportions, to produce a collection efficiency curve which conforms reasonably well to the desired acceptance curve.

　The design of personal respirable dust samplers presently used in the U.K. is usually based on a slightly modified version of the cyclone first developed by Higgins & Dewell (13). The cyclone performs in accordance with the BMRC separation curve, and hence this characteristic is reproduced both in the Safety in Mines Personal Dust Sampler (SIMPEDS) which is employed in underground workings and the Safety in Mines Quarry Dust Sampler (SIMQUADS) which is intended for use in quarries and general industry. The SIMPEDS and SIMQUADS both operate on the same principle, the only difference between the instruments being the type of battery which powers the pump unit, and the type of mounting used for attaching the cyclone unit to the wearer. The pump unit, which incorporates an air pulsation damper to ensure a smooth airflow, draws air through the cyclone elutriator at an accurately controlled flowrate of 1.9 l min⁻¹. The respirable particles which pass through the cyclone are collected on a previously weighed 37mm membrane or glass fibre filter contained in a cassette which is mounted on the top of the cyclone exhaust port. At the end of the sampling period the cassette is removed from the instrument and transported to the laboratory where the filter is weighed and, if required, the dust sample analysed.

Respirable dust fractionation

Although as a means of assessing the long-term health risks associated with the deposition of dust in the deep lung, the use of the two-stage sampler is very much superior to the simple measurement of total aerosol, there are occasions when it is desirable to obtain more detailed information than can be provided by a separation of particles into respirable and non-respirable fractions. It may, for example, be important to determine the distribution of particle sizes in a particular aerosol in order to predict the involvement of different compartments of the respiratory tract. Such data can be provided by a multi-stage sampler, and most practical instruments of this type use a series of impactor stages to separate and collect the particle fractions.

Dust capture by impaction, i.e. the forcible contact of particles with a collecting surface, depends on the fact that particulate matter sus-

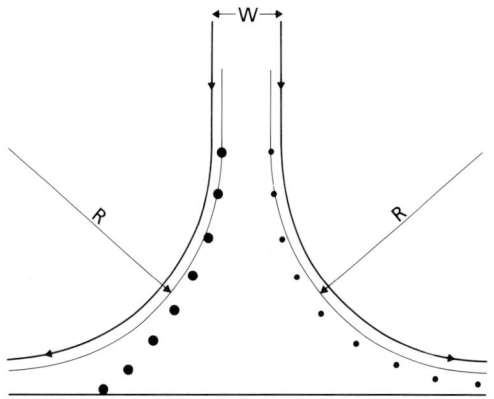

Fig. 2.6. Diagram showing trajectories of particles within a parallel-sided air jet directed against a flat plate.

pended in a moving airstream has a tendency, proportional to its mass, to resist a change in direction. This is illustrated in fig. 2.6 which is the two-dimensional representation of a parallel-sided aerosol jet of width w directed against a flat plate. On striking the plane surface, each half of the stream can be considered to make a 90 degree turn. If a particle of mass m and velocity v follows a streamline of radius R, then its path length of $\pi R/2$ in the turn will be travelled in time $T = \pi R/2v$, and a centrifugal force of mv^2/R exerted on the particle during the turn will move it away from the centre of rotation towards the plane surface at a terminal radial velocity V. For particles obeying Stokes' law

$$mv^2/R = 6\ \pi\mu rV$$

or

$$V = 2\varrho r^2 v^2/9\mu R$$

where ϱ = particle density, r = particle radius, μ = viscosity of gas

The radial distance S traversed by a particle in the turn is given by

$$S = VT = \pi\varrho r^2 v/9\mu$$

If S is the maximum distance a particle must travel to traverse the stream, then the minimum size of particle which will be efficiently removed by contact with the plane surface will be given by

$$S = w/2 = \pi \varrho r^2_{min} v/9\mu$$

or

$$r_{min} = \sqrt{(9w\mu/2\pi\varrho v)}$$

Stated in terms of the minimum particle diameter, d_{min}, this becomes

$$d_{min} = \sqrt{(18w\mu/\pi\varrho v)}$$

Particle minimum size impaction efficiencies predicted by the theory have been found to be in good agreement with the experimental values obtained for various impactors (25), particularly for low jet velocities and large particles. However, for high velocity, narrow jets such as are required for the impaction of very small particles, the observed efficiencies diverge from theory. These differences originate in the resultant effect on particle motion from, on the one hand, decreasing resistance to the radial movement of particles as their dimensions approach that of the mean free path of the gas molecules and, on the other, the increased linear velocity of the particles produced by the 'pinch' effect of the *vena contracta*. Thus the application of a correction factor to the impaction efficiency equation is necessary to predict the particle separation performance of the smaller jets.

In any event, it is observed that for a given size of jet, either rectangular or round, operating at a constant orifice velocity, there is a minimum particle size below which impaction does not occur and a maximum particle size above which all particles are impacted. The size range of particles which are partially impacted is sufficiently narrow to allow an effective separation of particles into two size classes.

Use is made of this characteristic feature in the design of cascade impactors which simultaneously collect and size airborne particles by drawing dust-laden air at a constant flow rate through a series of jets of decreasing size and increasing orifice velocity, each set of which is positioned at right angles to a collection plate to which the separated particles adhere. A multijet, multi-stage cascade impactor, such as the Andersen sampler shown schematically in fig.

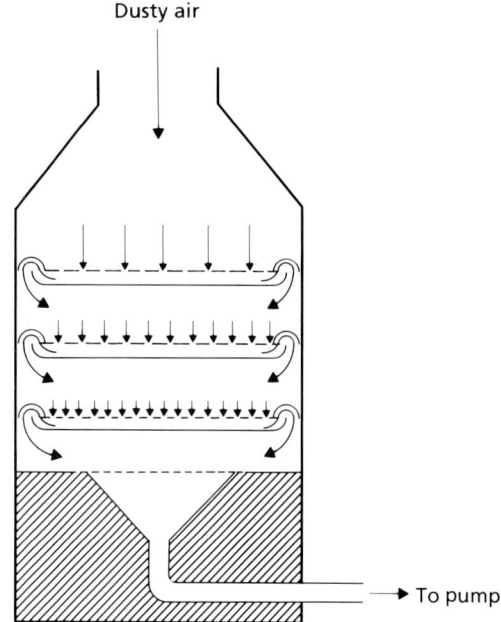

Fig. 2.7. Schematic diagram of the Andersen cascade impactor.

2.7, may incorporate from four to thirteen impactor stages depending upon the particle fractionation ranges required, and each stage will contain up to several hundred orifices. The particle size range collected at each stage will depend on the orifice velocity of the specific stage, the distance separating the orifice and collection surface, and the collection characteristics of the preceding stage. Particles too small to be impacted on the last collection plate are retained by a final filter.

The high volume flowrate through the multijet instrument, and the relatively large amounts of particulate matter that can be accommodated on the collection plates without introducing re-entrainment problems, help to increase the accuracy of the gravimetric analysis of the dust fractions. Further gains in weighing accuracy can be secured by the use of glass fibre, cellulose or metal foil collection plates rather than the standard glass or stainless steel plates. While the Andersen particle fractionating sampler is primarily intended for the static sampling of industrial plant atmospheres, a scaled-down version of the instrument consisting of four impaction stages and a terminal absolute filter, operating at 1.4 l min^{-1}, is available for use as a personal sampler.

Direct reading instruments

Although devices which provide an immediate indication of the atmospheric concentrations of gaseous contaminants have been in regular use for many years, it is only in recent times that comparable direct reading instruments for the field measurement of aerosols have been developed. These compact, portable devices which combine sampling and analytical functions are designed to measure respirable particle mass concentrations over both brief and extended sampling periods. The physical principles employed for the gravimetric analysis of aerosol samples are most usually the attenuation of β-radiation, the change in resonant frequency of a crystal oscillator, or the scattering of light.

β-*ray attenuation.* For its effective operation, the β-attenuation particle monitor relies on the fact that as a fast-moving electron travels through matter it loses energy, and its range or length of track depends mainly on its initial energy and the density of the material through which it passes. Thus, if a layer of respirable dust that has been collected on a low density membrane is interposed between a source of low energy β-radiation and a suitable β-particle detector, then the radiation will be attenuated exponentially as indicated by the empirical relationship

$$N/N_o = e^{-\mu_m \delta}$$

where N_o = β-count of incident radiation when no particulate is present on collection medium; N = β-count of emergent radiation when particulate layer is present on collection medium; δ = mass per unit area of particulate layer; μ_m = mass absorption coefficient (approximately equal to $0.002E_{max}^{-4/3}$ where E_{max} is the maximum β-energy of the source in million electron-volts); and the mass m of the collected dust layer is given by

$$m = A(\ln N_o - \ln N)/\mu_m$$

where A is the area of the collection medium covered by the dust layer. If the particulate material has been collected at a constant volume flow rate Q over a sampling time t, then the mass concentration C of the airborne particulate may be expressed as

$$C = A(\ln N_o - \ln N)/\mu_m Qt.$$

The practical sampling instrument uses a battery-driven pump to draw dust-laden air through an impactor nozzle which directs the jet against a thin, grease-coated Mylar impaction disc. This disc can be rotated in discrete steps to present a fresh impaction surface to the jet as required. A carbon-14 low β-energy source mounted on a stainless steel rod is positioned inside the impactor just upstream of the impaction nozzle, and the thin end-window of the Geiger tube β-detector is located directly below the impaction spot on the Mylar disc. A cyclone separator is attached to the inlet of the impactor to remove the non-respirable large particle fraction of the dust sample, essentially all particles larger than 10μm in diameter, while at the lower end of the respirable particle penetration size range the impactor cut-off size is approximately 0.7μm (17). The arrangement of the components of the two-stage sampling system is shown in fig. 2.8.

In operation the sampling pump, which is controlled by an electronic timing and program-

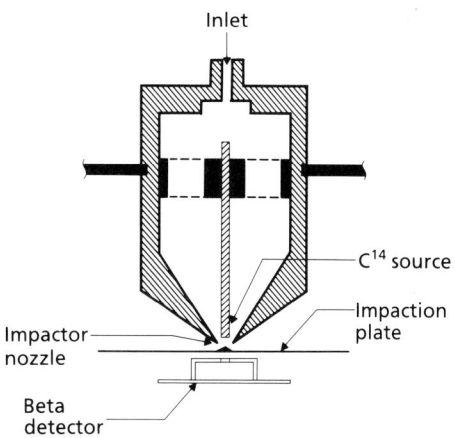

Fig. 2.8. Schematic diagram of the β-attenuation particle monitor sampling system.

ming circuit, maintains a constant flow rate of 2 l min⁻¹ through the impactor for exactly 60sec. Geiger counts are made for the first 20sec and final 20sec of the 1min sampling period. The signal processing sub-system of the instrument then computes the respirable dust mass concentration by subtracting the digitally stored product of the logarithm of the initial β-count and the system constant $(A/\mu_m Qt)$ from the logarithm of the final β-count multiplied by the same constant. A miniature digital display indicates the respirable dust concentration directly in mg m⁻³.

A recording version of the β-attenuation particle monitor incorporates a microprocessor which provides information on the short-term fluctuations of dust concentration as well as the average mass concentration over long periods of time. Thus at the end of each programmed sampling period in the series, the mass concentration of dust for that period, the cumulative mass of dust collected during all the previous sampling periods, and the total elapsed sampling time is digitally recorded on thermal printing tape which is stored for subsequent inspection. The use of a cyclone or, alternatively, a horizontal elutriator as a pre-collector allows respirable dust sampling conforming either to the ACGIH or BMRC criterion to be carried out.

Piezo-electric microbalance. The particle mass sensor in the piezo-electric microbalance consists of a 200μm thick crystalline quartz disc which can be made to oscillate at a stable resonant frequency in an electrical circuit. If particulate material is caused to adhere to the disc surface, the resonant frequency will decrease linearly with the total mass of the deposited particles. This effect is exploited in the Thermo-Systems Inc. portable instrument for measuring respirable dust (20). Air is drawn into the instrument (fig. 2.9) by a small pump, operating at a constant flow rate of 1 l min⁻¹, through an impactor which effectively separates particles greater in size than 3.5μm from the air stream. Particles smaller than 3.5μm remain airborne and are carried into the corona discharge of an electrostatic precipitator which deposits them on to a quartz crystal sensor oscillating at its natural frequency of about 5MHz. A second crystal which oscillates at a natural frequency slightly higher than 5MHz provides a stable reference frequency from which the sensor frequency is electronically subtracted in a mixer circuit to give the mixed or difference fre-

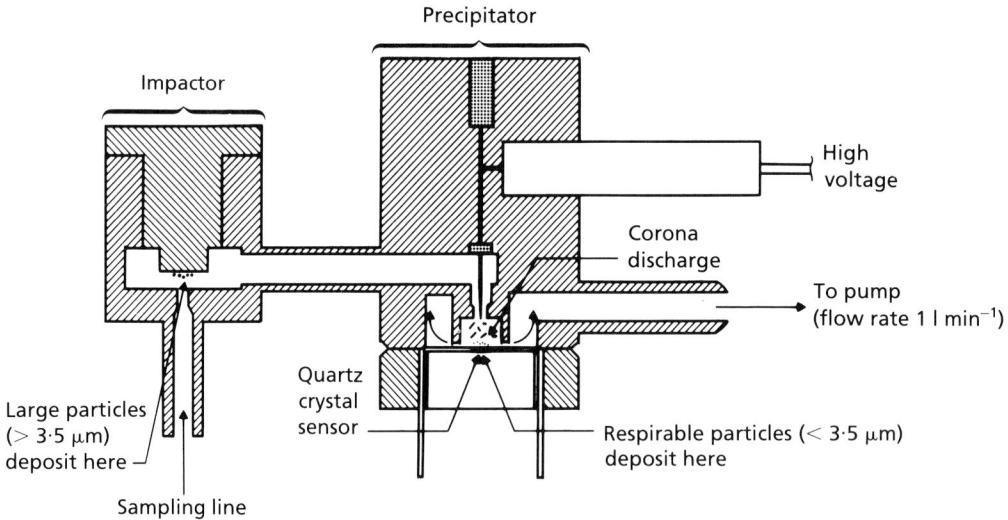

Fig. 2.9. Schematic diagram of the TSI piezo-electric microbalance.

quency. A shift in the difference frequency resulting from the deposition of particles on the sensor over the sampling period is related to the atmospheric concentration of respirable particles by the expression:

$$C = \frac{1}{SQ} \cdot \frac{\Delta f}{\Delta t}$$

where C = concentration of respirable particles, μg m^{-3}

f = resonant frequency shift, Hz
t = sampling time, sec
Q = sampling rate, m^3 sec^{-1}
S = mass concentration coefficient, Hz μg^{-1}, which accounts for crystal mass sensitivity, aerosol collection efficiency and particle sensing efficiency

Changes in difference frequency over the normal programmed 2min sampling period are measured and converted to concentrations which are presented by digital display in mg m^{-3} units. A cleaning device containing a pair of sponges charged with detergent and rinsing water can be manually operated to wipe the sensor crystal free of particles when the accumulated mass reaches the linear response limit of frequency shift.

Light-scattering. The intensity of light scattered by airborne particles larger than about 0.6μm (Tyndall scattering) varies directly with the surface area concentration of the particle suspension. This relationship is demonstrated particularly well in the measurement of light scattered at small angles to the direction of the incident beam.

The Tyndall light-scattering effect has been adapted to form the basis of the measuring system of the Safety in Mines Research Establishment respirable dust mass monitor, Simslin II (1). In operation, the rotary vane pump of the portable instrument draws dust-laden air at a flow rate of 0.625 l min^{-1} through a single channel horizontal elutriator which ensures that only particles complying with the BMRC penetration curve will be present in the airstream passing through the photometer unit. Within the photometer, a beam of coherent infrared radiation from a small laser diode is passed through the dusty airstream. A small fraction of the inci-

dent radiation is scattered by the dust, and light scattered within a cone of 20 degree angle in the direction of the incident beam is focussed by a lens system on to a detector which is shielded from the main beam by a light trap. The main beam radiation entering the trap is led away via a light pipe, made of energy-dissipating or lossy material, to a second detector which generates a reference signal proportional to the intensity of the incident beam. This reference signal is used to compensate for fluctuations in the light output of the laser source. The response of the scattered light detector is proportional to the surface area of the particles, which in turn is dependent on the square of the particle diameter. The mass of the particles, however, is proportional to the density and cube of the particle diameter and this means that the system must be calibrated for each type of dust cloud investigated. The calibration procedure is simplified by the provision of an internal filter, located immediately downstream of the photometer unit, which collects for subsequent weighing the same dust that has produced the scattered light reading.

Information on the mass concentration of respirable dust in mg m^{-3} units is presented by Simslin II either as an instantaneous reading on a liquid crystal display, or as a cumulative average concentration on a light emitting diode display which can be compared with the dust collected on the internal filter for the purpose of calibration. In addition, a detachable solid-state memory unit can store in digital form up to 12h of information which can subsequently be decoded on to a conventional chart recorder or analysed by other techniques.

Measurement of airborne fibres

Until recent times, the measurement of inorganic airborne fibres has been almost totally concerned with asbestos in its various forms. As with other biologically active aerosols, the hazardous asbestos particles are those whose dimensions permit them to enter and reside within the lungs. Unlike non-fibrous particles whose ability to penetrate into the pulmonary compartment is governed by their aerodynamic equivalent diameter, the respirability of fibres is principally a function of the actual diameter of the particle and is largely independent of its length up to the point where direct interception intervenes in the separation process. Fibres greater in diameter than about 2μm are unlikely to reach the pulmonary region although the maximum length of the penetrating fibres can be up to two orders of magnitude larger than the limiting thickness. The results of animal studies suggest that both the carcinogenicity and fibrogenicity of asbestos are associated with thin fibres which exceed about 8μm in length.

An appropriate method for measuring airborne asbestos dust must, therefore, take account of the size-related functions of respirability, retention and biological activity of fibres. While it would be desirable to use a respirable mass sampling technique, the inability of aerodynamic size selection to differentiate the fibrous from the non-fibrous portions of the sample, or to exclude irrespirable fibre aggregates from the sample, emphasizes the advantages of fibre counting as the method of choice.

The European Reference Method (11) for determining personal exposure to airborne asbestos dust and, with slight modifications, for static sampling applications, incorporates a standardized dust counting process and is now very widely employed. In this method, asbestos-contaminated air is drawn through a 25mm cellulose acetate membrane filter of pore size 0.8–1.2μm by means of a small, battery-operated pump. The filter holder is of the open face type fitted with an electrically conducting cylindrical protective cowl about 40mm in length which projects downwards from the filter (fig. 2.10). The flow of air through the filter must be smooth and must be maintained within ±10% of the selected flow rate throughout the sampling period. The latter should be representative of normal working exposure, and sampling is usually carried out for a period of 4h or for the whole of the period of exposure where this is less than 4h. A flow rate of 1 l min⁻¹ is usually selected for personal sampling applications although this rate may have to be doubled where short-term work activities are involved or intermittent peaks of exposure are anticipated. Clearance monitoring—the final step taken to confirm the decontamination of an area from which

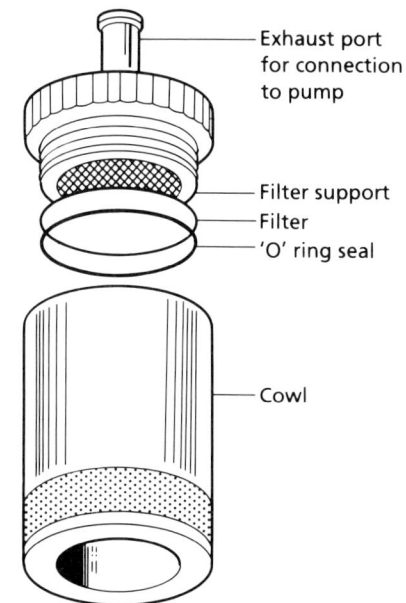

Exhaust port
for connection
to pump

Filter support
Filter
'O' ring seal

Cowl

Fig. 2.10. Asbestos sampling head.

asbestos has been stripped—normally involves static sampling using the same equipment as for personal monitoring but with an enhanced sampling flow rate up to a maximum of 8 l min⁻¹.

On completion of the sampling phase, the filter is transferred from the sampling head to a microscope slide and rendered transparent by treatment with hot acetone vapour followed by the addition of triacetin, or by the quicker procedure which involves application of triacetin and gentle heat to the membrane. The mounted filter is then examined by optical microscopy using a binocular phase contrast instrument with overall magnification of about 500×, and the fibres within a number of randomly selected areas of the filter are counted. A countable fibre is defined as any object which is more than 5μm in length, less than 3μm in width, and which has a length to width ratio greater than 3:1. The problems of counting particles of complex configuration such as split fibres, fibre clumps, or mixtures of fibres and other particles are resolved by the application of specific counting rules. In order to provide reference scales against which fibres can be assessed for length and aspect ratio, and to delineate the filter area within which fibres are counted, a Walton-Beckett graticule is inserted in one of the eye-pieces of the microscope. This provides a circular field with a nominal diameter of 100μm in the object plane of the microscope. An estimate of the total number of countable fibres on the filter is obtained by multiplying the mean count of the randomly selected graticule fields by the ratio of the exposed area of the filter to the area of the graticule field. For the evaluation procedure to produce estimates with acceptable limits of statistical error, a minimum of 20 graticule fields must be examined and the count continued until either 100 fibres or 100 fields (200 fields in the case of clearance samples) have been counted. The atmospheric concentration is given by

$$ND^2/Vnd^2 \times 10^3 \text{ fibres ml}^{-1}$$

where N = number of fibres counted, n = number of graticule fields examined

  D = diameter of the exposed area of the filter (mm)
  d = diameter of the graticule field (μm)
  V = volume of air sample (litres)

In an attempt to eliminate the drudgery and operator error involved in the manual counting process, research has been directed towards the development of automated counting techniques for the assessment of fibre densities on cleared membrane filters. The two most successful systems produced to date are based respectively on automated image analysis and magnetic alignment.

Automatic image scanning. The Magiscan system uses a sample prepared in the same manner as for manual counting, but the microscope image is viewed by a television camera and associated computer which converts it digitally into a 512 x 512 square grid of picture points, the brightness of each of which is ranked on a scale of grey levels. All potentially fibrous material is detected by first finding the darkest points in the image and examining the neighbourhood of each dark point to determine whether it forms part of a line structure. By deleting all points that do not form parts of lines the fibres are distinguished from the background. Next, the representation of the detected fibres is broken at all junction points between lines, leaving unconnected line-segments which are subsequently matched and rejoined according to programmed logical counting rules which permit the resolution of clumps of material into their constituent fibres. The fibres are then measured and those that do not meet the prescribed length, width and aspect ratio criteria are rejected. The remaining fibres are counted and, after an area of the filter comparable with that viewed in the manual method has been scanned, the fibre count and sample fibre density are printed out.

Magnetic alignment

It has been shown by Timbrell (1975) that in a strong magnetic field, respirable asbestos fibres in air or liquid suspension will align themselves either parallel with or at right angles to the direction of the field (23). This principle has been applied by Gale & Timbrell (1980) to the development of the Vickers M88 rapid asbestos counter for evaluating fibre densities on membrane filters (8). Samples that have been mounted and cleared in the normal way are placed between the poles of a powerful magnet and a reagent is added to the filter which releases the fibres and permits their alignment by the magnetic field. Subsequent evaporation of the reagent leaves the fibres fixed in their ordered arrangement. The sample is transferred to the motor-driven rotating stage of a microscope fitted with a light-detecting sensor and electronic data processing unit which provide a measure of the light scattered by aligned fibres. This scattering occurs in a plane transverse to the fibre alignment. As the stage rotates, the plane of scattered light also turns and in passing over the sensor produces an oscillating signal. The data processor separates this signal from the background noise and presents a numerical read-out which can be calibrated against visual fibre counts. The calibration factor is subject to considerable variation depending on the composition of the sampled dust, and for the successful application of the counting system it is necessary to establish the calibration for samples obtained from each type of industrial process or source examined.

Measurement of fumes

A fume consists of minute solid particles created by processes such as combustion, sublimation and condensation from the gaseous state. In the industrial environment, fume is often formed by vaporization of a metal, oxidation of the vapour and condensation of the oxide.

From the nature of the fume formation mechanism, it follows that the particle sizes involved are extremely small. The commonly accepted fume particle size range is from 0.01 to 1μm, but it has been observed that in the welding of metals, up to 99% of the particles in the fume have diameters less than 0.4μm. Thus the separation of fumes from the atmosphere requires a collector capable of retaining particles of sub-micron size. This rules out the use of inertial and gravitational collectors such as impingers and simple elutriators which are very inefficient against particles less than 1μm in diameter. Even wet impinger devices, in which the impinger nozzle and impaction surface are submerged in a liquid medium, are notoriously poor fume separators because of the difficulty encountered in wetting very fine particles. Much higher efficiencies may be expected from collectors which employ electrostatic or thermal precipitation techniques, particularly in the latter case where collection efficiency is virtually 100% down to a particle size of 0.01μm. While the electrostatic precipitator performs adequately as a static sampler for fumes, the low sampling flow rate of the thermal precipitator raises problems of chemical or gravimetric analysis because of the small sample collected, and neither type of instrument can be satisfactorily adapted for use as a personal sampler. In terms of collection efficiency and operational simplicity and flexibility, the filtration technique is undoubtedly the method of choice for fume monitoring.

Fume filtration

The removal of particles from an air stream passing through a filter involves a number of mechanisms, namely:

1. Direct interception. A collecting surface within a filter medium will intercept a particle moving with an air streamline whose distance from the surface is less than half the diameter of the particle. This mechanism is important only where the ratio of particle size to void or pore size of the filter is relatively large, and its role in fume filtration is consequently insignificant.

2. Inertial deposition. The streamlines of air flowing through a filter are forced to bend around obstacles in their path whereas entrained particles, because of their inertia, tend to continue moving in their original direction and may thus impinge on a collecting surface where they will be held by adhesive forces. Capture of fume particles will be favoured by high air velocities and close packing of collecting surfaces.

3. Diffusion. Fume deposition by Brownian diffusion depends on the existence of a particle concentration gradient in the air as it flows through the filter medium. Particles diffuse from the gas stream to the collecting surfaces where the concentration is zero, and capture is most effective for small particles at low flow rates.

4. Electrical forces. If filter collecting surfaces or fume particles carry a static charge, then collection efficiency may be enhanced.

5. Gravitational force. The sedimentation mechanism is of negligible importance in fume filtration.

The mechanisms which are of primary importance in the filtration of sub-micron particles are inertial deposition and diffusion, and the contribution which each makes to the overall collection efficiency is largely a function of the velocity of the air passing through the filter medium. This can be seen from fig. 2.11 which demonstrates the influence of sample air velocity on the penetration of 0.3μm particles through different types of filtration media. Starting from low flow rates, where particle deposition is almost entirely due to the diffusion effect, the collection efficiency of any given filtration medium will decrease with increasing flow until the point is reached at which the inertial mechanism takes over and reverses the trend. At high face velocities, inertial deposition becomes so effective that almost total fume capture is achieved irrespective of the type of filter involved.

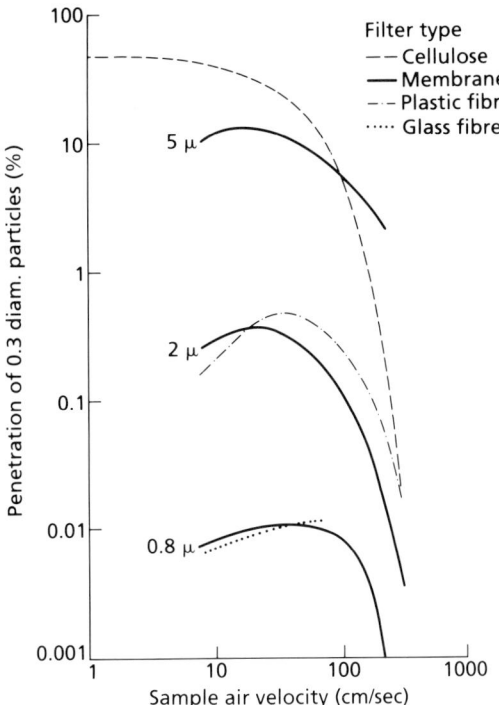

Fig. 2.11. The effect of sample air velocity on the fume collection efficiency of filtration media. (Curves based on the data of Lockhard *et al* (16) and Lippmann (15), courtesy of ACGIH).

Filter selection

The assessment of personal exposure to fume requires the use of a sampling head or filter holder loaded with a 25mm diameter filter through which the air sample is drawn by a small sampling pump at a maximum volume flow rate of about 2 l min⁻¹. At the linear flow rate through the filter medium imposed by the personal sampler, i.e. about 5cm sec⁻¹, only membrane filters with pore size less than 2μm, and glass fibre or plastic fibre filters possess the required collection efficiency (see fig. 2.11). For background or static sampling applications, fewer restrictions are placed on the size or weight of the air mover and much larger sampling pumps with high volume flow rates can be employed. These produce face velocities in the region of 200cm sec⁻¹ and enable alter-

native filter media, such as cellulose, to attain the desired collection efficiency.

Although of prime importance in the choice of filter for fume sampling, collection efficiency is not the sole criterion. The physical properties of the filter medium, the ambient conditions in the sampling location and the requirements of the analytical procedures may also need to be considered.

The mechanical strength of the filter material influences both the degree of support it requires in the filter holder and the general handling technique employed. A plastic fibre filter is weak and friable, glass fibre is moderately strong, while a cellulose filter possesses considerable tensile strength. Organic membrane filters tend to be rather brittle and may crack unless handled carefully, whereas silver membranes are tough and flexible. The electrostatic charge developed by gas flow through media such as polystyrene fibre or membrane makes the subsequent handling of the filter difficult and may cause gross errors in gravimetric analysis.

Fumes are normally generated by hot fabrication processes and filter media are consequently often exposed to hot gases. Under these conditions, plastic filters may sag or perforate whereas glass fibre remains intact. Ambient humidity may also interfere with fume assessment where small samples of collected fume are subjected to gravimetric analysis. Large weighing errors may be introduced as a result of the absorption of water vapour by the filter medium unless a precise constant weight moisture conditioning technique is adopted. It is extremely difficult to apply this technique to cellulose filters because of their rapid uptake of water vapour, but membranes present fewer difficulties in this respect and glass fibre media none at all.

The problems associated with the gravimetric estimation of fumes can be avoided by the use of chemical analysis, and this is normally the preferred assay technique where the mass of fume collected is small as, for example, in personal samples or where a chemically heterogeneous sample is collected requiring the quantification of individual constituents. An effective monitoring system should be capable of measuring the atmospheric concentration of a toxic substance down to 10% of the relevant hygiene standard concentration. Thus the required sensitivity of the analytical method employed may be expressed as:

$S = 0.0001\ QTL$

where S = analytical sensitivity (mg)

Q = sampling flow rate (l min^{-1})
T = duration of sampling (min)
L = hygiene standard concentration (mg m^{-3})

Because of the restricted sampling flow rates associated with personal samplers, and the corresponding low values of the required analytical sensitivity, the analysis of personal samples generally calls for methods with very low detection limits such as microcolorimetric techniques or atomic absorption spectrophotometry. In these circumstances it is important to eliminate errors which may be caused by interfering elements transferred to sample solutions from the filter medium during sample recovery processes such as acid digestion. Interference on a significant scale may result from the use of cellulose filters, but is usually negligible for membrane and modern glass fibre media.

Where larger sampling flow rates are compatible with the monitoring system, e.g. static sampling, then a much wider choice of analytical methods becomes available and filter interference presents no problems.

For the great majority of fume sampling applications, and particularly in the case of personal sampling, consideration of the selection criteria narrows the choice of filter medium to glass fibre and membrane of pore size up to 2μm. If direct measurement of sample mass is necessary, then glass fibre would appear to be the better choice, but if chemical analysis is the sole requirement then both glass fibre and membrane filters will perform satisfactorily.

Measurement of gases and vapours

A gas is a compressible, formless fluid whose molecules are practically unrestricted by cohesive forces, and which cannot be changed to the liquid form by pressure alone unless it is cooled to its critical temperature. A vapour is the gaseous form of a substance that is normally in the solid or liquid state and which can be changed to these states by the application of pressure alone. The distinction between gas and vapour is of no practical consequence as far as the measurement of these substances is concerned and the sampling methods employed are common to both.

A wide variety of sampling techniques is employed in the evaluation of gases and vapours, and careful consideration needs to be given both to the purpose for which the sample is required, and the chemical and physical properties of the gaseous contaminant itself, in order to select the most appropriate method. The collection technique will, in the first instance, be based on either reservoir or extractive sampling. The fundamental difference between the two procedures is that the whole of the air sample obtained by reservoir sampling is stored in a container until required for analysis, and no attempt is made to separate the gaseous contaminants at this stage, whereas in the extractive sampling procedure air sample collection and contaminant separation occur simultaneously.

Reservoir sampling

This procedure has in the past been exclusively associated with short-term sampling, the duration of which can vary from the few seconds required to obtain a so-called 'grab' sample up to 10min or so. The use of this form of sampling has therefore normally been confined to the measurement of transient exposures and peak emissions where gaseous contaminants are present in high atmospheric concentrations. Today, however, the ready availability of highly sensitive analytical techniques coupled with advances in the design of very low volume flow control systems have extended the application of reservoir sampling to both the short and long-term sampling of contaminants present in minute atmospheric concentrations. Sample receptacles used in reservoir sampling can be broadly classified as evacuated containers, displacement collectors, or gas-bags.

Evacuated containers. These are usually rigid-walled metal or glass vessels of less than 1 litre capacity, fitted with a tap which facilitates removal of the gaseous contents by means of a vacuum pump and subsequently permits the re-entry of a gas sample when opened in the sampling location. Depending on the rate at which air is allowed to flow into the container, the duration of sampling can vary from seconds to hours. As far as grab sampling is concerned, the attendant rapid variation in the rate of air flow into the receptacle is unimportant because the collected sample is meant to be representative of the momentary atmospheric composition in a specific location. The longer the duration of sampling, however, the more attention needs to be paid to the maintenance of a constant flow rate, particularly when the evacuated container is used for personal sampling and is consequently subjected to continuously changing locations and contaminant levels. An absolutely constant sampling flow rate, which will allow the estimation of time weighted average exposure, can be obtained by attaching to the tap of the sampling vessel a device containing a critical flow orifice through which the incoming air must flow. For as long as the pressure downstream of the orifice is maintained at a value less than 53% of the upstream (atmospheric) pressure, then the rate of flow through the restricted opening will remain constant. By using a critical flow device, it is possible to collect an air sample of about one half the volume of the container at a constant sampling flow rate over a period of hours, but it is necessary to filter the sample before it passes through the orifice to prevent the restricted opening becoming blocked by particulate material.

Displacement collectors. The simplest form of displacement collector consists of a bottle filled with liquid, usually water, which when emptied out at the sampling locale is replaced by the atmosphere under test. The grab sample collected in this way is retained by capping the bottle. The rate of sample collection by liquid displacement may be controlled by the use of glass bulbs fitted with end tubes which can be closed with stopcocks. The outflow of liquid through the lower stopcock can be adjusted to give the desired constant flow rate of the air sample through the upper. The same type of sampling bulb functions equally well as a gas displacement collector if a pump is used to draw the test atmosphere through it until the original gaseous contents have been completely purged, at which point the stopcocks are closed.

Gas-bags. Atmospheric sample gas-bags, which nowadays are invariably manufactured from thin, flexible plastic materials, are used to collect gaseous contaminants over a wide range of concentrations and sampling durations by inflation with the test atmosphere. By employing a low volume constant flow rate pump and a large capacity bag, long-term sampling can be carried out, while a small plastic bag coupled to manually-operated bellows is suitable for grab sampling. A useful feature of these containers is the ease with which accurately metered portions of the sample can be repeatedly withdrawn from the bag for analysis by means of a hypodermic syringe. These syringes themselves have been successfully used as atmospheric grab samplers.

While reservoir sampling suffers from a number of drawbacks such as the limitations imposed on sample size by the use of evacuated containers and displacement collectors, or the difficulty encountered in using a cumbersome gas-bag for personal sampling, it has compensating advantages in that collection efficiency is virtually 100% and the whole of the sample is readily available, without pre-treatment, for analysis by rapid and direct methods such as infrared spectrophotometry and gas/liquid chromatography.

Extractive sampling

In extractive sampling, the system most commonly used for the collection of gaseous contaminants in the workplace, a continuously moving atmospheric sample is brought into intimate contact with a collection medium which separates, and at the same time concentrates, the contaminant by the mechanism of absorption, adsorption, or condensation. Although a relatively large volume of the atmosphere is processed during long-term continuous sampling, it can be handled by a collector whose compact dimensions make it suitable for use as a personal sampling instrument as well as for static sampling applications.

Absorption. Absorbents employed for the

collection of gases and vapours are usually liquids in which the gaseous absorbate dissolves. The process of solution is often accompanied by a chemical reaction between absorbent and absorbate. For gases and vapours that are readily soluble in, or react with, the absorbing liquid in the collector, a simple gas washing device, such as an impinger which allows the air sample to bubble through a small volume of absorbent, is all that is required for efficient collection. Less soluble or reactive gaseous contaminants will require a substantial increase in the area and duration of contact between the gas and liquid phases for adequate separation. This may be achieved by introducing the air sample into the absorbing liquid through a porous glass plate which produces very fine bubbles; by using a sampler which incorporates a spiral baffle, thus forcing the air sample to take a tortuous path through the liquid; or by passing the air sample as the continuous phase through a column of glass beads wetted with absorbent liquid. If necessary, two or more absorber units in series can be used at the cost of some reduction in flow rate where the sampling pump is of the small personal type. The contaminant content of the absorbent liquid can be determined by standard micro-analytical methods including visible, infrared and ultra-violet spectrophotometry, and gas, thin layer, and high performance liquid chromatography.

Adsorption. When it is required to collect poorly soluble and unreactive gaseous substances, or, indeed, to sample for the majority of gases and vapours, the most convenient collection medium is a solid adsorbent. Adsorption is a physical process in which an extremely thin layer of gas or vapour is caused to adhere by molecular forces to the surfaces of an adsorbent. This effect is particularly marked when the adsorbing material is porous and has a very large surface area for a given mass. Gaseous substances that are highly soluble and easily liquifiable are also those that are most readily adsorbed and, consequently, all organic vapours and nearly all gases likely to be present as contaminants are adsorbed in preference to the oxygen and nitrogen of the air sample. In the practical application of the adsorption principle, the air sample is drawn through a glass or stainless steel sampling tube packed with a suitable adsorbent such as charcoal, silica gel or porous polymer granules (fig. 2.12). The adsorbent column normally consists of two separate sections, the smaller downstream section acting as an indicator of sample breakthrough from the main upstream section, and the collection efficiency of the adsorbent may be assessed by the extent of adsorbate migration. The adsorbed contaminants are recovered from the adsorbent by solvent stripping or thermal desorption and analysed, usually by gas chromatography.

Passive sampling, which also involves gas/vapour adsorption, possesses a distinct advantage over other forms of extractive sampling in that no external air mover or power source is required for it to function successfully. A passive sampler relies instead on molecular diffusion to bring gaseous contaminants into contact with an adsorbent medium. Two types of sampler, the badge monitor and the tube monitor (fig. 2.13) are in general use and, because of their small size and simplicity of operation, are favoured as personal samplers. In both types, a zone of stagnant air is maintained over the collection medium by means of a porous membrane stretched across the face of the sampler. The concentration gradient which exists between the outer surface of the membrane and the surface of the adsorbent layer induces a mass transfer of gas/vapour across the

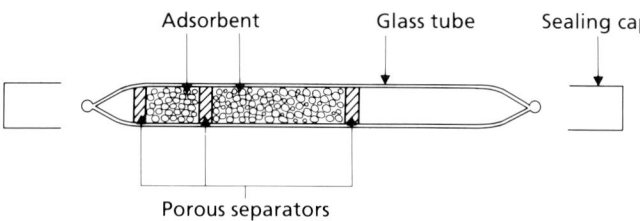

Adsorbent   Glass tube   Sealing cap

Porous separators

Fig. 2.12. Gas/vapour sampling tube.

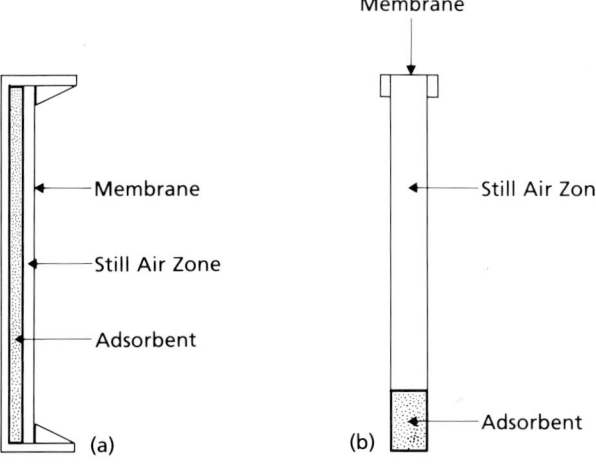

Fig. 2.13. Passive samplers: (a) badge monitor (b) tube monitor.

static air zone at a rate which the following equation, based on Fick's law of diffusion, gives as

$$J = \frac{DA}{L}(C_a - C_s)$$

where J = mass transfer rate (ng sec^{-1})

D = diffusion coefficient of gas/vapour in air (cm^2 sec^{-1})

A = cross-sectional area of sampler face (cm^2)

L = length of diffusion zone (cm)

C_a = ambient concentration of gas/vapour (mg m^{-3})

C_s = concentration of gas/vapour at adsorbent surface (mg m^{-3})

If, for practical purposes, it may be assumed that the concentration of the gaseous contaminant is zero at the adsorbent surface, then the mass transfer relationship reduces to

$$J = \frac{DA}{L}C_a$$

from which it can be seen that the mass transfer or collection rate is proportional to the ambient contaminant concentration, C_a. Thus, if the adsorbate is quantitatively analysed and the sampling period recorded, the time weighted average concentrations of contaminants in the atmosphere to which the passive sampler has been exposed can be calculated. On completion of the sampling process, gaseous contaminants collected on the adsorbent layer are usually recovered by solvent extraction and quantified by gas chromatography.

Condensation. Extractive sampling by the method of condensation involves the separation of gaseous contaminants from atmospheric samples by passing the air through a coil immersed in a cooling medium such as a mixture of dry ice and organic solvent, or liquid nitrogen. Despite the fact that it collects the contaminant in a highly concentrated form, this system can never be considered for use in personal sampling, and only in a few specialized applications is it practicable as a static sampling technique.

Direct reading instruments

Direct reading instruments for measuring gases and vapours are devices that sample the atmosphere either continuously or intermittently, quantitatively analyse the sample, and display the results, usually in a form that gives an immediate indication of the atmospheric concentration of the analyte. In many cases, however, these instruments are non-specific and, with one or two exceptions, are too bulky to be used as personal samplers. Among their more useful applications are the tracing of sources of contaminant emission, the immediate detection of unacceptable conditions, and the rapid assessment of the efficacy of hazard control procedures. Although portable, they are sometimes employed as fixed point continuous monitoring devices to provide permanent records of contaminant concentrations at work stations or, in conjunction with visual and audible alarms, to give warning of hazardous conditions.

Some of the more useful instruments, classified according to the physico-chemical principles on which they operate, are discussed below.

Photometry. Portable, direct reading devices based on the photometric principle make use of the selective absorption by solutions or air mixtures of gaseous contaminants of specific wavelengths of light in the ultraviolet, visible and infrared regions of the electromagnetic spectrum. The practical instrument operates by passing a collimated beam of monochromatic radiation, which has been selected from the lamp or energy source, through the air sample or through a solution of the contaminants, to a detector whose signal is amplified and fed to a meter or recorder.

In the direct measurement of mercury vapour, for example, an air sample is drawn into the absorption chamber of the instrument through which ultraviolet radiation of 253.7nm wavelength is beamed from a mercury vapour lamp light source. Any mercury vapour present in the sample will reduce the amount of light reaching the photo-electric cell in direct relation to the vapour concentration, the level of which is instantaneously displayed on a meter calibrated in units of mg m^{-3}.

The same principle of operation is employed in infrared analysers such as the MIRAN portable ambient air analyser (fig. 2.14). The interaction of infrared energy with a gaseous compound present in the air drawn into the sample cell causes vibrations and rotations of the molecules resulting in energy absorption. The vibration frequencies depend on the mole-

cular structure of the compound and correspond to specific wavelengths in the infrared. Selection of the appropriate analytical wavelength enables the photometer to identify and determine the concentration of a specific gas or vapour. The use of a variable infrared filter spanning an infrared spectral range from about 3 to 15µm, and a variable pathlength gas cell in which analytical sensitivity can be increased by multiplying the number of times the infrared beam passes through the sample prior to striking the detector, allows the instantaneous measurement of trace concentrations of several hundred organic and inorganic contaminants.

Chemiluminescence. The emission of light as a result of a chemical reaction at a temperature not normally associated with visible radiations is a phenomenon associated with certain oxidation processes such as the reactions between ozone and ethylene and ozone and nitric oxide. This effect forms the basis of operation of continuous air monitors which selectively measure atmospheric concentrations of ozone or nitric oxide. Photometric detection of the chemiluminescence produced by the gas phase reaction in the sample cell when ethylene from a bottled supply is mixed with the ambient air sample containing traces of ozone, or when nitric oxide in the air sample reacts with ozone supplied from an ozone generator, is capable of measuring with high specificity either contaminant at the parts per billion concentration level.

Electrochemical. Portable analysers incorporating voltametric sensors are available for the measurement of inorganic contaminants such as hydrogen sulphide, sulphur dioxide, nitrogen dioxide, chlorine and carbon monoxide. In operation, a small diaphragm pump continuously draws an atmospheric sample over the membrane seal of the sensor cell which contains a sensing electrode and a

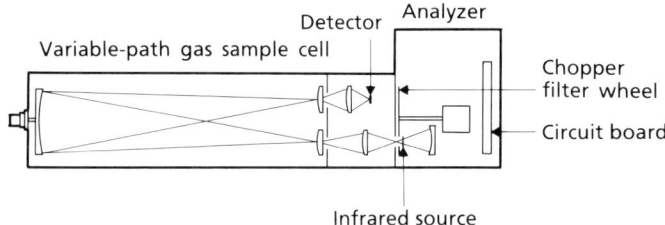

Fig. 2.14. Schematic diagram of the MIRAN ambient air analyser.

non-polarizable reference counter electrode separated by an electrolyte. Contaminant gas molecules diffuse through the membrane and are adsorbed on the sensing electrode where they are electrochemically reacted at an appropriate sensing electrode potential. This reaction generates an electric current which, because it is diffusion limited, is linearly proportional to the gas concentration above the membrane. The current is converted to a voltage for meter or recorder display.

Gas chromatography. The well-established laboratory gas chromatographic analysis system has been adapted for use in a number of portable, direct reading devices. These instruments are primarily intended to measure organic vapours in the workplace, and all function in a basically similar fashion. Mixtures of chemical compounds are separated from one another by selective partition between a stationary liquid phase and a mobile gas phase. In practical gaseous contaminant monitoring, a small ambient air sample is injected into a column through which a carrier gas is flowing. This column is packed with an inert solid support material, the particles of which are coated with a high-boiling liquid which constitutes the stationary phase. The sample components are separated from one another in the column by absorption, each component moving through the column at a different speed, and are detected separately in the effluent carrier gas as they emerge from the distal end. The output from the detector is channelled into a recorder which plots a graph of response versus time. The chromatogram thus obtained shows peaks, each of which corresponds to a component of the sample. The area under the peak is proportional to the concentration of the compound it represents, while the elapsed time between sample injection and component detection will, under controlled operating conditions, identify the compound.

Although a wide variety of detector systems is available, the use of the chromatograph primarily as a field instrument for the detection and measurement of a wide range of organic vapours tends to limit the choice to widely applicable and sensitive devices such as the flame ionization detector (FID) or photo-ionization detector (PID). The FID unit detects the separated component in the effluent carrier gas by burning it in a hydrogen flame. The resulting change in electrical conductivity of the flame is measured by two electrodes across which there is an applied voltage. The current carried across the electrode gap is proportional to the number of ions generated during the burning of the sample. In general, the sensitivity of the FID is less than 1ppm. In a similar fashion, the PID measures current flow between two electrodes caused by ionization of the separated organic component by ultraviolet radiation. The sensitivity of this detector is very high and, under the right conditions, permits measurement of gaseous contaminants in the parts per billion range.

Direct reading chemical detectors. Direct reading instruments of this type, as exemplified by gas detector tubes and tape samplers, make use of the chemical properties of the gaseous contaminant to promote a reaction between the gas or vapour and a specific reagent which results in the formation of a coloured product.

Gas detector tubes are filled with granular material, usually silica gel, which has been impregnated with an appropriate chemical reagent. When an air sample, usually of fixed volume, is drawn through the tube either with a hand-operated pump for short-term sampling or by means of a small battery-driven pump for long-term continuous sampling, a coloured stain develops in the solid phase as a result of the contaminant–reagent reaction. For this particular type of detector tube it has been found that the length of stain relates to contaminant concentration and air sample volume as follows:

$$\frac{L}{H} = \ln{(CV)} + \ln{\frac{K}{H}}$$

where L = length of stain (cm)

 C = contaminant concentration (ppm)
 V = air sample volume (cm^3)
 K = a constant for a given tube and gaseous contaminant
 H = a mass transfer proportionality factor (cm)

Thus, for a fixed sample volume, the stain length can be set against a logarithmic scale calibrated in ppm units to give a direct reading of contaminant concentration.

The tape sampler, shown schematically in fig. 2.15, uses an area on a reagent-impregnated paper strip as the sampling medium. The tape is advanced intermittently from a supply spool through the sampling head on to a take-up spool. The gaseous contaminant in the sampled air reacts with the specific reagent on the strip to form a discrete coloured spot. Simultaneously, a beam of light is played on the exposed area and as the amount of reflected light decreases due to stain development, the reduction is sensed by a photocell detector and this signal is converted by microprocessor to a contaminant concentration value which is displayed in digital form. This type of measuring instrument is capable of detecting many contaminants at low parts per billion concentrations.

Sampling strategy

As stated earlier, the primary purposes of air sampling are to assess risk to workers exposed to airborne contaminants and to determine the effectiveness and integrity of hazard controls. Sampling programmes designed specifically for engineering purposes are usually concerned with measuring changes in ambient levels of contaminants in order to follow trends of improvement or deterioration in air quality. The sampling instruments used in such exercises are located in fixed positions, normally in proximity to contaminant sources and not necessarily with reference to the actual or potential occupancy of the test site. On the other hand, air sampling for the purpose of assessing health risk is directed towards the measurement of personal exposure to airborne toxic substances. Despite their dissimilar objectives, the separate sampling programmes may, in some instances, provide complementary information. Thus, for example, a shift in the mean exposure of a group of workers may signal a change in the efficacy of hazard controls, or static sampling results from a particular area may indicate the severity of the potential health risk to persons visiting that space.

When atmospheric sampling is used to assess the levels of airborne contaminants in the workplace, it is inevitably observed that sequential samples taken in the same location or simultaneous samples from different locations yield results which differ from one another, sometimes to a surprising extent. This is merely a reflection of the fact that contaminant concentrations can fluctuate, sometimes wildly, over a short period or steep concentration gradients may exist over very short distances as a result of variation in the number, position, type and release rates of contaminant sources, and the random air movements associated with mecha-

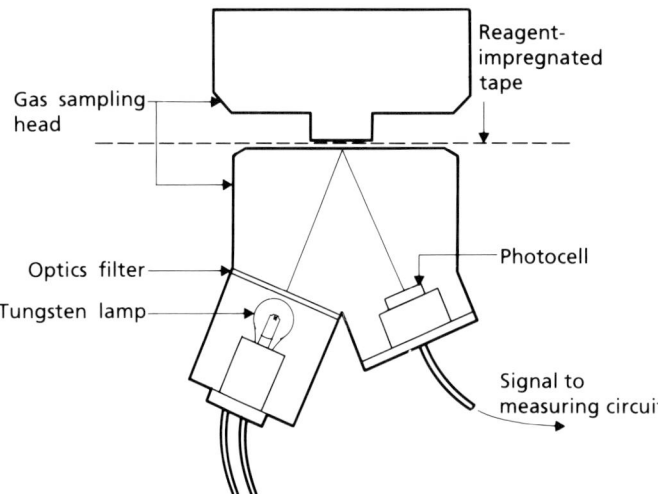

Fig. 2.15. Schematic diagram of the tape sampler.

nical and natural ventilation. Additional variation which will influence the assessment of personal exposure levels is introduced through the continual relocation of mobile workers and changes in their work practices. The sampling equipment and analytical methods are themselves subject to errors, both random and systematic in nature. While systematic error, or bias, is difficult to detect and eliminate, the random errors of the sampling/analytical system can be measured by means of laboratory calibration procedures. Typical values of coefficients of variation (CV) for sampling/analytical procedures fall within the range from 0.05 to 0.25.

Unless it is the specific intention to measure peak levels of contaminants, either to provide a guide to the performance of a control system or to gauge the risks associated with acutely toxic substances, the sampling programme employed should aim to reduce the variation in the sampling results so that a reliable estimate can be made of the time weighted average exposure concentration. An appropriate strategy to achieve this objective will, therefore, consider the deployment of sampling devices, the number of samples required and the duration of sampling.

Sampler deployment

In accordance with the broad classification of air sampling programmes into two groups, one concerned with contaminant emissions and the other with contaminant exposures, and leaving aside the qualitative or semi-quantitative procedures for tracing leaks, air samples are required to be taken by sampling devices located either at fixed points in the vicinity of contaminant sources or within the 'breathing zones' of exposed persons. While the siting of static samplers presents few problems, the region from which personal samples are drawn must be specified precisely if large errors are to be avoided. The logical choice of sampling location is at the point where airborne contaminants gain entry into the body, i.e. at the entrance to the nose. In order to overcome the practical difficulties associated with measurement at this point, it is common practice to locate the sampling device within the so-called breathing zone, either by maintaining the inlet of the sampler at an unspecified distance in front of the face or by attaching the inlet to the upper trunk or head.

The breathing zone is an ill-defined atmospheric region extending outwards from the face and chest within which it is assumed that the concentration of the contaminant is identical with that in the air which actually enters the nose. Although this assumption is now part of sampling orthodoxy, recent studies on exposure measurement suggest that the only sampler location which can be consistently used as a satisfactory alternative to the entrance to the nose is in the region close to the cheek (22). In contrast, depending on the mode of contaminant generation, the sampler mounted on the lapel (the commonest site) is capable of producing a result anywhere from one half to twice the actual exposure concentration.

Number and duration of samples

The results of exposure sampling are intended for eventual comparison with some form of hygiene standard such as Occupational Exposure Limits (12) or Threshold Limit Values (4). These standards, which are expressed in the same atmospheric concentration units as the samples, i.e. $mg\ m^{-3}$ or ppm, have been developed for a great many contaminants, usually from dose–effect relationships where the dose is the estimated body burden of the contaminant accumulated over a short time for a substance producing acute effects or over a long period for a substance giving rise to chronic effects. In order to predict the biological effects of exposure to a fast acting contaminant, it is necessary to sample over brief periods of time so as to detect the transient concentration peaks. Conversely, if the airborne substance only produces its effects in the long term after the build-up of a large body burden, then a series of measurements of atmospheric concentrations carried out over an extended time period will be appropriate.

From his studies (19) of the relationship between body burden and atmospheric concentration of the contaminant, Roach (1966) proposed a system of sampling in which the sample duration is related to the biological half-time, i.e. the time taken for the body burden to rise to half the contaminant uptake/elimination equilibrium value. A recommended sampling period of one-tenth the half-time was suggested, giving a range of sampling times for common air contaminants from 2min to ten workshifts. Notwithstanding the merits of this rational approach to the problem, sampling durations of the order of several workshifts are rarely contemplated in industry, mainly on the grounds of impracticability. While retaining the principle of brief sampling periods for contaminants with acute effects and extended sampling for those with chronic effects, current practice is based on sampling durations that will enable 8h time weighted average or 10min time weighted average concentrations to be estimated. These values may then be compared with the long-term and short-term occupational exposure limits which are themselves, respectively, 8h and 10min TWA values.

During the normal 8h working day or shift, the number of samples that may be obtained from a single location by either static or personal sampling can vary from one up to several hundred depending on the type of instrument and sampling period chosen. The number of samples is important because it has a direct bearing on the confidence that can be placed in the estimate of the contaminant concentration and its compliance with the relevant hygiene standard. The possible sampling systems are listed below; the confidence limits which may be set about the concentration estimate for each system widen with descending order in the list.

Full period consecutive samples. Consecutive sampling periods occupy the full 8h shift.

Full period single sample. One continuous sampling period occupies the full 8h shift.

Partial period consecutive samples. Consecutive sampling periods occupy the major portion of the 8h shift.

Grab samples. Short-term samples of 10min duration or less, taken at random and occupying in total only a small portion of the 8h shift.

The use of full period sampling, either by single sample or consecutive samples, gives a better estimate of the true contaminant concentrations as only the errors associated with

the sampling/analysis system must be taken into account, and these are much smaller than the environmental variations that affect short-term samples. As the number of consecutive sampling periods chosen for full period sampling increases, so the confidence limits move closer to the concentration estimate. It can be shown (21) that from two to eight sampling periods give reasonable confidence limits and four or five samples covering the full period are an acceptable compromise. If we are required to use partial period consecutive sampling, careful judgement of the unsampled period is necessary in order to determine whether ambient contaminant levels are likely to differ significantly from those in the sampled period. In any event, unless at least 70% of the full period is covered it is probably better to take grab samples. The grab sampling system tends to produce wide confidence limits, and in order to achieve reasonable results, about ten samples should be taken. Unless 10min samples are required for comparison with short-term exposure limits, the sample duration is determined by the requirements of the analytical method. The times at which samples are taken should be chosen randomly.

Interpretation of sampling results

The following procedures (5) may be used when comparing sampling results with the relevant hygiene standard to determine compliance. From the results of the sampling procedure, an estimate is made of the average concentration of the contaminant. To perform a compliance test the upper confidence limit (UCL) for this estimate is calculated at the required level of confidence (usually 95%).

Full period single sample

$$UCL \ (95\%) = \frac{X}{STD} + 1.645 \times CV$$

where UCL (95%) = upper confidence limit at 95%
X　　 = measured sample value
STD　 = hygiene standard
CV　　 = coefficient of variation for the sampling/ analytical method

Full period consecutive samples

(a) Uniform exposure:

$$\text{UCL (95\%)} = \frac{\text{TWA}}{\text{STD}} + 1.645 \times \text{CV} \times \frac{\sqrt{(T_1^2 + \ldots + T_n^2)}}{T_1 + \ldots + T_n}$$

$$= \frac{\text{TWA}}{\text{STD}} + \frac{1.645 \times \text{CV}}{\sqrt{n}} \text{ if } T_1 = T_2 = \ldots = T_n$$

(b) Non-uniform exposure:

$$\text{UCL (95\%)} = \frac{\text{TWA}}{\text{STD}} + \frac{1.645 \times \text{CV} \times \sqrt{(T_1^2 X_1^2 + \ldots + T_n^2 X_n^2)}}{\text{STD} \times (T_1 + \ldots T_n) \times \sqrt{(1 + \text{CV})}}$$

$$= \frac{\text{TWA}}{\text{STD}} + \frac{1.645 \times \text{CV} \times \sqrt{(X_1^2 + \ldots + X_n^2)}}{n \times \text{STD} \times \sqrt{(1 + \text{CV})}} \text{ if } T_1 = T_2 = \ldots = T_n$$

where $X_1, \ldots, X_n$ are n consecutive sample values
$T_1, \ldots, T_n$ are their durations
$$\text{TWA} = \frac{T_1 X_1 + \ldots + T_n X_n}{T_1 + \ldots + T_n}$$
CV   = coefficient of variation for the sampling/analytical method
STD = hygiene standard

Partial period consecutive samples

Calculate UCL (95%) as for full period consecutive samples and compare this limit to the standard. This assumes that the same concentration existed during the sampled and unsampled periods.
  Interpretation

$$\frac{X}{\text{STD}} > 1 \quad \text{non-compliance}$$

$$\text{UCL} < 1 \quad \text{compliance}$$

$$\frac{X}{\text{STD}} < 1 \text{ and UCL} > 1 \quad \text{indeterminate}$$

References

1 Blackford DB, Harris GW. Field experience with SIMSLIN II—a continuously recording dust sampling instrument. *Ann Occup Hyg.* 1978; **21**: 301–13.

2 Brown JH, Cook KM, Ney FG, Hatch T. Influence of particle size upon the retention of particulate matter in the human lung. *Am J Public Health* 1950; **40**: 450–8.

3 Committee on Threshold Limit Values. Threshold limit values of airborne contaminants for 1968. American Conference of Governmental Industrial Hygienists, Cincinnati, Ohio. 1968.

4 Committee on Threshold Limit Values. Threshold limit values for chemical substances in the work environment, 1985–86. American Conference of Governmental Industrial Hygienists, Cincinnati, Ohio. 1985.

5 Crosby T. Statistics and compliance testing. Statistics and Epidemiology, Institute of Occupational Hygienists, Report No. 2. 1982.

6 Davies CN. Dust sampling and lung disease. *Br J Industr Med* 1952; **9**: 120–6.

7 Dunmore JH, Hamilton RJ, Smith DSG. An instrument for the sampling of respirable dust for subsequent gravimetric assessment. *J Sci Instrum* 1964; **41**: 669–72.

8 Gale RW, Timbrell V. Practical application of magnetic alignment of mineral fibres for hazard evaluation. *Biological Effects of Mineral Fibres*, Wagner JC (ed). IARC Scientific Publications No. 30. 1980. Vol. I, pp. 53–60.

9 Hatch TF, Gross P. *Pulmonary Deposition and Retention of Inhaled Aerosols.* New York: Academic Press. 1964.

10 Health and Safety Executive. General methods for the gravimetric determination of respirable and total dust. MDHS 14. 1983.

11 Health and Safety Executive. Asbestos - Control Limits, and measurement of airborne dust concentrations. Guidance Note *EH10*. Revised April 1983.

12 Health and Safety Executive. Occupational exposure limits. Guidance Note EH40/86. 1986.

13 Higgins RI, Dewell P. A gravimetric size-selecting personal dust sampler. *Inhaled Particles and Vapours II.* Davies CN (ed), p. 575. Oxford: Pergamon Press. 1967.

14 Lapple CE. Processes use many collector types. *Chem Eng.* 1951; **58**: 144–151.

15 Lippmann M. Filter media for air sampling. In: *Air Sampling Instruments.* American Conference of Governmental Industrial Hygienists, Cincinnati, Ohio. 1972. Section N.

16 Lockhart LB, Patterson RL, Anderson WL. Characteristics of air filters used for monitoring airborne radioactivity. NRL Report No. 6054, U.S. Naval Research Laboratory, Washington D.C. 1964.

17 Marple VA, Rubow KL. An evaluation of the GCA respirable dust monitor 101–1. *Am Industr Hyg Assoc J.* 1978; **39**: 17–25.

18 Orenstein AJ. (ed). *Proceedings of the Pneumoconiosis Conference, Johannesburg.* London: Churchill. 1960.

19 Roach SA. A more rational basis for air sampling programmes. *Am Industr Hyg Assoc J* 1966; **27**: 1–12.

20 Sem GJ, Tsurubayashi K, Homma K. Performance of the piezoelectric microbalance respirable aerosol sensor. *Am Industr Hyg Assoc J.* 1977; **38**:580–8.

21 Soule RD. Industrial hygiene sampling and analysis. *Patty's Industrial Hygiene and Toxicology*, Vol. I. Clayton GD, Clayton FE. (eds). New York: John Wiley and Sons. 1978, pp. 707–69.

22 Steel J. Body location of personal samplers. Controversial Issues in Air Sampling, Institute of Occupational Hygienists, Report No. 4. 1984.

23 Timbrell V. Alignment of respirable asbestos fibres by magnetic fields. *Ann Occup Hyg* 1975; **18**:299–311.

24 Walton WH. Theory of size classification of airborne dust clouds by elutriation. *Br J Appl Physics*, 1954; Suppl 3:29–40.

25 Wilcox JD. Design of a new five-stage cascade impactor. *AMA Arch Industr Hyg Occup Med* 1953; **7**:376–82.

Chapter 3
Providing Clean Air
Part I: Dust Suppression and Control

Methods
Education
Inspection

The control of disorders due to inhaled substances usually begins with the appearance of clinical cases; the possibility of these having an airborne origin leads to study of the relationship to exposure and to the dose–response relationship. The latter in turn provides an objective basis for the hygiene standard which sets an upper limit for tolerable contamination of air breathed by the workforce. Within this standard the contamination should be reduced to a minimum. The technical success of the measures to achieve this is assessed by environmental monitoring (chapter 2), which may be supplemented by domestic criteria such as the dust visible on horizontal surfaces and the soiling of shirts and other clothing. The biological success of the measures in preventing respiratory disease is assessed from the medical and sickness records and by undertaking a respiratory survey (chapter 6). Once control has been achieved the identity of the remaining trace contaminants should be reviewed. The air should preferably not contain substances which might be harmful if the concentration rose due to failure of the control system. Even the best system breaks down occasionally so the feasibility of substituting a safer material should be examined.

Need for flexibility. Industrial processes usually develop in stages. The initial form is likely to have been determined in part by a principal raw material or other ingredient being available locally. Convenience, cheapness and chance will have contributed to the start and the attributes, quality and cost-effectiveness of the product will have determined that the process continued. Elsewhere a different combination of circumstances could have led to the same end-result being achieved in a different way. The aim of occupational medicine, hygiene and safety engineering is to ensure that the process, whilst remaining competitive, does not impair the health of those involved. This can be done in any of several ways.

The principles of suppression and control of dust are simple and are listed below with a brief commentary on each. The same principles apply to the prevention of occupational diseases whether they are caused by gas, fume, or dust, and whether toxic material enters the body through the respiratory tract, the alimentary tract, or the skin. The examples given below are, therefore, not limited to dusts, nor to materials which cause respiratory disease.

Abandon the process. The Carcinogenic Substances Regulations of 1967 prohibited the import, manufacture, or use of certain substances, mainly amines. The use of beryllium phosphors in fluorescent lights was abandoned in about 1949, the spraying of asbestos fibre stopped about 1970 and the industrial use of crocidolite asbestos, for example its addition to rubber in the manufacture of battery cases, ceased at about the same time. A report from the industrial medical officer that a process is too dangerous to be continued is likely to have been preceded by unsuccessful attempts to improve the situation, both in the factory and elsewhere. In addition management will have had to respond to the medical consequences of those failures and may have come to a similar conclusion. Thus there is often an unexpected willingness to abandon a process and either buy in the finished product or achieve the same result in some other way. Abandonment seems a disastrous step to take but it is often an easy and most effective way of eliminating a danger to health. In some instances it requires legislation or is a consequence of consumers choosing a safer product.

Change the process. It is sometimes possible to continue to use the same materials, but reduce the production of harmful dust, by introducing a small change in the process. For example, a guillotine produces much less dust than a circular saw, achieving a smooth finishing by fine casting, moulding or chemical coating eliminates a need for sanding or polishing, the making of silage in place of hay eliminates the risk of farmers' lung, and the flash-roasting of ores, in place of slow oxidation in a rotary furnace, greatly reduces the evolution of sulphur dioxide and metal oxide fumes. There is a possibility that the changes may themselves introduce new hazards, for example, the making of silage carries an increased risk from tractor accidents compared with making hay. Thus any change must be introduced with circumspection but this approach is often the easiest way of reducing a health hazard.

Substitution or replacement of a harmful substance by one that is less dangerous is the next line to pursue. Examples of successful substitution are the use of carborundum (corundum) in place of sandstone for grinding metals, zirconium silicate in place of sand for sand-blasting, rock wool for asbestos in high temperature thermal insulation, and glass fibre for asbestos at moderate temperatures. Some other examples are given in table 8.3 (page 162). The new material may carry its own dangers: silica flour has been used to replace diatomite, but materially increases the risk of disease. In most circumstances substitution is easy and makes no material difference to the end-product, though it may increase the costs of manufacture.

Segregation. Where the process is necessary but a potential hazard to those who live in the vicinity common sense dictates that it be carried out away from centres of population. Nuclear power stations, oil depots, factories making explosives or handling very toxic gases, and repositories and centres for study of harmful micro-organisms are obvious examples. The

segregation usually entails identifying very precisely the persons who work in the process and this facilitates their medical surveillance. Segregation is also practised within factories and installations, both to limit the dissemination of toxic material and to provide close medical surveillance of those persons who are at risk. The segregation of the handling of potentially infectious materials in hospitals to a small department of bacteriology is familiar to all doctors; it is often possible to segregate the handling of radioactive isotopes, or of potential allergens, in a similar way in industry. It is now common practice to isolate an area where asbestos insulation is to be removed by erecting temporary plastic sheeting around and above it. When this policy is adopted it is very important to carry out regular medical checks on those few workers who are employed within the segregated area, and these workers must, of course, be provided with personal protection (page 55). Segregation by time can sometimes also be used to reduce the number of persons exposed to a hazard. The potentially dangerous work is done during periods of low activity, for example meal breaks, or when few people are at work, for example in the evenings, at night or at weekends. Since relatively few people are at risk they can be closely supervised both in the work and in the performance of safety routines; this includes the use of personal protective equipment.

Suppression of dust at source. Dust is created by tearing, breaking, blasting, sawing, drilling, crushing, grinding, sanding, filing or otherwise abrading a material. It becomes airborne as a result of transfer of energy by an air current or through vibration, twisting, shaking, rotating and other agitation. Aerosolization may be reduced by slowing the rate of movement, especially if this leads to the material being broken into larger fragments which sediment rapidly and are not respirable in consequence. The dust may be prevented from becoming airborne by water applied at the site of energy transfer.

Traditionally wet tea-leaves were scattered in school corridors and in village halls before the sweeping up of dust, and water, sometimes mixed with detergent, is used extensively to suppress dust in coal mines. The coal faces are impregnated through 1–2m bore-holes, with water at high pressure before blasting, and sprays of water are directed onto the teeth of coal-cutters and onto the mined coal at those transfer points where it spills from one conveyor belt to another or from belt to wagon. Wet-drilling of siliceous rock has been obligatory in most countries for over 50 years, while Thackrah, in 1832, noted that knife-grinders, who used wet sandstone, lived longer than fork-grinders who did their grinding dry.

There are other ways of preventing a dust becoming airborne. Lead poisoning in painters became less common when pigments were retailed in paste form in place of cake or dry powder, and it is often possible to protect the end-user of other dusty products in a similar way. For example, bagasse may be packed wet instead of dry. Alternatively, the products can be sold in containers which do not have to be opened but can be added to a mixture of solvents in which they dissolve, or be thrown into a bath of molten chemicals in which they burn. Allergic reactions to alcalase (maxatase) during the manufacture of 'biological' detergents were almost eliminated by distributing the enzyme powder in the form of small compressed tablets (prills). The distribution of powders in large (1000kg) containers which can be attached directly to hoppers eliminates the evolution of dust during the opening of sacks.

However, water remains the chief material used for suppression of dust. The risk that this might cause outbreaks of Legionnaire's disease or allergic alveolitis seems to be entirely theoretical. Oil mists can harm the lung so should be avoided (pages 274 and 281).

Total enclosure accompanied by automation of the process should be considered when the previous methods are impracticable. It is common practice in the chemical industry (e.g. the nickel carbonyl method of purifying nickel) and in 'bag-houses' where sleeve-filters are used to separate fine dust, such as metal oxide, from air. The enclosure should be maintained at a pressure slightly below atmospheric to prevent leakage. If the enclosure must be entered for maintenance or repair it is usual for the maintenance staff to wear an impervious ventilated

suit or, at the very least, an airline respirator. The same principle of total enclosure applies, on a much smaller scale, to the glove-box used in laboratories to handle radioactive materials, and to the chambers used for the shot-blasting of small castings.

Partial enclosure should be considered where total enclosure is impractical. This will require the provision of local exhaust ventilation at points where materials pass into and out of the enclosure. A familiar example of this is the 'fume-cupboard' in many laboratories. But when a 'fume-cupboard' is used it is important to make certain that a forced draught is provided. It is surprising how often this is forgotten in industry, the only ventilation being a flue, sometimes opening into the laboratory. There should be an interlock on the fume-cupboard door so that it cannot be opened unless the exhaust fan is switched on, and when the door is open the aperture should not extend up above the faces of the operatives, a constructional error that is far from uncommon.

Local exhaust ventilation at the site of production of the dust should be advised when no form of enclosure is possible. Exhaust ventilation on grindstones, circular saws, chromium plating tanks, and at filling stations for bags of dry materials are familiar examples of this technique. Rather less effective are ventilated booths for welding, brazing, arc-air gouging and paint-spraying. In each instance the ventilation system should be correctly designed for the process that it is to control. Grindstones, saws and chip-hammers require a high velocity system to entrap the particles of dust which they evolve; a low volume may be all that is required. Fumes, such as those produced during welding, are often controlled by a high volume low-velocity system but a high velocity low-volume system is sometimes more effective. The exhaust system must be so sited that it draws the dust or fumes away from the operator's breathing zone. Commonly this point is overlooked so that the dust or fume is extracted from a work bench through an overhead cowl, a practice which is virtually useless. Thus if local exhaust ventilation is to be installed it must be designed by an engineer or industrial hygienist who is familiar with the pitfalls, and it must be tested after installation to make certain that it lives up to specification and achieves its aims.

Any harmful dust which is extracted by the system should not be vented to the atmosphere but must be trapped in a scrubber, in filter bags or by electrostatic precipitation. Which of these is appropriate depends on the nature of the dust or fume, and the choice of a suitable system, including the method of disposing of the accumulated dust, should be discussed with the Factory Inspector and the local Environmental Health Officer. The choice of method is particularly important when the air is to be recirculated into the general factory environment.

Further problems arise if exhaust ventilation is used in many sites throughout the factory. The volume of air extracted is large, so much heat is lost and must be replaced at extra cost unless a heat exchanger is used or the extracted air recirculated. The noise of the extractor fans reverberating along metal trunking may cause deafness or reduce efficiency inside the factory and disturb those who live beside it. The installation of extensive trunking may require the breaching of load-bearing walls and may interfere with lighting and with water, gas or electricity circuits. For these reasons the installation of exhaust ventilation is not an easy option, but requires the collaboration of hygienist, engineer, heating engineer, noise-control expert, architect, and the Factory Inspector or Environmental Health Officer. The utilization of such a system requires careful consideration for the health of those who repair or maintain it, and of those who dispose of the dust. It is clearly inexcusable to employ unprotected casual labour to sweep out trunking with brushes and compressed air-lines when the factory is closed at week-ends. Even the regular collection of the waste should be a carefully planned operation and the person who does it should be under supervision, both on the job and by regular medical examination.

Increased general ventilation may be the only way in which dust levels can be kept below danger levels. This, combined with dust suppression, is the policy adopted in coal mines and, until recently, in confined spaces in ships where welders and burners are working. It has the disadvantage that the dust is dispersed from its source; in coal mines this results in the con-centration of dust in the air being higher at the down-wind end of the face and in the 'up cast' road-way than elsewhere (fig. 9.1, page 167). Because of dispersion, increased general ventilation should not be used if the dust is carcinogenic (e.g. for asbestos).

Personal protection by use of a respirator or breathing apparatus can provide short-term protection for a repair or demolition during times of maximal dustiness, for example in a coal mine, or for an emergency, as when there has been a spillage of chemical or leak of toxic gas. Personal protection is unsuitable for long-term use because it requires close supervision, is seldom comfortable for long and interferes with speech. However, because more radical measures are expensive and often require extensive reorganization of a factory or of the manufacturing process, the provision of a dust respirator is the commonest way of attempting to deal with a dust problem. The subject is considered in detail later in this chapter.

Other measures. In addition to the specific techniques of dust suppression and control described above, there are a few extra measures which can and should be taken. Many of these come under the heading of good housekeeping. They include the use of clean work-clothes, shoes and head gear, tidying up operations and keeping the factory clean by washing, mopping, scrubbing, vacuum cleaning using an appropriate filter, laundering and dry cleaning. Dusting and sweeping are widely used but if performed dry are liable to spread the dusts. The state of the workshop or factory floor is often a good measure of the quality of management and morale of the workforce; it is also cost-effective in that fewer components get lost or broken and raw materials are conserved for future use. Vacuum line cleaning of accumulated dust on plant and ledges is particularly important as this prevents the spread of dust from one department to another. Transport leaving the factory should be hosed down to prevent spread of dust from factory road-ways to the outside environment. For the same reasons clothes used at work should not be taken home but should be laundered by or at the factory and employees should change out of work-clothes and shoes before entering the canteen. When the dust is

Table 3.1. Methods of obtaining clean air

Principle		Example
Substitution	Of safer material	Other abrasive for sand in blasting operations
	Of safer process	Other insulator for asbestos; silage for hay
Dust suppression	Less dust produced	Use non-abrasive processes
	Less dust airborne	Reduce energy transfer
	Dust removed	Apply water to source; filtration, precipitation centrifugation, scrubbing
Enclosure	Of plant	Many automated processes, e.g. NiCO
	Of individual machines	Making beryllium insulators
Segregation	With respect to time	Maintenance and repairs
Exhaust ventilation	Of enclosed process	As above
	At one site via cowl	Machine or process liberating dust
	Mobile with hose	Welding in confined spaces
General ventilation	Increased turnover of air	Any dusty process
Personal protection	Respirator	Servicing dusty equipment
	Breathing apparatus	Fire in confined space
Good housekeeping	Tidying, sweeping, vacuuming, washing	All places where work is done
Education	Recognized courses	Apprentices
	Pre-employment	All personnel
	Periodic	All personnel
Inspection	Safety Officer and representatives	Daily or weekly
	Inspectorate	When problems suspected

asbestos special arrangements for laundering should be made in order to protect the laundry workers from the risk of mesothelioma. Depending on circumstances similar arrangements may be needed for the clothes worn by beryllium workers.

Smoking at work is prohibited if it contributes to a risk from fire or explosion, as in coal mines. It should be discouraged in workers who handle asbestos (page 220) and polytetrafluoroethane. In the latter case the dust from the grinding, machining, filing, or sanding of PTFE (Teflon) breaks down to highly irritant gases if it falls onto a burning cigarette and can cause 'polymer fume fever' in the smoker (page 292).

Education in hygiene and safety. Those employees whose work may expose them to harmful dust should be warned of the danger and be given instruction and training in methods of work which will minimize the risk of ill-health. They also require supervision to ensure that these instructions are always carried out. In the U.K. the Health and Safety at Work Act lays this obligation on the employer (in Section 2), and imposes on the employee a duty to co-operate (in Section 7). These obligations are now imposed by legislation in most countries and similar legislation affects the handling of radioactive substances.

Education in hygiene and safety is an ingredient of training courses for apprentices and the introductory course which all major employers should now provide for new entrants of all ages and degrees of experience. The training is an ongoing process and it should be coupled with that for specific processes which now must have the safety aspect incorporated at the design stage.

Table 3.2.   Check list for factory visit

1. Nature of operation — raw materials, processes, products, by-products

2. (a) Number and sex of employees
   (b) Shift system and method of payment
       Hours of work and breaks. Weekend work. Overtime

3. (a) Geography of work place — where does each process take place?
   (b) Lines of movement between departments or processes

4. Environment — illumination, temperature, ventilation, smoke, steam, smells

5. (a) House-keeping — tidiness, cleanliness (who does it and how?), gangways
   (b) Smoking — when and where
   (c) Noise
   (d) Other general hazards

6. Special hazards — nature, monitoring, codes of practice, protective measures, enforcement, final responsibility

7. Training procedures

8. Safety committees, safety audits, safety representatives

9. Accident rates, sickness absence, labour turnover

10. Medical surveillance — pre-employment, post-illness, etc. Doctor, nurse, first aid, sick pay

11. (a) Welfare facilities — canteen, washing, changing rooms, protective clothing
    (b) Morale of workforce

Inspection of the workplace. The statutory requirements for safe conditions have led to the establishment of inspectorates whose duties and powers are discussed in chapter 1. Many of the inspections arise from specific incidents or from processes which have been found to be poorly controlled. However, the inspection should preferably embrace the whole plant as the problem may have ramifications outside the immediate process and may lead to contamination of the neighbourhood. A general inspection is more important for old than for new factories which have safety and hygiene measures incorporated in their design. Other factories will have had the hygiene measures added or these may have been overlooked in a rush to re-adapt old premises, change a process or make more efficient working arrangements.

The inspection should start with the objective, the general layout in relation to the natural drainage and the prevailing wind. The sources, nature and points of entry of raw materials, vehicles and personnel should be noted, also the sequence of operations including the extent to which lines of communication for materials and personnel and natural ventilation channels cross or inter-digitate. The crossing point may contribute to spread of contamination from one area to another by airborne spread or on clothing or vehicles. All processes should be inspected for the presence of the hygiene features listed in table 3.1 and any unsatisfactory aspects noted; the latter should be re-examined in the light of retrospective and prospective environmental measures. The inspection should continue through the process to the finished product and its disposal by storage, packing and dispatch. The output and disposal of waste and the servicing and cleaning operations should be inspected and the state of good housekeeping noted.

A survey along these lines leading to constructive recommendations is a major undertaking but may pay for itself many times over in better health and labour relations, increased productivity and conservation of valuable materials. A checklist of items which might be included is given in table 3.2.

Chapter 3
Providing Clean Air
Part II: Respiratory Protection

Respiratory protection
Filtration and absorption
Respirators and breathing apparatus
Personal protection
Management

Respiratory protection

The basic features of occupational respiratory hygiene are the preferred use of safe materials, elimination of dusty processes, suppression of dust and fumes at source, dust extraction and provision of clean air by appropriate ventilation at the workplace. These measures are described in the first half of the present chapter. They should be applied to the greatest possible extent using all available resources. Where resources are inadequate there may be a need for additional personal protection by respirators or breathing apparatus. The decision on their use should then be made as part of a comprehensive plan which takes into account all relevant factors of the process, equipment and operators so that safety can be ensured. Unfortunately this has not always been the case so a special responsibility rests with those who make the arrangements.

Filtration and absorption

Protection may be required against any harmful material capable of entering the respiratory tract, including particles, fibres, gases or vapours. These may be removed from the respired gas by appropriate means.

Particulate filters. Particles and fibres may be removed by impaction, sedimentation and diffusion (cf. page 62) as a result of the air passing through a pad or paper filter made of glass fibres or other material; this can have a filtration efficiency of 99.99% but at the cost of a high resistance to airflow unless the filtration area is enlarged by pleating. Alternatively or in addition the particles may be cleared by electrostatic precipitation in resin-impregnated wool which is electrically charged. The wool has a low resistance to airflow and the charge is not affected by storage. However, it is reduced by ionizing radiation and is lost if much oil mist is breathed as this forms an oil film over the fibres. The filtration efficiency deteriorates with use so the pads should be changed after an appropriate number of breathing hours. Alternative methods of producing the electrostatic charge are now being developed. In addition the life of the filter may be extended by the use of an inexpensive pre-filter. For total protection against particulate contaminants a liquid barrier filter may be used (7).

The efficiency of the filter may be tested using an aerosol of methylene blue or volatilized sodium chloride. These substances are analysed respectively by the colour of the stain on esparto paper and by flame photometry. In each case the maximal particle size is approximately 1 μm so the penetration is representative of that for spores of *M. faeni* (page 339) and other small particles but not for the majority of occupational dusts; however, the test is easily performed and provides a reproducible index of filtration efficiency. This may be expressed as:

$$\text{efficiency} = \frac{(C1 - C2)}{(C1)} \times 100\%$$

where C1 and C2 are the concentrations of test particles before and after filtration.

Adsorption of vapours. Vapours and gases are either inactivated chemically or they are removed by adsorption onto charcoal. Chemical inactivators include an alkaline solid for removing acidic vapour, an acid solid for removing alkali vapour and hopcalite for removing carbon monoxide by oxidation to carbon dioxide. Charcoal is a non-specific adsorbant and when appropriately prepared has a high adsorptive capacity. Formerly it was used as granules which were closely packed into canisters but the granules are now replaced by charcoal cloth woven from carbon fibres; the cloth, which was developed by the U.K. Chemical Defence Establishment, has a high adsorptive capacity which may be renewed by heating (1).

The efficiency of the adsorbant may be tested by monitoring the passage through it of a stream of air into which is injected a small amount of a suitable substance, such as 1-bromobutane. A sensitive halogen detector is used so the quantity of vapour needed is too small to materially reduce the capacity of the filter.

Efficiency of filters and absorbers. Tests of efficiency of filters and absorbers are described in the preceding sections. Items which meet the standards of the British Standards Institution and the U.S. National Institute of Occupational Health and Safety are very efficient but do not themselves confer protection. This comes about through their incorporation in protective systems which provide a connection with the respiratory tract via a face-piece or other device. These are described below.

Respirators and breathing apparatus

Respirators. These devices condition the ambient air by filtering out or absorbing harmful dusts and vapours. The driving force is usually the subject's own respiratory muscles sucking the inspired air through the filter; in these circumstances there is a need for an airtight seal at the interface between wearer and respirator and the design should be such that ability to work is not impaired. Alternatively a positive-pressure respirator may be used in which a portable electric fan draws air through the filters and supplies the face-piece. The fan can be carried together with batteries in a small back-pack or in a specially designed safety helmet. However, it requires additional equipment which must be carried and which may go wrong.

Breathing apparatus. This equipment provides the subject with gas which will support activity and is traditionally used when the atmosphere is deficient in oxygen or contains a harmful constituent such as carbon monoxide which cannot readily be removed. This is often the case in a rescue situation when the breathing apparatus should have its own built-in supply of oxygen and be self-contained; the technical specification must then be such that the equipment does not impede strenuous activity (table 3.3). In addition, to prevent inward leakage of contaminated gas, a positive pressure should be maintained inside the face-piece throughout the breathing cycle. When a ducted face mask is used (page 56) this may be done by feeding oxygen to the outer cavity of the mask independently of the supply to the user. As an alternative to portable oxygen the breathing apparatus may be supplied with clean air via a compressed airline. The air is delivered to a mask or hood which is either confined to the head and neck or forms part of a protective garment which may be a blouse or suit. The garment should be impervious to the relevant dust or fume. By this means good respiratory protection is readily achieved. In the case of garments the airflow should be at least 120 l min^{-1} to provide for ventilation and to disperse body heat, in addition the airline must be supported so that it does not drag on the face mask or garment, be protected against kinking, compression, or fracture and be supplied from a secure source of clean air. The air is preferably provided from a high pressure cylinder or compressor but a hose may be used provided its length is less than 10m. The air should contain minimal amounts of carbon monoxide (<5ppm), carbon dioxide (<0.05%) and oil mist (<0.5mg m^{-3}). Increasingly this type of equipment is being used in place of a respirator to provide protection against industrial dusts and vapours.

Overall efficiency. The weakest point in the protective system is usually the line of contact between face and face-piece or its equivalent. Discontinuities in contact leading to inward leakage of contaminated air occur frequently, either initially because the face-piece is unsuitable or because it moves during use. The overall

Table 3.3.   U.K. Standards for closed circuit compressed air breathing apparatus (3)

Weight	16kg
Leakage	Facepiece $\leq 0.05\%$ of inhaled air; no leakage when distended and immersed in water.
Resistance	Neither the inspiratory nor expiratory side of the circuit shall have a dynamic resistance greater than 3mbar, 5mbar and 16mbar at constant flows of 85, 125 and 300 l min^{-1}, respectively.
Relief valve	Opening pressure 1.5–4.0mbar $\leq$ 5mbar at 50 l min^{-1}. Leakage <0.0025% of external atmosphere.
Breathing bag volume	>5 litres.
Temperature of inspired air	<40°C.

Air composition	O_2 21%
	CO_2 Mouthpiece 0.75% average
	            1% maximum
	      Facemask 1% average
	            1.5% maximum

efficiency of the system takes this leakage into account. It may be assessed by the sodium chloride test described above or by exposure to ammonia gas in a concentration of 0.25–1%. The subject breathes the aerosol cloud or gas in a chamber and the extent of contamination of the inhaled air is estimated by analysing gas which has been sampled at the lips via a fine catheter. The nominal protection factor (NPF) is given by the following relationship:

$$NPF = \frac{atmospheric\ concentration}{concentration\ within\ face\ piece}$$

Under favourable conditions the protection factor ranges from approximately 7 for a disposable filtering face-piece respirator to 2000 for a self-contained or compressed airline breathing apparatus; under unfavourable conditions there may be no protection at all.

The inward leakage of contaminated air may alternatively be estimated using a tracer gas such as sulphur hexafluoride (SF_6), argon or helium and an appropriate detector. Results for argon and SF_6 are comparable with air but using helium the measured leak is larger by a factor of 1.3 on account of the low molecular weight of helium increasing its diffusivity. The leakage for air should not exceed 10% in the case of

general purpose dust respirators, 0.25% for gas respirators and 0.05% for a self-contained breathing apparatus. These limits determine the extent of atmospheric contamination against which protection is provided. Thus for a leakage of 10% the contamination should not exceed 10 times the acceptable level, for 1% leakage 100 times and for 0.05% leakage 2000 times the acceptable level. Atmospheres containing an unknown concentration of contaminant should not be entered except in an emergency.

Personal protection

Short-term personal protection. This is essential if work is to be undertaken in circumstances when safety cannot be ensured in other ways. Thus alternative protection may not be possible because the activity is undertaken on a single occasion, access may be difficult or circumstances may lead to a temporary rise in the environmental concentration of a harmful substance. Examples are the dismantling of old equipment lagged with asbestos, relining furnaces with silica brick, repairing equipment used to manufacture polyurethane foam and tackling an emergency leak in a pipe carrying nickel carbonyl or beryllium oxide powder.

Longer-term personal protection. This may be

used to supplement the environmental hygiene measures when the airborne concentration of harmful material fluctuates in a predictable manner, or when the process is only undertaken intermittently, either as short production runs or on repeated single occasions. Fluctuations in airborne concentrations occur in relation to specific events including emptying sacks and containers, cleaning equipment and during particular processes such as welding or giving hay to cows. Cyclical changes in exposure may occur as in mechanical coal-cutting when the operator down from the cutting engine but not the up operator is exposed to much dust; the exposures of the operators are then reversed with each change in direction of the engine.

As well as environmental factors a change in circumstances leading to increased dust deposition in the lungs may also be an indication for personal protection. Deposition may be influenced by posture via its effect on the thoracic gas volume. A supine posture is associated with a relatively small thoracic gas volume when the deposition is greater than under normal circumstances (page 74). Thus additional protection may be necessary if work is undertaken lying down instead of sitting or standing. The total pulmonary deposition also increases as a result of changing from nose to mouth breathing so the onset of mouth breathing during exercise might be considered as a warning sign. Unfortunately exercise may reduce the tolerance to breathing against resistance and increase the subjective discomfort of the respirator which may then be less acceptable to the intending user.

Difficulties in using protective devices. The difficulties mainly reflect the compromises which underlie the characteristics of the protective devices. Thus in the case of a dust respirator the resistance to airflow rises with increasing efficiency of the filter but a high resistance is subjectively unacceptable to the user. Leakage round the face-piece is a perpetual problem, particularly for bearded men, and persons with a flat bridge to the nose, are edentulous or wear spectacles (which should have flat side-arms). The problem is partly solved by use of a full face mask; this makes contact at the forehead, cheek and below the chin and provides a better seal

than one which makes contact around the bridge of the nose (half face mask) or beneath the lower lip (oronasal mask). However, the oronasal and half face masks, because they do not enclose the eyes, do not mist up and have a wider field of vision; they also have a smaller respiratory deadspace so that the wearer rebreathes less carbon dioxide. These advantages may be combined with those of the full face mask by having one inside the other when it is called a ducted face mask. Closed circuit breathing apparatus presents an additional problem on account of the heat which is generated during the absorbtion of carbon dioxide; the effect is greatest in hot environments when an inspired air temperature in excess of 40°C may occur unless additional cooling is achieved by fuelling the set with liquid oxygen. This in turn increases the cost and reduces the availability of the resulting protection compared with cylinder oxygen.

In general the design features of protective equipment which are usually satisfactory include particulate filters, vapour absorbers, canisters and valves. Difficulties may be experienced in achieving a good fit, low breathing resistance, thermal comfort, a wide field of vision and ease of spoken communication. Some devices are better than others in these respects and none are satisfactory in all of them. Many of the difficulties may be avoided by using an air-ventilated hood or suit or a positive-pressure respirator, but as indicated earlier these devices have other limitations, including in the cases of the hood or suit the purity and integrity of the air supply, and of the atmosphere-supplied respirator the bulk and cost of the equipment.

Management of personal protection

Choice of equipment. This is the resultant of all the aspects which have been discussed. (a) For work requiring unrestricted movement in an atmosphere which may not sustain life a self-contained breathing apparatus should be used (e.g. Siebe Gorman, Draeger). (b) For continuous work in a seriously polluted atmosphere, particularly when there may be a need to undertake moderately strenuous activity, an air-ventilated hood or suit is the best proposition (e.g. Martindale positive pressure powered respirator). (c) For continuous ambulatory work in an atmosphere which is moderately polluted and where there is also a need for head protection the atmosphere-supplied helmet respirator is highly recommended (e.g. Racal air stream helmet with high efficiency filter and visor assembly, fig. 3.1). (d) For intermittent use in circumstances where there may be transient serious pollution an individually fitted half-face or oronasal respirator is appropriate (e.g. Leyland, Baxter Pneuseal). (e) For continuous use in an atmosphere which is moderately polluted but where bulk of equipment, servicing and supervision may be a problem the disposable filtering facepiece is highly recommended (e.g. 3M 8800 respirator, fig. 3.1). (f) For protection against nuisance dusts which are unpleasant but not harmful a simple oral or oronasal filter is usually adequate (e.g. 3M 8500 filtering face-piece or Martindale disposable).

Practical considerations. These will determine the success or failure of any personal protection programme. The steps to be taken should be decided objectively by informed persons (e.g. hygienists, not line management) and each stage written down so that there is no ambiguity. First, the use of personal protective devices should be appropriate and should not be used as an excuse to evade installation of effective measures for removing or suppressing the offending material. Thus the reasons for using personal protection should be recorded. If personal protection is chosen as a short-term expedient, steps should be taken to ensure its replacement within a specified time. Secondly, the system which is adopted should be capable of providing the necessary protection and sufficient resources should be made available to ensure that it does so in practice. The arrangements should be supervised by one or more named persons who should be adequately trained. The arrangements include the issue and maintenance of equipment, continued monitoring of its use and training of those who use it.

The issue of equipment should include fitting and adjustments to ensure that the equipment effectively excludes contaminated air, is comfortable, does not impede vision and is altogether suitable for the individual who uses it. The size of any helmet, garment or face mask and the fit round the line of contact with the face should receive special attention; in the case of face masks more than one shape and size should be tried until one which is suitable is found. Fitting may be assisted by placing a card or piece of thin PVC film over the filter canister and asking the wearer to inhale then hold the breath;

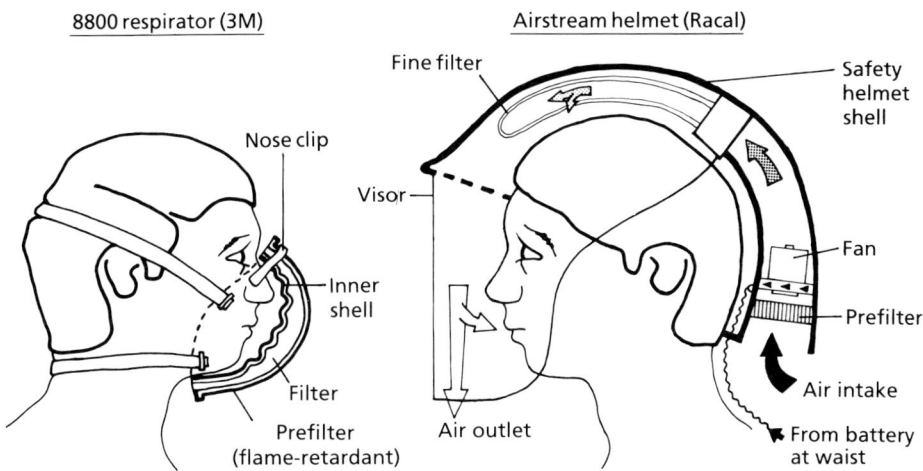

Fig. 3.1. Dust respirators. *Left.* Diagram illustrating the 8800 respirator (3M). *Right.* Air stream helmet (Racal).

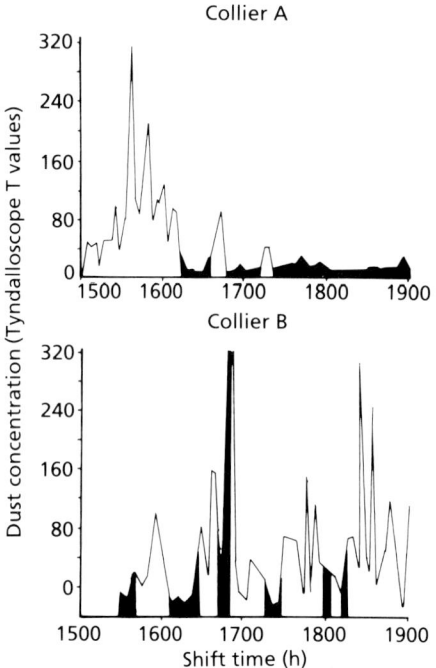

Fig. 3.2. Voluntary use of dust respirators by two colliers A and B; the graphs relate the dust concentration (Tyndalloscope T values) to time during the shift. Respirators were worn except where indicated in black; with one exception these were times of relatively low dustiness. (By courtesy of R. M. Howie and W. H. Walton (1), p. 294.)

the face-piece should adhere to the face and not fall off. Maintenance should include daily cleaning, a weekly check on all components, changing filters at specified times and checks to ensure that the equipment is used conscientiously. Training should include all aspects which have been mentioned; there should be a clear understanding of the circumstances when the equipment should be used.

Need for research. The design of face-pieces is a branch of ergonomics which has not kept pace with developments in filtration, air pumps and other components of respirators. As a result it is sometimes difficult to ensure a good face fit from among the respirators currently available; these seldom come in a range of sizes and when they do the differences are not always obvious. Current designs do not provide adequately for

people with short faces or for those with a shallow bridge to the nose.

The times when respirators should be used have received little consideration but it is important. Thus Howie and Walton have found that coal miners who voluntarily wear respirators do so on average for approximately 20% of the time but reduce their estimated dust intake by 40%. This is because the respirators tend to be worn at times of maximal dustiness (fig. 3.2). Protection is greatest during short periods of use so there is need for strategies which ensure that respirators are worn during heavy exposures.

The physiological aspects of personal protective devices have been investigated extensively. However, there is still need for simple tests of both the overall resistance of the equipment during use and the ability to undertake physically demanding tasks whilst using a respirator. The psychological aspects merit analysis as do the medical contraindications. In the absence of more information the latter should include any degree of cardiac insufficiency but not moderate respiratory impairment.

References

1 Ballantyne B, Schwabe PH. *Respiratory Protection: Principles and Application*. London: Chapman Hall. 1981.

2 British Standards Institution (1974a). Recommendations for the selection, use and maintenance of respiratory protective equipment. London: BS 4275. 1974.

3 Cotes JE. Advances in respiratory protection. *Ann Occup Hyg*. 1979; **22**:189–97.

4 Davies CN. (ed). *Design and Use of Respirators*. Oxford: Pergamon Press. 1962.

5 Pritchard JA. A guide to industrial respiratory protection. United States Department of Health, Education and Welfare (National Institute for Occupational Safety and Health) Publication (NIOSH). Washington: U.S. Government Printing Office. 1976; 76–189.

6 Raven PB, Dodson AT, Davis TO. The physiological consequences of wearing industrial respirators: A review. *Am Industr Hyg Assoc J*. 1979; **40**: 517–45.

7 Seufert WD, Bessette F, Lachiver G. The liquid barrier filter: total protection against particulate contaminants. *Br J Industr Med* 1984; **41**:1–5.

Chapter 4
Respiratory Defence Mechanisms

Deposition in the respiratory tract
Respiratory reflexes which protect the airways
Mucociliary clearance
Alveolar deposition
Fate of inhaled particles
Role of macrophages
Humoral defence mechanisms

Ambient air is seldom free from contaminants; instead it contains droplets and a variety of particulates, mainly pollen spores and debris from animal, vegetable and mineral matter in the local environment. Most of the substances are harmless in themselves but if allowed to accumulate in the airways would cause local damage. Some cause infection or are sensitizers. Protection is provided by respiratory defence mechanisms; these have evolved to cope with naturally occurring contaminants but are also effective against occupational ones. The occupational contaminants are in the form of gases, vapours, droplets, droplet nuclei and particulates (table 4.1). Of these, the vapours and gases cannot be filtered out so the defences only come into play following contact with epithelium. The contact can lead to the material being neutralised (for example, in the nose) or to its further entry being reduced by activation of respiratory or other reflexes. The larger inhaled particulates are removed from the airstream by deposition during transit through the nose and bronchi; these particles are excreted via the mucociliary escalator or by coughing. The remainder enter the alveoli where some deposit on the alveolar walls but the majority remain suspended in air and are subsequently exhaled. Alveolar deposition is usually a prelude to ingestion by macrophages, most of which subsequently migrate onto the mucociliary escalator; approximately 7% of particles enter the lung parenchyma. Here they come up against humoral defence mechanisms. Droplets are subjected to the same treatment as particles but the proportion which is deposited is larger due to droplets growing in size by absorbing water vapour. Droplet nuclei may absorb water or persist as such when the great majority remain in suspension and are eventually exhaled.

The magnitude of the problem presented to the defence mechanisms can be expressed

Table 4.1. Constituents and contaminants of air

Category	Normal constituents	Contaminants
Gases	Oxygen, nitrogen, carbon dioxide Rare gases	Carbon monoxide Oxides of nitrogen, ozone, sulphur dioxide
Vapours	Water	Volatile substances
Droplets	Water	Oils and other liquids
Droplet nuclei	Viruses, bacteria, oro-nasal secretions	Salts, amorphous chemicals, protozoa, etc.
Particulates	Pollen-spores, debris (animal, vegetable and mineral)	Condensates, products of combustion, occupational dusts and fibres

numerically. Alveolar ventilation is approximately 5 l min^{-1} at rest and 25 l min^{-1} doing what, in an occupational context, is usually regarded as hard work (oxygen uptake 60mmol min^{-1} or 1.3 l min^{-1}). Thus during a working lifetime of 40 years (40h per week, 48 weeks per year) the volume of workplace air which reaches the alveoli is in the range 23,000–115,000m^3. The content of respirable dust will normally be within the hygiene standard which is 10mg m^{-3} in the case of a nuisance dust, 4mg m^{-3} for coal mine dust and less for toxic dusts. Thus taking as an example a coal mine where the environmental conditions just meet the hygiene standard the miner who performs hard work for 25% of the time might have an average alveolar ventilation during the shift of 15 l min^{-1}. Over a working lifetime he might then inhale approximately 275g of dust, of which only about 20g would enter the lung parenchyma. The remaining 255g would have been exhaled or excreted. All parts of the respiratory tract contribute to this clearance, unlike in rodents where the nose is the principal organ of respiratory protection; thus the results of studies of clearance are species dependent. In man the deposition and clearance show large inter-subject variations in acute experiments; however, a link with long-term retention appears not to have been established.

Deposition in the respiratory tract

Mechanisms of deposition

Deposition occurs when particles or fibres make contact with the epithelium of the nasopharynx or tracheobronchial tree or alveoli. In the case of particles deposition occurs by impaction, sedimentation under the influence of gravity or diffusion (Brownian motion) when it is due to the particles being bombarded or jostled by adjacent gas molecules. Fibres deposit by any of these mechanisms or by making contact with the epithelium at a junction, bend or narrowing in the airway. This process has been described as interception (29); it is important for materials whose 'effective' diameter exceeds the actual diameter, for example fungal mycelium and the curved fibres of chrysotile asbestos.

The physical factors which contribute to deposition by impaction and sedimentation are reviewed by, amongst others, Gerrity, Hounam and Lippmann and their colleagues (10, 11, 15) and are described below. In the case of round particles the diameter and density are of prime importance. For irregular particles the diameter is not a definite measurement, whilst for fibres the deposition is also somewhat influenced by the length. These complicating factors may be taken into account by using instead of the actual diameter, the aerodynamic diameter. This is the diameter of a sphere of unit density having the same terminal settling velocity as the particle/fibre in question. For example, for amphibole asbestos fibres which are straight the aerodynamic diameter is approximately 3 times the actual diameter. In the case of spherical particles the aerodynamic diameter (D_e) is given by $D_e = \sqrt{\varrho}D^2$ where ϱ is the density of the particle and D is its diameter. For irregular particles and fibres the aerodynamic diameter may be determined using an aerosol spectrometer (page 33).

Inertial impaction occurs especially at points in the respiratory tract where the direction of air flow changes, in the anterior nares and bronchial bifurcations. The probability of impaction is proportional to the Stokes number. This is described by equation 4.1. The component terms for this and subsequent equations, which traditionally are expressed in c.g.s. units, are defined in table 4.2.

$$\text{Stokes number (N)} = \frac{\varrho D^2 \bar{V}}{9\eta d} \qquad (4.1)$$

Inertial impaction is an important cause for deposition of particles having an aerodynamic diameter in the range 3–20μm. The deposition is also proportional to the Reynolds number which is given by the relationship:

$$\text{Reynolds Number (Re)} = \bar{V}d\varrho_a/\eta \qquad (4.2)$$

hence the deposition is inversely related to the kinematic viscosity (η/ϱ_a).

Sedimentation occurs when the gravitational force acting on the mass of the particle exceeds the sum of the buoyancy of the particle and the resistance to fall offered by the surrounding air.

Table 4.2.   Symbols used in equations

Symbol	Definition	Units	
		c.g.s.	SI
N	Stokes number	–	–
Re	Reynolds number	–	–
D	Particle diameter	cm	m
De*	Equivalent for unit density	cm	m
d	Airway diameter	cm	m
V	Mean air velocity	$cm\,s^{-1}$	$m\,s^{-1}$
Vs	Settling velocity	$cm\,s^{-1}$	$m\,s^{-1}$
ϱ	Density of particle	$g\,cm^{-3}$	$kg\,m^{-3}$
ϱa	Density of air	$g\,cm^{-3}$	$kg\,m^{-3}$
η	Viscosity of air	$g\,cm^{-1}\,s^{-1}$ (poise)	$N\,s\,m^{-2}$
η/ϱ_a	Kinematic viscosity of air	$cm^2\,s^{-1}$ (Stoke)	$m^2\,s^{-1}$
g	Gravitational acceleration	981	–

* Aerodynamic diameter.

The particle then falls at a constant speed which is the terminal settling velocity. This is described approximately by Stokes law which may be represented as follows:

$$\text{Settling velocity } (V_s) = (\varrho - \varrho_a)\frac{D^2 g}{18\eta} \qquad (4.3)$$

In practice sedimentation is an important cause for deposition of particles of which the aerodynamic diameter exceeds 0.5μm. Diffusion contributes to the deposition of particles of aerodynamic diameter below 3μm thus accounting for some 1% of the total deposition. However, the contribution is material only at diameters of less than 0.5μm. In this size range the diameter is a poor guide to deposition. A long residence time in an air space of small diameter increases the probability that deposition will take place. The phase of respiration is of secondary importance. As well as these physical factors the deposition may be affected by any electric charges on either the particles or the walls of airways. But little is yet known about the role of electrostatic forces in the human respiratory tract.

Deposition in the nasopharynx

The nose is a remarkably accommodating organ; it is an important component of physiognomy, buffer against impact or assault, and organ of smell. It conditions the tidal gas passing to and fro and provides the first defence against polluted air. Some of its features are illustrated in fig. 4.1.

The nostrils or anterior nares have a combined cross-sectional area of approximately 1cm^2 and direct the incoming air upwards and backwards into the main horizontal passages of the nose. These are partially filled by the convoluted turbinate bones which are lined by specialized epithelium, comprising columnar ciliated cells, goblet cells and mucous secretory glands; the subepithelium is highly vascular tissue which can vary in thickness. The horizontal nasal passages are 5–8cm long and have a cross-sectional area of 50cm^2 but due to the convolutions the effective width is only about 2mm. This feature contributes to the nose warming and humidifying the incoming air and also to conserving heat and water vapour by receiving back a proportion of these ingredients as the air is exhaled.

The small cross-sectional area of the anterior nares has the effect that air enters the nostrils at a relatively high velocity. Swift & Proctor have estimated that even under resting conditions when the maximal volume flow rate during inspiration is only 12.5 l min^{-1} , the corresponding linear velocity is 2.3m s^{-1} (27). Since in an upright posture the direction of airflow is nearly vertical, the particles which enter the nose must have a settling velocity which is less than the

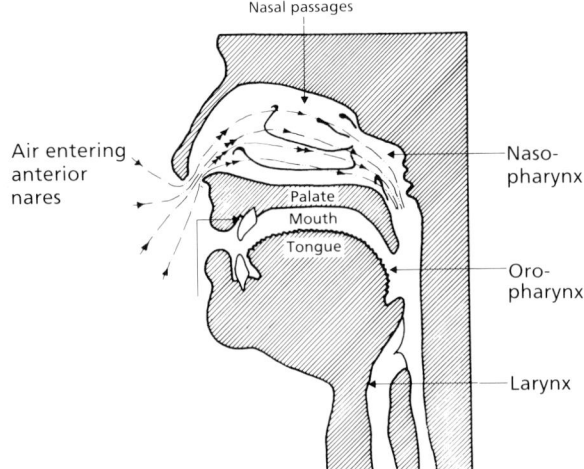

Fig. 4.1. The small cross-sectional area of the anterior nares results in a high linear velocity (indicated by arrows): this leads to the larger particles impacting on the anterior tip of the turbinate bones. (Adapted from D. L. Swift and D. F. Proctor (27), with permission.)

linear air flow velocity. At a velocity of 2.3m s^{-1} the critical particle diameter for spheres of unit density (1g cm^{-3}) is 0.6mm; this is the largest particle which can enter the nose by inspiration at rest. The high velocity imparts a momentum to the inhaled particles which causes them to impact on the anterior tip of the turbinate bones instead of flowing over them. Almost all particles down to a diameter of 7μm impact at this point. Some smaller particles also do so but below an aerodynamic diameter of 3μm the proportion is small (fig. 4.2). The process of impaction may be supplemented by the presence of hairs but their role appears to be of limited

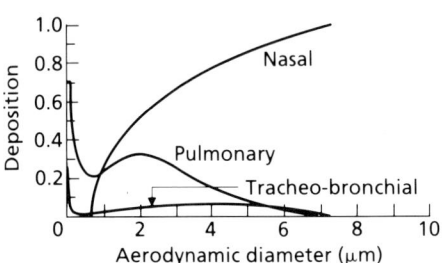

Fig. 4.2. Fractional deposition of particles in the respiratory tract: the deposition is calculated assuming a respiratory frequency of 15 per min and tidal volume of 1.45l: data of the task force on lung dynamics (28). (Reproduced from *Health Physics* Vol. 12, page 179 by permission of the Health Physics Society.)

importance in man. Impacted particles are removed by ciliary action and by blowing the nose.

On entry to the posterior nasal passage the rate of airflow slows considerably, creating conditions where clearance by sedimentation and diffusion can occur. However, due to the efficiency of the impaction mechanism, sedimentation in the nose makes only a small contribution. Gases and very small particles (diam. <0.01μm) are taken up by diffusion. In favourable circumstances, for example ammonia gas in low concentration, the clearance approaches 100% but for small particles the clearance is relatively small. It is likely to be influenced by the state of health of the nasal epithelium.

The nose is bypassed during mouth breathing so the nasal impaction mechanism is no longer operational. However, when the mouth is only slightly open the tongue takes over some of the functions of the nose by both creating conditions for impaction and contributing heat and moisture to the incoming air. These roles are lost during heavy exercise, singing and rapid speech when the oropharynx is wide open and the site of respiratory defence is entirely within the lung. The changeover from nasal to oral breathing occurs in response to a rise in the work of nasal breathing but the trigger mechanism and the factors which influence it are poorly understood. The level of ventilation at

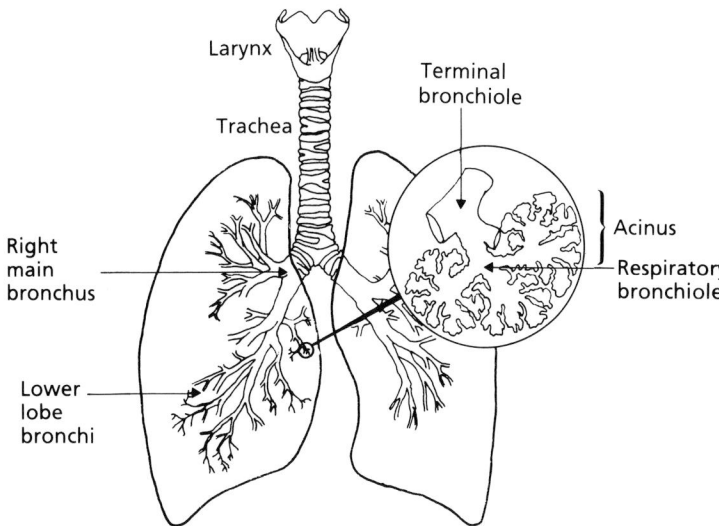

Fig. 4.3. Lower respiratory tract from larynx to alveoli. The insert shows three respiratory bronchioles coming off a terminal bronchiole. Each respiratory bronchiole supplies a cluster of alveolar ducts, atria and alveoli; this constitutes an acinus.

which the changeover occurs varies with circumstances, reflecting the extent to which the anterior nares collapse during inspiration and the relative engorgement of the vascular erectile tissue of the nose. The latter increases with cold and when breathing carbon dioxide or irritant substances including sulphur dioxide; it decreases with exercise and fear or anger.

Nasal dimensions and the lability of the nasal vascular tissue vary between individuals and cause some to do more mouth breathing than others; the mouth breathers incur the larger dust burden. Dust in the nose is mostly harmless. However, acute inflammation may be caused by inhaling corrosive vapours. Chronic ulceration of the nasal septum can follow prolonged exposure to chromate, arsenic or caustic soda dust, and nasal cancer is an occupational hazard of persons making hardwood furniture and leather footwear (1, 9, 16 and table 1.7, page 16). Vapours may also impair the sense of smell or damage the olfactory epithelium (17). Substances which may have one or more of these effects are discussed in chapters 12 and 13.

Deposition in the tracheobronchial tree

Air enters the trachea from the pharynx via the larynx where it acquires turbulent motion on account of passing through the vocal cords.

It has already been conditioned by passage through the nose or oropharynx and most particles of diameter $>7\mu m$ have been removed. The subsequent passage to the level of the alveolar ducts is by bulk flow. In the process the air has entered and emerged from some twenty to twenty-five intersections depending on whether it is on its way to the upper or lower lobe; the first intersection (fig. 4.3) is the bifurcation of the trachea into the two main bronchi and the last are the junctions between the different orders of respiratory bronchiole and the alveolar ducts with their attendant alveoli. At each intersection the combined cross-sectional area of the branches exceeds that of the common pathway so the linear velocity of airflow decreases progressively as the air is drawn into the lung. This pattern of flow largely determines the distribution of particulate material within the lung airways.

The process of cleaning by impaction which began in the anterior nares continues in the airways starting with the tracheal bifurcation (table 4.3). At this and each subsequent carina* particles are deposited both by linear impaction and secondarily to local turbulence associated

*The contour of the bifurcation resembles a ship's keel which in Latin is carina.

Table 4.3. Clearance of particles and fibres from the respired gas

Aerodynamic diameter	Principal mechanism	Main site*	Clearance (%)
> 20μm	Sedimentation	General atmosphere	100
20–7μm	Impaction	Nose, oropharynx, carina	100
7–5μm	Impaction, interception (fibres)	Nose, carina, bronchial bifurcation	80
5–0.5μm	Sedimentation	Alveoli, bronchioles	50†
0.5–0.05μm	Diffusion	Alveoli	25
0.05–0.01μm	Diffusion	Alveoli, bronchioles, bronchi	40

* Particles and most fibres which deposit in conducting airways are cleared via the mucociliary escalator.
† For mouth breathing. With nose breathing the clearance is greater but deposition in the acinus (alveolar deposition) is reduced to approximately 25%.

with vortices set up by the air stream dividing (fig. 4.4). The vortices also enlarge the area of epithelium on which deposition occurs. Impaction is greatest at the tracheal bifurcation where the linear velocity is highest; it becomes progressively less at each subsequent carina with rather more at the upper lobe than lower lobe bifurcations. The resulting uneven anatomical distribution of deposited particles is the probable cause of the similar anatomical distribution of bronchial carcinomata in the population as a whole (23).

The probability of a particle impacting at a bifurcation is related to the velocity of air flow and inversely related to the airway diameter (eqn. 4.1, page 62); on this account for a given minute volume the clearance by impaction will be greater if the airway calibre is reduced. This

occurs reflexly by contraction of smooth muscle in the bronchial walls as a result of particles stimulating irritant receptors in the airways (page 69). For a similar reason reflex narrowing of airways occurs in smokers compared with non-smokers whilst many bronchitic subjects have narrow airways because of thickening of the bronchial epithelium (chapter 17). Compared with asymptomatic non-smokers these changes contribute to more proximal deposition of particles: deposition in the periphery of the lungs is reduced in consequence.

Distal to the bronchi the linear velocity of airflow is low and impaction no longer occurs to a material extent. Sedimentation is the main reason for particles leaving the airstream in the peripheral airways. The proportion which does so is not known precisely but is probably less than 10% (fig. 4.5). Some fibres deposit by interception (page 62); the remainder are either exhaled or are deposited in the alveoli.

Deposition in the lung parencyhma

The structures distal to the terminal bronchioles constitute the lung parenchyma which is the gas exchanging part of the lung and includes the respiratory bronchioles, alveolar ducts, atria, alveolar sacs and alveoli. The lung tissue served by one respiratory bronchiole is called an acinus. Because of clearance in the nose and airways the particles entering an acinus have a diameter of less than 7μm. Of those that do so, some in the size range 7–0.5μm deposit by sedimentation whilst below this size deposition

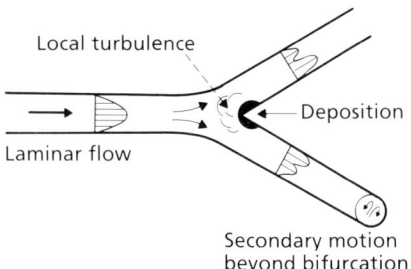

Fig. 4.4. Model airway showing flow profiles and deposition at a bifurcation. (Adapted from data of R. C. Shroter and M. F. Sudlow (24) with permission.)

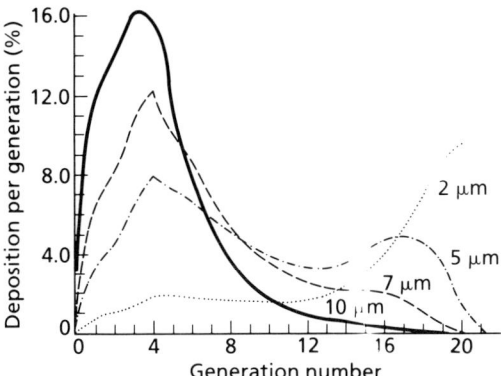

Fig. 4.5. Calculated deposition of inhaled particles by airway generation. (By courtesy of T. R. Gerrity and colleagues (10).)

can occur as a result of Brownian motion. The particle diameter 0.5μm is critical since at this aerodynamic diameter the root mean square displacement per second due to bombardment by gas molecules is equal to the terminal settling velocity. However, 0.5μm particles are too small for effective deposition by sedimentation and too large for there to be much impingement by diffusion so only about 20% are deposited. Smaller particles diffuse more rapidly and on this account have a higher fractional deposition (fig. 4.2). Deposition in the acinus is increased by any factor which increases the residence time for the particles in the lung including breath-holding and a low frequency of breathing. It is also increased by an increase in tidal volume and by breathing at a small lung volume. The deposition is important because it occurs distal to the ciliated epithelium of the lung airways. The particles are, therefore, not automatically removed on the mucociliary escalator and stand a chance of entering the lung tissue (page 74); they are a potential cause of occupational lung disease.

Respiratory reflexes which protect the airways

Nerve receptors

Receptors of a number of types are plentiful throughout the upper respiratory tract, larynx,

trachea and main bronchi. They also occur in the smaller airways and lung parenchyma. The majority are immediately accessible to inhaled materials whilst others may be stimulated by secondary reactions including interstitial oedema, diffuse fibrosis and release of chemical mediator substances. Stimulation of receptors initiates reflex responses which may protect the respiratory tract from further contamination, promote clearance of particles which are deposited and contribute to the clinical features of any resulting lung disease. However, contrary to common belief most receptors respond to more than one type of stimulus and contribute to more than one response. This complexity is clearly described by Widdicombe (31) but the subject is not helped by having an inappropriate nomenclature.

Simple nerve endings respond to the presence of particles or to local tissue damage; these endings occur throughout the respiratory tract. Those in the nose, pharynx, larynx, trachea and large airways (where they are called irritant receptors) may initiate the production of mucus. They also affect the airway calibre, but the response is not uniform. Endings in the larynx and large airways promote constriction and a reduction in airway calibre but stimulation of nasal receptors usually leads to bronchodilatation. More complex reflex responses also occur and are described below.

Stretch receptors served by myelinated nerves occur in the non-cartilaginous posterior wall of the trachea and main bronchi; these are the prototype of all lung receptors, their presence having been predicted by Hering & Breuer in 1868. Discharge from stretch receptors was first monitored by Adrian in 1933; their structure has only recently been described by Kraus. As well as responding to stretch the receptors are stimulated by hyperthermia and inhibited by carbon dioxide in a concentration of 10%; however, the reflexes are weak and these responses are not of clinical importance. Receptors served by non-myelinated fibres (C fibres) occur adjacent to alveolar capillaries; they were identified by Paintal who called them juxta-capillary receptors, hence J receptors (18). The receptors, now called C-fibre receptors, also occur in the bronchi. They are stimulated by interstitial oedema of the lung such as occurs in poisoning with phosgene (page 292); the response to stimulation includes shallow rapid breathing. Shallow breathing also occurs following stimulation of airway stretch receptors which reflexly cut short inspiration, and of irritant receptors which also cause augmented breaths. Stimulation of lung receptors is believed to be responsible for the altered pattern of breathing associated with inhalation of ammonia gas and other irritant substances (4) and the shallow breathing which has been observed in chronic beryllium disease (5).

Some features of the different classes of receptors are summarized in table 4.4. The defensive reflexes are described below; they have been reviewed by Richardson & Peatfield (22).

Apnoea reflex

Inhalation of an irritant substance into the nose or larynx can abruptly terminate that inspiration and close the larynx. At the same time the cardiac frequency decreases and the systemic blood pressure rises. The respiratory response limits the immediate exposure to the noxious

Table 4.4. Features of receptors of respiratory tract

Name/site	Type and location	Nerve supply	Stimuli	Responses
Nose	Little information	Trigeminal	Dusts, vapours Irritants	Sneeze, apnoea, bronchodilatation Secretion of mucus
Nasopharynx	Myelinated and non-myelinated	Glossopharyngeal	Pressure, etc.	Sniff and aspiration reflexes
Pharynx	Little information		Pressure, etc.	Swallowing reflex
Larynx	Free endings: (a) superficial (b) deep	Laryngeal (superior and recurrent)	Dusts, vapours Irritants	Swallowing (via epiglottis) Cough, expiratory effort (via vocal cords) Laryngeal broncho-constriction Secretion of mucus
Irritant receptors	Superficial and deep, rapidly adapting near carina and main bronchi	Vagus	Dusts, irritants, deep respn, decr. lung compliance, microemboli, etc.	Cough, raised BP, laryngeal and bronchial constriction, secretion of mucus, hyperpnoea
Stretch receptors (in airways)	Complex, slowly adapting. In muscular membranous posterior wall of trachea and main bronchi	Vagus	Stretch, inspn., decr. lung compliance, hyperthermia, low Pa_{CO_2}	Inspn. shortened, expn. often prolonged vocal chords abducted (reflex weak in man)
J receptors (pulm. c fibre receptors)	Juxtacapillary, also walls of bronchi	Vagus (non-myelinated)	Irritants, chemical mediators, interstitial oedema, microemboli	Apnoea, tachypnoea, tracheal and weak bronchial constriction, bradycardia, etc.

substance and gives time for further protective action including withdrawal from exposure. The receptors are nerve endings in the nasal septum including its posterior part, and in the larynx. The afferent pathway from the nose is via the trigeminal nerve and the effect on respiratory motor activity is probably mediated via the respiratory centres in the medulla. Substances which may have this effect depending on their concentration include tobacco smoke, sulphur dioxide, ammonia, ether, chloroform, benzol and water. Except in the new born, cold water applied to the face provokes a similar response when it is called the diving reflex.

Expiration reflex

Mechanical stimulation of the vocal folds of the larynx causes reflex narrowing or closure of the glottis and forced expiration. The nervous pathway overlaps with that for the cough reflex but is not identical since both the response is different and the two reflexes have different sensitivities to drugs. The expiration reflex has the effect of instantly expelling inhaled foreign material without prior inhalation which might otherwise draw the material further into the lung.

Bronchoconstriction

Inhaled particles and irritant chemical substances initiate bronchoconstriction by stimulating irritant receptors in the larynx and larger airways. There is then an increase in airways resistance and reductions in forced expiratory volume and other indices of forced expiratory flow. An example is given in fig. 4.6. The reflex is blocked by atropine which is evidence that it is mediated by the parasympathetic nervous system. The afferent and efferent pathways are via the vagus nerve (fig. 4.7). The bronchoconstriction increases the linear velocity of airflow and hence the proportion of particles impacting at bifurcations of the larger airways. Fewer particles then reach the lung parenchyma. This has been demonstrated using particles of uniform size (monodispersed) labelled with isotope (20). Tobacco smoke initiates the reflex and on this account an assessment of lung function should preferably not be undertaken

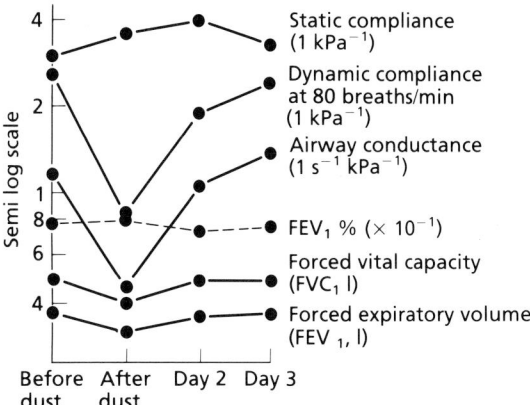

Fig. 4.6. Effect of mild bronchial obstruction caused by inhalation of cotton dust upon the lung function of a healthy subject studied by McDermott and her colleagues. To illustrate the relative magnitudes of the changes the data are plotted on a semi-log scale. The reproducibility (SD÷mean) is greater for the FEV and FVC than for the other indices. (From *Lung Function*, Cotes, J.E. (1979) 4th edn. Blackwell Scientific Publications, Oxford, p. 108.)

until at least 1h has elapsed after smoking a cigarette.

Sneeze

A sneeze is an explosive expiration through the nose. It is preceded by an inspiration or series of inspirations through the mouth; the glottis then closes temporarily whilst a positive pressure builds up in the lung. The reflex is initiated by stimulation of receptors in the nose which respond to mechanical deformation by accumulated mucus or dust and olfactory nerve endings which respond to ammonia and other irritant substances. The afferent information is conveyed to the respiratory reticular formation via the ethmoidal and olfactory branches of the trigeminal nerve; this is supplemented by information about lung volume from the vagi which contributes to the changeover from inspiration to forced expiration. The resulting expiratory flow rates resemble those in coughing but the manoeuvre differs both in the position of the palate which determines final direction of flow

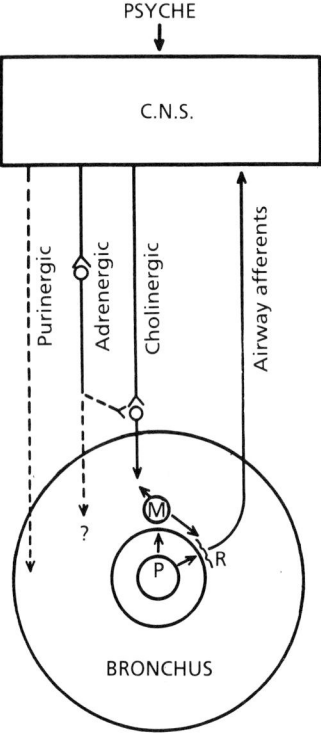

Fig. 4.7. Diagram showing bronchoconstrictor pathways. The particle (P) may stimulate the receptor (R) either directly or via a mediator substance (M). The main constrictor pathway is cholinergic. The interrupted lines indicate some hypothetical bronchodilator pathways. Recent evidence suggests that vasoactive intestinal peptide (VIP) may be the inhibitory neurotransmitter substance and not purines, opioids or prostaglandins (14, 31). (By courtesy of J. G. Widdicombe.)

and in the airway calibre which is relatively large during sneezing but narrow during coughing. The linear velocity of airflow through the nose is normally high enough to dislodge and expel the accumulated material but if the sneeze is partially inhibited the contents of the pharynx may be expelled via the mouth instead.

Cough

Coughing is a reflex forced expiration or series of expirations which have the effect of expelling

mucus and inhaled material from the wall of the tracheobronchial tree. It usually occurs in circumstances when the amount of such material is increased. The cough starts with a full inspiration which is followed by closure of the glottis and the development of a high positive pressure in the lung by contraction of the accessory muscles of expiration. Transient relaxation of the glottis then results in an explosive expiratory discharge of air. The air comes both from the periphery of the lung and from passive squeezing of the bronchi. The essential feature is a high linear velocity of airflow sufficient to shear mucus from the airway wall; the flow rate is increased by bronchoconstriction and the process of clearance is most effective when the bronchial mucus is both of low viscosity and in increased amount. Shearing is associated with the airflow becoming partly turbulent and ripples developing in the mucus. With a series of coughs the consequent clearance starts in the trachea and main bronchi, and then as the lung volume diminishes and the airways progressively narrow and collapse the clearance extends to small bronchi; there is no conclusive evidence that coughing also clears the bronchioles.

The cough is usually initiated by mechanical stimulation of receptors present in the wall of the airway between the pharynx and the bronchi; it can also be initiated voluntarily. The largest group of receptors is in the vicinity of the bifurcations of the trachea and lobar bronchi which are also the sites of impaction of inhaled material which the cough may then expel. The stimulus is usually mechanical deformation of mucosa but chemical stimulation by, for example, ammonia, sulphur dioxide or citric acid particles is also effective and can initiate cough from the peripheral airways. The receptors appear to adapt rapidly so a chemically induced cough is unlikely to be repeated unless the chemical stimulus is reinforced by dust, mucus or other factor. The afferent nerve pathway is via the vagus nerve to the medulla where the cough is co-ordinated. The responsible neurones or their connections are inhibited by codeine and other anti-tussive agents but are relatively insensitive to respiratory depressant drugs compared with the respiratory centre itself; this differential drug sensitivity is evidence for the two activities being to some extent distinct.

Mucociliary clearance

Particles depositing on the tracheobronchial tree are mostly removed by the action of cilia which propel them on a layer of mucus upwards from the airways to the pharynx; from here they are swallowed or expectorated. The process starts in the respiratory bronchioles. Ciliary action also clears material from the main nasal passages posteriorly to the same site. This important function depends on the remarkable properties of the epithelium of the respiratory tract; its attributes are reviewed by Brain and colleagues (3, 13).

Lining of respiratory tract

Squamous epithelium lines the anterior nares, the pharynx and parts of the epiglottis and larynx. The remainder down to the respiratory epithelium is covered by ciliated epithelium which is pseudostratified in the trachea and columnar elsewhere down to the level of the respiratory bronchioles where it becomes cuboidal: the epithelium contains secretory cells including goblet, serous and Clara cells, while the submucosa, down to the level of the

secondary bronchioles (diameter 1mm), contains mucous and serous glands. Other constituents of the epithelium are mast cells (page 349), brush cells whose microvilli may have an absorptive role in taking up surplus fluid from the respiratory tract, undifferentiated cells, basal cells, lymphocytes, Kultschitsky or Feyrter cells which may secrete serotonin, and nerve cells: some of these cells are illustrated in fig. 4.8.

Most epithelial cells are fused at their luminal surface by tight junctions which effectively seal the spaces between them. The junctions are formed of fibrils which may be discrete, interconnected or in the form of a mesh; the latter occur particularly between mucous cells and may become leaky when the cells secrete. Some cells are fused near to their bases leaving gaps at the luminal surface; these gap junctions enable secretions to reach the lumen from basal cells. They also provide a route whereby macrophages and foreign particles can penetrate the airway wall.

Cilia

Each ciliated cell has approximately 200 cilia which project into the airway lumen. Their features are reviewed by Sleigh (25, 26). Human cilia vary in length between 4 and 8μm, the shorter ones being those in the smaller airways.

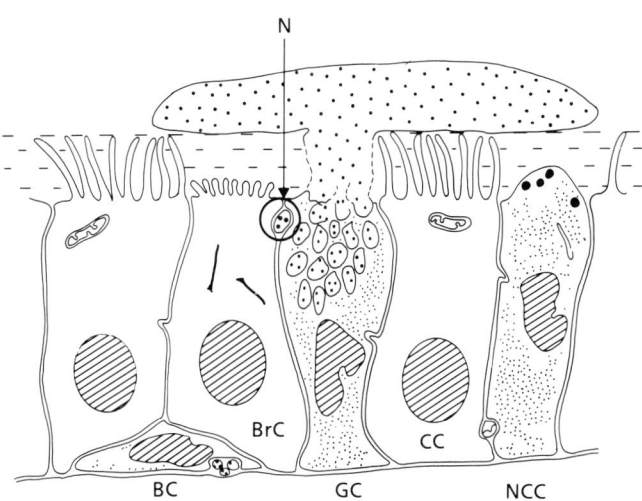

Fig. 4.8. Human bronchial epithelium traced from an electron-micrograph. BrC, brush cell; GC, goblet cell; CC, ciliated cell; NCC, non-ciliated cell; BC, basement cell; N, nerve cell with irritant receptor. (By courtesy of P. K. Jeffery (12).)

They are conical in shape, the base having a diameter of about 0.25μm, tapering to 0.1μm at the tip; this terminates in a cluster of claw-like projections. The shaft consists of a bundle of longitudinal fibrils; these slide over each other during the to and fro beating movements which occur at a frequency of 6–20Hz. The frequency is less in the small than the larger airways. The forward or effective stroke is made with the cilium more or less extended whilst for the slower return stroke the shaft is bent and nearer to the cell surface (fig. 4.9). Each cilium moves

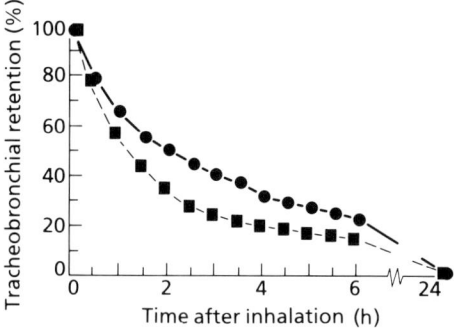

Fig. 4.10. Mean curves showing clearance of 5μm polystyrene particles (labelled with technetium 99) for ten healthy persons (●) and ten patients with impaired ciliary function due to obstructive azoospermia (■). (By courtesy of D. Pavia and colleagues (20).)

Secretion of mucus

Mucus is a mixture of substances including neutral and acid glycoproteins and mucopolysaccharides in which the acid radical may be sialic acid or sulphate. It is produced mainly by mucous acinar glands which are distributed with an average density of one per square millimetre throughout the greater part of the respiratory tract; the ducts mostly emerge in the gaps between fields of ciliated cells. The ducts are approximately 0.13mm long, lined with ciliated epithelium which is continuous with that of the airways. Each collecting duct is approximately 1mm long; it is supplied by about a dozen secretory tubules which also have branches. The tubules are about 0.5mm long and lined with densely packed secretory cells which mainly produce mucus. Some tubules are lined with serous cells which produce constituents of mucus whilst many mucous tubules have buds of serous tubules at their distal ends. The secretion from the serous cells passes over the mucous cells on its way to the collecting ducts.

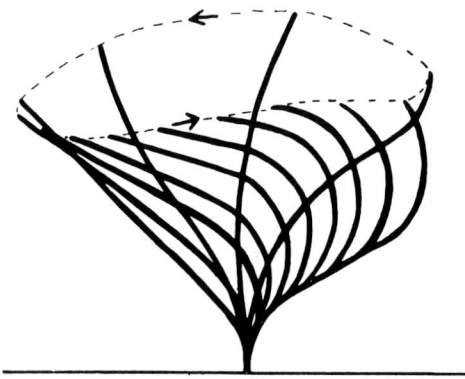

Fig. 4.9. Ciliary movement, showing the forward sweep and oblique return. (By courtesy of M. A. Sleigh and Marcel Dekker (25).)

in a two-phase liquid medium consisting of serous fluid near the cell surface with mucus floating on it. During the effective stroke the ciliary claws hook on to and propel the mucus layer whilst the return stroke is made through the serous layer which, therefore, oscillates but does not move down the length of the airway.

Ciliated cells are arranged in clumps or fields whose members all beat in the same direction towards the pharynx. The action is reduced or inhibited by acute infection, cigarette smoke, sulphur dioxide and cold. It is also reduced in inherited disorders associated with immotile spermatozoa (ciliary dyskinesia) (fig. 4.10). The factors which normally regulate ciliary action are largely unknown.

Secretion of mucus from the acinar glands is under the control of the autonomic nervous system via cholinergic nerves which are contained in the glands. The secretion is increased by stimulation of the vagus nerve or administration of acetyl choline, pilocarpine or carbachol; it is inhibited by atropine. Secretion may also be increased by stimulation of α and β adrenergic sympathetic nerve endings which have been observed in proximity to the mucous glands but the anatomical evidence is incomplete. The secretion is increased in chronic bronchitis, abnormally viscid in cystic fibrosis and absent in Sjögren's syndrome and other inherited disorders.

Inhibition of secretion is effected by non-adrenergic inhibitory nerves. These nerves have on their axons opaque vesicles which may contain biologically active peptides including substance P, vasoactive intestinal peptide and bombesin. Nerve endings containing these substances have been observed in human airways adjacent to mucous glands (7) but their role in the control of secretion is not yet known.

As well as the acinar glands, goblet cells contribute to the secretion of mucus especially in the peripheral bronchi but not normally in the bronchioles. The cells may be derived from intermediate cells or Clara cells: the mechanism by which their secretion is regulated is not at present established.

Hypertrophy of the acinar glands and an increase in the number of goblet cells occur in response to inhaled irritant substances and some drugs and bacteria. The increase in number of secretory cells is associated with an extension of their distribution to the larger and very small airways; there is also an increase in the number of dividing cells and hence in the mitotic index. Agents which enlarge the secretory capacity also stimulate the cells to synthesize and discharge at a faster rate so that the amount of mucus in the respiratory tract is increased. In the case of the acinar glands the secretion is at least in part a reflex response to stimulation of irritant receptors in the airway walls. Agents which act in this way include most inhaled dusts (21), irritant gases such as formalin, ammonia, chlorine, sulphur dioxide and nitrogen dioxide, tobacco smoke, drugs such as isoprenaline and pilocarpine (8) and local accumulation of bacteria as occurs with experimental inoculation of test animals.

Physical properties of mucus

Mucus exhibits viscosity (resistance to deformation), and elasticity (recovery after deformation).

However, the viscosity is not that of an ideal fluid in which the shear stress is proportional to the applied shear rate. Instead mucus is thixotropic in that it exhibits plastic flow which only begins when a certain shear rate has been applied; thereafter increasing the shear rate reduces the viscosity. This characteristic may contribute to the efficacy of clearance by coughing. The fall in viscosity produced by high rates of shearing may recover on standing or become increased as in some types of asthma. The viscosity may be reduced by an enhanced body fluid intake and increased by dehydration or by atropine.

Mucociliary flow

The tracheobronchial tree down to the level of the terminal bronchioles is lined by a liquid layer comprising mucus on a film of serous fluid. In the periphery the mucus occurs as discrete flakes: these are propelled proximally by cilia and coalesce as they converge in the larger airways to form first rafts and then a continuous film. In health the thickness of the film varies from about 0.1μm in the terminal bronchioles to 5μm in the trachea; the mucus is not conspicuous and cough is uncommon. The film becomes thicker in circumstances when the secretion of mucus is increased. The mucus flow rates are of the order 0.1mm min^{-1} in the terminal bronchioles, 1mm min^{-1} in the bronchioles and 5mm min^{-1} in the trachea but with wide variation (32). The flow rate in the main nasal passages resembles that in the trachea but it is of the order of 20mm min^{-1} in the region of the anterior tip of the turbinate bones. The flow rates are greater in circumstances when the secretion of mucus is moderately increased but reduced when the secretion is excessive. Changes in ciliary action may contribute to these responses.

In man clearance can be measured by the decline in radioactivity following the inhalation of radioactive particles of uniform size, for example, human albumen labelled with technicium 99 or iodine 123. The monodispersed particles may be of any diameter from 0.1 to 10μm, for example, 2μm for investigating clearance from small airways via the mucociliary escalator and 0.1μm for alveolar clearance. The radio-activity may be recorded over the mediastinum and the periphery of the lung using a gamma camera or sodium iodide crystals and scintillation counters. The count should preferably be continued intermittently for 48h. An example is given in fig. 4.10. The procedures are reviewed by Pavia (19).

An increase in mucociliary clearance occurs with cholinergic and adrenergic drugs (8), exercise, hyperventilation, inhaling cigarette smoke and after inhaling dust. The clearance is reduced by atropine and in attacks of asthma in which the response is independent of the bronchoconstriction and can persist for up to 7 days (2). An increased nasal flow rate occurs after drinking hot sweet fluid and this may be a factor in the expectorant action of a morning cup of tea.

The mucociliary mechanism is effective in removing from the lung the dust particles and some of the fibres which deposit on the tracheobronchial tree; its integrity is of the greatest importance for respiratory health in persons exposed to dust at work.

Alveolar deposition

Particles which penetrate the tracheobronchial tree to the level of the respiratory bronchioles can deposit in the lung parenchyma. On average approximately 25% of those in the size range 5–0.5μm do so by sedimentation whilst some 50% of particles of diameter 0.1μm deposit by diffusion (fig. 4.2). The fractional deposition is increased by circumstances which lengthen the time that particles remain in the lung and which reduce the size of air spaces. Thus respiratory frequency, tidal volume and expiratory reserve volume all influence the alveolar deposition but their effects are not independent. For example, an increase in tidal volume is usually effected by an increased inspiratory flow rate. This enhances tracheobronchial deposition and carries the particles by bulk flow relatively deep into the lung where the likelihood of alveolar deposition is greater. The deep breath also increases the lung volume and this reduces alveolar deposition. In addition when the increase in tidal volume is a result of exercise

the respiratory frequency is increased and the particle residence time reduced. The way in which the several factors interact has not been fully worked out. However, men exposed to dust when in a horizontal posture (which reduces the expiratory reserve volume) probably retain more dust than persons whose posture is upright; a similar reduction in lung volume may be a consequence of obesity and occurs in interstitial fibrosis and with pleural thickening associated with exposure to asbestos. Other factors must contribute to the observed inter-subject variations in deposition but what they are has still to be established. Alveolar deposition is important since a proportion of the material enters the tissue of the lung where it is a cause of occupational lung disease or enters the bloodstream and causes systemic poisoning.

Fate of inhaled particles: role of macrophages

Particles which deposit on the upper respiratory tract or on the tracheobronchial tree are mostly carried to the pharynx; they are then usually swallowed and and may be digested or inactivated by the gastro-intestinal enzymes or excreted in the faeces; some are expelled by coughing or sneezing.

Particles which deposit on the alveolar epithelium are not removed by mucociliary action or coughing. Instead they may be inactivated by substances present in the serous fluid lining layer of the lung. However, they are usually ingested by alveolar macrophages, many of which migrate along the tracheobronchial tree towards the mouth (fig. 9.3, page 169). Some alveolar macrophages remain in the alveoli but become incorporated into the lung parenchyma by realignment of the alveolar membrane. This occurs by proliferation of cuboidal (type 2) alveolar cells. Other phagocytic cells remain in the alveolar membrane or migrate through it to reach lymph nodes, especially those which occur in proximity to the respiratory bronchioles. The particles may then dissolve (as is the case with cement dust), or accumulate (as mainly happens with coal dust), or a more complex reaction may occur. This may be a specific cellular reaction as occurs with beryllium or type-specific as with extrinsic allergic alveolitis mediated by the reaction of IgG antibody with the relevant antigen (chapter 15). Alternatively the tissue macrophage may be so damaged by the ingested material that the intracellular enzymes and oxidants are released locally; they then digest the epithelium of the respiratory bronchiole causing centrilobular emphysema. This is a feature of tobacco smoke and a similar process may give rise to focal emphysema in coal miners (page 171). The damaged macrophages sometimes stimulate fibroblasts to lay down fibrous tissue. Fibrous nodules are formed in silicosis (page 148) whilst diffuse fibrosis, which initially is subpleural, occurs in asbestosis (page 204). In the latter condition the distribution of fibrosis is greatly influenced by the activity of macrophages since these remarkable cells can ingest and neutralize fibres up to 14μm long. The activated macrophages also attract neutrophils, generate and activate complement, secrete prostaglandins, which contribute to the inflammatory response, and initiate coagulation. Further information about the cellular responses is given in subsequent chapters.

Local humoral defence mechanisms

Organic material which has been deposited in alveoli may be inactivated by humoral agents; these are either non-specific in their action or antibodies which are specific to individual antigens. The antibodies will have been produced locally in the lung or in lymphoid tissue elsewhere in the body, travelling to the lung via the bloodstream. Inactivation of organic material may also be effected by cells of the reticuloendothelial system which are either resident in the lung or enter the lung for this purpose. These defence mechanisms are reviewed by Turner-Warwick (30).

The principal non-specific humoral agent present in the respiratory tract is possibly mucus itself which appears capable of neutralizing inhaled acid fumes and oxidizing agents including ozone (6). Bronchial secretions also contain proteolytic enzymes and oxidizing agents released from the lysosomes of macrophages: these substances immobilize and destroy micro-organisms, either by themselves or, in the case of lysozyme, in conjunction with complement and immunoglobulin secreted into the respiratory tract (secretory IgA). Interferon which inhibits the growth of viruses, lactoferrin (from bronchial mucous glands) which attacks iron present in micro-organisms, and complement are also present. The complement requires activation before it can exert an effect. Activation is achieved through a reaction between antigens which form part of the bacteria or other material, and antibodies which are secreted into the serous fluid layer of the airways; certain inhaled substances including the spores of *M. faeni*, bacterial endotoxins, silica, asbestos and other substances can activate complement directly. Activated complement exerts a direct destructive effect on bacterial cell membranes and also assists in their digestion by phagocytic cells.

The local specific immune defences are immunoglobulins and lymphokines which act in a number of ways to localize, immobilize, destroy and remove the foreign material. The substances are secreted into the serous fluid layer of the airways by lymphocytes which are present in or attracted into the lung. These local agents may be reinforced by others which are secreted by lymphoid tissue elsewhere in the body and carried to the lung by the circulation. Agents from the two sources differ both qualitatively and quantitatively because they are provoked by different stimuli; those present in bronchial secretions may be assayed in fluid obtained by broncho-alveolar lavage. At present the methods are semi-quantitative and there is need for better standardization of the procedure for sample collection.

The immunoglobulins (Ig) are secreted by lymphocyte B cells and by plasma cells. IgA comes from cells around the central airways and in the mucous and serous glands. The process of secretion is assisted by a protein fraction called the secretory piece; this attaches to and enlarges the IgA molecule to form secretory IgA (sIgA) which, therefore, differs from IgA present in serum. The sIgA is more resistant to digestion by proteolytic enzymes. It appears to block the adherence of bacteria to mucous membranes and hence the formation of bacterial colonies which might penetrate bronchial epithelium. A reduced level of sIgA has been observed amongst persons who are susceptible to recurrent infection but others have no IgA without apparent ill-effects. Thus its role is not essential.

IgE is produced by plasma cells in the tonsils, the central airways and the skin. In the former sites the production is provoked by inhalation of particulate material to which the subject is sensitized; some of the material has an aerodynamic diameter in the range 20–10μm so is small enough to enter the nose and lodge in the tonsils but not to penetrate into the lung beyond the tracheal bifurcation. Increased IgE production is a feature of atopic subjects, those with a relative deficiency of IgA and persons infected with some parasites. In the lung IgE attaches to mast cells and causes the release of histamine and leukotrienes C4 and D4, formerly identified as the slow-reacting substance of anaphylaxis (SRS-A) (table 16.1, page 351). In this way it contributes to the development of extrinsic allergic asthma, including many types of occupational asthma (chapter 16), but not to intrinsic asthma where no external antigen is involved.

IgG is secreted by cells in the peripheral airways and the acinus; both this immunoglobulin and IgM also enter the airways from the bloodstream. They facilitate the ingestion of microorganisms by phagocytic cells which form part of the local cellular defences of the lung (see below). They also contribute to hypersensitivity reactions including some forms of extrinsic allergic alveolitis and occupational asthma (chapters 15 and 16).

The lymphokines are produced in the lung by activated lymphocytes which originated from the thymus gland. These T lymphocytes may be present in large numbers in fluid obtained by broncho-alveolar lavage from patients with extrinsic allergic alveolitis. Many of the cells come from the circulating blood which may be relatively depleted in consequence. The cells combine with the inhaled antigen and in the process release lymphokines which have a direct cytotoxic action on the target cells. Lymphokines also promote the inflammatory response by attracting monocytes and inhibiting the migration of macrophages. Other T cells augment or inhibit the secretory activity of the B cells and on this account are called respectively helper and suppressor T cells. These reactions are controlled by complex processes not yet fully understood; they are at present the subject of much active research and this is adding almost daily to what is now the fastest growing aspect of respiratory medicine. The current literature should be consulted for further details.

References

1 Acheson ED, Cowdell RH, Rang E. Adenocarcinoma of the nasal cavity and sinuses in England and Wales. *Br J Industr Med* 1972; **29** 21–30.

2 Allegra L, Abraham WM, Chapman GA, Wanner A. Duration of mucociliary dysfunction following antigen challenge. *J Appl Physiol* 1983;**55**:726–30.

3 Brain JD, Proctor DF, Reid LM (Eds). *Respiratory Defence Mechanisms, Part I. Lung Biology in Health and Disease.* New York: Marcel Dekker 1977;**5**:1–488.

4 Cole TJ, Cotes JE, Johnson GR, Martin H De V, Reed JW, Saunders MJ. Ventilation, cardiac frequency and pattern of breathing during exercise in men exposed to o-chlorobenzylidene malononitrile (CS) and ammonia gas in low concentrations. *Quart J Exp Physiol* 1977; **62**:341–51.

5 Cotes JE, Johnson GR, McDonald A. Breathing frequency and tidal volume: relationship to breathlessness. In Porter R (ed). *Ciba Foundation Hering–Breuer Centenary Symposium: Breathing.* London: Churchill, 1970:297–314.

6 Cross C, Halliwell D, Allen A. Anti-oxidant protection; a function of tracheobronchial and gastrointestinal mucus. *Lancet* 1984; **i**:1328–9.

7 Dey RD, Said IS. Immunocytochemical localization of VIP-immunoreactive nerves in bronchial walls and pulmonary vessels. *Fed Proc* 1980;**39**:1062.

8 Foster WM, Bergofsky EH, Bohning DE, Lippmann M, Albert RE. Effect of adrenergic agents and their mode of action on mucociliary clearance in man. *J Appl Physiol* 1976;**41**:146–52.

9 Gerhardsson M, Norell SE, Kiviranta HJ, Ahlbom A. Respiratory cancers in furniture workers. *Br J Industr Med* 1985;**42**:403–5.

10 Gerrity TR, Lee PS, Hass FJ, Marinelli A, Werner P, Lourenco RV. Calculated deposition of inhaled particles in the airway generations of normal subjects. *J Appl Physiol* 1979; **47**:867–73.

11 Hounam RF, Morgan A. Particle deposition. In: Brain JD, Proctor DF, Reid LM (eds). *Respiratory Defence Mechanisms Part I. Lung Biology in Health and Disease.* New York: Marcel Dekker, 1977;**5**:125–56.

12 Jeffery PK, Reid LM. Ultrastructure of normal large bronchi. *Les Bronches.* 1973;**23**:368–80.

13 Jeffery PK, Reid LM. The respiratory mucous membrane. In: Brain JD, Proctor DF, Reid LM (eds). *Respiratory Defence Mechanisms, Part I. Lung Biology in Health and Disease.* New York: Marcel Dekker 1977;**5**:193–245.

14 Kirkpatrick CT. Nervous control of airways muscle tone. *Bull Europ Physiopath Resp* 1984;**20**:389–94.

15 Lippmann M, Yeates DB, Albert RE. Deposition, retention and clearance of inhaled particles. *Br J Industr Med* 1980;**37**:337–62.

16 Merler E, Baldasseroni A, Laria R, Faravelli P, Agostini R, Pisa R, Berrino F. On the causal association between exposure to leather dust and nasal cancer: further evidence from a case–control study. *Br J Industr Med* 1986;**43**:91–5.

17 Naus A. Smell, sense of. In Parmeggiani L (ed). *Encyclopaedia of Occupational Health* 1983;**2**:2065–9.

18 Paintal AS. Vagal sensory receptors and their reflex effects. *Physiol Rev* 1973;**53**:159–227.

19 Pavia D. Lung Mucociliary clearance. In: *Aerosols and the Lung.* Clarke SW, Pavia D (eds). London: Butterworths, 1984;127–55.

20 Pavia D, Bateman JRM, Clarke SW. Deposition and clearance of inhaled particles. *Bull Europ Physiopath Resp* 1980;**16**:335–66.

21 Peatfield AC, Richardson PS. The action of dust in the airways on secretion into the trachea of the cat. *J Physiol* 1983;**342**:327–34.

22 Richardson PS, Peatfield AC. Reflexes concerned in the defence of the lungs. *Bull Europ Physiopath Resp* 1981;**17**:979–1012.

23 Schlesinger RB, Lippmann M. Selective particle deposition and bronchogenic carcinoma. *Environm Res* 1978;**15**:424–31.

24 Schroter RC, Sudlow MF. Flow patterns in models of the human bronchial airways. *Respir Physiol* 1969;**7**:341–55.

25 Sleigh MA. The nature and action of respiratory tract cilia. In: Brain JD, Proctor DF, Reid LM (eds). *Respiratory Defence Mechanisms, Part I. Lung Biology in Health and Disease.* New York: Marcel Dekker, 1977;**5**:247–88.

26 Sleigh MA. Ciliary function in mucous transport. *Chest* 1981;**80**:6:791–5.

27 Swift DL, Proctor DF. Access of air to the respiratory tract. In: Brain JD, Proctor DF, Reid LM (eds). *Respiratory Defence Mechanisms, Part I. Lung Biology in Health and Disease.* New York: Marcel Dekker, 1977;**5**:63–93.

28 Task group on lung dynamics. Committee II. International commission on radiological protection. Deposition and retention models for internal dosimetry of the human respiratory tract. *Health Phys* 1966;**12**:173–208.

29 Timbrell V. Deposition and retention of fibres in the human lung. *Ann Occup Hyg* 1982;**26**:347–69.

30 Turner-Warwick M. In: Weatherall DJ, Ledingham JGG, Warrell DM (eds). *Oxford Textbook of Medicine.* Oxford University Press. 1983.

31 Widdicombe JG. Nervous Receptors in the Respiratory Tract and Lungs. In: Hornbein TD (ed). *Regulation of breathing, Vol. I. Lung Biology in Health and Disease.* New York: Marcel Dekker, 1981;**17**:429–72.

32 Yeates DB, Aspin N, Levison H, Jones MT, Bryan AC. Mucociliary tracheal transport rates in man. *J Appl Physiol* 1975;**39**:487–95.

Chapter 5
Screening and Examination Procedures

Introduction

The practice of occupational respiratory medicine begins in the workplace with consideration of the process, the potential hazards, and the roles of the workforce. The most important tool is advanced planning. This should be used to prevent the introduction of hazards or to isolate them from the work-force. The techniques are discussed in chapter 3. Where air pollution is unavoidable, or where a risk exists, it should be minimized by dust suppression and the other remedies described in the same chapter. The success of the measures should be checked by environmental monitoring which is described in chapter 2 and by biological monitoring of the work-force. The latter will be effected through medical examination of individuals, through recording and analysing sickness absences and through occupational surveys. This chapter describes some of the procedures which may be used. The conduct of occupational surveys is described in chapter 6.

Clinical interview and examination

A clinical interview and examination is usually undertaken for the diagnosis and management of a specific complaint. This may arise in the course of employment, for example respiratory symptoms following an acute exposure to fumes or tightness of the chest developing during the working day. The aspects which should then be considered are discussed in the relevant chapters. Pre-employment and periodic examinations are discussed below. This section considers the occupational aspects of consul-

tations in respiratory or general medicine and those occupational medical consultations where the diagnosis has still to be made. The clinical aspects of respiratory disease are considered by Crofton & Douglas (4). The diagnosis of the patient with a reticulo-nodular shadowing on the chest radiograph is discussed in chapter 15.

The first essential is to be aware that occupation may cause or aggravate the medical condition either directly or indirectly; a direct contribution can often be established or refuted by taking an occupational history. This should be done routinely. An indirect contribution which might be from a factory in the neighbourhood or contact with clothes from a person exposed to hazardous material is likely to be missed unless specific questions are asked.

The occupational history must include previous as well as current employment. If the history fails to reveal any clues but the medical condition suggests the possibility of exposure to noxious dust or fumes the subject should be specifically asked about this, perhaps using the checklist given in table 5.1. The possibility of exposure during childhood, during leisure-time activities and via other members of the household should be borne in mind; this might contribute to diagnosis in a suspected case of asbestosis, mesothelial tumour of the pleura, beryllium disease, occupational asthma or extrinsic allergic alveolitis.

If an occupational factor is suspected the occupational history should be expanded to include a list of jobs with dates when each began and ended, their nature and the circumstances in which they were undertaken. This may be prepared by the patient in consultation with the

Table 5.1. Brief check list of dusty occupations

Have you ever worked in:	coal mine
	other mine
	quarry
	foundry
	pottery
	cotton, flax or
	hemp mill
with:	asbestos
	animals or
	birds
	hay, grain or
	mushroom
	compost
in:	other dusty job
	(specify)
Have you ever worked exposed to:	irritant gas
	chemical
	fumes
	(specify)

spouse and then amplified at consultation. The sequence of dates should be consecutive and any gaps explored tactfully. The employment may appear to indicate the type of activity, for example, in a shipyard (shipbuilding) or for the National Coal Board (coalmining) but this is seldom sufficient information. Details should be obtained of what was actually done both for most of the time and occasionally. Thus the coal miner may have worked mainly on the coal face or screens where the predominant exposure was to coal dust, on development work including cutting roadways through rock containing silica, with pit ponies whose food or bedding might have included mouldy hay, with birds used as detectors of carbon monoxide (fire damp) or as a lagger, fitter, electrician or welder, these activities respectively entailing possible exposure to asbestos, oil mist, colophony and oxides of nitrogen. When contact with a known hazard is reported an attempt should be made to assess its severity in terms of the proportion of time spent in the particular environment, the extent of the exposure and what safety procedures were carried out with respect to suppression of dust at source, exhaust ventilation and personal protection by wearing a respirator or breathing apparatus. Activities undertaken only occasionally should be identified where possible

and, if likely to carry risk, should be considered in detail. Examples are cleaning and repairing equipment which normally operates in closed environments or protected by exhaust ventilation, servicing electrostatic precipitators, air conditioners and respirators, and disposing of the dust which has been collected in a dust extractor. Dust in the workplace, created by the activities of other workers, should also be recorded: for example, (i) a fitter may have been working alongside laggers whose job was to remove and/or install asbestos insulation, or (ii) the booth occupied by a clerk/timekeeper may have been in a shed where slate dressing was undertaken. A question should be asked about the occurrence of occupational lung disorders amongst other employees. Adequate answers about exposure often cannot be obtained when the subject works with mixtures of chemicals, on a new process, or with a new product, and in these cases it is often helpful to contact the employer. If the patient has worked in an air-conditioned environment this should be recorded.

The fumes and dusts which may present an occupational hazard also arise when the same or related activities are undertaken as hobbies or during maintenance of personal property and equipment. Thus, enquiries should also be made about leisure-time occupations and respiratory hazards possibly experienced outside working hours. Pigeon fancying and keeping a budgerigar are examples.

The clinical history should include the nature and intensity of any symptoms and the order in which they developed with approximate dates. The subject's present ability to undertake physical exertion should be compared with his previous ability illustrated by occupation and participation in competitive sport. Details of the award of industrial disablement benefit should be recorded. The smoking history should be recorded in detail (table 5.3 below).

The physical examination should record any stigmata of occupational origin including intradermal coal dust, asbestos corns, calluses and cutaneous thickening due to particular activities. With a view to interpreting the nature of any exercise limitation, the nutrition, the gait, the integrity of the locomotor system, the extent of development of the accessory muscles of respiration and any arthritis should be noted. A watch should be kept for the occurrence of breathlessness in relation to the consultation, including getting to and from the point of entry off the street and going to the canteen (page 400). When examining the respiratory system cyanosis should be looked for in the buccal mucosa. Finger clubbing should be noted. At one time clubbing was assessed quantitatively by measurement of volume of the terminal and mid-phalanges or by comparison with finger casts (18) but the extra information is of limited usefulness. On auscultation of the chest during deep inspiration a search should be made for fine crackles (râles or crepitations) and their timing noted with respect to the beginning of inspiration and whether or not they were cleared by coughing or influenced by posture: the common locations are below the scapula, at the bases posteriorly and in the mid-axillary line below the level of the nipples (19). As screening tests and with a view to assessing suitability for exercise testing the blood pressure should be measured and if ischaemic heart disease is suspected, a recording made of the electro-cardiogram.

Medical examinations in employment

Pre-employment examination

The pre-employment medical examination is the occasion for detecting respiratory conditions which put the applicant at increased risk in the event of subsequent dust or fume exposure. There may also be conditions which put other people at risk; pulmonary tuberculosis was formerly the prime example but is now amenable to treatment. Notably chronic bronchitis, emphysema, bronchiectasis, asthma or other established lung disease preclude employment in an environment where there is a risk of occupational lung disease, and also employments handling or preparing food. Atopic status including a history of childhood eczema, hay fever or asthma and a positive skin test response to common allergens is sometimes also considered to be a contraindication. However, there are few occupations where the risk of asthma is

materially greater for atopic subjects than for those who are not atopic. Thus the case for exclusion should be made on an individual basis (chapter 16). An individual decision should also be made in the case of the applicant with an asymptomatic occupational lung disorder who applies for work in another dusty occupation (14).

The pre-employment examination is an opportunity for obtaining baseline values for indices of lung function, especially the forced expiratory volume and vital capacity (q.v.). The results contribute to the immediate assessment and provide personal reference values against which subsequent measurements may be compared. For this reason the result should be stored for future reference. Work which is heavy or which intermittently may make heavy physical demands on the subject may also be an indication for an exercise test (chapter 18).

Periodic examination

Periodic medical examinations including measurements of lung function are recommended by the International Labour Organisation for persons in dusty occupations (12). Such studies provide invaluable information about the effects of respiratory hazards but their effectiveness on a routine basis depends on circumstances. In the case of mineral dusts an undue exposure can be detected radiographically before the onset of symptoms; surveillance is necessary if the exposure carries a material risk and should then be provided in the form of periodic chest radiographs. Workers exposed to coal dust, asbestos or silica fall into this category but tin-workers and welders do not. For the former the interval between radiographs after 10 years from first exposure might be respectively 5, 1 and 2 years. The films should be read on the ILO classification (page 86). Where the exposure gives rise to obstruction to airflow or disease of the lung parenchyma the development of breathlessness may lead the affected person to seek medical advice but not usually until the condition is advanced. Such cases should alert the medical department to the need for further scrutiny. This might take the form of a respiratory survey (chapter 6). The survey should reveal if there is a problem and suggest what additional information is needed to solve it. Once preventive measures have been installed periodic examinations are needed until such time as the measures have been shown to be effective and the hazard has been controlled.

Periodic examinations also provide an opportunity for assessing general health, and advising on the effects of smoking, overeating and drinking. The person's attention should be drawn to the risk from smoking, especially if exposed to asbestos and from alcohol, especially if working with solvents. Occupational deafness, diabetes, the state of the cardiovascular system including blood pressure and evidence of coronary ischaemia, musculo-skeletal disorders including back pain, and hernias should be noted. Such examinations are seldom cost-effective but they might be expected to be so for chronic respiratory and cardiovascular disorders in men above the age of 45 years. In practice the problems are usually tackled as they arise or at the time of return to work after a period of sickness.

Post-sickness examination

Return to work after a chest illness should be prepared for by rehabilitation and by taking steps to prevent recurrence. This usually entails going into all the factors which may have contributed to the illness and abandoning smoking.

Questionnaires on respiratory symptoms

Obtaining answers to questions is the basis of the clinical interview but in this situation the exchanges are influenced by interaction between the two parties; different interviewers might ask similar questions in ways which conveyed different shades of meaning to the person interviewed and come to slightly different conclusions in consequence. These sources of variability are removed by use of a questionnaire. The subject is presented with unambiguous questions to which the answer is normally yes or no, and the observer has little discretion as to how the replies are recorded. The person interviewed may also be asked to

choose between a number of realistic possibilities; there should then be no need for supplementary questions. The questionnaire should be tried out on persons similar to those for whom it is intended and any ambiguity or obscure feature corrected before use (1). The subjects will usually be groups rather than individuals for whom more relevant information may be obtained by personal interview. The questionnaire has a reproducibility of the order of 10% (15); the answers contribute to diagnosis and in the case of respiratory symptoms are significantly correlated with the exposure to respiratory irritants, the lung function and related findings in epidemiological surveys (chapter 6). The use of a questionnaire also simplifies the coding of information for computation.

A questionnaire on respiratory symptoms should be included in any survey of persons who may have breathlessness, bronchitis or wheeze. The MRC questionnaire (16) is usually employed and for this purpose has been translated into over 10 languages. The preamble and the first eleven questions are given in table 5.2 and the questions on smoking (numbers 13–21) are given in table 5.3. Question 12 is a checklist of past chest illnesses and related conditions (table 5.4). The interviewer need not be medically qualified but should be trained in both delicacy and interpretation; self-administration is also usually satisfactory except possibly for the questions on wheeze. The interviewer should use the questions as printed and ask them in a clear even voice which is only raised to emphasize the words in the questions which are printed in heavy type including 'Yes' or 'No' in the preamble and 'usually' in questions 1, 2, 4 and 5. The intonation should minimize the unintended choice which some subjects deduce from the alternative descriptions contained in questions 8a and 9. Chronic bronchitis may be diagnosed when cough and phlegm occur on most days for as much as 3 months each year (questions 3 and 6) but a stricter definition which is recommended by a committee of the European Coal and Steel Community and by the American Thoracic Society requires that the features should have been present for 2 successive years. 'Chronic bronchitis' is usually of greater consequence when accompanied by

Table 5.2. MRC questionnaire on respiratory symptoms (1976); questions 1–11 (16)

Preamble

I am going to ask you some questions, mainly about your chest. I should like you to answer **Yes** or **No** whenever possible. ☐

Cough

1 Do you **usually** cough first thing in the morning in the winter? ☐

2 Do you **usually** cough during the day – or at night – in the winter?

If Yes to 1 or 2
3 Do you cough like this on most days for as much as 3 months each year? ☐

Phlegm

4 Do you **usually** bring up any phlegm from your chest first thing in the morning in the winter? ☐

5 Do you **usually** bring up any phlegm from your chest during the day – or at night – in the winter? ☐

If Yes to 4 or 5
6 Do you bring up phlegm like this on most days for as much as three months each year? ☐

Periods of cough and phlegm

7a In the past 3 years have you had a period of (increased) cough and phlegm lasting for 3 weeks or more? ☐

If Yes
7b Have you more than one such period? ☐

Breathlessness

> If the subject is disabled from walking by any condition other than heart or lung disease, omit question 8 and enter 1 here. ☐

8a Are you troubled by shortness of breath when hurrying on level ground or walking up a slight hill? ☐

If Yes
8b Do you get short of breath walking with other people of your own age on level ground? ☐

If Yes
8c Do you have to stop for breath when walking at your own pace on level ground? ☐

Wheezing*

9a Does your chest ever sound wheezing or whistling? ☐

If Yes
9b Do you get this on most days – or nights? ☐

10a Have you ever had attacks of shortness of breath with wheezing? ☐

If Yes
10b Is/was your breathing absolutely normal between attacks? ☐

Chest illnesses

11a During the past three years have you had any chest illness which has kept you from your usual activities for as much as a week? ☐

If Yes
11b Did you bring up more phlegm than usual in any of these illnesses? ☐

If Yes
11c Have you had more than one illness like this in the past 3 years? ☐

* See also table 5.5.

Table 5.3. MRC questionnaire on respiratory symptoms (1976); questions on smoking (16)

	Additional observations
13a Do you smoke? □ **If No** 13b Have you ever smoked as much as one cigarette a day (or one cigar a week or an ounce of tobacco a month) for as long as a year? □	
If No to both parts of question 13, omit remaining questions	
14a Do (did) you inhale the smoke? □ **If Yes** 14b Would you say you inhaled the smoke slightly = 1, moderately = 2 or deeply = 3? □	
15 How old were you when you started smoking regularly? □	
16a Do (did) you smoke manufactured cigarettes? □ **If Yes** 16b How many do (did) you usually smoke per day on weekdays? □	
16c How many per day at weekends? □	
16d Do (did) you usually smoke plain [=1] or filter tip [=2] cigarettes? □	
16e What brands do (did) you usually smoke? □	
17a Do (did) you smoke hand-rolled cigarettes? □ **If Yes** 17b How much tobacco do (did) you usually smoke per week in this way? □	
17c Do (did) you put filters in these cigarettes? □	
18a Do (did) you smoke a pipe? □ **If Yes** 18b How much pipe tobacco do (did) you usually smoke per week? □	

Table 5.3 continued

19a Do (did) you smoke small cigars? **If Yes** 19b How many of these do (did) you usually smoke per day?	☐
20a Do (did) you smoke other cigars? **If Yes** 20b How many of these do (did) you usually smoke per week?	☐ ☐
For present smokers	
Have you been cutting down your smoking over the past year?	☐ *

For ex-smokers   Month   Year

21b When did you last give up smoking?   ☐☐   ☐☐   *

* It is often helpful to ask the reason for cutting down or discontinuing.

Table 5.4.   Checklist of past illnesses (16)

Have you ever had:

12a An injury or operation affecting your chest	☐
12b Heart trouble	☐
12c Bronchitis	☐
12d Pneumonia	☐
12e Pleurisy	☐
12f Pulmonary tuberculosis	☐
12g Bronchial asthma	☐
12h Other chest trouble	☐
12i Hay fever (or infantile eczema, food allergies, etc.)	☐

The questions on chest pain (Table 5.6) may be asked at this point.

recurrent chest illnesses (questions 11a–11c) but the term is emotive so is not used explicitly until a later stage in the interview (question 12c). It is then mainly of use for identifying wheezy bronchitis in childhood and previous bronchitis in ex-smokers; it does not substitute for questions 3 and 6 which describe the current situation.

The questions on breathlessness are used to obtain grades 1–3 of the clinical grade of breathlessness of Fletcher (table 5.2). For subjects who are obliged to stop walking at their own pace on level ground (yes to question 8c) it is often helpful to place them in grade 4 or higher by asking additional questions. These are contained in an extended version of the questionnaire which is given in table 18.11 (page 401). The absolute level of breathlessness is influenced by personality and mental attitudes to ill-health (page 399). Questions for use at the end of an exercise test are given on page 393. The questions on wheeze place the subjects in one of three categories but an additional refinement may be introduced by subdividing question 9b. These questions have also received the attention of the American Thoracic Society and a revised version is given in table 5.5. In neither version is reference made to asthma or chest tightness at this stage though asthma does appear in the

Table 5.5. American Thoracic Society and U.S. National Heart and Lung Institute respiratory questionnaire (1974): questions on wheeze (10)

Does your chest ever sound wheezy or whistling when:

1) you have a cold?	*any* yes	no
2) occasionally apart from colds?	*any* yes	no
3) most days or nights?	*chronic* yes	no

checklist; more detailed questions are needed for the investigation of occupational asthma (chapter 16) and byssinosis (chapter 14). Questions may also be used to elicit a diagnosis of angina of effort but in this condition, as in asthma, the symptoms may have been modified in response to treatment. Some questions which may be used are given in table 5.6. The questions on smoking are considered in chapter 17.

For longitudinal surveys additional questions designed to elicit changes in intensity of cough, phlegm and wheeze between surveys may sometimes be helpful (7). However, the standard questions should also be asked. In the case of those on breathlessness changes in grade of breathlessness between surveys are moderately

Table 5.6. Questions on chest pain

During the past 3 years have you had any pain or discomfort in your chest?

If yes

Do you get it when walking up hill?
Do you get it when hurrying?
Do you get it when walking at ordinary pace on level ground?

If yes

When you get the pain do you — carry on walking
　　　　　　　　　　　　　　 — slow down or stop
　　　　　　　　　　　　　　 — take a drug?
Is the pain relieved by this action?
How long does it take for the pain to be relieved
　　　　　　　　　　　　 — less than 10 min
　　　　　　　　　　　　 — less than 30 min
　　　　　　　　　　　　 — more than 30 min?

correlated with changes in other relevant features (table 18.10, page 400).

Chest radiography

The chest radiograph provides detailed information about the shape, size, expansion and appearance of the lung which is essential for clinical diagnosis and management. The radiograph also contains unique quantitative information relating to the extent of accumulation of dust in the lung and the type and extent of the tissue response; this information may be extracted by use of the international classification of radiographs of pneumoconioses of the International Labour Organisation (13, 20). The classification describes the appearance of the postero-anterior chest film but lateral and oblique views are often required for clinical purposes. Use of the classification requires training and experience which is likely to be found in an occupational chest unit but in only a few clinical departments of radiography. The process of learning is facilitated by the beautifully written guidelines to the classification and by reference to standard films of which copies are available from ILO. The resulting readings are the foundation of epidemiological studies of the mineral pneumoconioses (chapters 8–11) but they are primarily descriptive and in isolation are not diagnostic.

Radiographic technique

The radiograph should be of a consistently high quality which is best achieved by a regular dialogue between the radiographer and the x-ray reader. The overall quality of the films is the result of compatibility between all the stages in their production; some of these are considered below.

Equipment and exposure. The film to anode distance should normally be 1.8m (6ft). The anode should be of the rotating type and have a diameter of not more than 2mm. The collimator should be centred and adjusted so that irradiation is confined to the film; evidence for this should be visible as 'cone cuts' at the edges of the film. The film should be of medium speed and used with medium speed intensifying screens which should be comparable between cassettes where more than one is used. The screens should make good contact with the film. A grid should be used to cut down the effects of secondary radiation. In practice the anode should be centred horizontally in line with the middle of the film. The subject should be positioned symmetrically with the scapulae outside the lung fields. Exposure should be made at full inspiration and of duration less than 0.05s. For an average subject (anterior-posterior chest diameter 210–230mm) the exposure factors might be 5mA, 125kV and 0.017s. A lower kV is also appropriate though the dose of radiation is then somewhat higher. For obese subjects and those with larger chest diameters the exposure will need to be increased; this is usually done automatically by a photo-timer.

The processing should be automatic to ensure constant time/temperature and the strength of the processing chemicals should be maintained. The viewing screen should preferably have the dimensions 1600x400mm to accommodate four films and be illuminated by two matched 80W fluorescent tubes behind an opal screen.

The optical density of the exposed film may be checked using a portable micro-densitometer; this should show a maximum deflection over the lung fields of 1.8 units and a minimum in the hilar regions of 0.2 above fog. The contrast between these regions should be in the range 1.0–1.4 units of optical density. A well-exposed film should show the pulmonary parenchymal markings in great detail, both the costophrenic junctions should be included and the major pulmonary vessels should be visible through the cardiac shadow. After it is processed the film should be inspected and if these features are absent it should be re-taken. To this end the subject should, where practicable, remain in the vicinity of the x-ray set for 15min after the film has been exposed.

Reading the radiographs

Even when the radiographs are part of an occupational survey the films should be read as soon as possible in case they reveal tuberculosis, malignant disease or pneumothorax. For epidemiological purposes the reading for pneumo-coniosis should be made independently by two or three readers using the ILO classification. The extent of any small and large opacities, and any pleural or other abnormalities are recorded on a standard reading sheet (table 5.7). Depending on circumstances the number of films read per day by one reader plus assistant will be 100–400. The films should normally be in random order and with all identifying labels except the code number covered up in order to prevent the reader being influenced by the information they convey. As an aid to consistency some 2% of films whose x-ray category has been agreed between the readers should be inserted into the series; after each of these films is read the agreed reading is disclosed to the reader. Random-order readings are suitable for most applications but for assessing progression the films may also be read in pairs in date order.

Small opacities are graded for their profusion, extent, size and shape. The profusion relates to the part of the lung most affected by pneumo-coniosis: it is graded 'absent' to 'very profuse' in four mid-categories (recorded as 0/0, 1/1, 2/2 and 3/3) which are defined in terms of the appearance of standard radiographs. Eight intermediate categories are also recognized and with the mid-categories make up a 12-point scale; they are constructed by taking the reader's first and second choice of category in order. Thus a film for which the reader's first choice is 2 but where category 1 is a serious possibility is recorded as 2/1: if the first choice is category 2 but category 3 is possible then the film is recorded as 2/3 and similarly for the other categories. The lower limit of category 0 and the upper limit of category 3 are recorded respectively as 0/− and 3/+. The extent of the small opacities is indicated by their presence or absence in the upper, middle and lower zone of each lung separately. The shape of the small opacities is designated as round or irregular; each type is then designated by size as either small, medium or large. Small opacities (diameter or width <1.5mm) are recorded as p if they are round and s if they are irregular: the corresponding symbols for medium sized opacities (1.5–3mm) are q and t and for large opacities (3–10mm) r and u. In practice two symbols are used for each reading so that, for

Table 5.7. Reading sheet for radiographs of pneumoconioses with readings by three observers for a film showing asbestosis. The readings were made without knowledge of the case or of the other readings and were written down by assistants.

ILO 1979 INTERNATIONAL CLASSIFICATION OF RADIOGRAPHS OF PNEUMOCONIOSES

Film number ☐☐☐ ✗✗✗ 1-7
Date of Radiograph ✗✗✗✗✗✗ 8-13

	Reader 1	Reader 2	Reader 3	
Reader	✗✗	✗✗	✗✗	14-15
Date of reading	2 5 1 0 8 3	2 5 1 0 8 4	2 5 1 0 8 4	16-21
QUALITY 1 2 3 4	2	1	2	22
If not quality 1, record why			B	
Parenchyma clearly visible	2	1	M 2	23
Pleura *Yes = 1, No = 2*	2	1	2	24

SMALL OPACITIES 0/- 0/0 0/1 1/0 1/1 1/2 2/1 2/2 2/3 3/2 3/3 3/+

Profusion	2/3	2/3	3/2	25-26
Zones (Tick) Upper / Middle / Lower	R ✓ ✓ ✓ L ✓ ✓ ✓	R ✓ ✓ ✓ L ✓ ✓ ✓	R ✓ ✓ ✓ L ✓ ✓ ✓	27-28 / 29-30 / 31-32
Shape-size *p q r s t u* (2 symbols)	t t	s t	s q	33-34

LARGE OPACITIES	None	None	None	35
A B C	☐	☐	☐	36

PLEURAL THICKENING

	None	None	None	37
Type: Diffuse (Tick)	R ✓ L ☐	R ☐ L ☐	R ✓ L ☐	38-39 / 40-41
Plaques				
Width a b c	c c		a	42-43
Face on (Tick)	✓		✓	44-45
Extent 1 2 3	2 2		2	46-47
Diaphragm (Tick)	None R L	None R L	None R L	48-50
Costophrenic angles (Tick)	None R L	None R L	None R L	51-53

PLEURAL CALCIFICATION

	None	None	None	54
Site: Diaphragm	R L	R L	R L	55-56
Wall (Tick)				57-58
Other sites				59-60
Extent 1 2 3				61-62

SYMBOLS ax bu ca cn co cp cv di ef em es fr hi ho id ih kl od pi px rp tb

	None o d	None h i p L	None a ✗	63-65 / 66-67 / 68-69 / 70-71 / 72-73

COMMENTS	None	None	None	74-75 / 76-77 / 78-80
Continue overleaf if necessary - with reader's initials				

example, the presence of round opacities of medium size but no irregular opacities is recorded as q/q. If the majority of opacities are fine irregular ones interspersed with medium-sized round ones then the reading is s/q and so on (fig. 5.1). The scoring has the advantage of being logical, comprehensive and relatively easy to apply but the disadvantage that the profusions of round and irregular opacities are not recorded separately. The latter is helpful if the two types develop or regress at different rates as may occur in acute superimposed on chronic beryllium disease, and coal workers' simple pneumoconiosis complicated by emphysema.

Large opacities have a diameter of more than 10mm. They are categorized as A, B or C depending on whether the greatest diameter (or in the case of more than one large opacity the sum of the diameters) is less than or more than 50mm (A and B respectively). Category C indicates that the area or combined area of opacities exceeds that of the right upper zone. Illustrative chest radiographs showing these categories of progressive massive fibrosis in coal workers and men with silicosis are listed in table 5.8.

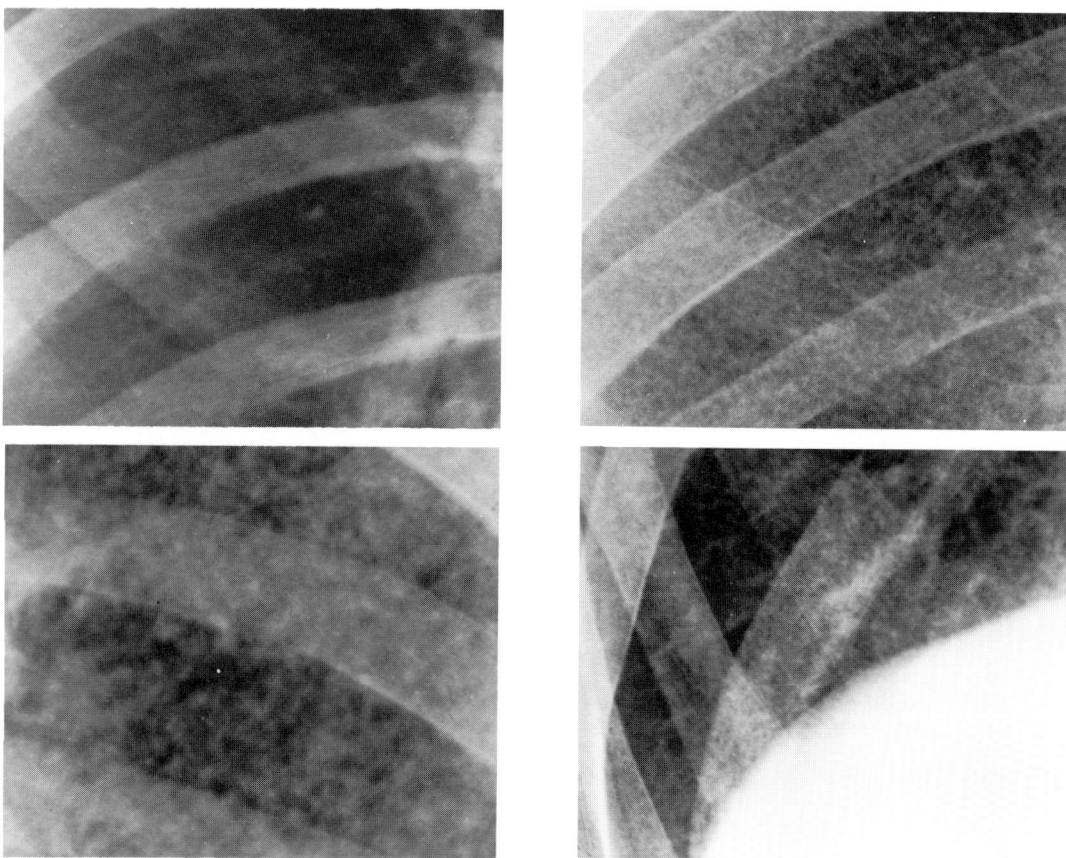

Fig. 5.1. Small opacities. Top left: category o. This patient's subsequent course is shown in fig. 11.5 (page 236). Top right: p type simple pneumoconiosis in a coalminer; this patient had a reduced transfer factor (cf. page 188). Bottom left: q type simple silicosis in a man who milled silica bricks: the subsequent progression is shown in fig. 8.9 (page 155). Bottom right: irregular opacities in the right costophrenic angle of a coal worker. The patient was later found to have centrilobular emphysema. (By courtesy of A. E. Cockcroft.)

Table 5.8. Illustrative chest radiographs of pneumoconiosis (figure and page numbers in text)

Small opacities

p type:	9.8 (175), 11.3 (234), 11.5 (236), 13.3 (279), 13.6 (297)
q type:	8.8 (154), 8.11 (158), 8.12 (159), 9.7 (174), 9.13 (182), 13.2 (268), 13.7 (302)
r type:	8.6 (152), 8.9 (155), 9.6 (172)
irregular:	9.9 (176), 9.16 (187), 10.8 (206), 10.9 (209), 11.3 (234), 15.3 (326)

Progressive massive fibrosis

	8.4 (150), 8.6 (152), 8.9 (155), 9.12 (179), 9.14 (183), 9.15 (184), 13.4 (280)

Normal films (category 0):	11.5 (236), 15.2 (323)

Pleural abnormalities are described as diffuse or circumscribed (plaques) and the presence of calcification is noted (12). For pleural thickening seen along the lateral chest wall the width is recorded in multiples of 5mm as a, b and c respectively; the extent either in profile or 'en face' is recorded in multiples of standard units of length of which 1 unit is a quarter of the overall length projection of the lateral chest wall (1–3 respectively, fig. 5.2). The presence of plaques on the diaphragm and of obliteration of the costophrenic angle is also recorded. In the case of pleural calcification both the site and the extent are recorded, the latter using the notation 1–3 to describe plaques of total length <20mm, 20–100mm and >100mm. Chest radiographs of asbestos workers showing some of these features are illustrated later (table 5.8).

Other abnormalities are reported as present or absent using the symbols given in table 5.9.

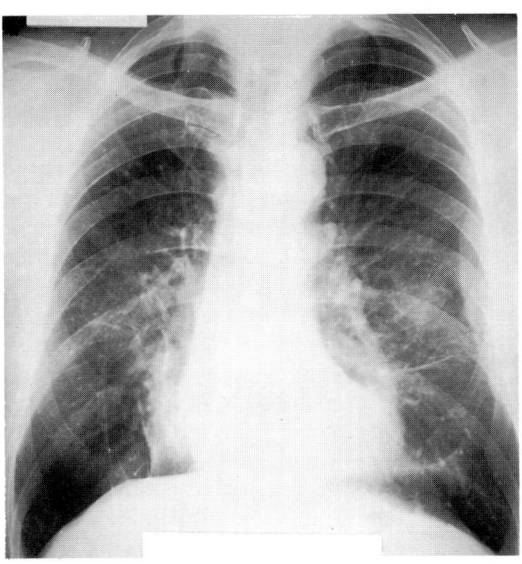

Fig. 5.2. Profile view of left pleural thickening (grade C2) on the chest radiograph of a painter who had worked with asbestos for 8 years. The parenchymal changes were read as 1t. The lung distensibility was reduced but the lung volumes and transfer factor were normal. (See also figs. 10.4–10.9, chapter 10.)

Table 5.9. Symbols for use in X-ray reading

ax — coalescence of small opacities	fr — fractured rib(s)
bu — bulla(e)	hi — enlarged hilar or other nodes
ca — cancer of lung or pleura	ho — honeycomb lung
cn — calcification in small opacities	id — ill defined diaphragm
co — abnormal cardiac size or shape	ih — ill defined heart outline
— costrophrenic angle obliterated	kl — septal (Kerley) lines
cp — cor pumonale	od — other significant abnormality
cv — cavity	pi — thickening of interlobular fissure or
di — marked distortion of viscera	mediastinum
ef — effusion	px — pneumothorax
em — definite emphysema	rp — rheumatoid pneumoconiosis
es — eggshell calcification of nodes	tb — tuberculosis

Learning to read chest radiographs. An original chest radiograph contains detailed information which cannot be reproduced exactly in a copy or in a black and white photograph; for this reason the lower categories of simple pneumoconiosis need to be seen in the originals. They are usually under-read by those whose experience is based on the ILO standard films and on textbook photographs. The learning process should be based on re-reading good quality survey films previously read by a panel of readers; subsequently those films where there is disagreement should be discussed.

Comment. Chest radiography is an essential tool for the physician concerned with almost any aspect of the mineral pneumoconioses or associated conditions; chapters 8–11 should be consulted for examples and details. Radiography also makes an invaluable contribution to the interpretation of lung function test results. The procedure is of limited usefulness for appraisal of bronchitis, byssinosis or asthma and sometimes contributes information which is potentially misleading as in siderosis or stannosis where the presence of pneumoconiosis may be irrelevant to the clinical problem. Thus chest radiography should be used with discretion in respect to when an x-ray is needed, how often it should be repeated and what it contributes to the file of information which is being built up. Approached in this way chest radiography is invaluable but in the context of occupational medicine a chest x-ray, unaccompanied by other information, may be a disaster.

Anthropometric measurements

Stature is an important reference value for interpreting tests of lung function, while sitting height is no longer recommended for this purpose. However, stature is usually measured inaccurately as a result of a failure to remove shoes, achieve uniform posture or allow for the fluctuations in thickness of intervertebral discs which occur throughout the 24h. Accurate measurement requires attention to all these points; the result is then noted by a colleague or read off the display of a digital stadiometer (e.g. Harpenden supplied by Messrs. Holtain, 21). The heels should be together and the subject as tall as possible with heels, calf, buttocks and back preferably all touching the stadiometer. The head is held in the Frankfurt plane with the lower eyelid on the same horizontal plane as the external auditory meatus; upward traction is applied by the hands cupped over the angles of the mandibles and mastoid processes (fig. 5.3). To do this effectively the operator may have to stand or kneel on a stool. The stadiometer should be calibrated regularly using a metal rod of known length and the result recorded.

Body mass is usually recorded, but unlike its subdivisions, fat free mass and percentage body fat, the body mass is of no importance unless it is abnormal. The mass is best measured using a beam balance or high quality spring balance which should be calibrated with weights. The shoes and top clothing should be removed first.

The fat free mass is an important reference variable for cardiac frequency during submaximal exercise (chapter 18). It is derived from body mass and percentage body fat which is in turn estimated indirectly from measurements of body skinfold thickness using the method of Durnin and Womersley (6): this is summarized in fig. 5.4. The measurements are made using calipers (e.g. Holtain) which are applied over the left biceps and triceps muscles, below the angle of the scapula and above the anterior superior iliac spine. The sites are marked with a skin pencil. The skinfold is picked up between the thumb and the forefinger and the readings are taken 2s after the calipers are applied (fig. 5.5). In the case of the upper arm, the olecranon process is marked with the elbow flexed and the arm then hangs free; the measurements are made at a level mid-way between this point and the acromion process with the blades of the calipers in the long axis of the limb. The measurement below the inferior angle of the scapula is made obliquely in the line of the ribs and that just above and medial to the anterior superior iliac spine in a line parallel to the external oblique muscle.

Assessment of lung function

Tests of function often provide the first objective evidence of damage to the lungs by occupational dusts and vapours. For this reason the tests are

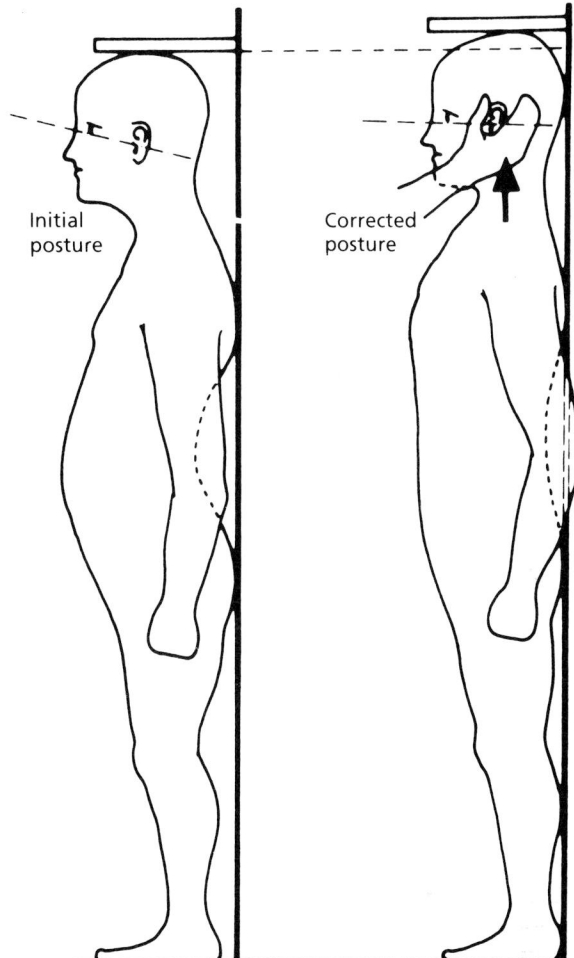

Fig. 5.3. Measurement of stature showing the error which can arise when the posture is wrong and no traction is applied. (Tracing from photographs; source: Cotes, J.E. (1979) *Lung Function*, 4th edn, Blackwell Scientific Publications, p. 50.)

used extensively in occupational surveys where very small changes may be detected by pooling the results for large numbers of subjects (chapter 6). The tests are also used for study of individuals; here it is usually only possible to identify relatively large deviations from the reference value. However, the results are often essential for diagnosis and clinical management, contribute to understanding of the underlying disorder and have a place in assessment of prognosis and disablement (12). The tests and average results for healthy persons are described in this section. Fuller details of calibration, measurement procedures, calculation of results

and ways of allowing for biological variation are given elsewhere (3). The interpretation of results is considered later in this chapter.

Lung function tests are most often used to describe the movement of gas by bulk flow (bellows function or ventilatory capacity), the distribution of gas within the lung (lung mixing) and the transfer of gas across the alveolar capillary membrane which takes place mainly by diffusion. The processes are described by indices whose magnitude is critically dependent on the size of the lung and the elasticity of the lung tissue; they are usually impaired if the subject is or has been a smoker. The lung size is

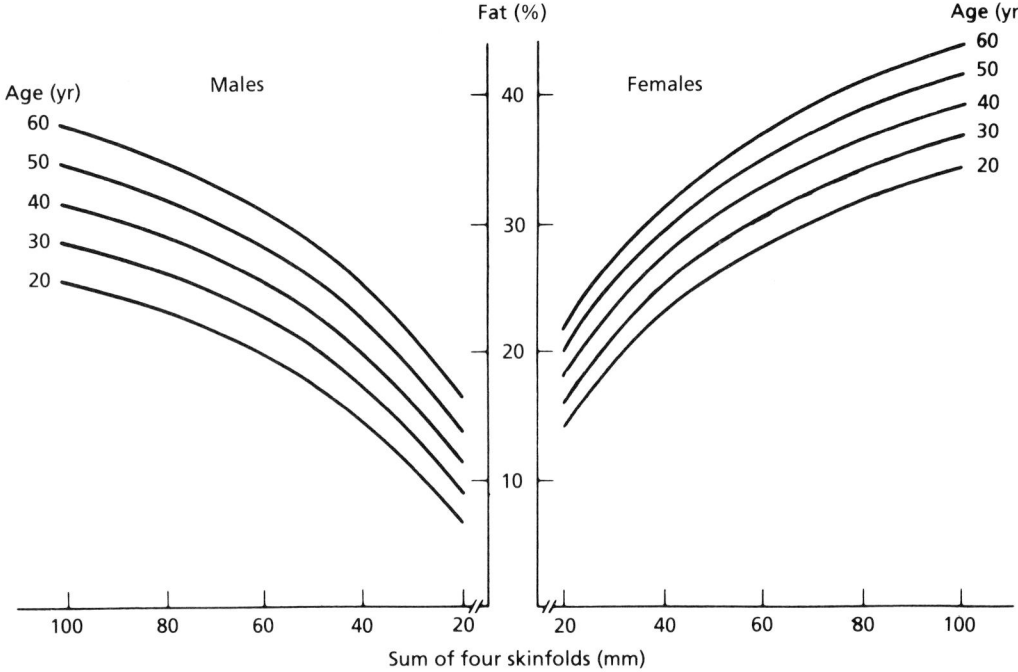

Fig. 5.4. Chart for obtaining from the sum of four skinfold thicknesses the percentage of body mass which is fat. For details see text. (Source: Cotes J.E. (1979) *Lung Function*, 4th edn. Blackwell Scientific Publications, p. 51.)

related to body size for which standing height (stature) is the most useful single index; its measurement is described above. Other determinants are gender, ethnic group, level of habitual activity and age. The last is important because lung elasticity, strength of respiratory muscles and amount of gas exchanging tissue all diminish with advancing years. The lung function is also influenced by the quantity and distribution of flow of alveolar capillary blood and hence by the vasomotor tone in the pulmonary circulation. Depending on circumstances some or all of these factors should be taken into account when assessing a person's lung function; this is usually compared with that of an asymptomatic individual having similar attributes. For any index of lung function the corresponding normal result is called the reference value. It is usually derived using the subject's gender, age and stature. Examples are given in table 5.10 and illustrated in figs. 5.7 and 5.8.

Ventilatory capacity and airflow resistance

The ability to move air rapidly in and out of the lungs is essential for normal activity; any diminution of more than minimal extent will usually cause breathlessness on exertion and hence reduce the capacity for exercise. Ventilatory impairment is usually caused by narrowing of lung airways which may be mainly structural as occurs with chronic bronchitis, or mainly functional as in emphysema and asthma. However, the ventilatory defect may also arise in the nervous system, the musculo-skeletal system, the soft tissues of the chest wall or, in the case of some divers and caisson workers, the inhaled gas. The detection of ventilatory impairment is the first stage in the assessment of respiratory function.

The peak expiratory flow rate (PEF). This is the maximal flow rate during a forced expiration starting from a position of full inspiration. It is

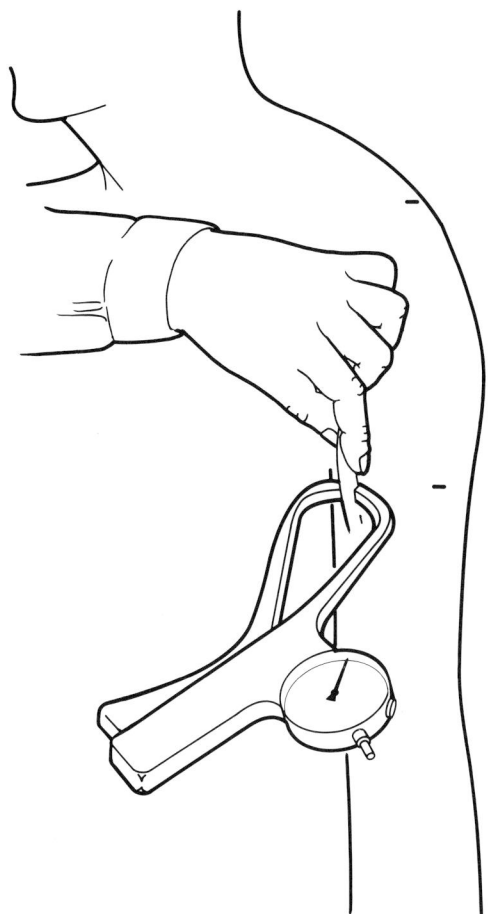

Fig. 5.5. Measurement of skinfold thickness. The fold is held between thumb and forefinger and the reading taken shortly after applying the caliper.

usually measured with a peak flow meter (e.g. Wright) but may be obtained during the registration of a maximal expiratory flow volume curve (see below). The mean result for an average man (age 40, stature 1.72m) is $9.6 \, l \, s^{-1}$ (SD 1.0). The index reflects mainly the calibre of the larger airways; it is particularly useful for the investigation of suspected occupational asthma since the equipment is very compact and may be used by the subject to provide serial measurements. A random read-out attachment may then be used to reduce deliberate manipulation of the results (11). Calibration of the

equipment is done either biologically or using a breath simulator (fig. 5.6).

Vital capacity and forced expiratory volume (FVC and FEV₁). The forced vital capacity is the volume of gas breathed out during a complete expiration delivered as rapidly and completely as possible starting from a position of full inspiration (fig. 5.9). It is usually measured with a waterless spirometer of the bellows or sleeve type (e.g. Vitalograph, McDermott or Morgan). The spirometer should be calibrated with a gas syringe (fig. 5.6) or by water displacement. The mean FVC for an average man (see PFR above) is 4.40 l (SD 0.58). The index reflects the size of the lung and is obtained in conjunction with measurement of forced expiratory volume. It is particularly useful for indicating the possibility of fibrosis of the lung parenchyma as may occur with asbestosis and extrinsic allergic alveolitis.

The forced expiratory volume is the volume of gas exhaled in the first second during the performance of the forced vital capacity manoeuvre described above. For this application the timing mechanism on the spirometer should be accurate and calibrated either in use, as is the case for the McDermott spirometer, or by an external calibrator (fig. 5.6). The mean FEV_1 for an average man (see PFR above) is 3.6 l (SD 0.5). The index reflects the average calibre of all generations of lung airways and is reduced in the presence of obstruction to airflow. In these circumstances the airflow resistance is increased and the FEV_1 is negatively correlated with the score for breathlessness (chapter 18). The index is very reproducible (coefficient of variation 1–3%). It should be obtained as part of the surveillance of all persons who are exposed to or affected by a respiratory hazard. The result is best expressed as absolute units and related to the reference value (figs. 5.7 and 5.8); it may also be expressed as a percentage of the forced vital capacity (FVC) when it is called the forced expiratory ratio (FEV%), i.e. FEV%=$FEV_1 \times 100/$FVC. The mean FEV% for an average man (see above) is 77 (SD 7.2)%. It is reduced if the FVC is increased, as in many divers, and if there is obstruction to air flow. The ratio is commonly used to confirm the presence of the latter condition. The ratio is relatively less sensitive than the FEV_1 for detecting early abnormality and is

Table 5.10. Regression equations for deriving reference values for selected lung function indices in adults of European descent. (Source: (3), page 369.)

Index	Units	Sex	Regression coefficients			SD
			Stature	Age	Constant term	
Vital capacity	l	M	5.20	−0.022	− 3.60	0.58
(VC and FVC)		F	4.66	−0.029	− 2.88	0.44
Forced expiratory volume	l	M	3.62	−0.031	− 1.41	≥0.50
(FEV_1)		F	3.29	−0.029	− 1.42	0.36
(FEV_1/FVC) × 100	%	M		−0.373	+91.8	7.19
		F		−0.222	+86.5	6.2
Peak expiratory flow rate	l s^{-1}	M	st x	(−0.025	+ 6.58)	1.0
(PEFR)		F	6.23	−0.035	− 1.88	1.1
Forced mid-expiratory flow	l s^{-1}	M		−0.057	+ 6.38	1.09
(FMEF)		F		−0.063	+ 6.14	0.77
Transfer factor	*	M	10.9	−0.067	− 5.89	1.71
(Tl)		F	7.1	−0.054	− 0.89	1.20
K_{CO}		M		−0.013	2.20	0.27
(Tl/V_A)		F		−0.007	2.07	0.20

* mmol min^{-1} kPa^{-1}.

useless for detecting short-term changes in airway calibre since in these circumstances the forced vital capacity may also vary. The sensitivity may be improved by using in the denominator the inspiratory or slow expiratory vital capacity and not the forced vital capacity (FEV_1 × 100/VC); the ratio is then called the Tiffeneau index.

The FEV_1 is obtained from the relationship of expired volume to time; the resulting spirogram is illustrated in fig 5.9. This type of analysis may also be used to obtain other indices, for example, the *forced expiratory time* (FET) which is the time to complete the forced vital capacity manoeuvre. It is normally less than 4.5s and is prolonged by airflow obstruction. The measurement may be made with a stopwatch and stethoscope and when combined with measurement of peak expiratory flow may contribute to clinical assessment.

The *maximal mid-expiratory flow rate* (MMEF) is the mean flow rate over the second and third quarters of the FVC manoeuvre (fig. 5.9). The MMEF is widely employed for detect-ing minimal obstruction to airflow but, whilst sensitive for this application, it is rarely used for clinical assessment so is a less versatile index than the FEV_1. A recently introduced index is the mean transit time (MTT) which is the mean time taken by gas molecules to leave the lung during the performance of the FVC manoeuvre; the index has several derivatives including the standard deviation of transit times and index of skewness. These indices show great promise but are not yet in regular use.

Forced expiratory flow. The forced expiratory flow rates at specified lung volumes during the performance of the forced vital capacity manoeuvre may be obtained concurrently with the FEV_1. The flow rate is usually related graphically to the lung volume when the resulting curve is called the maximal expiratory flow volume curve (MEFV, fig. 5.10). The resulting indices are the flow rates when 50% and 25% of the FVC remain to be expired (MEF50%FVC and MEF25%FVC respectively). The mean flow rates for an average man (see above) are 5.6 and 2.8 l s^{-1}. The flow rates are reduced by narrowing of

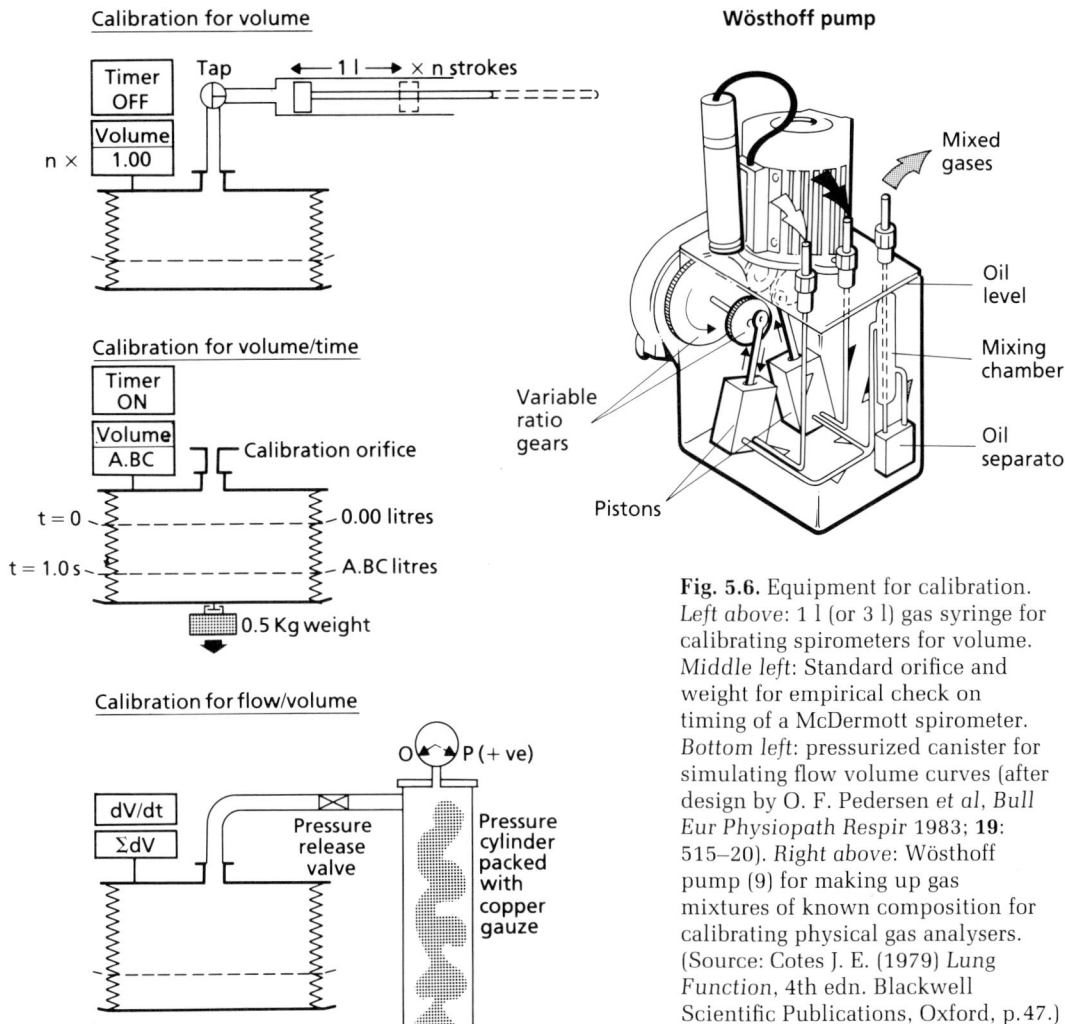

Calibration for volume

Calibration for volume/time

Calibration for flow/volume

Wösthoff pump

Fig. 5.6. Equipment for calibration. *Left above*: 1 l (or 3 l) gas syringe for calibrating spirometers for volume. *Middle left*: Standard orifice and weight for empirical check on timing of a McDermott spirometer. *Bottom left*: pressurized canister for simulating flow volume curves (after design by O. F. Pedersen *et al*, *Bull Eur Physiopath Respir* 1983; **19**: 515–20). *Right above*: Wösthoff pump (9) for making up gas mixtures of known composition for calibrating physical gas analysers. (Source: Cotes J. E. (1979) *Lung Function*, 4th edn. Blackwell Scientific Publications, Oxford, p.47.)

the smaller lung airways such as may occur in pneumoconiosis but they have a rather poor reproducibility (coefficient of variation in the range 5–10%) and this impairs their usefulness. The indices are measured using an accurate low inertia spirometer or a pneumotachograph and integrator which have been calibrated against an external calibrator. The curves may also be obtained while breathing helium but the difference from breathing air, though of theoretical interest, is of limited usefulness. A partial expiratory flow volume curve (PEFV) is obtained by starting the forced expiration after a normal and not a maximal inspiration; this procedure increases the sensitivity of the test but entails the concurrent measurement of lung volume in a whole body plethysmograph.

Airflow resistance (R_{aw}). The R_{aw} and its reciprocal the conductance (G_{aw}) reflect the calibre of the larger airways. These may be measured accurately by whole body plethysmography and, with rather less accuracy, by multiple brief interruption of airflow during expiration. The measurement is often used to control the assessment of bronchial reactivity and asthma challenge tests. For this application

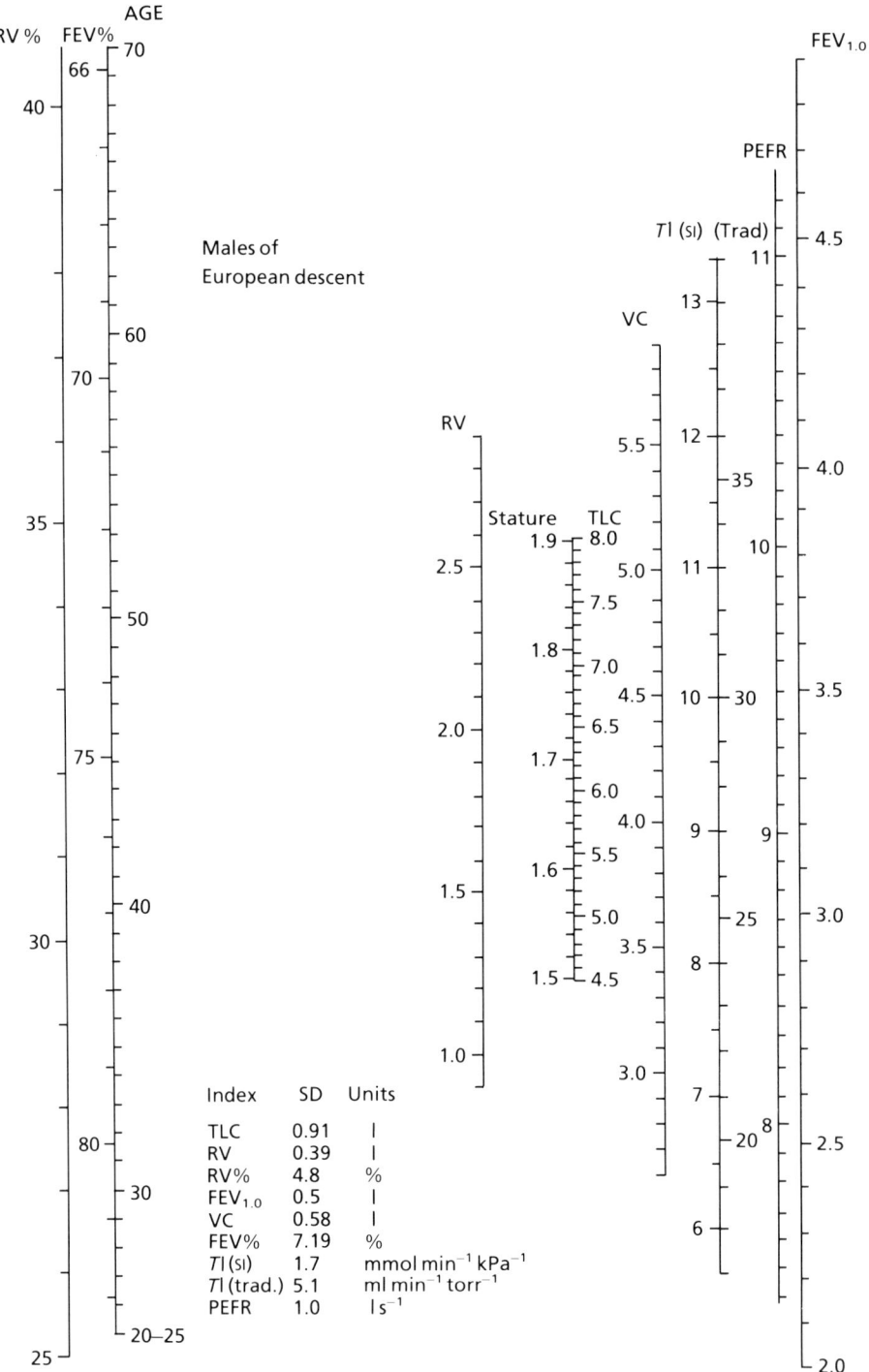

Fig. 5.7. Reference values for indices of lung function in males of European descent. A ruler is positioned at the age and stature of the subject and the indices are then read off. In males of Indian and African origin, the FEV_1, FVC and TLC are lower by approximately 13% and transfer factor by approximately 8% (Rossiter C.E., Weill H. *Int J Epidemiol* 1974; **3**: 55–61). (Source: Cotes, J.E. (1979) *Lung Function*, 4th edn. Blackwell Scientific Publications, Oxford, p. 377.)

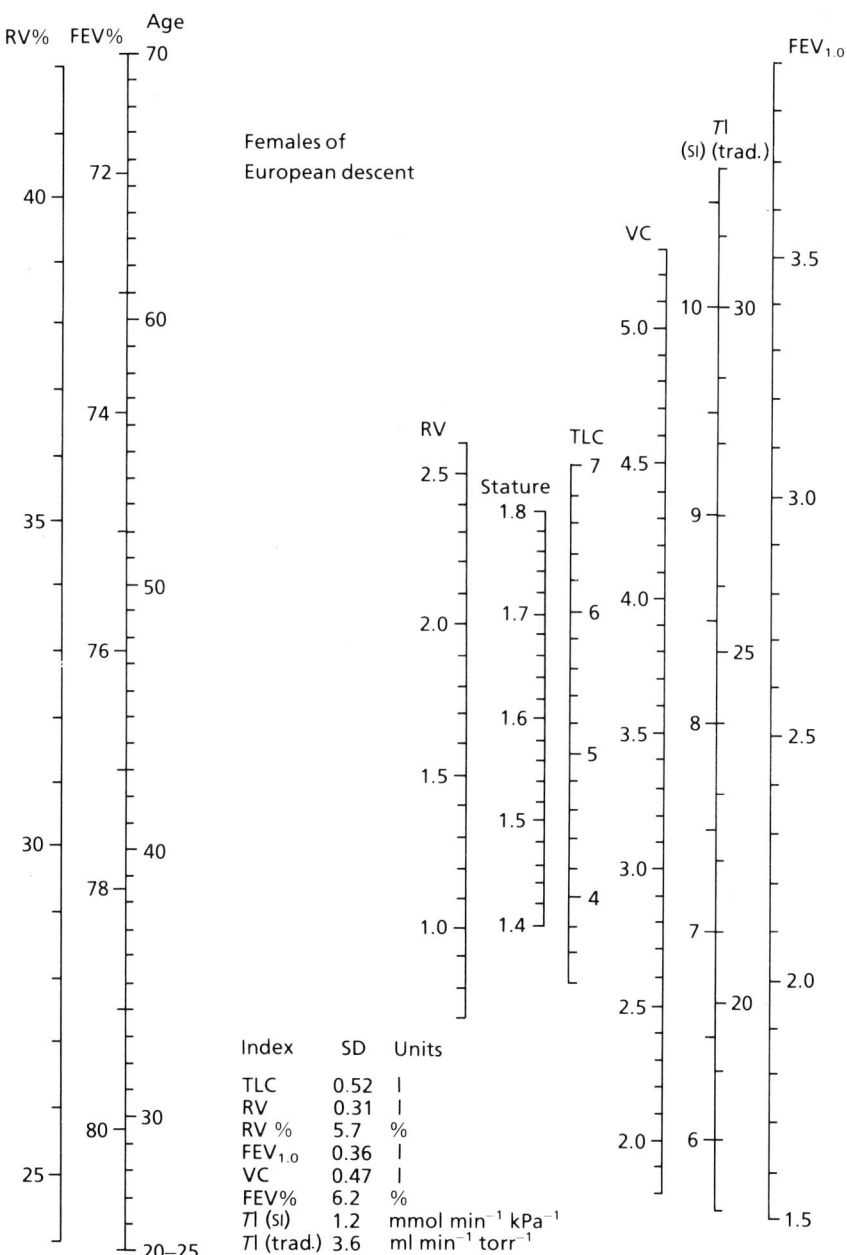

Index	SD	Units
TLC	0.52	l
RV	0.31	l
RV %	5.7	%
FEV$_{1.0}$	0.36	l
VC	0.47	l
FEV%	6.2	%
Tl (SI)	1.2	mmol min^{-1} kPa^{-1}
Tl (trad.)	3.6	ml min^{-1} torr^{-1}

Fig. 5.8. Reference values for indices of lung function in females of European descent. For females of Indian and African descent, the FEV$_1$ and FVC are lower by approximately 0.4 l and 0.6 l respectively. (Source: Cotes, J.E. (1979) *Lung Function*, 4th edn. Blackwell Scientific Publications, Oxford, p. 378.)

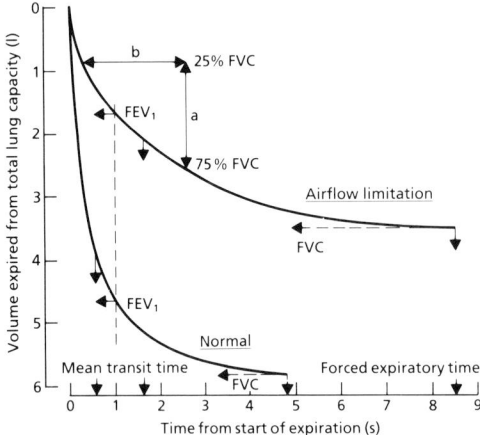

Fig. 5.9. Averaged forced expiratory spirograms (volume time curves) showing mean values for FEV_1, FVC, transit time and forced expiratory time in healthy subjects and patients with chronic airflow limitation (data of R. Bello *et al Thorax* 1980; **35**: 225). Maximal mid-expiratory flow rate (forced expiratory flow rate for expiration of the middle half of the forced vital capacity, FEF25–75%) is given by a/b. The starting point of expiration is defined either by backward extrapolation of the steep part of the curve to zero time or as the time when 50ml has been expired.

the FEV_1 is usually more convenient whilst the MEF50%FVC obtained from the partial expiratory flow volume curve may be more sensitive; however, in order not to bias the result the flow rate on each occasion should be taken at the same lung volume (usually 50% of the initial vital capacity).

Practical details. The measurement of ventilatory capacity is best made with the subject seated and wearing a nose clip. Any tight clothing is loosened and the procedure is explained and demonstrated by the operator who should have received some training; this should include comparing the results of measurements made on a group of naïve subjects with those made by an experienced operator. To perform the test the subject takes a full inspiration, places the mouthpiece within the mouth, closes the lips round it and exhales as rapidly and completely as possible. Two

practice attempts are usually made, then three blows are recorded. Any fault in the procedure, an atypical result or an unsatisfactory spirogram or flow volume curve constitutes a defective blow and should be repeated. Subsequently any breath is discarded where the FVC is less than the highest value by 5% or 0.3 l. The result for each index is then taken as the highest value from the breaths which remain. The methods for doing this are described elsewhere (17). Measurements should normally be made during working hours. Serial measurements should preferably be made at the same time of day by one operator and apparatus.

Distribution of gas

The distribution of ventilation within the lung is influenced by gravity, both directly and via

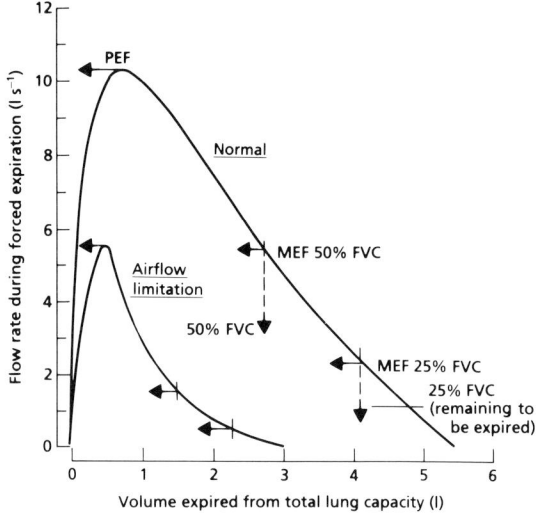

Fig. 5.10. Averaged maximal expiratory flow volume curves for the subjects whose volume time curves are given in fig. 5.9. Horizontal arrows indicate peak expiratory flow (PEF) and maximal expiratory flow, when 50% and 25% of forced vital capacity remain to be expired (respectively MEF50%FVC and MEF25%FVC). The indices are the highest values from three technically satisfactory expirations analysed either individually or after superimposition to obtain a composite curve. Individual curves are shown in fig. 7.5 (page 139).

control mechanisms; these have the effect of redistributing ventilation to match the perfusion which is greatest in dependent parts of the lung. The matching process is imperfect so the lung ventilation is distributed unevenly with respect to both regional lung volume and perfusion. The inequality is exaggerated by diseases of the lung, especially emphysema and narrowing of small lung airways. It may be detected by tests of uneven lung function which in some circumstances provide an early indication of abnormality. The following tests are amongst those which may be used:

Lung volume index of uneven ventilation (VA,eff/VA). This index is the ratio of the alveolar volume obtained by gas dilution following inhaling a single breath of inert gas (VA,eff) to that obtained by rebreathing or by whole body plethysmography (VA). Both the component volumes may be obtained during measurement by the breathholding method of the transfer factor of the lung for carbon monoxide (also called the diffusing capacity). This is described below. The index is convenient but not particularly sensitive.

Closing volume (CV). Closing volume is the lung volume above residual volume (see below) at which there is detectable closure of lung airways. The volume is usually reported as a percentage of inspiratory vital capacity (i.e. CV × 100/IVC). The index is abnormal in most smokers and on this account not a great help for studying whole populations. It may be obtained during measurement of the single breath inert gas index which is described below.

Single breath inert gas index. This index is the slope of the early part of the alveolar plateau for the concentration of an inert gas which is sampled at the lips during a full expiration. The inert gas is usually intra-thoracic nitrogen and the test expiration is then preceded by a full breath of 100% oxygen; the analysis is made with an ultraviolet emission spectrometer (nitrogen meter) or a mass spectrometer. Other inert gases including helium and xenon 133 may be used instead. The procedure is illustrated in fig. 5.11; it yields the inert gas mixing index, the single breath alveolar volume (VA,eff above) and the closing volume. The test was first described by Comroe & Fowler in 1951 and is still not widely used but this may change as it appears to provide a sensitive index of early narrowing of small airways.

Lung volumes and distensibility

Total lung capacity (TLC) is the volume of gas present in the lung at the end of a full inspiration: it may be represented as the sum of the vital capacity (page 93) and the residual volume (RV) which is the volume present in the lung at the end of a complete expiration. TLC is

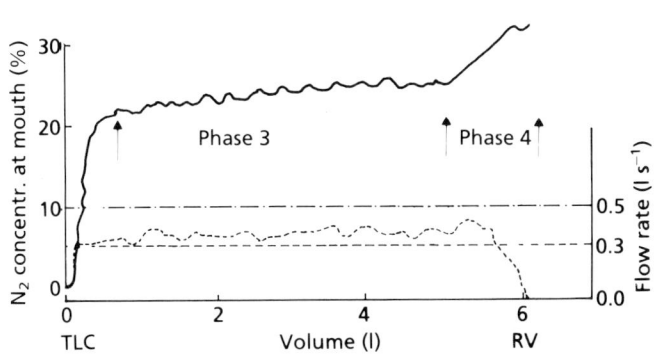

Fig. 5.11. Nitrogen washout curve and corresponding expiratory flow rate following a full breath of oxygen up to total lung capacity (TLC). Inspiration was started from 1 l below functional residual capacity and the flow rate was within the range 0.3–0.5 l s⁻¹. The nitrogen index is the slope of the alveolar plateau (phase 3); the volume expired from the onset of phase 4 to residual volume (RV) is the closing volume. This is expressed as a percentage of vital capacity. (By courtesy of F. M. El-Gamal *Clin Sci* 1985; **68** (Suppl. 11); 6p.)

reduced by all processes which reduce the size of the lung or limit the expansion of the lung or chest wall; it is increased in physically active subjects and in some patients with emphysema, asthma and acromegaly. The distribution of lung volume as between vital capacity and residual volume also varies. The measurement of total lung capacity is an essential component of a full assessment of lung function. The residual volume is usually measured by rebreathing gas containing helium from a closed circuit spirometer, but it may be measured by whole body plethysmography. The total lung capacity may also be derived from postero-anterior and lateral chest radiographs taken at full inspiration; the measurements and calculations can now be made by computer.

The distensibility of the lung is described by the static lung compliance which is the change in lung volume induced by a unit change in the pressure difference across the lung. The latter is the elastic pressure or recoil pressure of the lung and, in the absence of airflow, is approximately equal to pleural pressure. The pressure may be measured indirectly using a soft latex balloon swallowed into the oesophagus; with a view to serial measurements the placement should be made by a skilled operator. The compliance is reduced by fibrosis of the visceral pleura or diffuse disease of the lung parenchyma, including interstitial fibrosis and extrinsic allergic alveolitis; it is increased in the presence of emphysema, either in isolation or as a material component of some other condition. The measurement is sometimes invaluable for making a functional diagnosis, especially in cases where the pathology is in doubt.

Lung gas exchange; transfer factor

Defective gas transfer is a feature of disease processes which affect the lung parenchyma including extrinsic allergic alveolitis, pulmonary granulomas, diffuse interstitial fibrosis and emphysema. In all these conditions the transfer factor (diffusing capacity) is likely to be reduced. Its measurement is an essential component of surveillance of personnel with suspected disease of the lung parenchyma and is described below. The transfer defect has the consequence that during exercise of progressively increasing intensity the quantity of oxygen in the arterial blood usually falls and the exercise ventilation increases in consequence. The latter changes may be detected by measuring the physiological response to exercise which is described in chapter 18.

The transfer factor (diffusing capacity) is the rate of transfer of oxygen or carbon monoxide from alveolar gas to arterial blood in unit time for unit gas pressure difference across the alveolar capillary membrane. The results are usually expressed in standard international units (mmol min^{-1} kPa^{-1}) but sometimes in traditional units (ml min^{-1} mmHg^{-1}). The mean result for an average man (see page 93) in S.I. units is 10 (SD 1.7) mmol min^{-1} kPa^{-1} and in traditional units 30 (SD 5.1) ml min^{-1} mmHg^{-1} (i.e. conversion factor is $\times 3$). The measurement is usually made for carbon monoxide which has a high affinity for haemoglobin, so the dissociation of the resulting carboxyhaemoglobin is effectively zero. Hence for this gas the pressure difference across the alveolar capillary membrane is nearly equal to the partial pressure in the alveolar gas. The measurement may be made during regular breathing (steady state method) or during a single expiration but is usually made by the breathholding method of Forster and colleagues; the procedure is summarized in fig. 5.12. This may appear complicated on first confrontation but the measurement can now be made using automatic apparatus.

The subject inhales and holds in the lung for a minimum of 5s a nearly vital capacity breath of test gas which includes carbon monoxide in low concentration and helium or other insoluble gas not normally present in the body. During the subsequent exhalation a sample of alveolar gas is obtained and analysed for both gases. The result is calculated from the inspired and alveolar concentrations of helium and carbon monoxide together with the time of breathholding and the volume of gas in the lung during the period of breathholding (VA). The latter is the sum of the residual volume measured by the closed circuit helium dilution method and the volume of test gas inspired; it yields the transfer factor (Tl). An effective alveolar volume (VA,eff) may be calculated from the dilution of the helium pres-

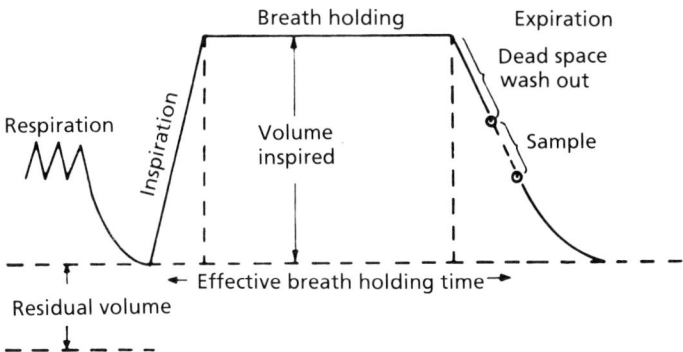

Fig. 5.12. Spirogram illustrating the procedure for determining the transfer factor for the lung by the single breath (breath-holding) method. The subject breathes out to residual volume, inhales a vital capacity breath of the test gas, holds the breath for 10s, then exhales slowly; after the exhalation of 750ml, a sample of 0.5 or 1.0 l of alveolar gas is collected for analysis. The effective duration of breathholding is taken to include two-thirds of the time of inspiration and the time of expiration up to half-way through the period of sample collection. Alveolar volume is the sum of volume inspired and residual volume. (Source: Cotes, J.E. (1979) *Lung Function,* 4th edn. Blackwell Scientific Publications, Oxford, p. 235.)

ent in the test breath. This yields an alternative index of transfer (Tl,eff) which is derived solely from information obtained during the test breath and for this reason is often used for occupational surveys. The two indices are nearly identical in subjects with normal gas mixing but in the presence of uneven lung function VA,eff is reduced compared with VA. Hence Tl,eff is reduced compared with Tl. The latter more nearly reflects the capacity of the lung to transfer gas, except in emphysema when neither index is correct because it is not possible to obtain a representative alveolar gas sample. Use should then be made of the transfer factor per litre of alveolar volume which is the Kco (i.e. Kco = Tl/VA = Tl,eff/VA,eff).

The transfer factor should be measured at a time remote from a heavy meal or strenuous exertion with the subject in a relaxed, upright seated posture. The ambient temperature should be in the range 16–25°C. A high blood concentration of carbon monoxide will lead to an erroneously low result and to avoid this the subject should preferably not have smoked on the day of the test. In addition, since anaemia or polycythaemia affect the quantity of haemoglobin which is available to combine with carbon monoxide, the colour of the conjunctiva should be noted and, if it appears to be abnormal, the haemoglobin concentration estimated; the transfer factor may then be corrected to what would obtain at a normal haemoglobin concentration (3). A correction is also necessary if the measurement is made at high altitude since the consequent reduction in alveolar oxygen tension increases the quantity of haemoglobin not combined with oxygen which is, therefore, immediately available for the carbon monoxide.

Interpreting the lung function results

Indices of lung function are liable to technical error and to biological variation both within and between individuals: after allowing for these factors the results usually conform to a recognizable pattern of abnormality which relates to the clinical and other features. Thus the results should be interpreted at several levels. At the technical level the instruments should have been calibrated and their mechanical parts should have been functioning satisfactorily. The subject should have performed the requisite manoeuvres correctly (e.g. fig. 5.13). There should be consistency to within 0.3 l in the results of the several vital capacity manoeuvres which are performed in the course of the

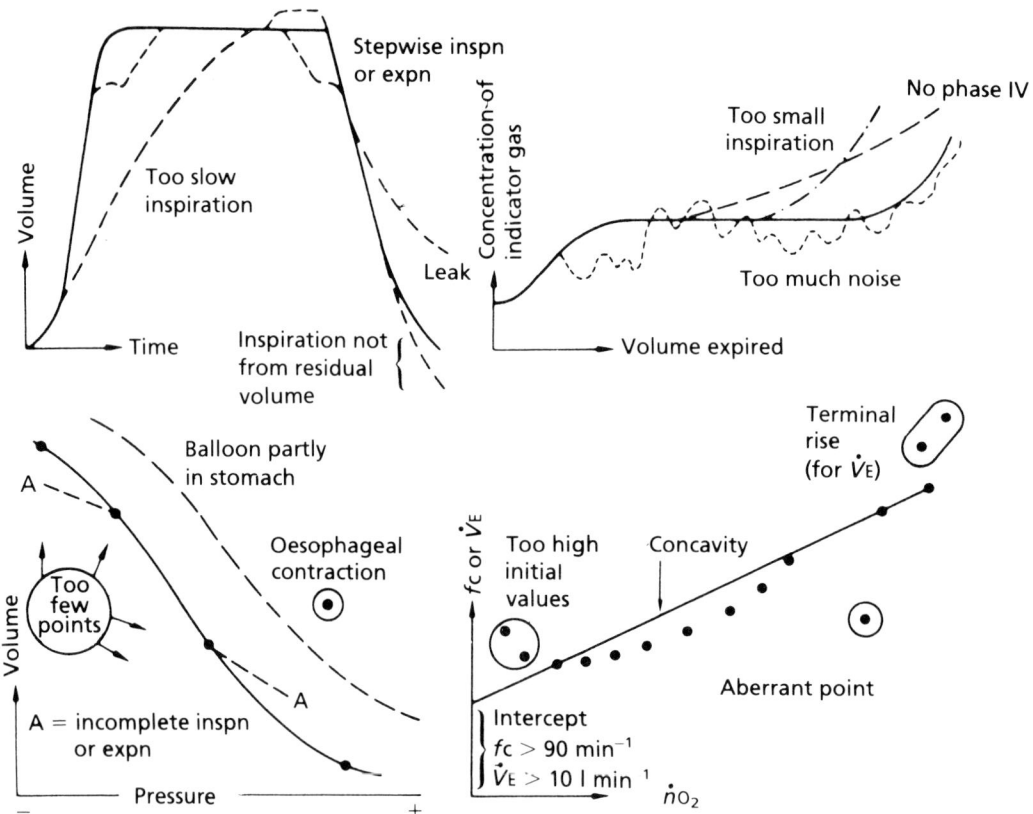

Fig. 5.13. Faults which can arise during the performance of tests of lung function; in most instances they are grounds for rejecting the result. (Source: Cotes, J.E. (1979) *Lung Function*, 4th edn. Blackwell Scientific Publications, p. 328.)

different tests; in addition, where the manoeuvre is recorded on a chart this should show a slowing down in the rate of airflow as the lung approaches the limiting volume, either total lung capacity or residual volume. Discrepancies may reflect inadequate instruction or unfamiliarity with the procedure but they may be due to non-co-operation. This is uncommon in a clinical context or during occupational surveys but may occur when the assessment is in connection with a claim for compensation. Ways in which the distortion may be detected are given in chapter 18. At the biological level the conditions of measurement should have been appropriate and the relevant anthropometric and other information should have been

obtained with a view to calculating the reference values. If the result passes both these scrutinies the next step is to assess whether or not it is abnormal. This is usually done in the broad categories excellent, normal, possibly normal, abnormal and very abnormal. The categories are determined by comparison with the expected or reference values; in ideal circumstances these are the previous results for the subject in question but usually they are average results for healthy persons who are similar with respect to the appropriate reference variables including age, stature, gender and ethnic group. The way in which the reference variables are used for purposes of constructing reference values is indicated in chapter 6: in general the reference values vary directly with stature, exhibit deterioration with increasing age, are less in women than in men and in the case of the lung volume and forced expiratory volume are less in other ethnic groups compared with Europeans. However, in the decade 16 years rising to 25 years, for young men the size of the lung and the magnitude of indices which depend on lung size show a small increase while for young women the lung function is relatively constant. The normal variation about the reference value is defined by the residual standard error of the prediction equation: after standardizing for gender and ethnic group this is approximately 15% of the mean value. A result will usually be abnormal which deviates adversely from the mean by more than 1.64 standard deviations. The standard deviations are given in the charts of reference values and a way in which these may be used to categorize the result are given in table 5.11. The categories are appropriate for diagnosis, including the possible effect of an occupational exposure, but not for assessing present ability to undertake physical exertion; for the latter application the absolute level of lung function is more important. A result which is possibly abnormal should alert the observer to scrutinize the other evidence carefully but by itself it is not a cause for concern. Having assessed the results individually they should next be looked at corporately to see if they are consistent with the level of breathlessness (chapter 18) and to identify patterns of disordered function which may illuminate the diagnosis and/or underlying pathology. For this purpose results which differ from the reference

Table 5.11. Categories of respiratory impairment applicable to FVC, FEV, and Tl (5)

Impairment category	Criterion — with respect to reference value
None (normal)	Within 1.64 SD*
Slight	Not normal but > 60%
Moderate	In range 59–40% (50% for FVC)
Severe	< 40% (< 50% for FVC)

The American Thoracic Society's criterion is ≥ 80% and for FEV% ≥ 75% (page 405, ref. 1).

value by 1 standard deviation and, therefore, are possibly abnormal should be given due weight. Some syndromes of abnormal lung function are described below.

Limitation to airflow. This is the principal cause of breathlessness occurring in association with chronic bronchitis, emphysema, asthma and related disorders. The limitation is usually due to narrowing of airways throughout the respiratory tract but may be due to reduced elastic recoil leading to collapse of airway walls. The main feature is inability to move air rapidly out of the lungs; hence there are reductions in all indices of forced expiratory flow including the forced expiratory volume. Gas which is inhaled mixes unevenly with that present in the lungs so the mixing indices V_A,eff/V_A and nitrogen slope are abnormal. On complete expiration the airways close prematurely so the closing volume and residual volume are increased. The uneven lung function leads eventually to hypoxaemia, pulmonary hypertension and, ultimately, death which may be from infection, pulmonary heart disease, hypoxaemia or hypercapnia. Flow limitation which is due to increased bronchomotor tone is partly or completely reversed by bronchodilator drugs (chapter 19); in smokers, limitation from all causes is helped by abandoning smoking.

Narrowing of small lung airways. Most types of airflow limitation affect all classes of airways; however, in the early stages of disease the limitation may be confined to the small airways (diameter <3mm). There is then a reduction in forced expiratory flow at small lung volumes (e.g. MEF 25%FVC), impaired gas mixing and an increased residual volume; the changes are often small and only demonstrable in groups of subjects, for example, those exposed to the same environmental agent.

Restriction to lung expansion. Fibrosis of the lung or pleura, lesions of the chest wall or its nervous connections, obesity, pleural effusion and other abnormalities reduce the size and limit the expansion of the lung. In these circumstances the vital capacity is reduced and this results in a proportional reduction in forced expiratory volume. Unless the restriction is accompanied by airflow limitation other indices of forced expiratory flow are usually normal while the residual volume is reduced. When the changes are due to pulmonary fibrosis the compliance of the lung is reduced, the elastic recoil pressure is increased and the patient usually exhibits the features of defective gas transfer. The reduction in vital capacity is associated with a diminution in tidal volume and increase in respiratory frequency during exercise; these changes contribute to breathlessness.

Emphysema. A proportion of patients with emphysema suffer a loss of lung tissue; the transfer factor is then reduced, the static compliance of the lung is increased and the recoil pressure is reduced, usually to below 1.2 kPa at total lung capacity. These changes indicate reduction of elastic recoil in the lung. The chest then enlarges and in doing so maximizes the traction which is exerted on airway walls by the lung tissue. If, despite this, the traction is insufficient to prevent narrowing of airways during expiration, the patient exhibits the features of limitation to airflow. In addition, the loss of alveolar capillary membrane results in the features of defective gas transfer.

Transfer defect. Oedema, cellular proliferation, fibrosis or emphysema interfere with gas exchange by slowing the rate at which oxygen is transferred from alveolar gas to blood in alveolar capillaries. The change is detected as a reduction in transfer factor (diffusing capacity) or Kco (transfer factor per unit of lung volume). The measurement is routinely made at rest but recent work suggests that measurements on exercise may be more informative (2). Defective gas transfer becomes apparent during progressive exercise as a fall in the saturation of oxygen in the arterial blood (chapter 18). The exercise hypoxaemia stimulates breathing to cause hyperventilation which contributes to breathlessness and may lead to hypocapnia. The changes in the lung parenchyma may also stimulate pulmonary J receptors to cause rapid shallow breathing. The damage to the lung parenchyma is associated with loss or obliteration of small pulmonary vessels and a progressive reduction in size of the pulmonary vascular bed; the resulting pulmonary hypertension and cor pulmonale are often relatively resistant to therapy.

Mixed defects. Restriction of lung expansion reduces the ability of the lung to transfer gas so the transfer factor is diminished whilst the Kco is increased to a proportionally smaller extent. However, a lung which is constrained by pleural thickening may be well perfused and in these circumstances the Kco increases unless damage to the lung parenchyma coexists. Conversely, in emphysema in which the total lung capacity is increased, the transfer factor calculated on the assumption that the whole of the lung contributes to gas exchange may be normal for the patient's age and stature, but still less than would be expected for a healthy lung of the same size. On this account, in emphysema, the Kco is reduced relative to lung size. In these circumstances it may be helpful to correct the transfer indices to a standard lung volume before attempting an interpretation (8). Fibrosis and emphysema occur together in the condition cystic or honeycomb lung; there may then be some airflow limitation, a relatively normal total lung capacity and features of defective gas transfer. The compliance and recoil pressure may help to indicate if it is the fibrosis or the emphysema which predominate.

Comment. The assessment of lung function is an essential component of the practice of occupational respiratory medicine including occupational surveys, screening procedures and assessment of individuals; for the last application it will often be combined with measurement of the physiological response to exercise. This is described in chapter 18. Further information is given in references 3 and 17 and the chapters describing individual occupational lung disorders.

References

1 Bennett AE, Ritchie K. *Questionnaires in Medicine. A Guide to their Design and Use.* Oxford University Press, 1975.

2 Chu SS, Cotes JE. Lung transfer factor and Kco at cardiac frequency 100 beats/min as a guide to impaired function of lung parenchyma. *Thorax* 1984;**39**:524–8.

3 Cotes JE. *Lung Function*, 4th ed. Oxford: Blackwell Scientific Publications, 1979.

4 Crofton Sir J, Douglas A. *Respiratory Diseases* 3rd ed. Oxford: Blackwell Scientific Publications, 1981.

5 De Coster A. Respiratory impairment and disablement. *Bull Eur Physiopath Respir* 1983;**19**:1P–3P.

6 Durnin JVGA, Womersley J. Body fat assessed from total body density and its estimation from skinfold thickness: measurements on 481 men and women aged from 16 to 72 years. *Br J Nutr* 1974;**32**:77–97.

7 Field GB. The application of a quantitative estimate of cough frequency to epidemiological surveys. *Int J Epidem* 1974;**3**:135–43.

8 Frans A, Francis CH, Stanescu D, Nemery B, Prignot J, Brasseur L. Transfer factor in patients with emphysema and lung fibrosis. *Thorax* 1978;**33**:539–40.

9 Frans A, Veriter C, Nullens W, Brasseur L. Préparation de mélanges gazeaux à l'aide pompes Wösthoff. *Bull Physiopath Respir* 1969; **5**: 409–23.

10 Helsing KJ, Comstock GW, Speizer FE, Ferris BG Jr, Lebowitz MD, Tockman MS, Burrows B. Comparison of three standardized questionnaires on respiratory symptoms. *Am Rev Respir Dis* 1979;**120**:1221–31.

11 Higgs CM, Richardson RB, Lea DA, Lewis GTR, Laszlo G. Influence of knowledge of peak flow on self assessment of asthma: studies with a coded peak flow meter. *Thorax* 1986;**41**:671–5.

12 International Labour Organisation. *Respiratory Function Tests in Pneumoconioses*. Occupational Safety and Health Series No. 6. Geneva: ILO, 1966.

13 International Labour Office. *Guidelines for the Use of ILO International Classification of Radiographs of Pneumoconioses*. Occupational Safety and Health Series No. 22. Geneva: ILO. 1980.

14 Kelman GR. The pre-employment medical examination. *Lancet* 1985;**ii**:1231–3.

15 Lebowitz MD, Burrows B. Comparison of questionnaires. The BMRC and NHLI respiratory questionnaires and a new self completion questionnaire. *Am Rev Respir Dis* 1976;**113**:627–35.

16 Medical Research Council. *Questionnaire on respiratory symptoms*. London: Medical Research Council. 1976.

17 Quanjer PhH. (ed). Standardization of Lung Function Testing. *Bull Europ Physiopath Respir* 1983;**19**(Suppl 5):7–92.

18 Regan GM, Tagg B, Thomson ML. Subjective assessment and objective measurement of finger clubbing. *Lancet* 1967;**i**:530–2.

19 Shirai F, Kudoh S, Shibuya A, Sada K, Mikami R. Crackles in asbestos workers: Auscultation and lung sound analysis. *Br J Dis Chest* 1981; **75**: 386–96.

20 UICC/Cincinnati classification of the radiographic appearances of pneumoconiosis: A co-operative study of the UICC Committee. *Chest* 1970;**58**:57–67.

21 Weiner JS, Lourie JA. *Practical Human Biology*. London: Academic Press. 1981.

Chapter 6
Occupational Respiratory Surveys

Types of survey
Number and definition of subjects
Information which may be obtained
Approaches to management and unions
Other preparations
Conducting the survey
Analysis of results
Comment

Occupational respiratory surveys

The health of persons in occupations may be investigated from national mortality statistics, social security returns (including those for disablement benefit attributable to pneumoconiosis), health service records, company medical records and occupational surveys.

National mortality statistics have the advantages of extending over many years and of including a record of occupation. Their main use is as pointers to where to look more deeply. Due to the way the information is collected the statistics are of limited usefulness for investigating diseases of occupations in detail. The stated occupation is often the most recent one and not the principal occupation during the working lifetime. The classification is under broad headings which may not indicate what the person actually did. The cause of death may have been recorded incorrectly. In addition the mortality experience of each occupational sub-group within the population is to some extent unique and not comparable with that of other groups. The occupation may require particular physical or mental characteristics and a pre-employment medical examination or at least freedom from chronic disease. Thus the person who is taken on for employment initially enjoys above average health. Subsequently this healthy worker effect (15) may be offset by other attributes of industrial workers including their possibly higher consumption of tobacco, alcohol and food stuffs thought to be associated with vascular disease compared with other groups within the community. Additional unrecorded selection factors which influence the exposure to respiratory and other hazards operate within occupational groups. Thus national mortality statistics, whilst valuable for showing long-term trends, are of limited usefulness.

Returns for industrial injuries benefit provide a measure of the burden imposed on the community by an occupational hazard: they are a poor indication of prevalence or attack rate since many eligible persons prefer not to apply (14) and long-term comparisons are influenced by changes in legislation.

National Health Service statistics have similar limitations but may provide the first indication that an occupation is the cause of a particular disorder (1). Company medical records and sickness absences monitor the day to day health of the work force; in conjunction with information from the personnel department they may provide a complete retrospective picture. The medical department may be the first to detect that all is not well; this could be the starting point for a detailed enquiry. The company records usually cease on termination of employment: in some circumstances the subsequent health is recorded by the trade union.

A survey of the respiratory health of people engaged in a particular occupation or industry is usually the best way of establishing the extent and cause of a respiratory problem and identifying those who are affected; it is also the first step towards correcting what has gone wrong. To achieve this the survey requires careful planning including the integration of contributions from a number of disciplines: depending on circumstances these are likely to include occupational medicine, epidemiology, occupational hygiene, radiology, applied respiratory physiology and statistics.

The exact objective must first be defined: this is likely to be to identify or exclude an abnormality in the group and, if present, to relate it to the occupational exposure. Secondary objectives are to describe the natural history of a particular occupational disorder, to establish the effectiveness of preventive measures or, if possible, to assess the role of individual susceptibility. Once the objectives have been established the steps needed to achieve them should be considered. The type of survey and the optimal nature and size of the study population should be decided and an assessment made as to whether or not what is practicable is also likely to provide a useful answer. It may be that it will not! A strategy for undertaking the study should then be worked out; this is likely to include detailed consideration of what is required, consultation with colleagues who might contribute, approaches to management and unions, consultation with the local ethical committee and application to the industry or a grant-giving body, research director or finance department for the requisite funds. In the case of research based on an academic department the parent university will also need to be consulted. These stages usually take longer than might reasonably be expected. However, they should be tackled systematically and in depth since an omission or wrong decision may prove hard to correct, either in relation to the project itself or to any follow-up or subsidiary study which may subsequently prove to be necessary.

Types of survey

These are listed in table 6.1. They may conveniently be divided into morbidity and mortality surveys though the latter may arise as a sequel to the former.

Cross-sectional morbidity surveys

In a cross-sectional survey all the members of a defined group are seen at one point in time. The group may be defined in terms of occupation when it may include former as well as current employees or of domicile when it becomes a community survey. Former employees should usually be included in a mortality survey. Their inclusion in a cross-sectional survey often presents difficulties but should be attempted if the abnormality may have been a cause for discontinuing employment or prolonged sickness absence or if, as is usually the case, the objectives of the study relate in part to environmental conditions in the past. Alternatively if the group

Table 6.1. Occupational surveys

Type	Feature/Objective	Comment
Cross-sectional	Prevalence	Criteria for selecting subjects different from those of a longitudinal study
	Relation to exposure	
Longitudinal		
Short-term	Variation over day or week	Technically demanding
Prospective, morbidity	Dose–response relationship	Requires meticulous planning, conduct and analysis
Prospective, mortality	Used for establishing carcinogenicity (cf. table 12.1)	Technically easy (in U.K. and U.S.A.). Criterion unambiguous but causes of death may be unreliable
Cohort	Avoids bias due to secular trends	May not apply to other age groups
Case reference	Natural history of condition	Should be followed to post-mortem

is a large one a sub-sample may be drawn for study; the sampling may be done by random selection from the whole workforce, by stratified sampling from selected groups (strata) or by a mixture of both processes. The study of sub-samples may lead to some employees feeling that they have been 'left out' or that something will be missed by not including everybody. For these reasons the study of the whole population is good for public relations within the company. However, to undertake such a survey is un-economical if the same information can be obtained by studying smaller numbers, particularly those who are at the extremes of the spectrum of likely exposure. The heavily exposed subjects are usually the older ones who also have the most symptoms. In most instances they should all be included in the study population, together with a representative sample of the younger groups. The selection is made by stratified sampling. Other persons can be accepted as volunteers who are investigated and reported on individually but not included in the analysis. The cross-sectional survey is used for establishing the prevalence of abnormality and the relationship to exposure. For this purpose it is a common fallacy to assume that there should be a control group of persons who have not been exposed to the presumed hazard. Theoretically there should be but in practice the proposed controls are usually persons in other trades or office staff or personnel from an adjacent factory; such people often differ from the primary population in a number of respects besides exposure including their physique, academic record, habitual activity, domicile, smoking habits or diet and their inclusion in the study may contribute to a misleading result. Instead use should be made of the wide range of exposures which is almost always present within the primary population. If the approximate exposures are not known in advance a dose–response relationship should be constructed from within the primary population. This mode of operation has the advantage that it is usually effectively 'double-blind'. Alternatively if strata of exposure are already known the best approach is usually to compare subjects who are heavily and lightly exposed. This may take the form of a case-reference study.

A *case-reference study* (formerly called case-control study) is one in which persons with a known high exposure or clinical feature are compared with others who lack this feature. If the selection criterion is exposure each member of the heavily exposed group is matched with a lightly exposed reference subject whose characteristics are in other respects similar: matching should ideally be done with respect to gender, age, smoking habits and other confounding variables. Since the analysis will now take the form of a direct comparison between groups, care must be taken to avoid bias both in the identification of 'cases' and in the information which is to be compared (clinical, radiographic, lung function, etc.). The information should preferably be obtained without knowledge of exposure or ideally of age. A case-reference study may be cross-sectional or longitudinal.

Converting to a longitudinal study

The cross-sectional survey may be used subsequently as a starting point for a longitudinal study. If so, this decision should be made at the start to ensure that standards and methods can be maintained unchanged for a second occasion. This is not easily done. In addition an early decision is more likely to be supported by workforce and employer than one which appears to be an after-thought. However, depending on the objectives a cross-sectional survey is usually stratified to include all the older employees whereas a prospective longitudinal study often addresses persons who have many years of employment ahead of them. This may be an obstacle to converting from a cross-sectional survey but where longitudinal information is subsequently needed it may be obtained more readily from a follow-up survey than by making a fresh start. This is particularly the case for a mortality survey.

Surveys to study short-term changes in response

A variant of the cross-sectional survey is the short-term longitudinal survey in which observations are made over a defined period such as one working shift or over specified days of the week; such surveys have proved useful in the study of airflow obstruction in cotton workers (chapter 14). They are necessary for the investigation of occupational asthma (chapter 16) and extrinsic allergic alveolitis (chapter 15).

Prospective longitudinal morbidity surveys

A prospective longitudinal survey is the best way of establishing the effectiveness of hygiene measures for preventing or controlling an environmental hazard. The index of effectiveness is then the biological response to the hazard and sensitivity is achieved by using the initial measurements on each participant to establish the individual starting points. This use of the subjects as their own controls eliminates the component of overall variability in response which is due to initial differences *between* subjects; such variability is almost always larger than that between replicate measurements *within* subjects even when made on different days. In addition for some indices including FEV_1 and to a lesser extent respiratory symptoms, the reproducibility is subject to seasonal and circadian variation and to the time interval since the last cigarette. These aspects should be recorded and, so far as possible , standardized. The biological response should preferably be related to the environmental conditions over the period of the survey. A positive association is then evidence for causality. However, an association might be obscured by the late effects of exposure before the survey began. To avoid this the study could be confined to new entrants, or better to apprentices with no previous occupational exposure.

Cohort study

A cohort study is a prospective longitudinal study in which the group is defined by date of birth. This reduces the variation introduced by confounding environmental factors such as the weather, fashions in diet or environmental air pollution but except in a very stable environment the results are unique to that cohort. The term cohort is sometimes also used to describe groups defined in other ways, for example, by the year of starting employment but this usage is incorrect.

Longitudinal case reference study

This approach is used to investigate the aetiology and natural history of an occupational disorder and ideally spans the whole period from first exposure to death. The study may be done either prospectively by entering cases on exposure or at certification as in the Beryllium Case Register founded by Harriet Hardy (page 232) or retrospectively by starting from hospital case notes or post-mortem returns. In a prospective study the interest is mainly clinical and the reference cases are usually non-exposed persons matched for age, smoking and other confounding variables. The retrospective approach is used for investigating aetiology. The previous occupational history of the affected persons is obtained and compared with that of the reference cases; the latter are usually the next consecutive hospital or post-mortem cases. The sensitivity of this method of investigation is limited by the quality of the information which is available. This is sometimes better than at first sight appears likely (16) and will be increased when employment and medical records are retained for 30 years as is now proposed (page 4).

Mortality surveys

Any occupational survey may be completed by establishing the date and cause of death of the exposed persons compared with reference subjects. To make this possible the full name, address and date of birth should be recorded, together with an appropriate identifying number. In the U.K. the National Health Service number can be used to trace a person's general practitioner or, if the person has died, to secure a copy of the death certificate. During life the National Insurance number can also be used for tracing.

Death is a reliable end-point for a study but the causes given on the death certificate may be only approximate (page 214). Either an underlying condition may be omitted or diagnosed in error (e.g. mesothelioma) or a condition present during life which did not contribute to the death may be entered incorrectly as a supplementary cause (e.g. pneumoconiosis). Oldham has suggested that the non-contributory conditions should be recorded systematically under a separate heading (*The Times*, correspondence, 28 September 1984). Meanwhile scrutinized and possibly amended certificates of death for exposed subjects should not be compared with unamended certificates for reference subjects.

Mortality surveys are used for establishing carcinogenicity, for monitoring the effectiveness of hygiene standards and for checking on risks that have been overlooked or suggested rather tentatively on the basis of laboratory tests of mutagenicity. These objectives are mostly met by prospective longitudinal study of exposed persons but retrospective case reference studies can yield invaluable information, especially about conditions which are uncommon, hence few persons are affected. Criteria for establishing carcinogenicity from epidemiological evidence are given in table 12.1 (page 244). The studies have the constraint that lung cancer seldom develops less than 10 years and often more than 30 years from first exposure so long-term follow-up is essential. The long period contributes to errors and bias in the information which is collected. The collection should preferably be in the same way for all subjects and special care taken to trace lapses. The reference group should be either lightly exposed persons from the same works (page 108) or matched for socio-economic and general environmental factors as well as for age. The principal uncontrolled factor is then whether or not the subjects smoked and if so, how much. This information should be obtained if possible. It is helpful to know that differences in smoking habit are unlikely to account for a relative risk from lung cancer that is more than 50% above the national average (11). However, the effect of smoking and other contributory factors may not be linear with time (even if the first 10 years are discounted) so the results of the study cannot be considered completely reliable until all subjects have been followed up to an appropriate endpoint. For investigating causes of lung cancer this may be old age or premature death but where post-mortem evidence is needed, as for establishing the role of emphysema in coalworkers' pneumoconiosis, the information should not be limited to those who die early.

Thus whilst limited information on causes of death can usually be obtained with relative ease (certainly in the U.K. and the U.S.A.) the interpretation put on the evidence can as easily be incorrect.

Number and definition of subjects

The number of subjects to be included in the survey will depend on its type and on the number of people who are at risk. In different circumstances ten or 10,000 may each be appropriate. Ideally the number should be decided by the magnitude of the minimal relevant effect and by the variability of the measurements; in practice these quantities often only emerge as a result of undertaking the survey. Thus a more empirical approach is usually necessary; this will nonetheless be based on the premise that an occupational disorder which is known to exist in the population will be assessed satisfactorily using smaller numbers than are needed for an abnormality where the link with occupation is only suspected. Occupational asthma and the pulmonary effects of welding illustrate the extremes. Numbers will similarly be smaller if the recorded indices are specific and reproducible compared with circumstances where only non-specific information is available such as sickness absences. In practice where large numbers of people are at risk a sample size of 100–500 is usually satisfactory; the former number is probably the minimum for a longitudinal survey where the principal index is the forced expiratory volume: for this index Berry has pointed out that the optimal time of follow-up is 5 years (4). Five years is also optimal in most other circumstances since with a shorter interval the disturbance to work schedules is obtrusive whilst with a longer interval the loss from changing jobs and other factors leads to a high lapse rate.

The identification of individuals for study starts with definition of the population. The criteria should be unequivocal and any subsequent sampling should be made from all who are included in the definition. This might be in terms of work in a particular industry, plant or workplace, at a particular trade or on an identified process. The qualifying date might be recent or at some time in the past and additional features might be with respect to age, gender or duration of employment (see types of survey above). The criteria need careful choice, precise statement and rigid application in both survey and analysis as they greatly influence the result.

Information which may be obtained

The observations which it is proposed to make should contribute to diagnosis and assessment of severity of the suspected disorder (12); there will be few circumstances when they will be unique. Tests should be chosen which identify a high proportion of persons with the disorder in question (i.e. the tests should be sensitive, table 6.2) and there should be a minimum of false positives (i.e. the tests should be specific). Thus the respiratory symptom questionnaire includes questions on breathlessness which is a sensitive indicator of respiratory impairment; it includes questions which indicate whether or not the

condition is 'asthma'. The specificity is further increased by the addition of questions about angina (table 5.6, page 85), since that disorder can also give rise to breathlessness on exertion. The information should ideally be independent of the extent of participation of the subject and the personality of the operator (i.e. the tests should be objective); the information should also be capable of description in genuinely quantitative terms. In practice both objective and subjective information can be useful. There is a range from lung function results which are objective and numerical, through x-ray readings which are subjective but semi-quantitative, to symptoms and sounds in the chest which are at present subjective but are increasingly become semi-quantitative (e.g. visual analogue scales, page 400). At present numerical scores are used for the x-ray category of pneumoconiosis and the grade of breathlessness of byssinosis. Chronic bronchitis and wheeze are usually scored on a 3 point scale (absent, mild, severe),

Table 6.2. Criteria for tests

Aspect	Criterion	Expression
Acceptability	Safe, simple and not unpleasant for subject	Arbitrary
Reproducibility	Within and between sessions, occasions, observers, laboratories, etc.	Coefficient of variation
Accuracy	Extent of any systematic error (estimate affected by reproducibility)	Percentage
Validity	Relevance or discriminative power of the test; now replaced by sensitivity and specificity	
Sensitivity	Proportion of affected persons who are identified by the test	Percentage
Specificity	Proportion of unaffected persons who are correctly identified	Percentage
False positives	Subjects who are wrongly identified as having the condition	May be reported as percentage
False negatives	Subjects who have the condition but are not identified by the test	
Technical considerations	Time for the test, bulk of equipment, convenience in use, output (analogue or digital), time for intermediate analysis	Arbitrary

whilst other features are absent or present, for example the flu-like illness of extrinsic allergic alveolitis or an occupational cancer. Indices of mortality and sickness absence are referred to above and indices of environmental exposure on page 117.

Where there are several indices of equal discriminative power and objectivity the choice between them may be made on the basis of their reproducibility and their acceptability to the subjects. Reproducibility is the extent to which the result differs on different occasions between different observers and in different laboratories; reproducibility is enhanced by the use of equipment which meets a suitable specification (page 91), by training the observers and by procedures for calibration which can be applied at the beginning and end of each measurement session. It is also improved by standardizing the results for time of day and other nuisance variables (table 6.3). In favourable circumstances the overall reproducibility is to within 3–5% for lung function tests used in surveys and 10% for questionnaires of respiratory symptoms. For these procedures the acceptability to the subjects is high. It is intermediate for measurement of compliance and usually low for re-breathing tests and tests of maximal exercise. The criteria for tests and some which are commonly used are given in tables 6.2 and 6.4.

Table 6.3. Variables to be taken into account when analysing lung function measurements obtained in an occupational survey; they should be allowed for at planning stage if possible

Nuisance variables
   Observer, time of day, season,
   time after exercise, meal or cigarette,
   gender and ethnic group of subjects.

Confounding variables (to be allowed for in analysis)
   Stature, thoracic dimensions, habitual activity,
   body mass, body fat, fat free mass,
   age, smoking history (but see below),
   socio-economic group,
   angina of effort

Variables of prime interest
   Exposure, x-ray category,
   age and smoking interactions with exposure,
   respiratory symptoms,
   previous pleurisy, pneumonia, etc.

Approaches to management and unions

The approach to management and unions should be preceded by detailed consideration of the questions which it is proposed to answer and the methods which should be used. Both parties will require a simple but accurate

Table 6.4. Information commonly obtained in occupational morbidity surveys (for details see chapter 5)

Category	Essential	Optional
Personal details	MRC Questionnaire	
Symptoms (including those related to exposure)	with additional questions	
Smoking history		
Previous illnesses		
Occupational history	Yes, in full	
Clinical examination	No	? Finger clubbing, loose cough, râles, electrocardiogram
Anthropometry	Stature, body mass	Four skin folds
Lung function	Spirometry	Mixing indices, transfer factor, exercise, etc.
Chest radiography	Postero-anterior film	Obliques or a lateral
Environmental monitoring		Personal/static sampling
Body burden or specific sensitivity		Usually on subsample

explanation of the position, including the benefits which they might expect from the study being undertaken. The discussion should include reference to the uncertainties in the situation since if a complete answer could be guaranteed the study would not be necessary! The possible need for subsequent studies or supplementary investigations should be clearly indicated at this stage. Possible difficulties for the management include the direct costs of the survey, the disruption of work schedules, the congestion caused by the presence of the survey team, the effects of any remedial action which might be necessary and the risk that the findings would be used by the trade union to influence wage bargaining. For the unions the difficulties include the suspicion that circumstances might be worse than they actually were or that employees found to be in poor health would lose their jobs. In addition whatever their personal opinions the union representatives need to be guided by the views of their members on whose behalf they are rightly cautious. Both sets of difficulties should be discussed and the ways of overcoming them agreed. These are likely to include that the study be broadly based, discussed with the line management and shop-stewards and carried out efficiently with adequate back-up facilities to overcome technical difficulties as they arise. Individuals who are found to be in poor health should be informed quickly but confidentially and referred to their medical practitioner for treatment. A formal agreement to this effect should be made with the union. The overall findings of the survey, which should not include information on individuals, should be reported to all concerned as soon as practicable. However, flexibility is necessary as in the event of a problem being identified the management might wish to outline the remedial action at the same time. Ideally the action for each of the possible outcomes should have been decided in advance of the study jointly by management and unions. The amount of detailed information to be included in the survey report should also have been decided. Such forward planning is seldom achieved in practice!

The agreement which precedes the survey should include that the management provide a suite of rooms for the survey work or space for a trailer, a telephone and appropriate electrical supply. Management should also agree to the results being published in an appropriate scientific journal for which the editorial scrutiny would provide independent corroboration of reliability. During this process of discussion and negotiation the investigator demonstrates his integrity and competence and builds up the good relations which must be preserved throughout if the survey is to be successful.

Other preparations

The approach to the ethical committee may precede or follow the discussions with the industry; either way round the one will help smooth the path of the other. Circumstances will also dictate the timing of the approach for funds: the amount requested should cover the basic costs but should be competitive and should be seen to be value for money. Depending on circumstances this may require that the investigator should identify a subsidiary aspect of the project which can be funded separately. An extension of knowledge on biological variability or on one of the test procedures which it is proposed to use may be achieved in this way.

Conducting the survey

Once the details are settled the project is set up, local publicity is arranged and any additional staff are recruited and trained. The help of the local industrial nursing officers is usually invaluable. The subjects are identified and told individually about the survey. They are provided with an opportunity to ask questions on all aspects and participation should be seen to be in their best long-term interest. They are then given appointments which should be realistically timed and adhered to. The appointments often carry more weight if they are made by shop-stewards rather than representatives of management. At this stage, in order to achieve a valid result, it should be the firm intention of the investigator to make observations on 100% of the designated persons so there is a need to persist in persuading potential subjects to attend for assessment until this figure is reached. The strategy should be worked out in advance: depending on circumstances it may involve personal approaches to reluctant participants from shop-stewards and members of the survey team including finally the medical officer. A good response is assisted by the subjects being fully informed along the lines outlined above and by the first subjects responding favourably to the procedures including the time taken, the privacy and the absence of difficulty or discomfort in what is entailed. Subjects who are unable to or refuse to participate fully should be encouraged to contribute partial information, for example by completing part or all of the MRC Questionnaire of Respiratory Symptoms and performing spirometry at home. At the final count the proportion of subjects on whom there is no relevant information should be less than 5%.

During the study the results should be scrutinized for clinical abnormality and action taken along the lines agreed previously; this will usually include sending a standard summary card to each participant containing a brief comment on the findings and the offer of a personal interview on request. A notification may be made to the general practitioner. The results should also be examined for their completeness and for technical failures and repeats made as necessary; these should be accompanied by a full explanation as to the reason.

Analysis of results

Preliminary scrutiny

After the study the results are coded for recording on a tape or disc and an analysis undertaken. In the first instance this will be directed to detecting rogue results which have eluded the checking and verification procedures; to this end the ranges for each of the variables and graphical displays of each index against an appropriate reference variable should be scrutinized. For example, forced vital capacity divided by (stature)^2 might be plotted against age (fig. 6.1) and exercise cardiac frequency (e.g. fC45, page 395) against the reciprocal of fat free mass. Radiographic category of simple pneumo-

coniosis might similarly be plotted against an index of exposure but the correlation is usually too low for this to provide a useful check on the results. Once the data are considered satisfactory the main analysis is undertaken, starting with a search for differences between observers, instruments, time of day and other identifiable sources of error (table 6.3). Frequency histograms should be prepared in order to establish whether or not the variables are distributed in a normal (Gaussian) manner. If they are not, an attempt should be made to normalize the distribution; the ways of doing this are described by Oldham (20). If the attempt is not successful the method of analysis should be of the nonparametric type. The means and standard deviations of the results for the principal sub-groups of subjects in the study should then be prepared; the means can be compared between groups including any control group which may have been incorporated in the study. If the distributions are satisfactory the significance of any possible differences can be tested using a Student's t-test. With a view to comparison the results should, if appropriate, be standardized for any nuisance or confounding variables. These are factors which influence the variables of main interest but are not themselves relevant to the objectives of the study. The effect of nuisance variables (table 6.3) can often be allowed for in the design of the study, for example by randomization of subjects between observers or time of day. In other instances the effect should be allowed for in the analysis. For measurements of lung function the confounding variables include stature and body mass which affect the indices in a manner which is now well documented. Age and gender may also be confounding variables but age provides a measure of exposures undetected by questioning, whilst gender may influence the response to the exposure and in this event should not be eliminated from the analysis. If the survey population is appropriate the standardization for confounding variables is made in the manner described below but if not, correction factors from the literature can be used instead. Alternatively in the case of stature use may be made of the proportional relationship between lung function and (stature)^2 to produce standardized indices

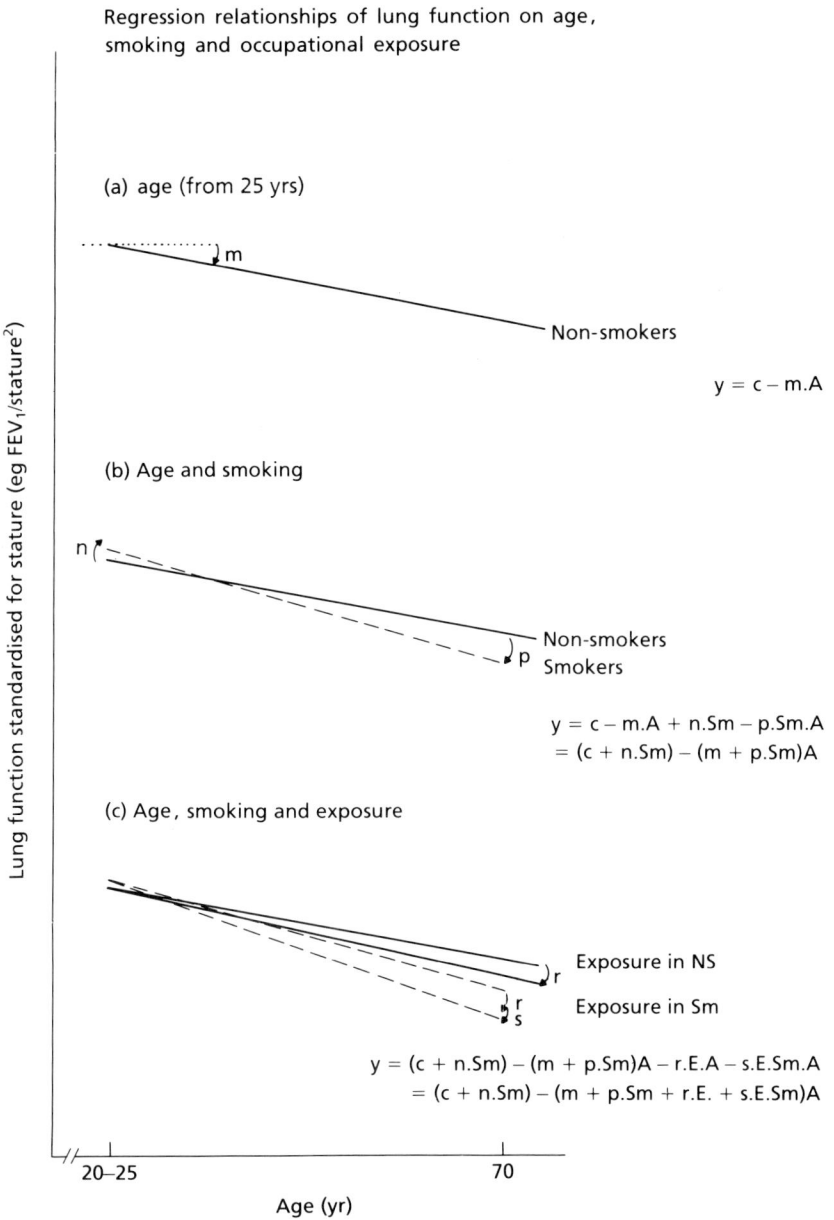

Regression relationships of lung function on age, smoking and occupational exposure

Lung function standardised for stature (eg FEV$_1$/stature^2)

(a) age (from 25 yrs)

} m

Non-smokers

$y = c - m.A$

(b) Age and smoking

n {

Non-smokers
} p   Smokers

$y = c - m.A + n.Sm - p.Sm.A$
$= (c + n.Sm) - (m + p.Sm)A$

(c) Age, smoking and exposure

} r   Exposure in NS

} r   Exposure in Sm
  s

$y = (c + n.Sm) - (m + p.Sm)A - r.E.A - s.E.Sm.A$
$= (c + n.Sm) - (m + p.Sm + r.E. + s.E.Sm)A$

20–25   70

Age (yr)

Fig. 6.1. In this simplified diagram the relationship of lung function standardized for stature (y) on age (A) is represented by a simple linear equation. Smoking (Sm) is scored 1 for smokers, 0 for non-smokers. Smokers are represented as initially having superior lung function compared with non-smokers because the latter group includes most of those with childhood wheeze, etc.; hence the term nSm is positive. However, the lung function of the smokers declines with age at an increased rate so the term pSm.A is negative. The effect of exposure is represented as increasing the decline with age in all the subjects (hence the negative term r.E.A), but with an additional effect in smokers (the term s.E.Sm.A). On re-arrangement the age term includes a direct effect, separate interactions with smoking and exposure and a complex interaction between all three variables.

which are then used as primary variables in the subsequent analysis. Thus

$$FEV_1 \propto St^2$$

hence

$$FEV_1 . st = \frac{FEV_1}{St^2} \times \bar{St}^2 \qquad (6.1)$$

where $FEV_1.st$ is forced expiratory volume standardized for stature, St is the stature of the subject in question and $\bar{St}$ is the mean stature for the group whose lung function is being investigated. This procedure is due to Cole and to Berry. Smoking habit might be a confounding variable but should preferably be treated separately since not all smokers are affected to the same extent; in addition for both this variable and for age the effect may interact with that of the pollutant under investigation. The demonstration of such an association is an important part of the result. For some studies the analysis will stop at this point but most probably it will be continued to look for a quantitative dose–response relationship; this will usually be done by multiple regression analysis. The analysis will begin with construction of a cross-correlation matrix which will indicate which of the measured variables are likely to contribute usefully to the result (table 6.5).

Multiple regression analysis is a statistical procedure for describing a quantity in terms of the variables which might influence it. The quantity under investigation is the dependent variable; its possible determinants are the independent variables. They are either continuous variables on a numerical scale or dummy variables which are included in the analysis as present or absent. In men exposed to an airborne pollutant the dependent variable might be breathlessness on exertion, radiographic category of simple pneumoconiosis or an index of lung function. These variables are scored respectively on a 6 or 8 point scale (page 401), a 12 point scale (page 86) and as a continuous variable. If the dependent variable is forced expiratory volume (FEV_1) the independent variables should include the continuous variables, age (A), stature (St), and a function which describes the subject's exposure to an airborne pollutant either now or in the past (E); the latter is the variable of interest and care should be taken that it is expressed in an appropriate way. Some examples of exposure scores are given in table 6.6. The dummy variables might be for a specified observer (Obs), whether or not the subject smoked (Sm) and the ethnic group (Eth). Questions on smoking are given in chapter 5 and some effects of smoking are considered in chapter 17. Other dummy variables might be religion, place of residence or keeping racing pigeons. Depending on circumstances there might be a case for including in the analysis some relevant symptoms, for example persistent cough and phlegm or regular wheeze, but care must be taken that an effect of the occupational exposure is not then wrongly attributed to intrinsic abnormality or to smoking. In the simplest form of multiple regression equation the effects of all the independent variables

Table 6.5. Cross-correlation matrix for FEV_1, age, smoking (yes or no) exposure (accumulated years, Table 6.6) and their interactions for 409 shipyard welders and other tradesmen. FEV_1 was significantly correlated with all the other variables. The higher inter-correlations between the independent variables in lines 3–6 were evidence for collinearity. (Cotes & El-Gamal, in preparation)

	Exp	Age	Sm	A.Exp	Sm.Exp	A.Sm
Exposure	1.0					
Age (A)	0.45	1.0				
Smoking	0.06	0.21	1.0			
A.Exp	0.98	0.59	0.10	1.0		
Sm.Exp	0.79	0.43	0.58	0.79	1.0	
A.Sm	0.23	0.60	0.88	0.33	0.67	1.0
FEV_1	−0.27	−0.62	−0.20	−0.36	−0.32	−0.43

Table 6.6. Exposure scores (18)

Exposure	Yes or no
Time since first exposure	Years
Years of exposure	$n_1 + n_2$ years
Total dose	$n_1 x_1 + n_2 x_2$
Average exposure	Total dose $\div$ Years of exposure
Accumulated years	$(1 + 2 + \cdots + n_2) + [(n_2 + 1) \cdots + (n_2 + n_1)]$
Accumulated exposure (weighted by time elapsed)	$(x_2 + 2x_2 + \cdots + n_2x_2) + [(n_2 + 1)x_1 + \cdots (n_2 + n_1)x_1]$
Discounted exposure (weighted for recent exposure)	$x_2 (1 - \exp(-Bn_2)) + x_1 \exp(-Bn_2)(1 - \exp(-Bn_1))$

Where n_1 and n_2 are number of years of exposure to environmental concentrations x_1 and x_2. B is the proportional rate at which the lung heals such that if half the damage is repaired in 5 years $B = \log_e 2/5$; it is estimated by trial and error (5).

are considered to be additive: this implies that the relationship to the dependent variable of one independent variable is the same for all values of the others. In practice this is not so, for example the decline of lung function with age is usually greater in smokers than non-smokers (fig. 6.1) and not independent of smoking as the simple model implies. The difficulty is overcome by including in the regression equation terms for interaction between smoking, age, occupation and any other relevant factors. The multiple regression equation might then take the following form:

$$FEV_1 = d.St + e.Obs + f.Eth + m.A + n.Sm \\ + o.E + p.Sm.A + q.Sm.E + r.E.A \\ + s.E.Sm.A + c \qquad (6.2)$$

where d to s are partial regression coefficients and c is the residual term which should be normally distributed. The multiplicative terms having the coefficients p to s are interactions. Additional terms may also be included, for example for ex-smoking. This has been omitted here for convenience but in a recent study of shipyard welders proved to be the most important of the dummy variables investigated (9). The continuous variables are entered as their numerical value whilst the dummy variables are entered as 0 if absent and 1 if present. Using this convention the term, $e.Obs$, if it is significant, indicates that measurements of forced expiratory volume made by one observer were systematically higher or lower than those made by another observer. The term $p.Sm.A$ indicates the extent to which the decline in lung function with age $(m.A)$ is modified by smoking whilst $s.E.Sm.A$ indicates the contribution to the age decline in smokers of their occupational exposure. For example, if the coefficient p was negative and significantly different from zero this would indicate that the decline in FEV_1 with age was greater in smokers than in non-smokers; a significant negative value for s would indicate that the decline with age in smokers was greater in exposed than in non-exposed persons. A simplified version of this equation is illustrated in fig. 6.1. The analysis is usually made by the method of step-wise multiple regression; the steps may be made forwards by including variables one at a time if they are significant, or backwards by excluding variables from the whole set, one at a time, if they are not significant. Eventually only the terms with significant coefficients remain. The result must be scrutinized before it is accepted since the failure of a term to appear as significant may be due to the presence of another or vice versa. In addition, where an interaction such as $q.Sm.E$ is significant the terms for the constituents, in this case those with the coefficients n and o, must be included even if they are not themselves significant. The interacting terms often contain very important information and if used with due regard to logic may indicate both the magnitude of an effect and if it is primary or secondary. Thus breathlessness on exertion associated with impaired lung function can be a risk shared by all the exposed persons or affect preferentially those who are atopic: in this event the breath-lessness could be secondary to the development of wheeze.

Problem of multicollinearity

The inclusion of interaction terms in the multiple regression greatly increases its descriptive power. However, any interactive (multiplicative) term is usually correlated with its components which for completeness should also be included in the analysis. A high correlation (collinearity) leads to the partial regression coefficients having large standard errors;* in equation 6.2 the coefficients m, o, r and s will be most affected since age and exposure score are often themselves correlated. These partial regression coefficients are likely to have wide confidence limits, hence a significant effect may be missed. In addition the coefficients are un-stable so if, as is often the case, one coefficient is over-estimated the other is under-estimated, or of opposite sign in consequence (10).

Collinearity is present when two or more 'independent' variables are highly correlated ($r \geqslant 0.5$, table 6.5); in the case of a pair their intercorrelation is then greater than that for the entire regression equation. Where there are three or more independent variables the determinant of the matrix (Rx) (scalar product of the matrix Rx) is close to zero instead of approaching unity as is the case when the independent variables are truly independent. Collinearity may be reduced by collecting more data, by choosing one of the intercorrelated variables to represent the common underlying dimension or by creating new variables which are independent.

The practice of omitting all but one of a number of intercorrelated variables eliminates collinearity at the expense of useful information. The loss can sometimes be avoided by

---

*The standard error (SEb_1) is given by

$$\frac{SD(Y)/x_1 \cdot x_2}{[\Sigma(x_1 - \bar{x}_1)^2 \, (1 - r_{1,2})^2]^{0.5}}$$

where $SD(Y)$ is the standard deviation of Y, $r_{1,2}$ is the correlation between components x_1 and x_2. If $r_{1,2}$ approaches unity the standard error becomes very large.

submitting the intercorrelated variables to a preliminary principal component analysis; this yields a series of factors which contain the same information. In favourable circumstances most of the information is contained in the first factor which can then replace the constituent variables in the analysis. For example, airflow limitation independent of lung size can be expressed by the indices FEV%, RV% and VA eff/VA (page 99). In one study (8) the first factor of a principal component analysis using these variables was the basis for an obstruction index (OI):

$$OI = 75 + 0.5 \, RV\% - 40 \, VA \, eff/VA - 0.3 \, FEV\%$$
$$(6.3)$$

This index has proved to be of great practical use. The method may be applied to any groups of intercorrelated variables. It may also be extended to all the independent variables which it is proposed to include in what is then called principal component regression analysis. For this application the factors are rotated in order that each may relate to a single subgroup of intercorrelated variables (17). However, the interpretation is seldom clear cut and the procedure is not recommended for routine use.

Collinearity usually arises because elements of age, smoking history, body size or lung size are present in two or more of the independent variables. Age is correlated with many indices of exposure if, as is usually the case, the majority of men started their exposure on entering the industry from school (see table 6.6). This source of collinearity can be reduced by expressing both age and exposure about the mean values for the study population. Age is usually also correlated with exposure to tobacco smoke expressed as pack years; the correlation can be eliminated by reporting current smoking as absent or present (0 or 1). However, smoking is then correlated with ex-smoking. The resulting error can be avoided by analysing the results for smokers and ex-smokers separately. Alternatively either all the ex-smokers or the recent ex-smokers can be included with the smokers and the others treated as non-smokers. The partitioning can be further refined by introducing intermediate scores (between 0 and 1) for ex-smokers depending on how long ago they gave up smoking.

Table 6.7. Collinearity and how it can be avoided

Intercorrelated variables		Alternative
Duration of exposure	Age	Express variables about their means
Smoking (pack years)	Age	Use—current smoker—yes or no
Ex-smoker	Smoker	Analyse separately or partition ex-smokers
Body mass or fat free mass	Stature	Express as mass/(stature)^2
Thoracic dimensions	Stature	Use linear regression
Forced expiratory volume	Stature	Use FEV_1/(stature)^2 (in adults)
Forced expiratory volume	Forced vital capacity	Use FEV% (similarly for RV%)
Specific airway conductance	Lung volume	Use linear regression
Ventilation equivalent	Oxygen uptake	Use linear regression or $\dot{V}_{E45}$ (page 394)
Oxygen pulse	Cardiac frequency	Use linear regression or f_{C45} (page 396)
Maximal O_2 uptake per kg	Mass	Use uptake/(mass)$^{0.67}$

These and other examples of collinearity and ways of correcting it are given in table 6.7.

Cross-sectional surveys

The results of the cross-sectional survey should be submitted to a preliminary analysis and probably also to a multiple regression analysis as described above. Illustrative results are given on pages 188, 391 and 394 whilst the effects of smoking and of the nuisance variables are described respectively on pages 376 and 102. The subsequent report will be based on the analysis. It will also include an account of the lapses indicating the reasons and the extent to which the lapses may have differed from the participants in age, years since first employment or other attribute which could have influenced the result.

Longitudinal surveys

Results become longitudinal when two or more sets have been collected. By this time the material from the initial survey may have been analysed on a cross-sectional basis in the manner described above. If so, pointers to the longitudinal analysis will have been uncovered. This starts with a scrutiny of the material including the changes in the interval between the two surveys. The changes are recorded either as rates per annum (based on decimal dates for the two surveys) or in the case of attributes which exhibit a quantitative change as 'yes' or 'no'; the latter include the development of a new respiratory symptom or physical sign (e.g. fine râles on auscultation of the chest) or abandonment or taking up smoking. These indices can then be submitted to analysis of variance. Longitudinal changes in the continuous variables should be related to the mean level of results over the period of the survey and not to the initial levels. This aspect of longitudinal analysis is considered by Fletcher and colleagues (13) and by others (5, 21). The changes may be analysed along the lines indicated in the preceding section including making allowance for collinearity. If external reference values for decline in lung function with age are included in the analysis they should be from longitudinal and not cross-sectional studies (7).

Dose–response relationship

A relationship between the biological response to a respiratory hazard and the estimated exposure is both strong evidence for causality (table 12.1, page 244) and the basis for the hygiene standard: its establishment is the principal objective of most occupational respiratory surveys. The response is usually in terms of respiratory symptoms, lung function, x-ray category of pneumoconiosis or death from lung cancer. The exposure should ideally be that obtained by personal sampling over the working lifetime but except for some exposures to radiation this information is seldom available. The exposure to asbestos of some factory workers is available from static samplers and that of

U.K. coal miners from the results of gravi-metric sampling of the return air but in most instances the exposure can only be estimated semi-quantitatively (table 6.6).

Biological monitoring can also provide quantitative evidence of exposure. The x-ray category of simple pneumoconiosis reflects the lifetime exposure to coal dust, and the amount of ferromagnetic dust, measured by magnetop-neumography, the environmental exposure to welding fumes. Over a shorter time space the concentrations in blood or urine of many inhaled dusts and vapours similarly reflect the environmental concentrations. If the process has existed for a number of years the concentration in body fluid can be used to estimate the expo-sure (e.g. fig. 12.1, page 247). Where there are no environmental measurements and where bio-logical monitoring is not relevant the exposure can still be estimated semi-quantitatively (e.g. table 6.4). However, subdivision in three categories, ever high, ever medium or always low, exposure may be the best that can be achieved (11). The relationship of response to dose is looked for using multiple regression analysis; the presence of such a relationship is indicated by significant partial regression coeffi-cients for the exposure terms (e.g. coefficients o, q, r and s in equation 6.2 or the equivalent principal component terms). The other terms in the multiple regression equation allow for the effects of any nuisance variables (e.g. stature when forced expiratory volume is the depen-dent variable) and of some confounding vari-ables including age.

Other confounding variables are smoking, ex-smoking and secondary occupational exposures, for example oxides of nitrogen as well as ozone, sulphur dioxide as well as arsenic, radon gas as well as lead or cadmium as well as nickel. These multiple exposures may interact; they can be included in the multiple regression either using a model of their likely behaviour or factors from a preliminary principal component analysis. The model approach is intuitively attractive but should only be used where there is supporting evidence; in other circumstances a preliminary factor analysis is more likely to yield a realistic result. The difficulty is practical for studies of occupational lung cancer; here the use of years since first exposure and years of exposure as guides to dose, the use of standardized mortality ratio (SMR) as a measure of response and the interactive model for the confounding effects of smoking are increasingly coming under scrutiny (10). SMR may be replaced by the excess death rate defined as the number of deaths per person per year at risk (3). In addition the absence of adequate smoking histories and exposure records is often a major obstacle to accuracy. The error is less for longitudinal morbidity studies in which the smoking history and other data for the analysis are obtained direct from the subjects and the period of follow-up is much shorter. Some problems in interpreting the dose–response relationship are discussed in the context of asbestos lung cancer on page 223.

Comment

The occupational survey is a powerful tool which has contributed unique information about the prevalence, aetiology and control of occupational lung disorders and some are con-sidered in subsequent chapters. The procedures are outlined above. They require considerable resources and where there is failure it is usually due to insufficient attention to one or more of the stages. Of these the most precarious are often the initial definition of the population, the estimates of environmental exposure and the subsequent statistical analysis. Thus an epide-miologist, an industrial hygienist and a statis-tician are all essential members of the team. The statistician and the occupational physician should consider very carefully the variables to be included in the analysis as the wrong choice may result in a misleading conclusion. The analysis is likely to require some mathematics and statistics to supplement a standard statis-tical package (e.g. 2, 19). It also needs both time and a sense of urgency if the result is to appear within an acceptable interval after the comple-tion of the survey. Many of the best studies are distinguished by the excellence of the statistical analysis and there is a need to maintain among statisticians an interest in this type of work.

References

1 Acheson ED, Cowdell RH, Rang E. Adenocarcinoma of the nasal cavity and sinuses in England and Wales. *Br J Industr Med* 1972; **29**:21–30.

2 Alvey NG, Banfield CF, Baxter RI, *et al A general statistical program.* Harpenden: Statistics Department, Rothamsted Experimental Station 1977.

3 Bell CM, Coleman DA. Predicted mortality patterns in cohort study populations exposed to different types of hazard: Can SMRs show a dose-response? *Statistics in Medicine* 1983; **2**:363–71.

4 Berry G. Longitudinal observations. Their usefulness and limitations with special reference to the forced expiratory volume. *Bull Eur Physiopathiol Respir* 1974;**10**:643–56.

5 Blomqvist N. On the relation between change and initial value. *J Am Stat Assoc* 1977;**72**: 567–9.

6 British Thoracic and Tuberculosis Associated Research Committee. Opportunist mycobacterial pulmonary infection and occupational dust exposure. An investigation in England and Wales. *Tubercle* 1975;**56**:295–310.

7 Burrows B, Lebowitz MD, Camilli AE, Knudson RJ. Longitudinal changes in forced expiratory volume in one second in adults. *Am Rev Respir Dis* 1986;**133**:974–80.

8 Cotes JE. Lung volume indices of airway obstruction: a suggestion for a new combined index. *Proc Roy Soc Med* 1981;**64**:1232–5.

9 Cotes JE, Feinmann EL, Male VJ, Rennie F. Respiratory health of shipyard workers. *Thorax* 1984;**39**:691 (abstract).

10 Darlington RB. Multiple regression in psychological research and practise. *Psychol Bull* 1968;**69**:161–82.

11 Doll R. Occupational cancer: problems in interpreting human evidence. *Ann Occup Hyg* 1984; **28**:291–305.

12 Ferris BG (chairman). Guidelines as to what constitutes an adverse respiratory health effect, with special reference to epidemiologic studies of air pollution. *Am Rev Respir Dis* 1985;**131**:666–8.

13 Fletcher C, Peto R, Tinker C, Speizer FE. *The Natural History of Chronic Bronchitis and Emphysema.* Oxford: Oxford University Press. 1976.

14 Glover JR, Bevan C, Cotes JE, Elwood PC, Hodges NG, Kell RL, Lowe CR, McDermott M, Oldham PD. Effects of exposure to slate dust in North Wales. *Br J Industr Med* 1980;**37**:152–62.

15 Hernberg S., Fact and fiction in occupational epidemiology. *J Roy Coll Physicians Lond* 1983;**17**:139–43.

16 John LR, Marsh GM, Enterline PE. Evaluating occupational hazards using information known only to employers: a comparative study. *Br J Industr Med* 1983;**40**:346–52.

17 Massy WF. Principal components regression in exploratory statistical research. *J Am Stat Assoc* 1965;**60**:234–56.

18 Musk AW, Cotes JE, Bevan C, Campbell MJ. Relationship between type of simple coalworkers' pneumoconiosis and lung function. A nine-year follow-up study of subjects with small rounded opacities. *Br J Industr Med* 1981;**38**:313–20.

19 Nie NG, Hull CH, Jenkins JC, Steinbrenner K, Bent DH. *Statistical Package for the Social Sciences,* 2nd ed. New York: McGraw-Hill, 1975.

20 Oldham PD. *Measurement in Medicine: the Interpretation of Numerical Data.* London: English Universities Press, 1968.

21 Rossiter CE. Law of initial values: In: discussion following paper by Kauffman F, Brille D, Lellouch J. *Scand J Respir Dis* 1976;**57**:315–6.

Further Reading

Cohen J, Cohen P. *Applied Multiple Regression/ Correlation Analysis for the Behavioural Sciences.* Hillsdale, New Jersey, Lawrence Erlbaum, 1983.

Schilling RSF (ed). *Occupational Health Practice,* 2nd ed. London: Butterworth. 1981.

Weill H, Turner-Warwick M. (Eds). *Occupational Lung Diseases: Research Approaches and Methods. Lung Biology in Health and Disease.* **18.** New York: Marcel Dekker. 1981–18.

See especially articles by G. Berry, J. C. McDonald and G. B. Field.

Chapter 7
Abnormal Conditions of Temperature and Barometric Pressure

Cold
Heat
High Altitude
Aviation
Diving

Cold

Inspired air is normally fairly cool and dry compared with alveolar gas and is warmed during its passage through the respiratory tract into the lungs. For this purpose the nose has excellent heat-exchanging properties, including the turbinate bones and cartilages which provide a large irregular surface covered with highly vascular epithelium. The shape of the passages ensures that air comes into close contact with the epithelium by which it is both heated and humidified (chapter 4). This process is continued in the pharynx and trachea so that by the time the air reaches the larynx it is warm and humid and under resting conditions is considered to be in thermal equilibrium with the alveolar gas. However, during maximal ventilation of air at 20°C the tracheal air is raised to only about 30°C (2) and when cold air is breathed the thermal deficit is likely to be even larger; under these conditions the convention that measurements of respired gas are reported at 37°C saturated with water vapour is no longer valid.

The heat which passes into the tidal air during inspiration is to some extent returned to the respiratory tract during the subsequent expiration but the process of recovery is incomplete. Loss occurs because the expired air is both warmer and of higher humidity than that inspired; the dry respiratory heat loss is a function of the temperature gradient and the ventilation, which is related to the metabolic rate (m). The dry heat loss (L) may be described by the relationship:

$$L = 1.6 \times 10^{-3} \, m \, (34 - t \text{ insp.air}) \, W$$

where the term within the parentheses is an estimate of the temperature gradient from inspired to expired gas (°C). Similarly the evaporative heat loss (E_{ve}) is proportional to the product of the ventilation and the difference in water content of expired and inspired air. This simplifies to:

$$E_{ve} = 2.7 \times 10^{-3} \, m \, (44 - P_{H_2O}, \text{insp.air}) \, W$$

where P_{H_0O} is aqueous vapour pressure (3). Normally the respiratory heat loss is less than 10% of the total body heat loss. However, for subjects wearing insulated clothing the dry gas and evaporative heat loss, together with loss from the skin of the face, may represent one-third of total heat loss in these circumstances.

The thermal capacity of respired gas is increased by the presence of water mist as occurs in fog. On this account, during exercise in a cold misty environment, the temperature of the airways may fall sufficiently to impair the function of the ciliated, goblet and mast cells in the bronchial epithelium. Constriction of smooth muscle in the airways or at the level of the acinus is also a possibility and may affect gas exchange (4). In horses and amongst sledge dogs performing strenuous exercise, frost bite to the lung and pulmonary oedema have been reported. Thus extreme cold does damage the lung and may contribute to the respiratory impairment and pulmonary hypertension which has been reported amongst physically active males in very cold climates (8). It is probable that lesser degrees of cold lower resistance to secondary infection of the lungs following coryza and influenza. These effects may be aggravated by smoking or by passive smoking if the ventilation of dwelling places is reduced; they can be prevented by the heating of offices, shops and other buildings to a minimum of 16°C and by ensuring adequate ventilation (7).

Cold causes cutaneous vasoconstriction which reduces heat loss, and shivering which increases the metabolic rate. The vasoconstriction raises the blood pressure (5) and diverts blood from cutaneous vessels into central blood compartments including the lung; the transfer factor of the lung for carbon monoxide is then increased. Shivering also increases the pulmonary ventilation. In the nose there is vasodilatation and this leads to partial nasal obstruction which is reversed by exercise or a decongestant spray (1). Extreme cold leads to stiffening of joints and weakness of skeletal muscle including the muscles of respiration and these changes may contribute to a reduction in ventilatory capacity. Cold air also causes airflow obstruction in persons with labile airways, including most asthmatics and some who are atopic. Breathing cold air during exercise is the principal cause of exercise-induced asthma (2) and cold mist can have a similar effect. The mechanism is discussed in chapter 16.

These observations have practical applications for employment in occupations which entail exposure to severe cold either acutely or over periods of time. Persons with asthma should be advised against such work. Those with a history of asthma during childhood should be questioned carefully for evidence of cold-induced airflow obstruction and a provocation test performed if there is doubt (chapter 16). The cold-induced vasoconstriction may present as or aggravate hypertension, angina (6), acute myocardial ischaemia, intermittent claudication or Raynaud's phenomenon. Persons with these conditions should not expose themselves to cold unnecessarily. Exposure to extreme cold for short periods in cold stores and refrigerators appears not to damage the lungs. However, improvements in the design of insulating clothing now allow personnel to expose themselves for longer periods without the danger of frost bite or hypothermia; in these circumstances the risk to the lungs is increased. Respiratory protection may be achieved by the use of a respirator or mask which does not freeze up; the

mask acts as a heat exchanger. Protective clothing should be used as well. In addition the air to the respirator can be heated but whilst this is a statutory requirement in some circumstances it is seldom necessary in practice.

Heat

Breathing very hot air or steam may scald the respiratory tract but in other respects a high environmental temperature does not harm the lungs. The main adverse effect on the rest of the body is that the high heat load causes hyperthermia (10). The heat load is a function of both the dry bulb temperature and the conditions which influence the evaporation of sweat; these are reflected in the wet bulb temperature and the air movement. Unacclimatized subjects can perform moderate exercise of a few minutes duration under conditions of 100% humidity, at dry bulb temperatures of up to about 40°C. These conditions have no direct adverse effect upon the lungs and none can be detected during longer exposure to less intense heat such as occurs during residence in the tropics. However, the high temperature profoundly influences the cardiovascular system (12), and hence indirectly other organs, by augmenting the skin blood flow and the production of sweat. The pulmonary component includes a reduction in the volume of blood in the alveolar capillaries, hence in the transfer factor (diffusing capacity) and an increase in ventilation minute volume; the latter is a response of the central nervous system to the rise in body temperature. The increase is effected mainly by a rise in the frequency of breathing which becomes shallow and rapid (9). This change is reflected in the tidal volume at a minute volume of 30 l min^{-1} (Vt_{30}) which as a proportion of the vital capacity is less than in other circumstances (chapter 18). The circulatory effects include a reduction in central venous pressure which results in a fall in stroke volume and a high cardiac frequency relative to the uptake of oxygen. These effects of exposure to heat may be aggravated during prolonged exercise by dehydration secondary to loss of fluid by sweating. The changes have the effect of reducing the blood flow to the active muscles so that the capacity for exercise is reduced (13).

These effects must not be forgotten when interpreting the results of exercise tests performed in a hot environment (chapter 18); a possibly misleading result may be avoided by maintaining the laboratory temperature in the range 18–23°C. Alternatively the tachycardia caused by excessive heat may be estimated with a view to making an empirical correction (11) but the validity of this approach has not been confirmed.

Repeated exposure to a hot humid environment sufficient to raise the deep body temperature induces the changes of heat acclimatization (10); even 4h per day for 10 days has a marked effect and this may be enhanced by concurrent exercise which also raises the deep body temperature. The principal change is an increase in production of sweat; at the same time the concentration of sodium chloride in both sweat and urine is usually reduced. The blood volume is increased. The changes are associated with an increase in secretion of aldosterone by the adrenal glands during the first few days of heat exposure. Subsequently, if the intake of salt is adequate the secretion returns to normal but a low serum sodium with a corresponding increase in potassium are usually found amongst indigenous herbivorous people.

Most of the adverse effects of work in conditions of high environmental temperature may be overcome by heat acclimatization, the provision of ample drinking water with salt and the use of loose-fitting garments made from absorbent cloth of light weight and colour. For more extreme conditions with a high radiant heat load, for example near furnaces and ovens, insulated and protective clothing with air or water cooling may be used instead. If there are fumes associated with the process a respirator may be needed but is often poorly tolerated.

High altitude

The ambient pressure is reduced by ascent to high ground or into the air or by reduction in pressure in a closed space (decompression). All three circumstances, depending on their extent, may expose the subject to hypoxia and in some circumstances to cold. Ascent to high ground may lead to mountain sickness whilst decompression if undertaken rapidly will cause

bubbles of nitrogen to form in the nervous system, blood or other tissue and these may give rise to the features of decompression sickness (see below). The mean barometric pressure at different altitudes and the corresponding pressures of oxygen and carbon dioxide in alveolar gas under quiet resting conditions are given in fig. 7.1 and table 7.1. Some constraints to human exploration at high altitudes are given in fig. 7.2.

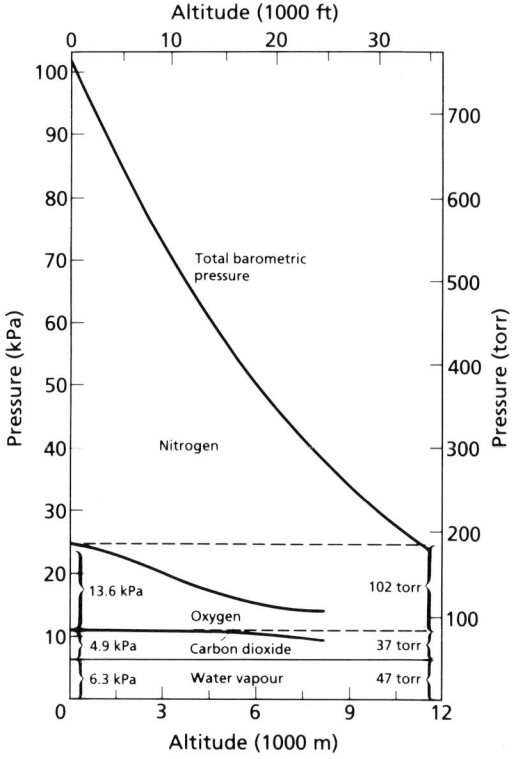

Fig. 7.1. Composition of alveolar gas in unacclimatized subjects breathing air at reduced barometric pressure. The upper curve is barometric pressure; the vertical distance between curves indicates the partial pressure of the alveolar gases. For a person breathing 100% oxygen (nitrogen partial pressure zero), the alveolar oxygen tension falls to its sea level value breathing air at an altitude of approximately 10,300m (34,000ft); this is the point of intersection of the pressure curve and the upper interrupted line. (Source: Cotes, J.E. (1979) *Lung Function*, 4th edn. Blackwell Scientific Publications, p. 460.)

Table 7.1. Conditions of equivalent alveolar oxygen tension for unacclimatized subjects breathing mixtures of oxygen and nitrogen at altitude and at sea level. Source: Cotes J. E. (1979) *Lung Function* 4th edn. Blackwell Scientific Publications, page 463

Altitude ($\div$ 1000)		Barometric pressure		P_{A,H_2O} $\div P_B$ (%)	P_{A,O_2} breathing air at altitude		$F_I O_2$ in inspired gas	
							(a) At sea level equivalent to air at altitude	(b) At altitude equivalent to 1500m breathing air
m	ft	kPa	torr		kPa	torr		
0	0	101	760	6.2	13.6	102	0.209	—
1.5	5	84	632	7.4	10.9	82	0.17	0.209
3.0	10	70	523	9.0	8.1	61	0.14	0.26
4.6	15	57	429	11.0	5.9	44	0.11	0.32
6.1	20	46	349	13.4	4.7	35	0.09	0.41
7.6	25	38	282	16.7	4.4	33	0.07	0.52

Exercise physiology of high altitude

The proportions of oxygen, carbon dioxide and nitrogen in air are not much affected by altitude so a reduction in barometric pressure is accompanied by a proportional reduction in the tension of oxygen in respired gas. In the alveolar gas the oxygen tension is further influenced by two factors: first, the partial pressure of water vapour is related to body temperature, not barometric pressure so it represents a progressively increasing proportion of the total pressure as the subject ascends; the dry gas pressure and the alveolar oxygen tension are reduced in consequence (figs. 7.1 and 7.2). Second, the oxygen enters the alveolar capillary blood by diffusion, not active secretion, so the tension in the arterial blood is even less than that in alveolar gas. The hypoxaemia stimulates the receptor cells in the carotid body to augment the chemoreceptor drive to respiration. This leads to an increase in the total and alveolar ventilation of the lung and hence to the alveolar oxygen tension being higher than would otherwise be the case. The hyperventilation causes the excretion of additional carbon dioxide which reduces the arterial CO_2 tension. The resulting alkalaemia sets in motion compensatory adjustments to acid–base balance whilst the hypoxaemia both stimulates erythropoiesis and increases the efficiency with which oxygen is utilized in the tissues. These aspects of acclimatization are referred to again below. The hyperventilation becomes increas-

ingly conspicuous on exercise in proportion to its intensity and to the altitude; as a consequence the subject attains his maximal breathing capacity at levels of oxygen uptake which at sea level would be asymptomatic. Lactacidaemia is not a conspicuous feature (23). Thus exercise is limited by ventilatory capacity and not by the ability of the circulation to deliver oxygen to the active muscles, as is the case at sea level. However, the limiting level of ventilation (expressed at ambient pressure) is higher at altitude than at sea level due to the air being less dense; this reduces the resistance to flow of air within the lung and permits an increase in maximal breathing capacity (fig. 7.3). The maximal breathing capacity is further increased through training of the respiratory muscles by increased use. However, despite these compensatory mechanisms an ascent to altitude entails reductions in the capacity for exercise and the amount of physical work which can be performed. Some situations where this may be important and some hazards of the ascent and altitude are considered below.

Work at high altitude

An altitude of 1500m (5000ft) is associated with a reduction in barometric pressure of 17% to 84kPa (632mmHg). Throughout the world many towns and cities served by airports are at this altitude which has no detectable effect on long-term residents who are fully acclimatized. New-

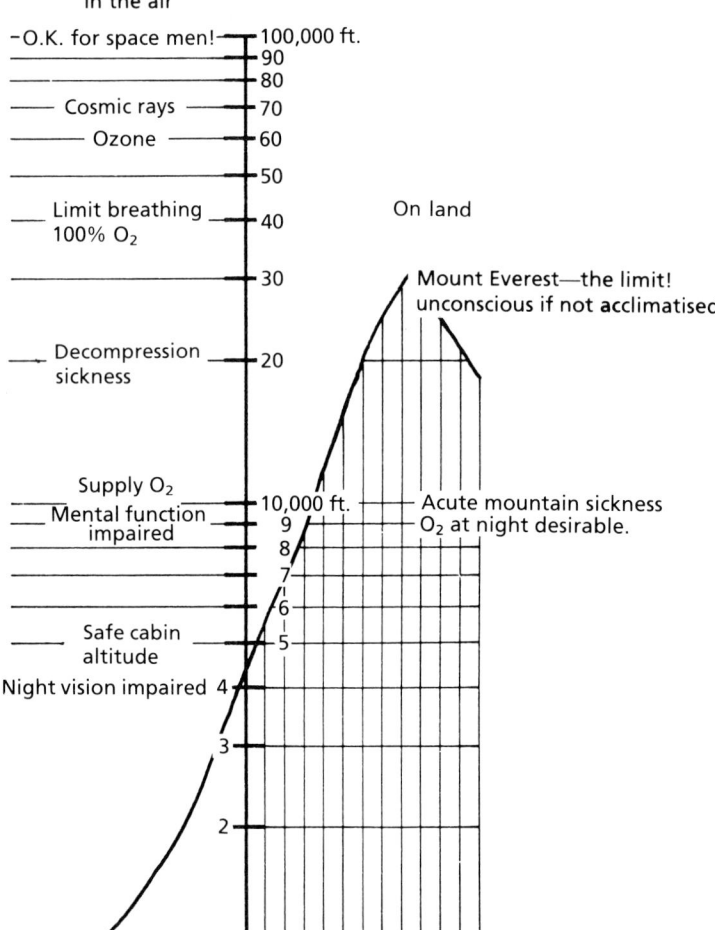

Limitations to human exploration of high altitude

In the air

-O.K. for space men!——100,000 ft.

Cosmic rays

Ozone

Limit breathing 100% O$_2$

On land

Mount Everest—the limit!
unconscious if not **acclimatised**

Decompression sickness

Supply O$_2$
Mental function impaired

Acute mountain sickness
O$_2$ at night desirable.

Safe cabin altitude

Night vision impaired

1,000 ft.

Fig. 7.2. Limitation to human exploration of high altitude. Note: To convert altitude from feet to metres multiply by 0.3.

comers are generally unaffected but may experience breathlessness on severe exertion. Thus persons who on account of their occupation make a brief visit requiring a high level of physical activity may find that their performance is unexpectedly reduced on this account. Ballet companies, sports teams and some industrial personnel fall into this category. The handicap disappears after a few days' acclimatization. The breathlessness may be relieved by breathing oxygen. At 3000m (barometric pressure 70kPa) newcomers are notably breathless and after a

rapid ascent are at risk of developing acute mountain sickness; this is described below. There is some impairment of cerebral function including visual discrimination, night vision and performance of psychomotor tasks. Ability to learn new skills may be particularly affected (16). It is only with difficulty that quality control in electrical and mechanical engineering workshops is maintained (22) and problems are experienced with servicing sophisticated equipment. At night sleep is light and can be disturbed by violent dreams; there is Cheyne—

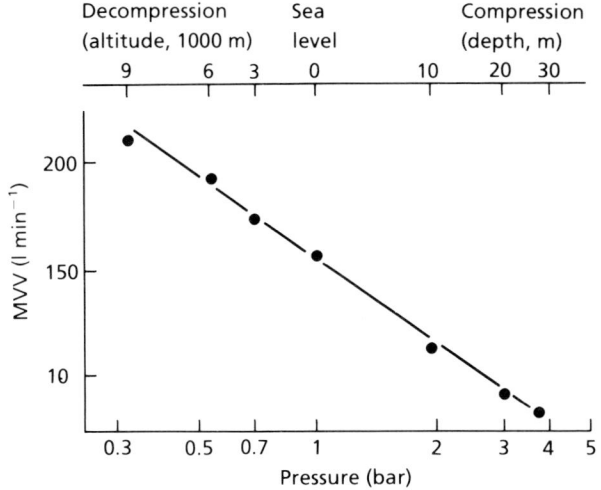

Decompression
(altitude, 1000 m)
Sea
level
Compression
(depth, m)

Fig. 7.3. Maximal voluntary ventilation (MVV) at different ambient pressures in healthy subjects breathing air. The slope of the regression line reflects the inverse relationship between ambient pressure (hence gas density) and the work done in overcoming airway resistance due to turbulent flow in the lung airways. (Source: Cotes, J.E. (1979) *Lung Function*, 4th edn. Blackwell Scientific Publications, p. 91.)

Stokes breathing with cyclical fluctuations in tidal volume between apnoea and hyperventilation. Appetite and digestion may be impaired and giddiness may occur, particularly during exercise. The exertional dyspnoea is accompanied by tachycardia which may switch to bradycardia at high rates of work on account of a rise in parasympathetic tone. These features become more prominent with increasing age and are aggravated by ethanol and by the carbon monoxide in inhaled tobacco smoke; they contribute to altitude fatigue in personnel undertaking exacting work in mountainous regions, including telecommunication centres, and may be a factor in the development of flight fatigue amongst air crew. The latter should be protected by maintaining the cabin pressure at not less than 84kPa (1500m) but in practice this is not always achieved. Aviation is discussed below.

Acute mountain sickness

Rapid ascent to above 3000m especially when accompanied by a high level of physical activity predisposes to acute mountain sickness (19, 21). The symptoms usually develop on the day after arrival but may come on within 8h or be delayed for 3 or 4 days. On arrival at altitude the subject often feels light-headed but euphoric, then becomes lethargic, sleeps badly with dreams

and periods of breathlessness. On waking there is a headache which is often severe and not responsive to aspirin; on trying to stand up there may be dizziness. There is also nausea, anorexia, vomiting (which accentuates the dehydration associated with ascent to high altitude), and accompanying misery. Hallucinations, blurred vision, visual field defects, difficulty with speech and other effects of cranial nerve palsies may also occur. On auscultation of the chest râles (crackles) may be heard; there are few other physical signs. In 95% of cases the condition responds to rest and leaves no sequelae but it may recur if the ascent is resumed too rapidly. Peripheral oedema of the legs, hands and face may complicate acute mountain sickness in some circumstances. In a few cases the condition progresses to high altitude pulmonary oedema or occasionally to cerebral oedema.

As *pulmonary oedema* develops the patient's condition deteriorates with increasing breathlessness, dry cough, tachycardia and mild fever. The breathlessness may be periodic with accompanying orthopnoea and the patient becomes very anxious. Pulmonary hypertension and coarse râles are invariable and there may be expectoration of frothy sputum which is sometimes blood-stained. This may be evidence for pulmonary vascular thrombosis which is a common complication. It is often accompanied by thrombosis elsewhere in the body and by thrombocytopenia (17). At this point, if not before, the patient's life is at risk and descent to a lower altitude is imperative.

Acute mountain cerebral oedema also arises from acute mountain sickness as a progression of the cerebral features of that condition: it may or may not be accompanied by pulmonary oedema. The patient becomes incoherent and hallucinated, increasingly ataxic and drowsy, then comatose with flaccid paralysis. There is urinary incontinence or retention with overflow and mild papilloedema. The latter should be distinguished from the retinal vasodilatation and raised retinal blood flow which also occur at high altitude and may give rise to retinal haemorrhage.

Treatment of acute mountain sickness and its complications is primarily by descent to a lower altitude and this should be undertaken in the event of moderately severe symptoms which do not respond to rest and aspirin. A descent of 300m is often sufficient but when there is ataxia or mild pulmonary oedema a 600m or 900m descent should be undertaken without delay. Specific treatment for pulmonary oedema should include oxygen in dosage sufficient to reduce the central cyanosis, frusemide 20–40mg by mouth and morphine 15mg intravenously. Tracheal intubation and suction or positive pressure ventilation (e.g. via hand-operated bellows) may also be necessary. For cerebral oedema intravenous dexamethazone and hypertonic solution such as mannitol should be administered and the bladder emptied via a urethral catheter.

Mechanism. The features of acute mountain sickness and its complications are due to hypoxaemia. The hypoxaemia causes cerebral vasodilatation and a redistribution of body fluid from the interstitial fluid compartment into the cells. In subjects who develop mountain sickness the hypoxaemia is of above average severity; this is due to the susceptible individuals having a below average ventilatory response to hypoxia. The hypoxaemia probably initiates minimal cerebral oedema sufficient to cause headache and vomiting. It may also lead to increased secretion of antidiuretic hormone

which aggravates the fluid retention, but why this occurs in some subjects more than others is unclear. Milledge and colleagues suggest that it may reflect disturbance to the renin–aldosterone system. Normally the activity of angiotensin-converting enzyme is reduced by hypoxia. However, in persons who acclimatize poorly the activity does not fall to a normal extent; the levels of angiotensin II and aldosterone, and hence the fluid retention, are increased in consequence (20). The cause of the pulmonary oedema is also not known for certain but localized cerebral oedema causing reflex changes in the lungs together with hypercapnia causing pulmonary vasoconstriction may contribute. Once pulmonary oedema has set in this aggravates the hypoxaemia and hence the risk of development of severe cerebral oedema.

Distribution and prevention. Acute mountain sickness was formerly most prevalent in the Andes where the principal mining towns and highland pastures at an altitude of about 4000m could be reached from the coast by foot in a few days or by train or car in a few hours. It was less common in Kenya where few people were at risk and in the Himalayas where the ascents were longer and more gradual. However, the availability of air transport for trekking holidays in Nepal and Kashmir has altered the geographical distribution of the illness. The incidence is in the range 10–60% depending on circumstances. Predisposing factors include a relatively young age, a rapid ascent, a high mean altitude and, independent of these, a high level of energy expenditure. Persons making a re-ascent after a visit to low altitude are at particular risk. In addition some persons, like some cattle, are far more susceptible than others. Thus 'Brisket disease' occurs in Aberdeen Angus cattle exported to South Dakota. In the summer they are driven to the high grass-lands around 1800m and develop symptoms of mountain sickness with oedema of the brisket area. The high susceptibility appears to be related to the possession of a brisk pulmonary vasoconstrictor response to hypoxia and this is probably the case in man (18). A reduced ventilatory response to chemoreceptor drive has also been incriminated but does not appear to be sufficient explanation. The subject is of great practical importance for persons who work in the high mountain ranges of the world and more information is needed.

Prevention is best achieved by arranging that ascents above 3000m are made gradually, preferably not more than 300m per day with pauses after every third day. If there is urgent need for work to be done at a higher altitude this should be on a daily basis with sleeping quarters at lower altitude. Alternatively during nights spent at altitude oxygen may be administered at the flow rate of 1 l min^{-1} or 2 l min^{-1} via nasal prongs. Administration of oxygen during the performance of some skilled tasks may also be desirable; this may often be achieved by the use of an oxygen concentrator run off a small generator (15). Acetazolamine (diamox) and spironolactone may have a place in prophylaxis (14, 19). However, except in emergencies, it is better to secure acclimatization by graded exposure to altitude and to abstain from smoking, alcohol and hypnotic or sedative drugs. In addition members of a party should carefully observe each other with a view to identifying and controlling the earliest manifestations of the condition.

Business trips to high altitudes

The executive going to high altitude will usually ascend rapidly, make important decisions and either entertain or be entertained with alcohol. Energetic sightseeing and other activities may be included in the visit which may well be stressful and induce a desire for increased smoking. Relative seniority in age, latent atherosclerosis and obesity may increase the risk; these factors may interact with the hypoxia to cause a personal or company disaster. Therefore, persons with known chronic respiratory or cardiovascular disease should be discouraged from going to high altitude, or there should be provision of extra oxygen for them. Screening tests should include assessment of lung function (chapter 5) and stress electrocardiography during hypoxia; appropriate gas mixtures are given in table 7.1. Artificial acclimatization by breathing the same gas mixture at sea level for 15h each evening and night for the week prior to the visit might theoretically be helpful but is unlikely to be a realistic proposition. Advice to the traveller should include the points made in the preceding paragraph. In addition, where the ascent is from sea level to above 2000m (6500ft) the spouse should be encouraged to go as well in order to reduce the stress to the working partner. Oxygen should be provided in the bedroom for use at night in the event of sleep being disturbed.

Sojourn at high altitude

The processes of acclimatization include changes in acid–base balance of the blood to permit sustained hyperventilation, erythropoiesis leading to moderate polycythaemia which increases the oxygen capacity of the blood, increased concentration of cellular enzymes and the growth of new capillaries in muscles, including cardiac muscle. These changes make possible relatively normal physical performance at altitudes which were initially almost incapacitating. Intellectual capacity will also be restored by acclimatization but residual defects will remain: some common ones are described above. The acclimatization inevitably weakens the body's responses to further hypoxia and has its own complications. Thus the hypoxaemia increases the pulmonary arterial tone; this has the consequence that any further increase due to an episode of chronic bronchitis or the onset of occupational lung disease increases the pulmonary arterial pressure to a greater extent than at sea level and hence the incidence of right heart failure (chapter 15, page 342, ref. 30). The polycythaemia increases the incidence of intravascular thrombosis. In addition, in some persons over periods of years the normal physiological responses become distorted and fail to maintain an adequate level of alveolar ventilation. The hypoxaemia then returns accompanied by hypercapnia; there is irritability, depression, headache and somnolence which may progress to coma. The patient is cyanosed, grossly polycythaemic, has right ventricular hypertrophy and may develop congestive cardiac failure. These are the features of Monge's disease or chronic mountain sickness for which the only satisfactory treatment is return to living at sea level.

Aviation

The environment

The difficulties associated with ascent to high altitude occur in an acute form during flight in unpressurized aircraft in which the crew and passengers are exposed to oxygen at ambient pressure; this is reduced compared with sea level, mainly because the barometric pressure is lower (fig. 7.1) but as described above the constancy of the water vapour pressure in the lungs also makes a small contribution. The air is colder with the temperature decreasing by approximately 2°C per 300m (1000ft) ascent above sea level. In addition, at very high altitude the atmospheric oxygen is exposed to ultra-violet light which reacts to form monatomic oxygen and ozone:

$$3 \ O_2 + \text{ultra-violet light} \rightarrow$$
$$O + O + 2 \ O_2 \rightarrow 2 \ O_3$$

The atmospheric concentration of ozone at an altitude of 40,000ft is approximately 1ppm and at 100,000ft 10ppm; this is well in excess of the hygiene standard of 0.3ppm (chapter 13). The ozone does not constitute a hazard for aircraft flying at below 40,000ft but at materially higher altitudes ozone should be removed from the ambient air before it enters the cabin. In modern aircraft the occurrence of hypoxia is avoided by the skin of the craft forming an airtight shell within which the air pressure is maintained at an acceptable level. This is higher than that outside the aircraft but lower than at sea level. The minimal cabin pressure is determined by the structural limits on the fuselage. For example, in the Boeing 747 the maximal differential pressure is approximately 7.5psi and the equivalent cabin altitude when the aircraft is cruising is 1850–2150m (6–7000ft). In Concorde the maximal differential pressure is 9.25psi and the equivalent cruise altitude is approximately 1500m (5000ft). The cabin air is bled from the compressor stage of the jet engine. The temperature is then in the range 300–500°C depending on the phase of flight. The air passes through a cooling system before entering the cabin where the temperatures should be between 22 and 27°C. The air has a very low humidity, below 20% after 2–3h flight, as any water vapour is condensed by cooling.

Risks to passengers from hypoxia

The air pressure within the cabin is normally maintained at approximately 84kPa equivalent to 1500m (5000ft) falling to 2500m (8000ft) in some older aircraft at high altitude, but the pressurization may not be properly adjusted or it may fail altogether. In either event the passengers and crew may be exposed to hypoxia and require supplementary oxygen; in the case of the pilot and co-pilot oxygen equipment capable of supplying enough oxygen under pressure to meet the full respiratory demand is available on the flight deck. For passengers in most aircraft a sudden loss of cabin pressure to less than 446mmHg (14,000ft) leads to the release of oxygen masks from lockers above the seats. At altitudes of above 25,000ft these should be used without delay as the time before loss of consciousness is relatively short, ranging from 2 to 4 min at that altitude down to 15s at 37,000ft. Partial loss of cabin pressure does not release the masks and is usually not announced to the passengers unless it is intended to descend to lower altitude. Moreover the associated symptoms whilst sometimes distressing are often trivial and may not be recognized, so the passengers, unless they carry an altimeter, have no means of knowing that they are at increased risk: the exposure may none the less be harmful.

Conditions which carry an increased risk from hypoxaemia during flight include chronic lung disease or congenital heart disease sufficient to lower the arterial saturation below 90% at sea level, degenerative arterial disease and sickle cell anaemia (table 7.2). Persons with these disorders may require supplementary oxygen which should then be given at a flow rate of 2–4 l min^{-1} via nasal prongs or oronasal mask. The likelihood that oxygen may be needed can be assessed before the flight by using the gas mixtures given in table 7.1. Alternatively or in addition the duration of the flight and the exposure to hypoxia in excess of that prevailing at 5000ft may be reduced by flying Concorde.

Table 7.2. Medical conditions which may contra-indicate flight (see references 30 and 31 for details)

Hypoxia	Expansion of gas
Respiratory failure (walking distance <50m)	Acute otitis media

Anaemia
  Hb <7.5g dl^{-1}
  Sickle cell HbC
    or β thalassaemia
	Recent stapedectomy or other ear surgery

	Abdominal surgery within 10 days
	Gastro-intestinal haemorrhage within 3 weeks
Cardiac failure	
	Pneumothorax
Myocardial infarction within 2 weeks	
	Thoracic surgery within 3 weeks
Stroke within 3 weeks	
	Air encephalography within 7 days
Atherosclerosis with nocturnal confusion	
	Fracture affecting ear or sinus
Epilepsy	
	Plaster cast (unsplit)

Other
  Psychiatric disorder
  Terminal illness
  Copious sputum
  Incontinence (urinary or faecal)	

Barotrauma

According to Boyle's law the volume of a given quantity of gas is inversely related to the pressure. During ascent the pressure decreases by half for every 18,000ft increase in altitude; the volume doubles in consequence. Converse changes occur during descent. There are corresponding movements of gas out of and into the lungs, middle ear and nasal sinuses. During a normal ascent the cabin pressure may fall by 35% to the equivalent of 8000ft over a period of some 30min; the volume changes take place slowly and are usually not noticed by the subject. However, if an airway is occluded the lung distal to the occlusion will expand and may rupture. In the rare event that the eustachian tube is completely blocked the eardrum may rupture. A tension pneumothorax may seriously compress the underlying lung whilst if the ostium to a sinus is occluded the gas pressure inside the cavity will remain high relative to the environment; the blood flow to the sinus will then cease and the wall may rupture. On descent the volume changes and the corresponding gas movements are in the reverse directions; obstruction to an airway may then cause atelectasis. Obstruction to an ostium may lead to a partial vacuum with consequent aspiration of tissue fluid and blood into the cavity; similar changes may take place in the middle ear or a dental cavity. These manifestations of barotrauma are often extremely painful, a failure to maintain pressure within the middle ear during descent being the commonest.

Acute barotrauma is best avoided by adopting a rate of pressure change of less than 0.15 bar per min and by the subject opening the eustachian tubes by swallowing, singing or yawning at regular intervals during the time when the pressure is changing. If symptoms develop during descent, the subject should inhale methedrine or a similar decongestant drug, then take a deep breath, shut the mouth, close the nose with one thumb and forefinger and attempt to exhale. The manoeuvre will usually force air into the middle ear or the sinus which is affected. If it is unsuccessful it is best to consult an otolaryngologist who will apply a solution of 0.5% ephedrine in saline over the ostium of the appropriate sinus by suitable positioning of the head. If this treatment fails resort may be made to politzeration or myringotomy.

The need for these measures may be avoided by changing the time of a flight until after recovery from an upper respiratory infection which is the usual cause of the difficulty. In addition patients with gross airflow obstruction or a pneumothorax should not fly except by special arrangement, for example in a private aircraft at low altitude.

Decompression sickness (bends)

This condition is due to bubbles of nitrogen which form in some tissues as a result of reduction in barometric pressure. The nitrogen is already present in solution in the body fluid and for its liberation requires a reduction in pressure of at least 50%: in aviation this is equivalent to ascent to 18,000ft. The risk is positively correlated with the proportional drop in pressure in excess of 50%, the age, the quantity of body fat and other variables. The condition does not occur during normal flights (cabin altitude 5000–8000ft) by persons resident at sea level but might affect those who have recently been exposed to higher ambient pressures during underwater diving. Professional and amateur divers including some holiday makers are at risk on this account; they should not have dived immediately before the flight. Decompression sickness is also a complication of failure of cabin pressurization or rupture of an aircraft window or door in flight leading to explosive decompression. The condition is treated by recompression either *in situ* by descent to a higher ambient pressure or on the ground by transfer to a compression chamber (24). It is considered further under diving medicine below.

Other complications of flight

Civil air crew are subject to stress on account of the uncertainties and exacting nature of their occupation, including the need to assimilate large quantities of information of various types, make responsible decisions in a restricted and potentially hazardous environment, adjust to different time, climate and food at staging posts, and other factors. Passengers are subject to some of these difficulties; they may also take unsuitable food and drink in flight or develop motion sickness. Military air crew are subject to additional stresses including acceleration (g) and vibration.

Effects of acceleration (g)

Acceleration of the body mass in a cranial direction is attributed to positive g and in a negative direction to negative g. However, the blood and internal organs, because they have inertia and are mobile, accelerate slowly. If already moving they also decelerate slowly. As a result positive g causes pooling of blood in the legs and hence cerebral ischaemia. Negative g causes cerebral congestion. Cerebral ischaemia is also caused by vibration through the sequence hyperventilation, hypocapnia and cerebral vasoconstriction. The cerebral function is impaired in consequence. Positive g displaces the liver and other viscera; this lowers the diaphragm so the functional residual capacity increases. The expansion takes place mainly in the alveoli of the upper zones where the ventilation is increased. By contrast the perfusion is redistributed in favour of the lower zones with a reduction in blood flow to the apices. These changes aggravate the slight mismatching of ventilation and perfusion which is a feature of the normal lung and cause hypoxaemia. Part of this may be due to blood transversing non-ventilated regions; the remainder is corrected by breathing oxygen. However, 100% oxygen should be avoided because of a risk of *atelectasis*; this occurs from absorption of oxygen continuing in alveoli distal to an airway which is temporarily blocked by distortions due to the acceleration. The condition may be corrected by a single deep inspiration or prevented by the routine use of oxygen in a maximal concentration of 0.70 (70%). Established cases exhibit the radiographic and other features of atelectasis.

Pooling of blood in the legs is prevented by applying counterpressure with a partial-pressure (anti-g) suit; this protects against the effects of positive g.

Respiratory and cardiovascular health of air crew

Despite modern technical advances air crew require all their mental faculties unclouded by hypoxia, fatigue, carbon monoxide, ethanol or other handicap. They should be free from 'any abnormality, congenital or acquired, any acute, latent or chronic disease and any injury or sequelae from operation such as would entail a degree of functional incapacity likely to interfere with the safe handling of an aircraft at any altitude throughout a prolonged or difficult flight (28). They should not need to take drugs and not be at risk of developing acute illness whilst on duty. These considerations have led the International Civil Aviation Organisation to require a very high standard of physical health and visual and auditory function for all airline and commercial pilots and air traffic control officers; a slightly lower standard is acceptable for flight navigators, engineers, radio officers and private and student pilots (27, 28). In the U.K. the assessments are supervised by the Civil Aviation Authority. The class 1 certificate which is renewed every 6 months requires freedom from acute, chronic or intermittent disorders of the respiratory tract including chronic bronchitis, emphysema, asthma, hay fever and sinusitis. Atopic status is not itself a bar to certification. The chest radiograph should be normal on entry and at 5-yearly intervals or when indicated thereafter. Normal spirometry is not specified in the regulations but it is implied. The resting ECG should be recorded on entry and at intervals of 5 years up to age 30, then at shorter intervals down to every six months at age 50 years onwards. Any evidence of myocardial ischaemia or undue hypertension disqualifies. For the latter purpose the blood pressure should be less than 140/80mmHg at age 20–29 years rising to less than 160/98 at age 50 years. A standard for physical fitness is not included in the regulations but a reasonable level is implied (25, 26, 29).

Diving

Divers commonly start as amateurs who select and equip themselves for what is a rewarding but often dangerous hobby. Some go on to become professionals; they are highly self-selected, well-trained, and conform to a high medical standard. Unlike in aviation the general public are seldom involved. This is fortunate as, despite his probable evolution from a lagoon ape, man is poorly adapted for a marine environment. Similarly diving-medicine abounds with difficulties for the uninitiated doctor. For the diving doctor his speciality is a very logical if exacting discipline where dramatic cures may often be predicted with confidence in circumstances which appear impossible to non-specialists. Using modern communication technology the cures may even be effected in distant parts of the world by careful instruction of local diving personnel in the procedures they should follow. Non-diving surgeons and physicians, including thoracic physicians may, however, make a contribution; that of thoracic medicine is considered below. The subject is reviewed in references 34, 41 and 51 and some constraints to human exploration of the sea are summarized in fig. 7.4.

Physical aspects of the marine environment

The shore around most of the land masses is relatively shallow forming a continental shelf which slopes gradually from sea level down to about 250m. The sea above the shelf is warmed by the sun, enriched with minerals from the sea bed and capable of supporting plants, fishes and other animals. Outside the continental shelf the sea bed descends steeply to the Abyssal plains: these are vast expanses of soft mud at a depth of 3–6km. The plains are mostly flat but traversed by ridges, mountain ranges and deep chasms which go down some 11km below sea level. The surface of the sea may be traversed by high waves in excess of 2m which hinder entry and exit. It may be moved by currents flowing too fast for man to swim against (maximal swimming velocity approximately 80m min^{-1} or 2.5 knots). The daylight only penetrates to a depth of 80m at midday and vision is further impeded by turbulence, debris and the limitations imposed by visors. The sea is cold with an average temperature at a depth of 200m of not more than 4°C, or less in the Arctic and Ant-

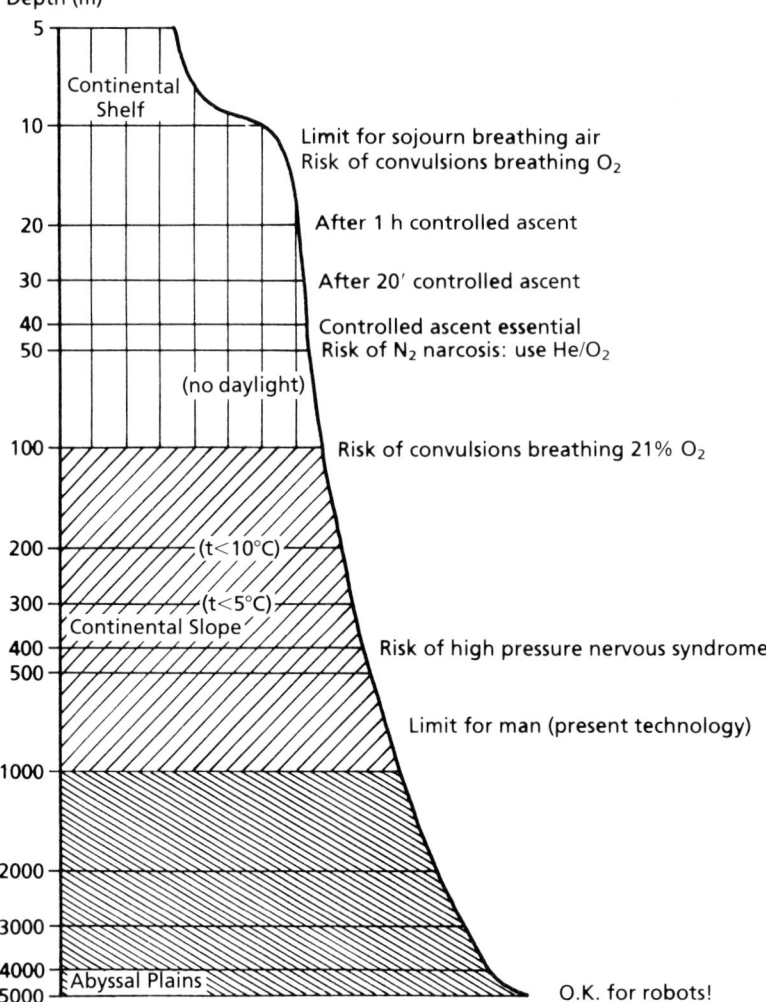

Fig. 7.4. Limitations to human exploration of the sea. Note: The temperatures are for the tropics. They are lower further away from the equator. To convert from depth in metres to absolute pressures in atmospheres divide by 10.3 and add 1.

arctic. It readily conducts heat and sound, and shock waves from explosions, impedes all bodily movements and, during submersion, compresses the body and creates a neutral buoyancy which eliminates the accustomed effects of gravity. The increased thermal conduction in this cold, wet environment leads to rapid loss of heat; this is associated with a reduced limb temperature, hence loss of manual dexterity, and deep body temperature, hence mental torpor and risk of death from hypothermia. The increased velocity of sound waves and associated loss of air conduction reduce auditory acuity and ability to identify the direction from which a sound is coming. Transmission of shock waves may damage the lungs, intestines and other organs. The high viscosity of water compared with air impedes the movement of the body in performing external work (33). The relatively high density of water, because it approaches that of the body, eliminates the stability which is conferred by gravitational force when the subject is standing in air. Thus the force generated by a push or a pull with an arm or leg will be partly dispersed by contra-directional movement of the body and the maximal sustained thrust during swimming under water is reduced to about 5kg.

The buoyancy of the body in the sea is approximately neutral at functional residual capacity with a range from plus 2.5kg at total lung capacity to minus 2.5kg at residual volume so the maximal swimming force is not much in excess of that which is needed to maintain position with little to spare for vertical movement.

These physical aspects of the marine environment create obvious difficulties for man; however, he is even less well equipped to cope with others which arise from biological interactions with the environment.

Effects of changes in gas volume

The effects of changes in gas volume consequent upon changes in barometric pressure during aviation are considered under the heading 'barotrauma' above. In diving the pressure change is proportional to the depth and increases by approximately 1 atmosphere (atm) with every 10m of descent. Since man can now descend to a depth of some 700m the possible pressure and volume changes are vastly greater during diving than during aviation. The corresponding risk of damage to ears and sinuses is qualitatively similar to that in aviation and is discussed above. The risk to the lungs is much greater. On descent the compression is such that if there were no ribs and without additional gas a vital capacity breath taken just before descent would disappear into the residual volume at a depth of 20m (i.e. by Boyle's law, 6 l x 1atm = 2 l x 3atm). In practice the thoracic cage can support a large pressure difference; this enables Japanese pearl divers (Ama) to make breathholding dives to a working depth of 44m. The maximal depth attained in this way is approaching 100m

(Jacques Mayoz, 94m in September 1983). The associated circulatory adaptations are poorly documented in man. The compression of gas has the further effect of reducing the buoyancy progressively as the depth increases and this may cause difficulty at the start of a free ascent.

During ascent from depth the gas in the lung expands. The volume changes are such that gas trapped behind an occluded airway will usually rupture the affected part. In healthy subjects ascending under controlled conditions this is uncommon. Rupture of peripheral alveoli leading to pneumothorax occurs occasionally and has been attributed to local scar formation with emphysema (36). However, the evidence is inconclusive and there is need for more information. Air embolism may also follow alveolar rupture; the incidence is greater in persons of linear than of stocky physique and may be associated with the former group having larger alveoli at the apices of the lung. In addition, a healthy lung will rupture if the subject fails to exhale during the ascent. The risk is enhanced by the progressive increase in buoyancy which occurs as the lung gas expands since this makes more difficult the control of the ascent. The speed should be controlled so as not to exceed that of the bubbles which the diver is exhaling. The problem arises mainly during emergency ascent and may be mitigated by training.

Rupture of air spaces near the root of the lung may cause surgical emphysema of the mediastinum. The rupture commonly involves a pulmonary blood vessel and leads to bubbles of gas entering the circulation as emboli. The bubbles may be big enough to interrupt immediately the blood supply to a part of the body. Unfortunately this is not the end of the matter; the displaced gas continues to expand and causes additional damage during the rest of the ascent. The initial symptoms are local pain and breathlessness, with or without cough, and haemoptysis. There may be disturbance to speech and a sensation of fullness with accompanying subcutaneous crepitations. On examination there may be typical features of pneumothorax or surgical emphysema of the mediastinum: the latter may involve the head and neck and interfere with the venous return to the heart and other structures in the mediastinum. There may be shock and signs attributable to vascular emboli. Death is not uncommon. Treatment should preferably be by recompression and this is mandatory in the event of vascular emboli. To prevent their spread the subject should be on the left side with the head below the level of the buttocks. Mild cases may be treated by aspiration of the pneumothorax and/or the administration of 100% oxygen. The oxygen should be given at atmospheric and not positive pressure. This treatment accelerates the elimination of nitrogen. The clearance from different tissues varies inversely with their blood supply and also with their content of fat, in which the solubility of nitrogen is 5 times as great as it is in serum. Older subjects usually have a reduced tissue blood flow but more fat compared with younger ones, so their clearance times are prolonged. In young men, during the inhalation of oxygen, the nitrogen is cleared very rapidly from the blood and those organs such as the kidney and the thyroid gland which have a large blood flow in relation to their size (half-time 1–2min). For the abdominal viscera, but not the lumina of the intestines, for the grey matter of the brain and spinal cord and for the organs which are well perfused with blood the half-time is approximately 5min. The nitrogen in the muscles and the connective tissues of the body is cleared more slowly with a half-time of 15–30min, whilst the nitrogen in the depot fat is cleared very slowly with a half-time of 1–4h. The clearance from a large bubble may take even longer. Thus oxygen therapy is not a substitute for recompression as a treatment for air embolism or symptomatic surgical emphysema.

Biological interactions with the environment

Decompression sickness. In aviation any decompression sickness is due to bubbles forming from nitrogen which is already present in the body; the nitrogen is in equilibrium with air at a pressure of 1atm at sea level and the bubbles are formed when the environmental pressure is reduced. In diving the source of the bubbles is additional inert gas which, as the environmental pressure rises during descent, dissolves in the fat and aqueous compartments of the body. The rate of uptake of a tissue is determined by the blood supply and the chemical composition (see above). The responsible gas is usually nitrogen but during deep saturation dives it is helium or occasionally hydrogen (see below). The bubbles are formed during return to sea level. They may be identified using a Doppler technique and are present without symptoms at the end of most decompressions from pressures in excess of 2atm. The subsequent repair process involves the blood platelets of which the blood concentration falls during the period 1–4 days after the dive. The cause of bubble formation is not known. Explanations which have been proposed include that bubbles may be present as micro nuclei before the dive; they may form at sites of turbulent flow in blood vessels or where there is local tissue ionization caused by the impact of cosmic rays. During brief dives only well-perfused tissues are at risk of decompression sickness but during prolonged or deep dives the risk extends to all tissues. In the case of nitrogen, which is highly soluble in lipid, the tissues with a high fat content are most affected.

The sites of bubble formation vary depending on the characteristics of the dive. The commonest site is the limbs which become painful and cause the subject to double up (hence the bends); this is designated Type I decompression sickness and usually comes on a few hours after decompression has been completed. Type II decompression sickness is less common: it develops during the decompression and may present with any of a number of symptoms and signs depending on which organ is affected. Lesions of the spinal cord, especially the lower cervical, thoracic or upper lumbar segments, may cause paraplegia. Other parts of the central nervous system may be involved concurrently. The skin may become blotchy and develop paraesthesiae. Bubbles at the root of the lung may cause the central thoracic symptoms of cough, dyspnoea and chest pain. The latter signs are colloquially called the chokes and are evidence for pulmonary intravascular accumulation of bubbles; these may give rise to gas embolism to all organs including the brain. The bubbles carry a risk of immediate death.

A long-term complication of exposure to hyperbaric conditions is aseptic bone necrosis. This commonly affects the lower femoral shaft or the upper tibia when it rarely causes disablement. Of greater consequence is necrosis of the hip joint which is a serious cause of disablement in compressed air workers in tunnels, hence caisson disease. Divers more often experience necrosis of the elbow or shoulder joints but the condition is fortunately uncommon. The cause of aseptic bone necrosis is not known; it was formerly considered to be a bubble interrupting the local blood circulation. However, the persistence of ischaemia would seem to require the local presence of a vasoconstrictor substance.

A reduction in pressure by at least 50% is usually needed to cause symptoms of decompression sickness. This important observation of Haldane's was the basis for decompression schedules until the 1930s. Modern schedules take into account the properties of the inert gas (usually nitrogen or helium) and the time and pressure profile of the dive. On a dive to 10m there is virtually no risk from decompression sickness; for a 20m dive breathing air the risk develops after about an hour and for a 30m dive after about 20min. After longer times at these depths or at greater depths the return to sea level must be by controlled ascent; for this purpose the environmental pressure is usually halved by decompression or ascent and the diver then stays at the resulting intermediate pressure for a specified time before the decompression is resumed. During the latter part of the decompression, oxygen may be given in controlled amounts to promote the elimination of inert gas. The decompression may take place by physical ascent in the water but usually it is performed in a pressure chamber. For relatively brief dives the subject may ascend rapidly to sea level, transfer quickly to a chamber, be recompressed and subsequently decompressed at the recommended rate. However, the risks involved in such a 'bounce dive' are greater than when the initial decompression is controlled. Greatest care is necessary at the end of saturation dives in which the diver is maintained at pressure for a period of days. During this time the tissues come into equilibrium with the gaseous environment which usually contains helium (see below). During saturation the diver lives in a complex of chambers on a diving support vessel and transfers under pressure to a diving bell for work at depth. The pressure during the excursions should be similar to that during storage but need not be identical; thus when storage is at 250m the excursions can deviate from this by up to 50m. Decompression from saturation usually takes 7–10 days depending on the saturation pressure and on the associated partial pressure of oxygen. Thus decompression from 250m takes 12.5 days at an oxygen partial pressure of 0.22bar but only 6.75 days at a partial pressure of 0.6bar; however, the procedure then carries a risk of oxygen toxicity (see below). In practice a compromise is reached, for example, 9.1 days at a partial pressure of 0.42bar (48), but faster rates are sometimes used. Decompression is performed in a chamber on shore or on the diving support vessel.

The treatment of decompression sickness is by recompression usually to 50m, then slow decompression over 42h or less depending on the severity of the symptoms and the previous diving exposure. In addition if the subject has 'chokes' or evidence for cerebral gas emboli he should be postured appropriately.

Dehydration. Immersion leads to displacement of body fluid from peripheral veins into the thorax where it distends the right atrium; this stimulates stretch receptors which promote diuresis; on return to ambient pressure the subject is dehydrated and in need of fluids by mouth.

Oxygen toxicity. Oxygen in a concentration in excess of 2atm causes epileptiform convulsions; these may be preceded by muscle twitching, often seen first around the lips which may be a warning sign of an oncoming major convulsion. There is apprehension and often other symptoms. A reduction in vital capacity occurs and may be used as an indicator. The time of onset varies from a few minutes to one or more days depending on the pressure above 2atm and other factors, of which some are discussed below. At lower pressures down to 0.5atm the oxygen also damages the alveolar epithelium and capillary endothelium in the lungs and other organs including the glomeruli, carotid bodies and choroid plexus. The central nervous system, endocrine glands and special senses are also affected.

Hyperoxia suppresses erythropoiesis but does

not prolong the life of formed red blood corpuscles so exposure for a period of weeks, as in a saturation dive, can cause anaemia. Pulmonary oxygen toxicity is due to inactivation and cessation of production of surfactant and destruction of endothelial and type I alveolar cells and invasion of the tissue by macrophages. At this stage the subject experiences cough and retrosternal pain, there is a reduced velocity of mucus flow and changes in lung function including reductions in vital capacity, transfer factor and lung compliance; there is no change in airflow resistance and the expiratory reserve volume may be increased. This phase occurs within 5–48h depending on the concentration of oxygen above 0.50atm; it is reversed by breathing air at 1atm pressure for a period of days or weeks depending on the intensity of these symptoms. If exposure is continued the changes progress to pulmonary oedema and death or in chronic cases to proliferation of type II cells and ultimately pulmonary fibrosis.

Oxygen poisoning is due to the oxidation of substances which contain reduced sulphydryl groups, unsaturated carbon chains and other combinations which may be disrupted by free super oxide anions. The anions act either directly or via hydrogen or lipid peroxides. Tissue enzymes and lipid structures including cell membranes are at particular risk. The superoxide radicals are normally scavenged by superoxide mutase which is present in the cells of all aerobic organisms; production of the enzyme is increased by subclinical exposure to hyperoxia. Oxygen poisoning is aggravated by any circumstance which raises the metabolic rate including exercise, hyperthermia, shivering, administration of corticosteroid and sympathomimetic drugs, thyroxine and other agents; a raised ambient concentration of carbon dioxide such as might occur in a confined space is an additional risk factor. Oxygen poisoning is prevented by not exceeding an oxygen pressure of 2atm in any circumstances and by limiting the duration of exposure to oxygen at concentrations in excess of 0.5atm. This requirement effectively limits to 10m the depth for overnight visits to the sea bed breathing air.

Inert gas narcosis: Use of helium or hydrogen/ oxygen mixtures. Inert gas narcosis occurs during compressed air dives to depths in excess of 50m. At this pressure the membrane of nerve cells takes up a large quantity of nitrogen molecules in solution. The membrane becomes thicker in consequence and this impairs its ability to conduct nerve impulses. Many anaesthetic agents act reversibly in this way and the condition may be prevented by use of helium instead of nitrogen for dives in excess of 50m as the molecules are smaller and less numerous so do not thicken the nerve membranes to the same extent; as a result the narcotic potential of helium is less than 1% of that of nitrogen. However, the helium interferes seriously with speech. Compared with nitrogen the helium conducts heat more readily and this predisposes to hypothermia: the helium is also more expensive. These disadvantages are reduced by using the minimal concentrations of helium necessary to prevent narcosis; in addition during saturation dives the underwater living accommodation is maintained at a temperature of approximately 30°C and a heated suit is used during excursions. For sojourn at a depth of 60m the following gas mixture has been found satisfactory: FIO_2 0.04, He 0.80, N_2 0.15. At greater depth the nitrogen is eliminated altogether; however, speech then becomes almost unintelligible. It could be improved by substituting hydrogen which has a higher viscosity than helium. However, the narcotic potential is 25% of that of nitrogen and hydrogen forms an explosive mixture with oxygen; its useful role has still to be established.

High pressure neurological syndrome. Exposure to depths of the order of 400m may give rise to high pressure neurological syndrome (HPNS). This is characterized by tremor, dizziness, nausea, vomiting and loss of attention (micro sleep) which may progress to convulsions. The condition is probably due to a direct effect of pressure on the structure and enzyme activity of the nervous system. The effect may be minimized by adopting a very slow rate of pressurization. It may also be helped by the property of anaesthetic gases that their narcotic action is reversed at very high pressure; the thickening of nerve cell membranes referred to above then appears to be beneficial. These observations suggest that HPNS may be avoided by increasing the pressure over weeks rather than days and by judiciously incorporating nitrogen into the respired gas (trimix). Until these procedures have been fully developed the HPNS appears likely to limit man's diving ability to 700m below sea level.

Respiratory physiology of diving

Exposure to a high environmental pressure compresses the respired air and increases its density. A higher driving force is then needed to move the air along the majority of airways of the lung where the flow is at least partly turbulent (45, 46, 53). Thus for a given maximal force developed by the respiratory muscles the ventilatory capacity expressed as maximal voluntary ventilation is reduced by pressurization (fig. 7.3). The reduction affects particularly the peak flow rates during both inspiration and expiration (fig. 7.5); there is also a diminution in forced expiratory volume. On mechanical grounds the ventilation during exercise is reduced in consequence. These changes reduce the maximal exercise ventilation and hence the maximal oxygen uptake (32, 52).

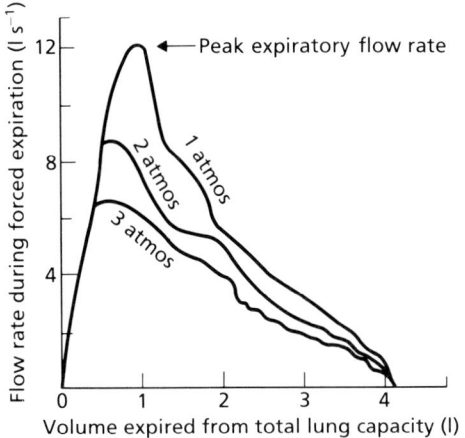

Fig. 7.5. Effect of an increase in barometric pressure upon the maximal expiratory flow volume curve of a healthy subject breathing air. Pressurization reduces the peak expiratory flow rate because this is associated with turbulence in the lung airways; there is little effect upon flow at small lung volumes which is mainly laminar.

The ventilation is further reduced by the rise in environmental pressure increasing the partial pressure of oxygen in the respired gas. This reduces the hypoxic chemoreceptor drive to breathing which is normally effected via the carotid body. It also reduces the chemoreceptor component of the drive from hypercapnia since the magnitude of the latter response is greatly influenced by the prevailing oxygen tension. These effects interact with the increased gas density to reduce the ventilation during exercise. The ventilation may also be reduced voluntarily by some divers using underwater breathing apparatus (scuba divers) who introduce pauses between the inspiratory and expiratory phases of respiration in order to conserve gas. In addition to these physiological causes for hypoventilation there is also the mechanical constraint imposed by the surrounding water which is displaced as the thorax expands. This is an important factor when in the water but not in a hyperbaric chamber.

The reduction in ventilation relative to oxygen uptake reduces the excretion of carbon dioxide and this is associated with a rise in the tension of CO_2 in arterial blood (Pa,co_2). Under normal circumstances the increased Pa,co_2 would stimulate breathing sufficient to nearly restore the ventilation but under hyperbaric conditions the response is often feeble. This mainly reflects the increased work of breathing. Additional contributory factors are the extra deadspace and resistance of the breathing apparatus and accumulation of carbon dioxide in the hyperbaric environment as a result of incomplete removal by the CO_2 absorbant. The distribution of gas by diffusion within the lung may also be disturbed (31, 37, 52). The resultant of these processes is to reduce the respiratory sensitivity of divers to carbon dioxide (44) and this in turn further reduces the ventilatory response to exercise. The reduction in CO_2 sensitivity is greatest during saturation dives when many of these factors are operating for long periods and the sensitivity returns towards normal following ascent. Some divers are more affected than others and these persons, on account of associated hypercapnia, are at increased risk of oxygen poisoning and nitrogen narcosis. They may also develop symptoms of

CO_2 intoxication including headache, dizziness and light-headedness with accompanying tachycardia and peripheral vasodilatation. The symptoms may include breathlessness and may progress to confusion and loss of consciousness. They need to be distinguished from those due to oxygen toxicity, nitrogen narcosis and high pressure neurological syndrome which are described above.

Medical examinations of divers

Formidable obstacles exist to exploring the sea bed which are summarized above. They make it essential that divers are well trained, in excellent physical condition and supported by the best available technology. However, despite such provisions the casualty rate is high and there is a significant long-term morbidity. Recruitment as professional divers is confined to those who are of above average health and stamina; many of them gain their first experience as amateur divers. In the U.K. the health standard is set by the requirements for commercial divers of the Health and Safety Executive (42, 43). This requires freedom from acute recurrent and chronic disease including all diseases of the cardiovascular and respiratory systems, ears and sinuses. The electrocardiogram at rest and after exercise should be within normal limits and the subject should be lean, normotensive (B.P.<140/90mmHg) and physically fit; fitness may be assessed using an exercise test (chapter 18). The forced vital capacity should exceed 3.5 l and the forced expiratory volume as a percentage of the forced vital capacity (FEV%) should not be less than 75% on first examination or 70% on subsequent examinations. These characteristics are assessed in an annual medical examination by doctors approved by the HSE. An extensive radiographic scrutiny for evidence of aseptic bone necrosis is carried out either annually or at longer intervals depending on the type of dives.

Other countries have different requirements which in some instances are graded by the depth to which it is proposed to descend. Thus for dives in excess of 300m the Norwegians require serial observations of vestibular and cardiorespiratory function including direct measurement of maximal oxygen uptake ($\dot{n}o_2$max), the respiratory sensitivity to carbon dioxide and a version of the Flack test in which the subject exhales against a column of mercury. A different version of the Flack test is required for deep dives based in France. The Norwegian threshold of physical fitness is $\dot{n}o_2$max $\geqslant$ 2.0mmol kg^{-1} min^{-1} (45ml kg^{-1} min^{-1}) up to age 30 years and thereafter 1.8mmol kg^{-1} min^{-1} (40ml kg^{-1} min^{-1}). This level or its submaximal equivalent (chapter 18) might be adopted more widely. For amateur divers the British Sub-Aqua Club (BSAC) sets medical standards for entry into Sports Diving and for surveillance by chest radiography and medical examinations at regular intervals. Most other amateur diving organizations follow the BSAC Medical Standards.

Lung disorders in divers

Asthma or the respiratory effects of smoking developing in a diver may be detected during the annual medical at a stage when the condition is reversible. Latent asthma is associated with a risk of airflow obstruction developing during exposure to cold water; if there is any doubt a test of bronchial hyperreactivity should be carried out (page 356). Difficulty may also arise in assessing the medical significance or the risk of barotrauma associated with a low FEV%, a small vital capacity or a linear opacity on the chest radiograph. A low FEV% is usually due to the diver having a large vital capacity: this is partly a consequence of self-selection for diving since a large vital capacity increases the buoyancy of the body and hence performance at swimming. In addition the increased respiratory work associated with swimming and breathing dense air develops the accessory muscles of respiration; there is then an increase in vital capacity without a corresponding increase in forced expiratory volume (f 7.6). In these circumstances a low FEV% is normal (35). However, the low ratio may also reflect narrowing of small lung airways (39, 40). There is then a reduced forced expiratory flow at small lung volumes (MEF25%FVC), poor lung mixing (N_2% and Va.eff/Va) and a large residual volume; these aspects should be assessed using standard methods (chapter 5). A below average vital

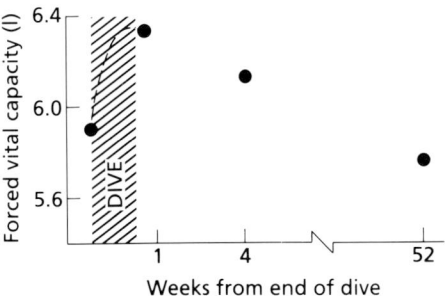

Fig. 7.6. Mean results for seven men showing the increase and subsequent recovery of forced vital capacity (FVC) associated with a single saturation dive to 300m for 3 weeks (38). On the assumption that the recovery is exponential the half time is approximately 4 weeks.

capacity may be evidence for a relatively stiff lung (36) in which the compliance is reduced relative to the reference value and the maximal recoil pressure increased. These changes developing after a saturation dive may be evidence of oxygen toxicity. The presence of radiological features of emphysema or a linear opacity are indications for a full assessment which should include measurements of transfer factor (diffusing capacity) and lung compliance. Ventilation studies with radioactive gas can be very helpful, by demonstrating areas of reduced ventilation. The physiological factors which predispose to pulmonary barotrauma are not known for certain but generalized emphysema and local scar emphysema around an area of fibrosis are probably amongst them (36). This possibility should lead to the preferential recruitment of divers from amongst non-smokers and to the exclusion from diving of men with a material previous exposure to coal dust (chapter 9).

Changes in diving exposure affect the state of training of the respiratory muscles and hence the vital capacity and FEV%. On this account these indices reflect the diving history. A progressive decline may also reflect the development of chronic airflow obstruction. A fall in transfer factor may indicate the development of emphysema. However, in a man who has recently emerged from saturation it may be due

to oxygen toxicity or to anaemia secondary to hyperoxic depression of the bone marrow. If the former, the ventilatory cost of exercise is likely to be increased and the distensibility of the lung reduced (fig. 7.7).

Medical emergencies in divers. Any of the specific complications of diving including barotrauma, decompression sickness, oxygen toxicity and inert gas narcosis may present as a medical emergency during the dive or in some cases afterwards. Their nature, correction and treatment are described in the preceding section. The causes are well documented so their occurrence is a result of culpable ignorance, mechanical failure, human error or unforeseen circumstances. The human contribution may arise at any stage in the complex process of preparing for a dive, launching the diver and securing a safe return. The commonest failing is impatience leading to an urge to skimp the times for decompression. The urge must be resisted! The commonest faults are misreading a pressure gauge, using an incorrect gas mixture and recording time incorrectly. The likelihood of

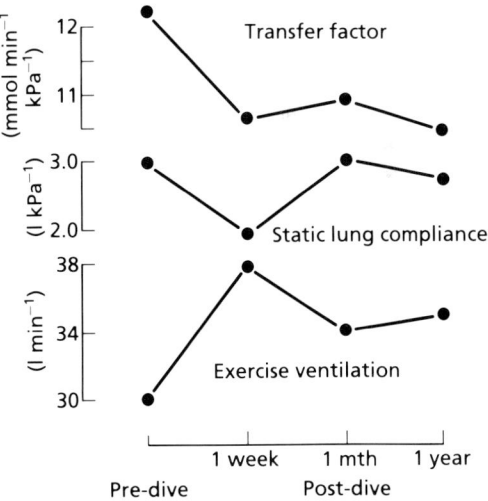

Fig. 7.7. Lung function in a man who developed symptoms of oxygen toxicity in association with a saturation dive. Individually the changes were within their standard errors; in combination they were suggestive of temporary respiratory impairment (38).

these faults occurring is reduced by measures to ensure and maintain vigilance, use of standard procedures and of gas mixtures which are prepared in advance, not on site. An alarm which indicates deviation of oxygen pressure outside the safe limits would also be an advantage (49). Other emergencies arise from trauma, asphyxia and drowning. The latter is described below.

Drowning

Submersion in water has a number of effects upon the lungs, both indirect through cold or stimulation of cutaneous receptors and direct when the response depends on the type and quantity of water which is inhaled. The changes are reviewed by Keatinge (47).

Cold immersion may induce a gasp reflex with attendant risk of water inhalation; it may give rise to acute bronchoconstriction in an asthmatic or to peripheral vasoconstriction which may displace sufficient blood into the lungs to cause pulmonary oedema. The cooling of the skin may stimulate the release of noradrenaline which may cause ventricular fibrillation whilst the cold stimulus to the face augments vagal tone to cause reflex bradycardia with attendant risk of unconsciousness. Thus cold immersion may set in motion a potentially lethal chain of reactions before any water has entered the lungs.

Entry of a small quantity of water into the larynx and larger airways stimulates local irritant receptors: there is then apnoea, reflex laryngeal spasm and reflex bronchoconstriction. Passage of water further down the airways may cause bronchiolar obstruction. This may be followed by atelectasis and other changes including delayed pulmonary oedema which may occur up to several hours after rescue.

The apnoea and spasm due to submersion may persist for up to 5min after which there is massive inhalation of water into the lungs. This causes ventricular fibrillation but the mechanism depends on the type of water which is inhaled. In the case of sea water the fibrillation is due to calcium and magnesium ions which are absorbed into the blood, whilst with fresh water the fibrillation is due to potassium ions which are liberated into the plasma by

haemolysis of red blood corpuscles. The prognosis depends on which of these mechanisms is responsible. In the case of sea water drowning, comprehensive treatment applied within 5min will usually lead to absorption of the alkali metal ions into the tissues and restoration of respiration and normal cardiac contractions. With potassium-induced fibrillation the recovery is slower and unlikely to be successful unless complicated by hypothermia which protects the brain from anoxia. The hypothermia is a function of water temperature, body size, subcutaneous fat thickness and insulating clothing; it is usually greater in children than adults and males than females. Against expectation the prospect for recovery is better with a water temperature of 1°C than 20°C but for the reasons given earlier the likelihood of drowning is greater with the colder water.

Treatment is initially by clearing the airway, lifting into a jack-knife posture to drain out as much fluid as will come quickly, then applying both external cardiac massage and mouth to mouth or positive pressure ventilation. As soon as is practicable a tracheal catheter should be inserted to permit further aspiration of fluid from the lungs and the stomach should be emptied with a gastric tube. The catheter may be used for positive pressure ventilation (50). In advanced cases these remedies may preserve life whilst arrangements are made for exchange transfusion and electrical defibrillation of the heart. The treatment may continue with positive end-expiratory pressure ventilation to reduce or prevent pulmonary oedema, barbiturate drugs and other measures to control a raised intracranial pressure and prophylactic antibiotics.

References

Cold

1 Cole P, Forsyth R, Haight JS. Effects of cold air and exercise on nasal patency. *Ann Otol Rhinol Laryngol* 1983;**92**:196–8.

2 Deal EC Jr, McFadden ER Jr, Ingram RH Jr, Strauss RH, Jaeger JJ. Role of respiratory heat exchange in production of exercise-induced asthma. *J Appl Physiol* 1979;**46**:467–75.

3 Edholm OG, Weiner JS (Eds). *Principles and Practice of Human Physiology*. London: Academic Press. 1981;111–190.

4 Guleria JS, Talwar JR, Malhotra OP, Pande JN. Effect of breathing cold air on pulmonary mechanics in normal man. *J Appl Physiol* 1969;**27**:320–2.

5 Hartung GH, Myhre LG, Nunneley SA. Physiological effects of cold air inhalation during exercise. *Aviat Space Environ Med* 1980; **51**:591–4.

6 Hattenhauer M, Neill WA. The effect of cold air inhalation on angina pectoris and myocardial oxygen supply. *Circulation* 1975;**51**:1053–8.

7 Jones WT. *The Health and Safety at Work Act. A practical handbook.* London: Graham and Trotman. 1975.

8 Schaefer O, Eaton RDP, Timmermans FJW, Hildes JA., Respiratory function impairment and cardiopulmonary consequences in long-term residents of the Canadian Arctic. *Canad Med Assn J* 1980;**123**:997–1004.

Heat

9 Cunningham DJC, O'Riordan JLH. The effect of a rise in the temperature of the body on the respiratory response to carbon dioxide at rest. *Quart J Exp Physiol* 1957;**42**:329–45.

10 Edholm OG, Weiner JS (Eds). *Principles and Practice of Human Physiology.* London: Academic Press. 1981:111–90.

11 Miller GJ, Martin HdeV. Effect of ambient temperature between 21°C and 35°C on the responses to progressive submaximal exercise in partially acclimated man. *Ergonomics* 1975;**18**:539–46.

12 Rowell LB. Human cardiovascular adjustments to exercise and thermal stress. *Physiol Rev* 1974;**54**:75–159.

13 Williams CG, Bredell GAG, Wyndham CH, Strydom NB, Morrison JF, Peter J, Fleming PW, Ward JS. Circulatory and metabolic reactions to work in heat. *J Appl Physiol* 1962;**17**:625–38.

High Altitude

14 Bradwell AR, Dykes PW, Coote JH, Forster PJE, Milles JJ, Chesner I, Richardson NV. Effect of acetazolamide on exercise performance and muscle mass at high altitude. *Lancet* 1986; **i**:1001–5.

15 Cotes JE, Douglas-Jones AG, Saunders MJ. A 60% oxygen supply for medical use. *Br Med J* 1969;**4**:143–6.

16 Denison DM, Ledwith MA, Poulton EC. Complex reaction times at simulated cabin altitudes of 5000 feet and 8000 feet. *Aerospace Med* 1966;**37**:1010–3.

17 Dickinson J, Heath D, Gosney J, Williams D. Altitude-related deaths in seven trekkers in the Himalayas. *Thorax* 1983;**38**:646–56.

18 Hultgren HN, Grover RF, Hartley LH. Abnormal circulatory responses to high altitude in subjects with a previous history of high altitude pulmonary oedema. *Circulation* 1971; **44**:759–70.

19 Milledge JS. Acute mountain sickness. *Thorax* 1983;**38**:641–5.

20 Milledge JS, Catley DM. Angiotension converting enzyme response to hypoxia in man: the role in altitude acclimitization. *Clin Sci* 1984;**67**:453–6.

21 Rennie D. Diseases of high terrestrial altitudes. In: Weatherall DJ, Ledingham JGG, Warrell DA (Eds) *Oxford Textbook of Medicine.* Oxford University Press. 1983:57–64.

22 Tichauer ER. Operation of machine tools at high altitude. *Ergonomics* 1963;**6**:51–73.

23 West JB, Boyers J, Graber DJ, Hackett PH, Maret KH *et al.* Maximal exercise at extreme altitudes on Mount Everest. *J Appl Physiol* 1983; **55**:688–98.

Aviation

24 Dhenin G, Sharp GR, Ernsting J. (Eds). *Aviation Medicine: Vol. 1. Physiology and human factors.* London: Tri-med Books. 1978.

25 Dhenin G, Whiteside TCD, Price TJG, Taylor JG, Ernsting J. (Eds). *Aviation Medicine, Vol. 2. Health and clinical aspects.* London: Tri-med Books, 1978.

26 Goodwin JF (Chairman). The cardiovascular fitness of airline pilots. *Br Heart J* 1978;**40**: 335–50.

27 Harding RM, Mills FJ. Aviation Medicine: licensing requirements for air crew. *Br Med J* 1983;**287**:114–6.

28 ICAO. *Manual of Civil Aviation Medicine*, 2nd ed. Document 8984. Montreal: ICAO. 1985.

29 ICAO. *International Standards and Recommended Practices. Personnel Licensing.* Annex 1 to the Convention on International Civil Aviation. 7th ed. Montreal: ICAO. 1982.

30 Mills FJ, Harding RM. Aviation Medicine: fitness to travel by air. *Br Med J* 1983;**286**: 1269–71, 1340–1.

31 Preston FS, Denison DM. Aviation Medicine. In: Weatherall DJ, Ledingham JGG, Warrell DA (Eds). *Oxford Textbook of Medicine.* Oxford University Press. 1983;**6**:64–76.

Diving

32 Anthonisen Nr, Utz G, Kryger MH, Urbanetti JS. Exercise tolerance at 4 and 6 ATA. *Undersea Biomed Res* 1976;**3**:95–112.

33 Bell DG, Wright GR. Energy expenditure and work stress of divers performing a variety of underwater work tasks. *Ergonomics* 1979; **22**:345–56.

34 Bennett PB, Elliott DH. (Eds). *The Physiology and Medicine of Diving.* 3rd ed. London: Balliere Tindall. 1982.

35 Bouhuys A, Beck GJ. Large lungs in divers? *J Appl Physiol* 1979;**47**:1136.

36 Colebatch HJH, Smith MM, Ng CKY. Increased elastic recoil as a determinant of pulmonary barotrauma in divers. *Respir Physiol* 1976; **26**:55–64.

37 Christopherson SK, Hlastala MP. Pulmonary gas exchange during altered density gas breathing. *J Appl Physiol* 1982;**52**:221–5.

38 Cotes JE, Davey IS, Reed JW, Rooks M. Respiratory effects of a single saturation dive to 300 m. *Br J Industr Med* 1987:**44**:76–82.

39 Crosbie WA, Reed JW, Clarke MC. Functional characteristics of the large lungs found in commercial divers. *J Appl Physiol* 1979;**46**:639–45.

40 Davey IS, Cotes JE, Reed JW. Relationship of ventilatory capacity to hyperbaric exposure in divers. *J Appl Physiol* 1984;**56**:1655–8.

41 Denison DM. Diving medicine. In: Weatherall DJ, Ledingham JGG, Warrell DA (Eds). *Oxford Textbook of Medicine.* Oxford University Press, 1983:6.76–6.83.

42 Diving operations at work regulations. *Statutory Instruments. Health and Safety.* London: HMSO. 1981:No.399.

43 Employment Medical Advisory Service. The medical examination of divers. A guide to the diving operations at work regulations. Health and Safety Services booklet HS(R) 8. London: EMAS. 1981.

44 Florio JT, Morrison JB, Butt WS. Breathing pattern and ventilatory response to carbon dioxide in divers. *J Appl Physiol* 1979;**46**:1076–80.

45 Hesser CM, Linnarsson D, Fagraeus L. Pulmonary mechanics and work of breathing at maximal ventilation and raised air pressure. *J Appl Physiol* 1981;**50**:747–53.

46 Hickey DD, Lundgren CE, Pasche AJ. Influence of exercise on maximal voluntary ventilation and forced expiratory flow at depth. *Undersea Biomed Res* 1983;**10**:241–54.

47 Keatinge WR. Heat, cold and drowning. In: Weatherall DJ, Ledingham JGG, Warrell DA (Eds). *Oxford Textbook of Medicine.* Oxford University Press. 1983;6.52–6.57.

48 Leitch DR. Complications of saturation diving. *J Roy Soc Med* 1985;**78**:634–7.

49 Levack ID. Oxygen hazards in divers breathing helium and oxygen mixtures. *Br Med J* 1983;**287**:1594–5.

50 Pearn J. The management of near drowning. *Br Med J* 1985;**291**:1447–52.

51 Strauss RH. Diving medicine. *Am Rev Respir Dis* 1979;**119**:1001–23.

52 Van Liew HD. Mechanical and physical factors in lung function during work in dense environments. *Undersea Biomed Res* 1983;**10**:255–64.

53 Vorosmarti J Jr. Influence of increased gas density and external resistance on maximum expiratory flow. *Undersea Biomed Res* 1979; **6**:339–46.

Further Reading

Cotes JE. *Lung Function: Assessment and Application in Medicine,* 4th ed. Oxford: Blackwell Scientific Publications. 1979.

Weatherall DJ, Ledingham JGG, Warrell DA (Eds). *Oxford Textbook of Medicine.* Oxford University Press, 1983.

Chapter 8
Silicosis

Sources of silicosis

Silicon is the second most abundant element in the earth's crust after oxygen. It is the main constituent of the igneous rocks, granite and feldspar (respectively mainly SiO_2 and $KAl Si_3O_8$) and occurs in sedimentary rocks formed from them including shale and sandstone.

From the day when man first used tools and dressed stone for buildings, he has been exposed to a risk of silicosis. Primitive man broke flint to make pointed weapons, iron age man used sandstone for grinding and sharpening, and throughout the ages rocks containing free silica have been tunnelled into, quarried and dressed for buildings and other uses (e.g. 30, also fig. 8.1). Faults in granite rock have been searched out and mined for the gold and other mineral which they contained, while uses for crushed siliceous rocks have multiplied over the years, to include incorporation in refractories and ceramics, as a filler in paper and plasters, for cleaning, smoothing and polishing, in electronics and for producing laser beams (table 8.1). Any of these activities may generate atmospheric dust containing crystalline silicon dioxide which if inhaled in sufficient quantity may cause silicosis. The commonest crystalline form is quartz. This is the harmful constituent of most of the substances listed in table 8.1. In the case of flint, chert and some ornamental stones, including cornelian and agate (chalcedony) the crystals are very small and cemented with amorphous silica (hence their name crypto-crystalline silica). Even smaller crystals occur in coesite which is only slightly fibrogenic and stishovite which

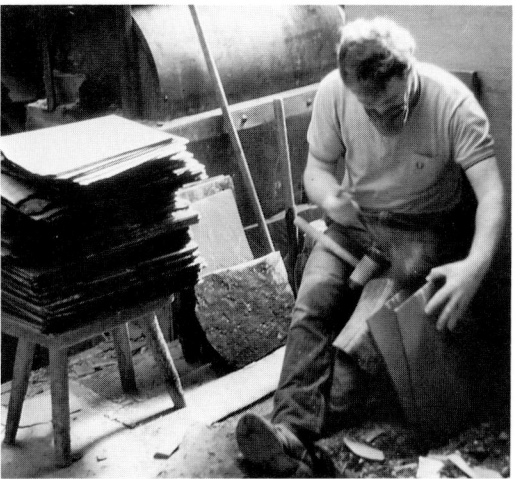

Fig. 8.1. Slate quarry worker splitting slate: the risk of quarry men and slate makers developing silicosis is given in fig. 8.13. (By courtesy of J.R. Glover.)

does not cause silicosis. The fibrogenicity of quartz is enhanced by heating which, depending on temperature, converts the quartz into tridymite or cristobalite; the latter substance is formed during calcining, e.g. in refractories and in foundries where sand is still sometimes used in moulds or as parting powder to assist the separation of the casting. Amorphous silica also occurs as diatomite. In this form it is inert but becomes fibrogenic on heating due to conversion to cristobalite. Whatever type of silica is inhaled the resulting silicosis usually takes the form of small fibrotic nodules throughout both lungs.

Table 8.1. Sources of silicosis

Substance	Process	Uses and related occupations
A. Potentially high risk from crystalline SiO_2		
Granite (rock)	Q, (44), cutting, dressing, tunnelling (16,17,18)	Construction, monuments (28), grinding (33), building roads, railways, water courses, sewers, laying cables, etc.
Sandstone	Q, cutting, dressing, crushing, etc., tunnelling (18)	Construction, monuments, sandblasting (22,25,37), refractories, foundries (27,32), abrasives, scouring powders, polishes, boiler scaling, manufacture of carborundum (35), fibre glass, optical equipment, etc.
Flint	Separation from chalk, calcining, milling	China ware (36), filler, abrasive, as 'flints', for facing, etc.
Slate	M/Q, sawing, splitting, cutting, trimming, polishing (15)	Construction work, tabletops, electric panels, pencils (23)
Shale	M/O-C, grinding, etc.	Ceramic, aggregate, extraction of oil (39)
Silicon metal	Vapourization of quartz (43)	In electronics, lasers, etc.
B. Risk from variable contamination with SiO_2		
Granite contaminating or containing other mineral ores	Mining gold (6,7), silver (30), copper, mica, platinum, iron, (taconite, 9), tungsten (wolframite), fluorine (fluorspar*), barium (40)	
China and fire clays	M, Q, crushing, milling, wet mixing	Paper, paint, china and stoneware, refractories
Feldspar	M, crushing, milling, etc.	Ceramics, filler, enamel (14)
Bentonite	Q, crushing, milling (34)	Crayons, filler, lubricant
Diatomite	O-C, crushing, screening, calcining (forms cristobalite, 10,13)	Refractories, abrasives, (also filler, filter and for insulation), may affect local animals

M = mining; Q = quarrying; O-C = open-cast mining; *Ca fluorite.

Related substances

Diatomaceous earth (Kieselguhr). This material is amorphous silicon dioxide formed from the compressed shells of unicellular algae (diatoms); it is present in sedimentary deposits which are mined by the open cast method in many countries, including the U.S.A. and Western Europe. Diatomite has a wide range of uses which are listed in table 8.1. The stone is friable and during its preparation is crushed and screened to liberate a fine dust which is, how-ever, harmless in its raw state. The particles have a lattice structure and on this account are readily identified by microscopy. The process of treatment entails calcining and formation of crystalline silica which is mainly cristobalite but also contains quartz and tridymite. These substances are highly injurious and in the absence of precautions may cause diffuse fibrosis or acute silicosis (10,13).

Shale. This is a clay containing kaolinite, mica, silica and other minerals which is present as sedimentary rock often in the vicinity of coal deposits. Quartz is present in the dust in concentration of the order of 7% and may give rise to both chronic bronchitis (chapter 17) and diffuse pulmonary fibrosis. Progressive massive fibrosis may also occur (39). Some shales contain oil, which form the world's largest reserves, but the concentration is low, hence extraction is expensive. The oil may cause cancer of the skin, especially the scrotum in shale miners and users of shale oil. On this account scrotal cancer was formerly an occupational hazard of mule spinners in Lancashire cotton mills.

Bentonite and other clays. Bentonite is a clay containing sodium montmorrillonite. It occurs in deposits formed of airborne volcanic ash and is mined by the open-cast method in Wyoming, U.S.A. It is used as a filler in crayons, for manufacture of concrete and a lubricant in drilling oil wells. The clay is contaminated with silica in the concentration of 1% to 24% and with cristobalite formed from the quartz by heat prior to the volcanic eruption. The dust is a cause of silicosis amongst the production workers (34). Fuller's earth, which is either the related substance calcium montmorrillonite or attapulgite, rarely contains quartz. China clay (kaolin) occasionally does so but the quartz concentration seldom exceeds 1%. When it does the dust is capable of causing silicosis but the condition is seldom observed in practice. The processing, uses and medical effects of these substances are reported on page 273.

Biological effects of silica

Silicon is present in many items of diet including hard water, wheat fibre, soya bean and pectin and on this account is freely ingested. It is a constituent of complex acid mucopolysaccharides such as glycosaminoglycan–protein complexes which occur in connective tissue throughout the body, including the lung, skin and arterial walls where the content decreases with age. Silicon is also present in bone and cartilage. Organo-silicon compounds contribute to the regulation of connective tissue, the growth and strength of hair and nails and the cohesion of keratin; they are present in non-steroid antigens in semen and may have a role in atherosclerosis. The enzyme silicase present in pancreatic mitochondria liberates silicic acid from appropriate substrate and in the lung the inhalation of quartz (SiO_2) leads to the formation of complex substances containing phosphosilicate with a single oxygen atom $>Si–O–P<$ which is highly catalytic and reactive (5). It is possibly this substance which initiates the chain of events leading to silicosis. However, the active component is not known. Alternative candidates are silicic acid itself and biologically active surfaces created by the cleavage of SiO_2 crystals to form freshly fractured silica. The active agent differs in potency as between different types of SiO_2 (page 145).

The first stage in silicosis is ingestion of SiO_2 crystals by alveolar macrophages (8); the crystals are engulfed into the cytoplasm by encapsulation to form secondary lysosomes. The silica reacts chemically with the adjacent phospholipid; this disrupts the lysosomal membrane and releases enzymes which then kill the macrophage (1). When this happens the macrophage disintegrates and the quartz is taken up, possibly by several macrophages which then share the toxic burden between them. There is evidence that silica may move about in the lung by this process (20). The reaction with phospholipid can be prevented by coating the silica with one of several substances (page 158).

The ingestion of an amount of quartz which is insufficient to kill the macrophage stimulates it to release a substance which promotes activity in fibroblasts; the number of fibroblasts is increased and they produce hydroxyproline which is an essential step in the formation of fibrous tissue. At the same time the quartz has been shown to have other actions which, individually, are capable of influencing the tissue response; how they interact is still a subject for research. There is increased local production of prostaglandin E and this can assist the migration of macrophages by increasing the permeability of alveolar capillaries. At the same time the alveolar type II cells are stimulated to produce phospholipid. In high concentration this causes lipidosis which is a feature of acute silicolipoproteinosis. The lipid appears to (i) stimulate the production of monocytes by the bone marrow, (ii) disrupt the pavement epithelium of the alveoli to permit passage of macrophages through to the alveolar surface, and (iii) physically separate the quartz from the macrophages, thereby interrupting the sequence which leads to formation of fibrous tissue. These hypotheses and the evidence on which they are based are reviewed by Heppleston (21). However, we still do not know why massive exposure to quartz has such a powerful stimulant action on the type II cells, whereas smaller intermittent exposures cause mainly fibrosis. Mixtures of quartz and relatively inert dusts including coal and haematite cause less fibrosis than that due to quartz alone (fig. 8.2). The resulting condition is called mixed dust fibrosis (page 149). Complete coating of the quartz by iron particles renders it inactive; this accounts for there being relatively little silicosis amongst workers in the Kolar gold mines in India (6).

Macrophages which have ingested a sublethal quantity of quartz as well as releasing inflammatory mediators and hydrolytic enzymes have other abnormal features. Activated macrophages release hydrogen peroxide and related lipid peroxides; they appear to suppress the immunological function of lymphocytes and they lose the ability to inactivate or restrict the growth of mycobacteria, including tubercle bacilli (29). This may account for the increased incidence of tuberculosis amongst subjects with silicosis.

The actions of silica described above are mainly direct chemical responses but evidence is increasing that some may be immunologically mediated. Thus circulating antinuclear antibodies are a feature of many cases of silicosis, especially those with mainly confluent lesions. Immunoglobulins and cells which secrete them are present in and around the silicotic nodules and silicosis may be accompanied or followed by auto-immune diseases, including scleroderma in which the presence of antinuclear antibodies is almost invariable (24). This was the case in the patient described in fig. 8.11 (page 158). However, no causative association between antibodies or lymphocyte responses to mutagenic substances and fibrosis has been demonstrated in man unlike in other species (38). Thus the role of immunological mechanisms remains uncertain and there is need for further work.

Pathology of silicosis

Inhaled particles of quartz which evade the respiratory defence mechanisms and reach the alveoli have a diameter less than 7μm (chapter 4); those which are most biologically active are in the size range 1–5μm. Following deposition on the alveolar epithelium a few particles pass through pores to enter the interstitial tissue:

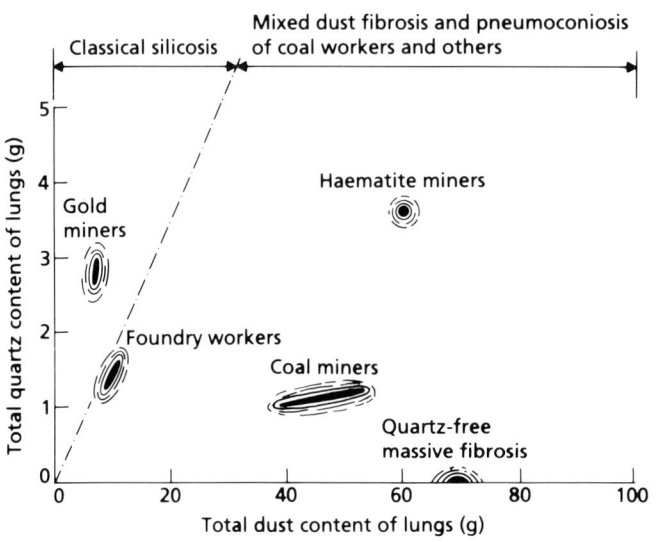

Fig. 8.2. Relationship of quartz to total dust content of both lungs for men with advanced dust disease. The oblique line separates cases of classical silicosis from mixed dust fibrosis and pneumoconiosis. The findings suggest that haematite miners are to some extent protected from silicosis by the inert dust. Data of G. Nagelschmidt (31).

some more are taken up by type II cells in the alveolar wall. The majority are engulfed by macrophages which fill the affected alveoli, usually those in the walls of respiratory bronchioles. The macrophages react in the ways described in the preceding section with resulting cell death, proliferation of fibroblasts and deposition of reticulin fibres which subsequently convert to collagen. This process leads to the formation of silicotic nodules having concentrically arranged fibres, of which those in the middle may become hyalinized or calcified, whilst the outer ones form a capsule; this in turn may be surrounded by macrophages and plasma cells but not giant cells (fig. 8.3). Thus the lesions are formed by

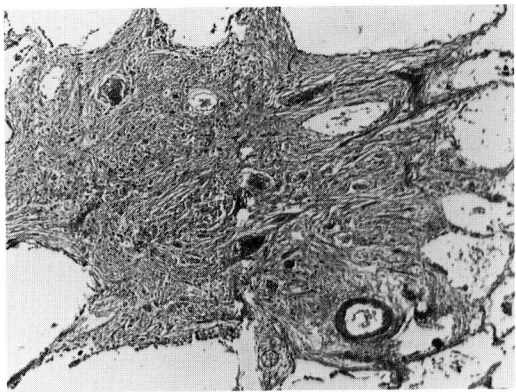

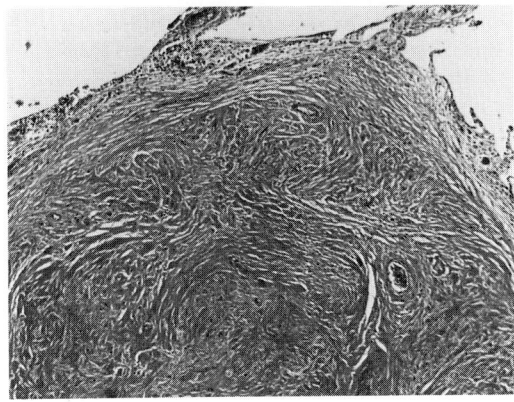

Fig. 8.3. Silicotic nodule. Above: Early lesion. Below: Part of a mature lesion showing concentric strands of fibrous tissue (low power views) (By courtesy of T. Ashcroft.) The appearance on paper-mounted lung section is shown in fig. 8.4.

cells which come together in response to the quartz; the lesions contain some mineral sufficient to ensure their persistence but much less than in coal macules where the quantity of mineral is high (page 170).

Silicotic nodules occur initially in the periphery of the upper zones but later are distributed throughout the lung. The nodules arise in the walls of respiratory bronchioles and may obstruct their lumens. They are usually discrete, of diameter 2–6mm and readily palpable in unfixed tissue; nodules frequently occur in clusters. The overlying visceral pleura may be thickened and fibrosed, probably on account of spread of macrophages containing silica via the subpleural lymphatics. The pleural and nodular lesions may coalesce to form a sheet resembling armour plating (cuirass) or the nodules may coalesce to form conglomerate lesions (fig. 8.4). These usually retain a nodular pattern; the nodules often become hyalinized but seldom cavitate, possibly because unlike in progressive massive fibrosis the fibrous capsule of the necrotic area prevents break out into a bronchus (page 182). Tuberculosis may occur as a complication (page 152).

As well as spreading to the pleura, the macrophages containing quartz particles may travel in the lymphatics to the hilum of the lung, the mediastinum and even the neck and abdomen. On the way they form nodules which may obstruct and eventually obliterate the bronchial blood vessels and lymphatics and cause enlargement of affected lymph nodes. These contain silicotic nodules or sheets of fibrous tissue and have a fibrous capsule which may hyalinize and become calcified. The resulting egg-shell calcification is referred to on page 159. Calcification appears to be most common in persons having a relatively small exposure to nearly pure quartz dust and presumably reflects the final distribution of the dust; why calcification occurs in some more than others is unclear.

Mixed dust fibrosis. In foundry workers, haematite miners and some coal miners, inhaled quartz interacts with the other dust to produce a mixed dust fibrosis. The typical silicotic nodules are then accompanied or replaced by more diffuse stellate lesions in which the fibrous tissue radiates out from the centre of

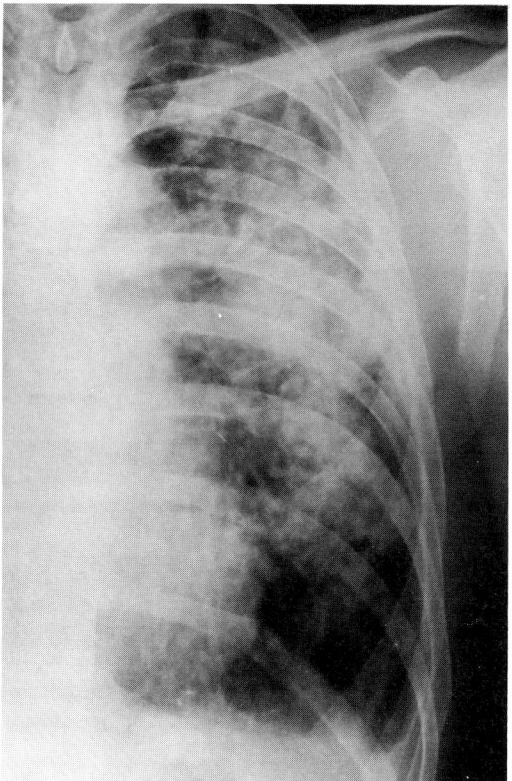 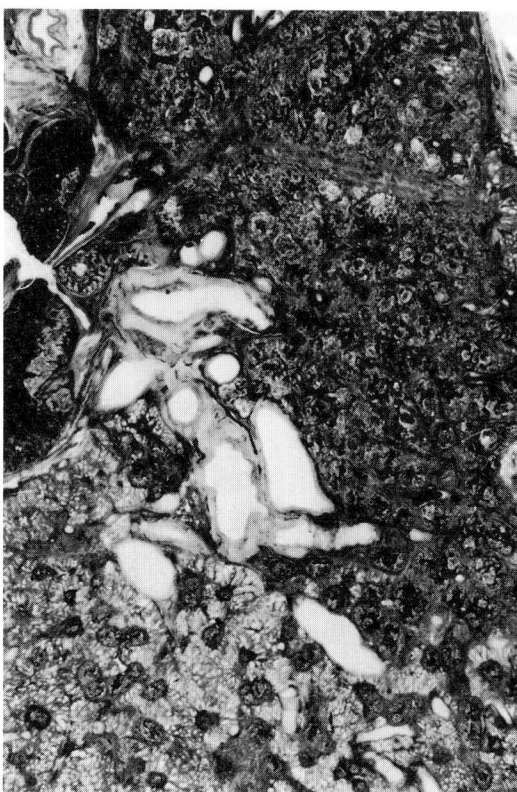

Fig. 8.4. Radiograph of the left lung a year before death showing pneumoconiosis (category 3q/C) and detail from the paper-mounted lung section of a barytes miner with advanced massive silicosis. From the age of 13 until he was 31 the patient worked on a farm. In the mine he spent a year tramming, then for 12 years was drilling through sandstone. He gave up work on account of breathlessness on exertion and died 4 years later at the age of 48. At post-mortem the upper zone of the left lung was occupied by a massive lesion formed by the coalescence of silicotic nodules, many of which were calcified. The lower zone contained discrete nodules of simple silicosis. Similar changes were present in the right lung. (By courtesy of J.E.M. Hutchinson.)

the nodule and is not arranged concentrically. The fibrosis is sometimes accompanied by emphysema (table 9.2, page 173). Similar lesions can also occur in the late stages of classical silicosis (fig. 8.5). Coal miners who have been exposed to respirable dust with a high quartz content often show rapid radiological progression (fig. 8.6); in these men the amount of emphysema at post-mortem is lower than in other coal miners (chapter 9).

Rheumatoid 'silicosis'. A rheumatoid type of silicosis has been reported in which the nodules are relatively large and have necrotic centres. They resemble other rheumatoid nodules in having clefts containing cholesterol crystals (fig. 9.11, page 178) and also differ from normal silicotic nodules in having a 'pallisade' layer of polymorphonuclear leucocytes in the surrounding tissue. The lesions are accompanied by other features of the rheumatoid syndrome, including arthritis and a raised plasma titre of rheumatoid factor. The condition was at one time thought to be Caplan syndrome as occurs in coal miners (chapter 9); but amongst the latter it is not related to a high silica content in the dust. Caplan syndrome appears not to be linked to

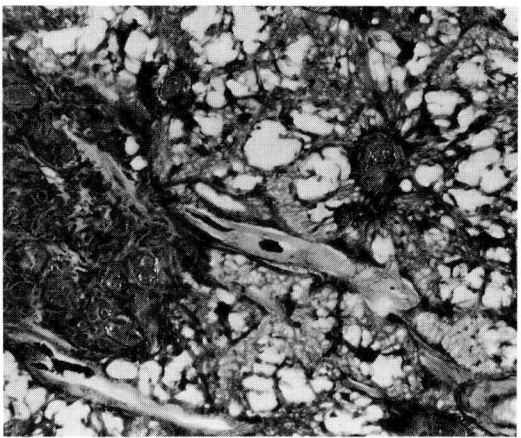

Fig. 8.5. Stellate nodule in silicosis. Detail from paper-mounted lung section showing a stellate silicotic nodule with fibrous centre and radiating strands of fibrous tissue interspersed with emphysematous spaces. To the left of the nodule is an area of confluent silicosis. Details of the patient are given in fig. 8.9 (page 155).

quartz but definite rheumatoid arthritis predisposes to an increased attack rate and progression of silicosis (41).

Acute silicolipoproteinosis. Massive exposure to quartz may lead to the lung filling up with neutrophils and numerous alveolar cells containing spherical inclusions and some quartz (11). The cells are probably degenerate type II pneumocytes and they release amorphous pink hyaline fluid resembling surfactant. The fluid contains cholesterol, fat and protein and it occupies alveoli and plugs small airways to cause the clinical features of alveolar proteinosis; these include fever, malaise, increasing cough, expectoration, breathlessness on exertion and radiographic evidence of widespread loss of airfilled lung; the opacities may then be small and discrete or coarse linear or rounded, becoming confluent when they resemble pulmonary oedema (45). The diagnosis may be made from the history, for example of sandblasting, plus the characteristic microscopic appearance of the sputum or fluid from bronchial lavage (fig. 8.7). The condition appears to be a non-specific reaction to a massive dose of dust and may respond to repeated therapeutic bronchial lavage (12).

Clinical features

Silicosis usually presents as simple nodulation on a chest radiograph taken for purposes of surveillance (page 161, figs 8.6–8.12); the diagnosis is based on the radiographic features (page 156), the history of exposure to silica (commonly 6 or more years) and the absence of a tenable alternative. The patient is initially asymptomatic and may remain so, but if there is extensive nodulation, or if the nodulation progresses to form confluent lesions (fig. 8.9), the condition may give rise to symptoms. In non-smokers the first symptom of silicosis is breathlessness on strenuous exertion (44). It is due to impaired function of the lung which is discussed below. If the exposure is slight, the breathlessness may be so trivial as to be attributed to age or wear-and-tear, but if very heavy, such as occurs during unventilated tunnelling in granite rock or sandblasting without use of protective equipment (37), the breathlessness may develop over a period of months and rapidly become incapacitating. There is every gradation in between. The rapidly progressive illness is called acute silicosis (or acute silicolipoproteinosis). The radiographic appearance is of pulmonary oedema, not nodulation; other features are given above.

In smokers the pattern of breathlessness resembles that in non-smokers but it may be preceded by chronic cough, with or without the production of phlegm (15). The prevalence of cough and phlegm is greater than that associated with smoking alone and is evidence for interaction between the dust and tobacco fumes; this was apparently so for the patient whose case is summarized in fig. 8.8. Interaction between smoking and dust also occurs in other occupations and is discussed in chapter 17.

Irrespective of smoking habits, cough and phlegm are common in the confluent form of silicosis; however, they sometimes indicate the presence of an associated tuberculous infection of the lung. The results of one study in which these factors were investigated is given in table 8.2. The chronic cough and phlegm may be accompanied by the presence of coarse râles and rhonchi in the chest.

Tuberculosis in patients with silicosis may take one of several forms: (a) clinically active

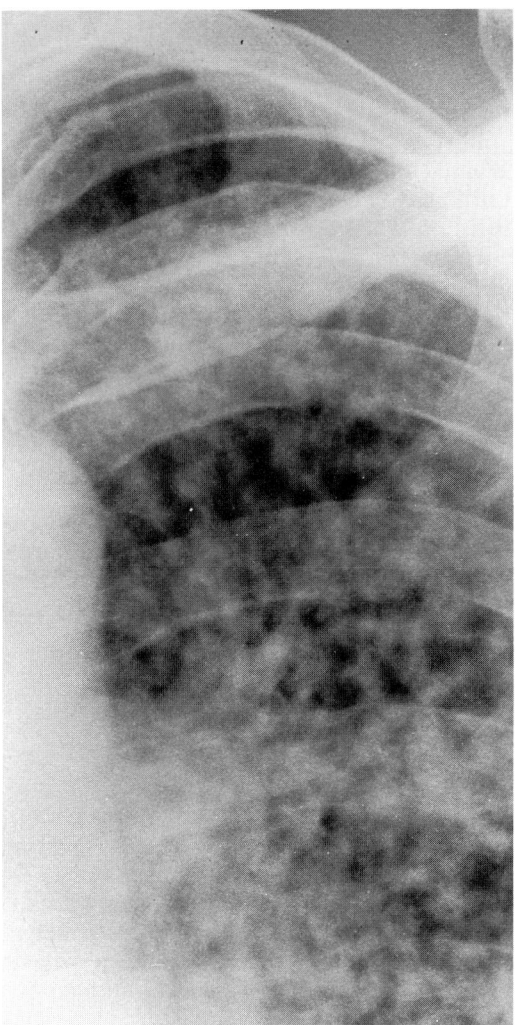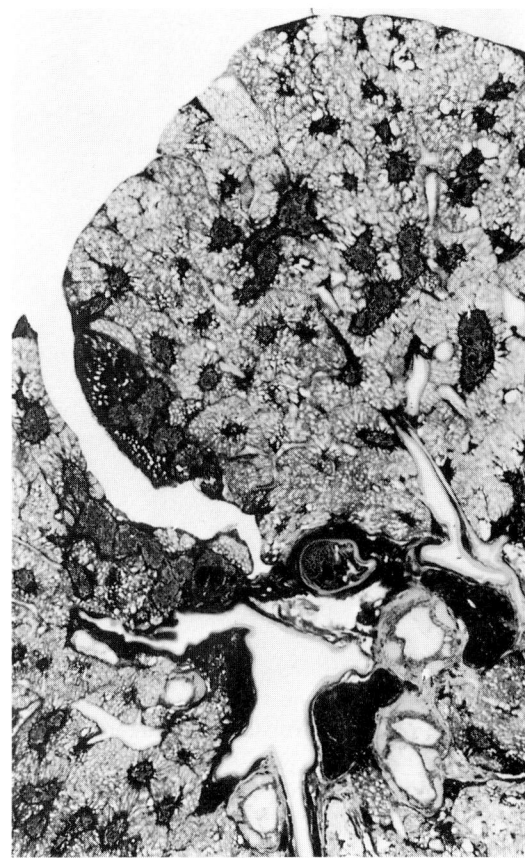

Fig. 8.6. Silicosis in a coalminer. Radiograph of the left upper zone 15 months before death showing pneumoconiosis (category 3r/A) and corresponding area of paper-mounted lung section from a man who worked as a coal miner for 37 years from the age of 23. As well as hewing coal, he spent much time drilling into rock (stone work). Death occurred at age 61 from respiratory and congestive cardiac failure. At postmortem he was found to have nodular and confluent silicosis. The hilar lymph nodes contained coal dust. (By courtesy of J.E.M. Hutchinson.)

acute disease with haemoptysis, positive sputum and symptoms of toxaemia, (b) chronic lesions with or without cavitation visible on the chest radiograph, or (c) quiescent fibrotic lesions (42). Some of the infections are with *M. kansasii* and other opportunist mycobacteria (2) and occur on account of reduced resistance to myco-bacteria. Cavitation of a tuberculous lesion may give rise to copious offensive-smelling sputum but this is not jet black and cannot be confused with melanoptysis from breakdown of a massive lesion of pneumoconiosis of coal workers (page 182). Confluent silicosis rarely cavitates (see below). The nodular form of silicosis may

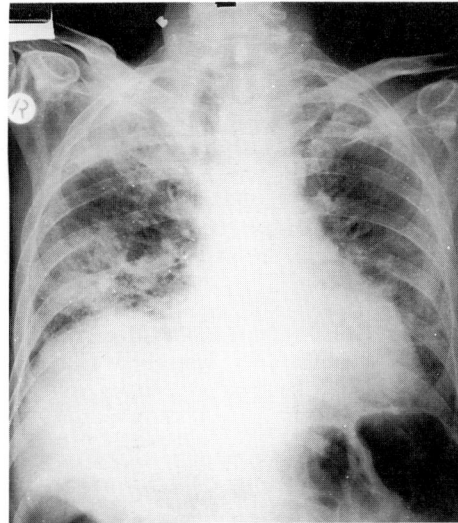

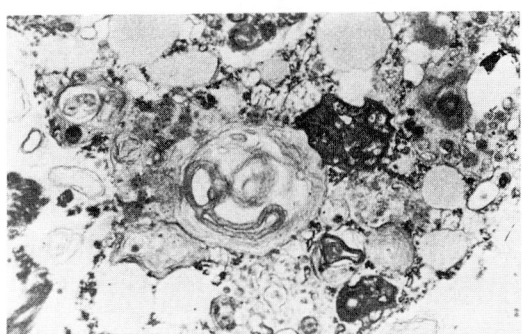

Fig. 8.7. Acute silicolipoproteinosis. The patient spent 7 years milling quartz and developed respiratory symptoms shortly after the introduction of a compressed air supply for cleaning the machines. At that time the chest radiograph showed enlarged hilar shadows and simple silicosis (category 2q). A year later (left), the radiograph exhibited generalized abnormality with shrinkage of the right lung. Death occurred 3 years after the onset of symptoms. At post-mortem the alveoli contained eosinophilic PAS positive exudate which stained with IgM anti-serum. There was proliferation of type 2 pneumocytes, mononuclear cell infiltration and some interstitial fibrosis. The type 2 cells (right) contained weakly osmiophilic lamellar bodies and fragments of silica (top right). (By courtesy of J.M. Xipell (45).)

remain unchanged over many years, especially when it is due to mixed dust from a foundry or coal mine containing a relatively low proportion of free silica (page 149). Alternatively, there may be a progressive increase in profusion of the nodules. Factors which predispose to progression include heavy exposure to quartz or its derivatives (page 145) at a young age, the occurrence of relatively large nodular opacities on the chest x-ray and continuing to work in a contaminated environment after developing simple silicosis (22). The progression may be gradual and fairly uniform or more rapid and patchy when the nodules coalesce to form confluent lesions (fig. 8.9); these become consolidated by extension and shrinkage of the fibrous tissue present in the nodules. The shrinkage causes overstretching of other parts of the lung and predisposes to emphysema; this is then called compensatory emphysema but the aetiology is almost certainly multiple (chapter 17). Fibrosis may also occur round the pleural

surface of the lung and extend into the mediastinum which may itself be distorted by enlargement and fibrosis of lymph glands draining the lung. A rim of hyaline tissue round the glands may then calcify leading to egg-shell calcification which, when it occurs, is a conspicuous feature of the chest radiograph (fig. 8.10). The extension of fibrosis and of compensatory emphysema causes severe disturbance of the function of the lung and of circulation through it. Very often one is surprised by the total absence of abnormal physical signs in the presence of marked radiological abnormality. Alternatively there may be flattening and reduced expansion of the chest usually in the upper zones, tracheal displacement, impaired percussion and harsh or reduced breath sounds over an area of fibrosis. Very occasionally there are inspiratory and expiratory rhonchi in association with compression of a major airway or the supraclavicular lymph glands may be slightly enlarged. Extensive disease causes pro-

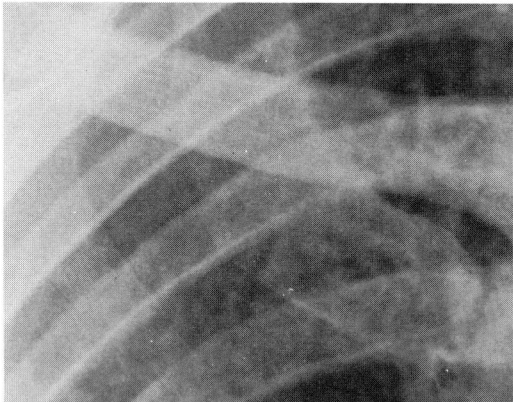

Fig. 8.8. Silicosis. Chest radiographs showing the right upper zone of a man who for 13 years from age 21 was employed in the manufacture of silica bricks. At age 46 he was diagnosed as having simple silicosis (category 3q, top); this progressed to complicated silicosis with apical pleural thickening (lower left) which subsequently contracted (lower right). By this time the patient was aged 61 and had discontinued smoking, was breathless on mild exertion (grade 4), had a chronic productive cough and wheezed on most nights. The FEV_1 was 1.8 l (expected 2.88 l) with an 11% improvement after salbutamol. The total lung capacity and transfer factor were reduced by approximately 20% compared with the reference values.

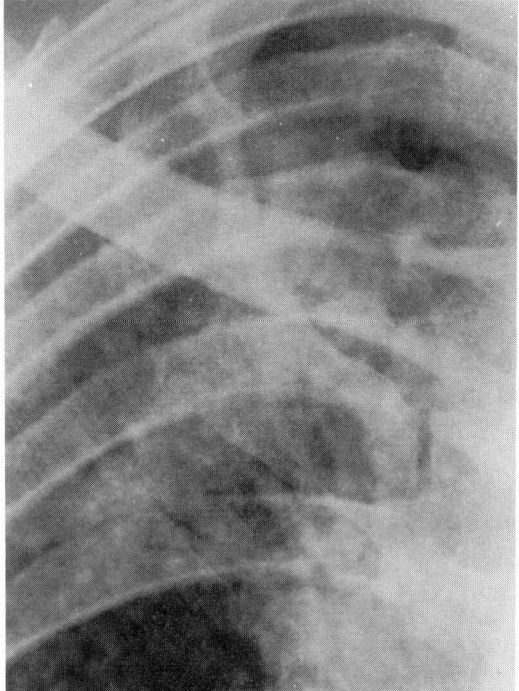

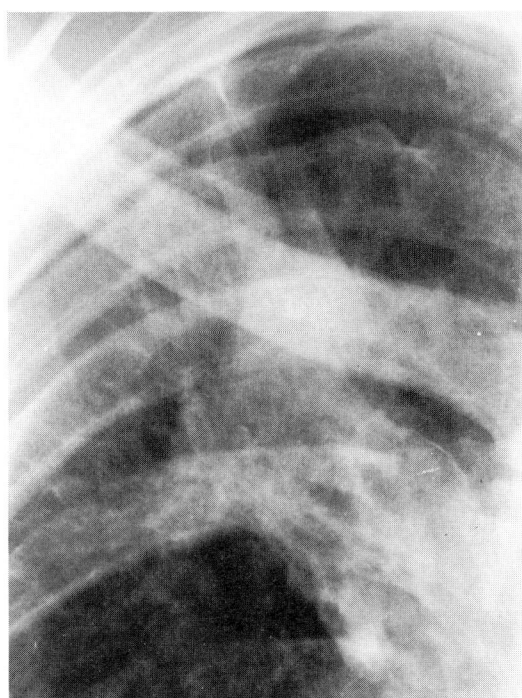

gressively increasing breathlessness on exertion and recurrent chest infections, both chronic and acute; the loss of pulmonary vascular bed leads to pulmonary hypertension and sometimes to right ventricular failure. The disturbance of pulmonary function causes hypoxaemia and this affects the function of every organ and metabolically active tissue in the body, including the conducting tissue of the heart. Thus, whilst death may be due primarily to the changes in the lung, it often occurs peacefully from unheralded cardiac arrest. However, most men with silicosis

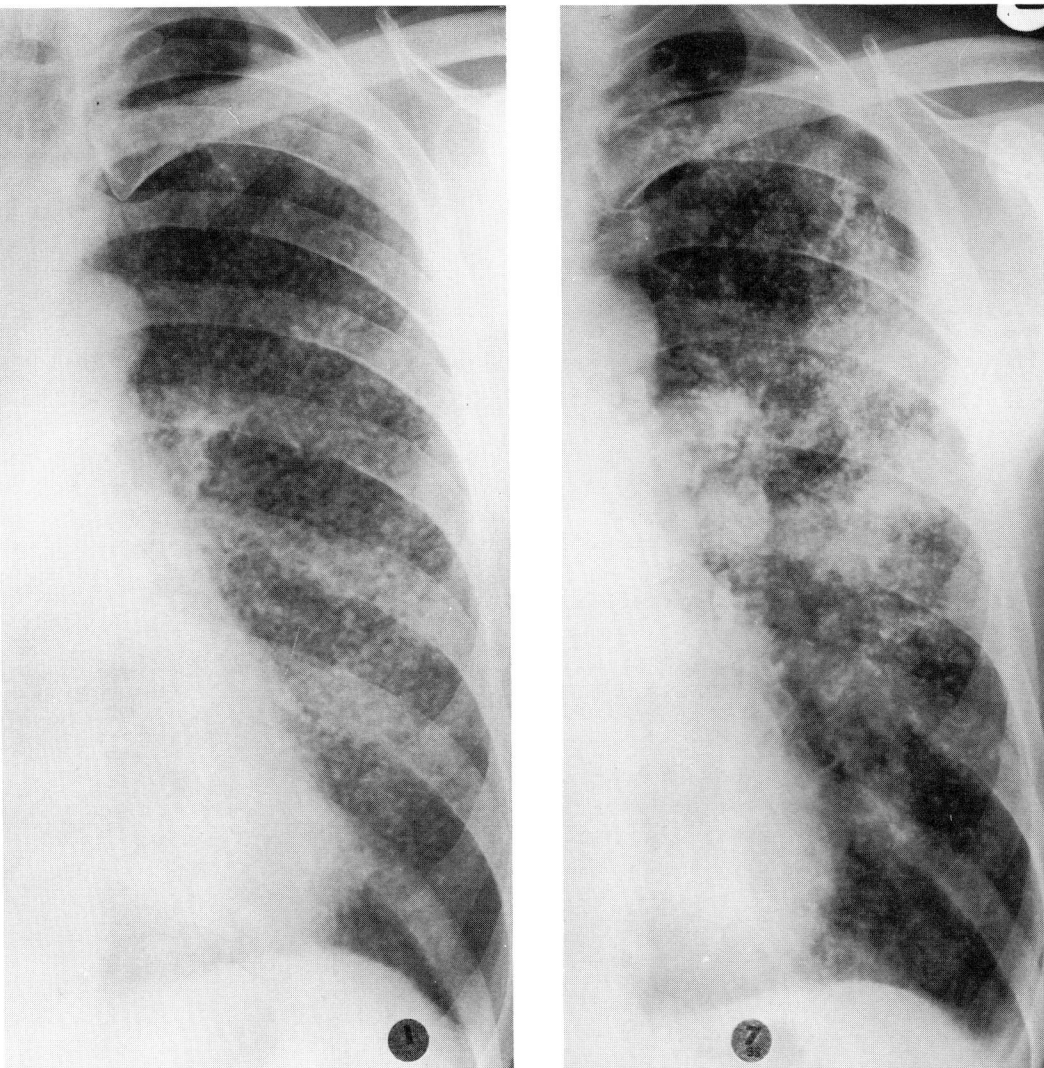

Fig. 8.9. Progression of silicosis. Radiographs showing the left lung of a man who from the age of 14 was milling and cutting silica bricks. By age 38 years (left) he had advanced simple silicosis (category 3r) and the disease progressed despite his giving up work. At age 46 there was extensive massive silicosis (right) and death occurred 5 years later. The large lung section showed confluent lesions, interspersed with cystic spaces (fig. 8.5). (By courtesy of J. E. M. Hutchinson.)

Table 8.2. Prevalence of chronic respiratory symptoms amongst North Wales slate workers and other men from the same community. (Reproduced from Glover *et al.* (15) with permission.)

	Exposed (n=547)		Non-exposed (n=402)	
	Smokers	Non-smokers	Smokers	Non-smokers
Mean age (years)	45.5	47.1	48.0	43.5
Prevalence (%)				
Cough	39 CXR	19 tb	27 a	5
Phlegm	30 CXR	17 tb	20	4
Dyspnoea	18 CXR, a	17	12 a	4

CXR = significant association with x-ray category; a = significant association with age; tb = high prevalence associated with evidence for previous tuberculosis.

die from unrelated causes, including ischaemic heart disease and carcinoma of the lung (7) for both of which the main risk factor is smoking. The inhalation of silica dust does not contribute to malignancy. However, carcinoma of the lung occurs amongst miners and quarry men who are exposed to radon 222 (page 254). This gas is formed during the radioactive decay of uranium 235 and is present in significant quantities in uranium mines. It also occurs in some predominantly granite rock which is mined for other minerals, including haematite in Cumbria, tin in Cornwall, fluorspar in Newfoundland and zinc, lead and silver in Sweden. It is only in these circumstances that silicosis may be complicated by an increased incidence of lung cancer. Work with granite is not a cause of peptic ulceration, but there is an association with rheumatoid arthritis (see rheumatoid silicosis above). The actively progressive form of silicosis is rarely, but significantly frequently, accompanied by clinical collagen vascular disease, including scleroderma and systemic lupus erythematosis (page 148).

Radiographic appearances

Silicosis typically presents as diffuse small round opacities in the outer half of the upper zone of both lung fields, usually the right before the left (e.g. fig. 8.8). The opacities are initially soft and difficult to distinguish from the background; they become more contrasting with passage of time and may subsequently calcify (fig. 8.11). Their diameter is usually in the range

2–6mm which is type q of the international classification (chapter 5). With continuing exposure the number and distribution of opacities may extend to include all rib spaces. The size of the individual nodules may also increase (category q becomes category r, fig. 8.12). In addition the opacities may coalesce to form conglomerate lesions almost always bilateral: these differ from those in typical progressive massive fibrosis in retaining initially their discrete nodular character (fig. 8.9). At this stage pleural thickening at the apices or upper zones is common (fig. 8.8), there may be a reduction in lung size and compensatory emphysema may be conspicuous (fig. 8.9). Pneumothorax may occur as a complication. Enlarged lymph glands may be present in the hilum or mediastinum and there may be distortion or narrowing of the trachea. The glands may exhibit egg shell calcification (fig. 8.10). The calcification usually occurs subsequent to the pulmonary lesions but may precede them. Tuberculosis, sarcoidosis and histoplasmosis may produce similar appearances but in contrast to most cases of silicosis these may progress rapidly; they may also regress. The diagnosis of silicosis is usually made radiographically but depends on establishing that appropriate exposure to silica has occurred. Rarely silicosis presents as a single massive lesion (silicoma). However, a unilateral mass should be regarded as bronchial carcinoma until this is disproved. There may be complicating tuberculosis for which there will usually be clinical or bacteriological evidence. The radiographic features may then include rapid appear-

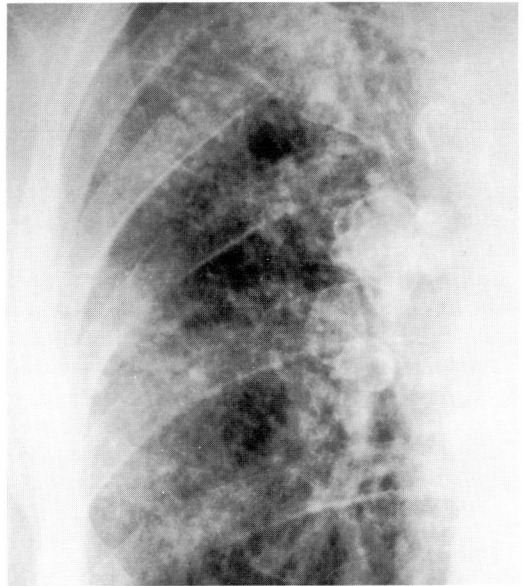
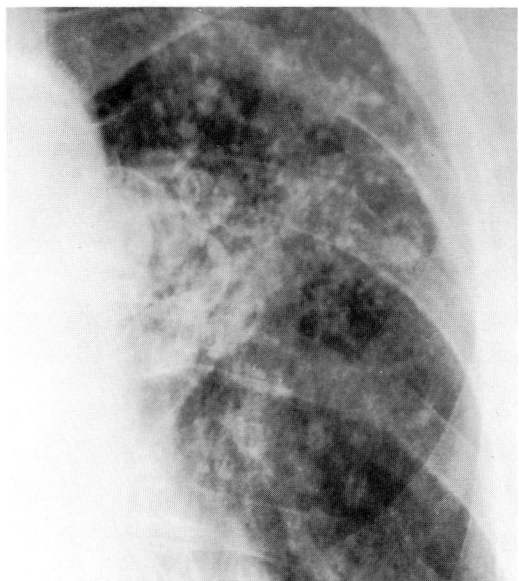

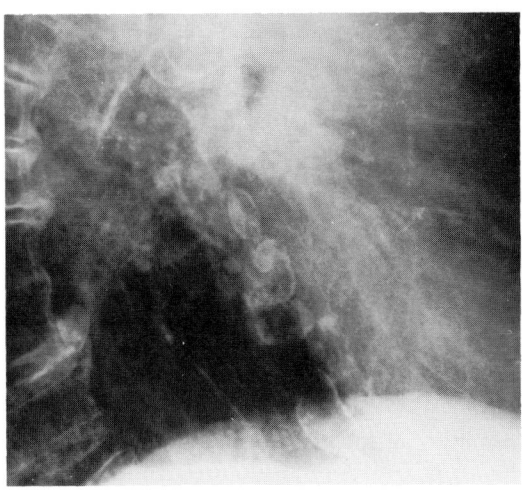

Fig. 8.10. Chest radiographs showing egg shell calcification associated with complicated silicosis in a man who for 30 years worked as a metal dresser. He had only minor respiratory symptoms. (By courtesy of G. L. Leathart.)

ance of new infiltrates, especially in the upper zones, progression out of proportion to the exposure, and coalescence of nodules or formation of discrete massive lesions which may cavitate. These masses, unlike PMF do not extend across interlobar fissures and the cavities have an irregularly shaped inner wall (42). Pleural effusion may accompany tuberculosis and there may be bronchial narrowing or stenosis.

Lung function

Simple silicosis, unlike pneumoconiosis of coalworkers, is associated with impaired ventilatory function of the lung. Except in advanced disease the degree of impairment is usually small and detectable only in population studies or longitudinal studies of individuals, not from laboratory assessments made on a single occasion (e.g. fig. 8.11). Thus, amongst North Wales slate

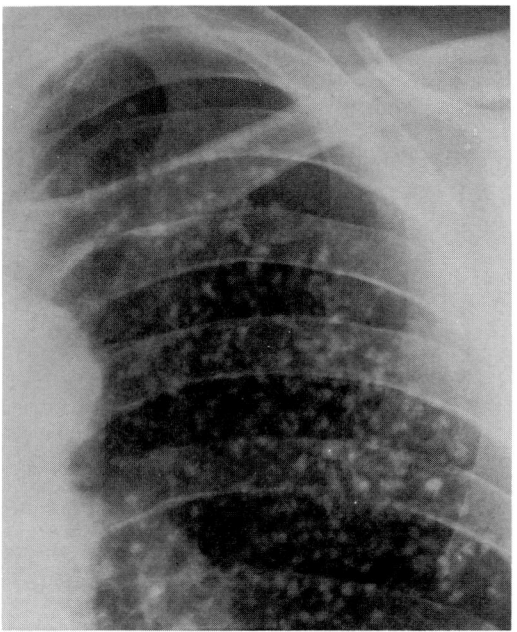

Fig. 8.11. Radiograph of left upper zone showing calcified simple silicosis (category 3q) in a man aged 51 who for 14 years worked as a tunneller through hard rock on hydro-electric schemes and to open up new coal faces. He was breathless on mild exertion (grade 4) despite a normal FEV$_1$ (2.78 l compared with 3.07 l predicted). The breathlessness was associated with an enlarged physiological deadspace and reduced transfer factor and Kco (both approximately 65% of predicted). The patient subsequently developed scleroderma.

workers the forced expiratory volume and vital capacity were on average reduced respectively by 0.24 l and 0.3 l per radiological category of simple silicosis (15). The reductions were larger in lifetime non-smokers than in current smokers, possibly as a consequence of some smokers who experienced breathlessness becoming ex-smokers. There was no additional impairment associated with years of working with slate. Studies of Vermont granite workers have come to a less certain conclusion, possibly on account of the poor technical quality of some of the measurements (16). The ventilatory impairment may be unevenly distributed through the lung, leading to a fall in arterial

oxygen tension and increased physiological deadspace during exercise. Other changes are uncommon, gas mixing, lung compliance and the transfer factor for carbon monoxide having all been reported as normal in simple silicosis. But, in conglomerate disease with B or C shadows on the chest radiograph, all these indices are usually abnormal (4). The features may then be primarily of an obstructive type or of a restrictive type, with or without impaired function of the lung parenchyma (25, see also fig. 8.8). In acute silicosis and in acute silicolipoproteinosis, there is more marked impairment of function, including a reduced transfer factor. In the late stages of silicosis, there is gross impairment of all aspects of lung function and notable disablement.

Treatment of silicosis

Fibrous tissue formed in response to silica cannot be dissolved away so to this extent there is no specific treatment. Attempts have been made to modify the process of fibrogenesis but without much success. Greater success has been achieved in ameliorating the effects of silicosis and in managing acute silicosis. The fibrogenic action of silica can be modified by the presence of non-fibrogenic dusts of which coal and haematite are naturally occurring examples (page 148). Fibrogenesis is also affected by metallic aluminium powder and by polyvinyl pyridine-N-oxide (PVPNO) and related compounds, including poly-2-vinyl pyridine-1-oxide which is reputedly less toxic. These substances in effect coat the silica particles and reduce the solubility of the surface layer. They have been found to confer protection against silicosis in most animal studies. Aluminium dust is used as a prophylactic measure in Canada but whilst benefit has been claimed no controlled trial has been conducted. Aluminium therapy was assessed by Kennedy. In a controlled study he found no significant benefit compared with dummy treatment which itself had a placebo effect (26). The toxicity of quartz particles for macrophages is reduced by coating them with serum protein but no way has yet been found for harnessing this action therapeutically. Thus specific treatment at the time of exposure to

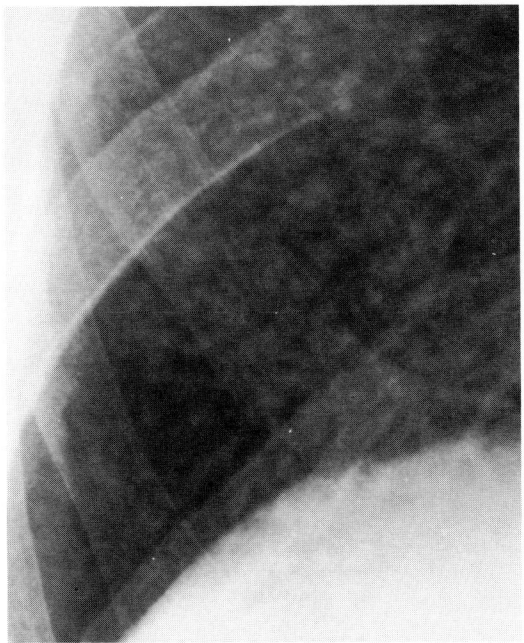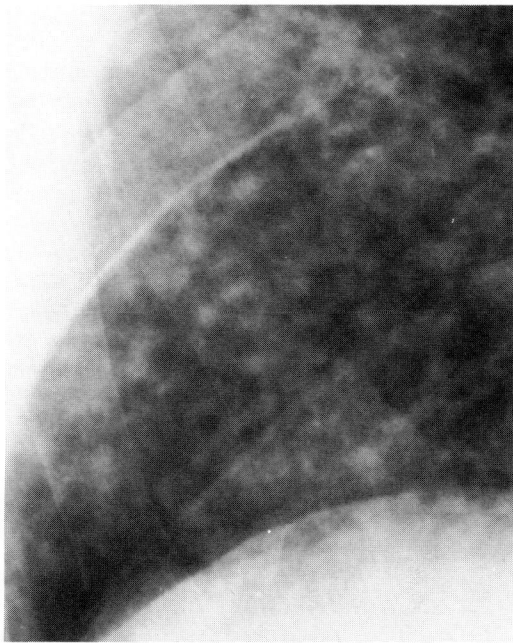

Fig. 8.12. Radiographs showing the right lower zone of a man who for 5 years from age 20 was grinding fire bricks. At age 36 years he was diagnosed as having simple pneumoconiosis, category 2q (left); over the next 13 years the condition progressed to category 3r (right). At this time, despite having abandoned smoking 11 years earlier he was breathless on moderate exertion (grade 3), had a chronic productive cough and wheezed on most nights. The FEV$_1$ was 1.4 l (expected 3.1 l) and increased by 19% after salbutamol. The transfer factor was 49% of predicted but hypoxaemia was not observed during exercise. The clinical diagnosis was silicosis and chronic bronchitis.

silica is not yet possible. The subsequent laying down of fibrous tissue might theoretically be inhibited by substances which prevent cross linkages developing within tropocollagen molecules. One such substance is β-aminoproprionitrile which has been shown to be effective in acute experiments in rats. However, the substance cannot be given over the whole period of exposure to silica and does not affect mature collagen.

The absence of specific treatment for silicosis places a great responsibility on the physician to explain, to generate and maintain hope, to prevent complications and to ensure that the affected person makes full use of his residual lung function. This is usually an easy task since most instances of silicosis of the nodular type are only slowly if at all progressive and are accompanied by only moderate breathlessness on exertion. Confluent silicosis is more serious. The management is then as for progressive massive fibrosis in coalworkers (chapter 9) and for chronic respiratory disease generally (chapter 19). Silico-tuberculosis is treated by antitubercular chemotherapy with isoniazid, rifampicin, ethambutol and pyrazinamide. A successful outcome can be expected even when the organisms are resistant to one or more of the drugs. Acute silicosis should be treated by repeated bronchopulmonary lavage (12), with steroid therapy to suppress the inflammatory reaction. Cardiopulmonary transplantation can be performed as a last resort.

Epidemiology

The prevalence of silicosis in the U.K. has fallen steadily since the condition became certifiable

60 years ago (e.g. 19). Before that the prevalence in some occupations had approached 100%; this was the case for knife grinders in Sheffield and men who built the railway through the Pennines. Even in the decade 1971–80, amongst a representative sample of 725 North Wales slate workers, 10% had simple pneumoconiosis categories 2 or 3 (15). In the U.S.A. in 1954 the prevalence amongst mill workers processing diatomite, who were exposed to cristobalite, was 48%; some of these men had progressive massive fibrosis (10). High prevalences were also observed amongst foundry workers and some men may still be at risk at the present time (27). The problem is world wide. For example, quite recently amongst unselected Nigerian grindstone cutters, the prevalence was 40% (44) and amongst Indian stonecutters and slate pencil workers it was respectively 35% and 56% (18, 23). A few years earlier silicosis was reported amongst Bedouins living in the desert (3) and a 10% prevalence from grinding mealie flour between stones was observed at pre-employment examination amongst nursing applicants in Transkei (33).

The individual *dose–response relationship* appears to be linear with silicosis developing within a few months or over a lifetime depending on the environmental exposure. Thus the relationship for North Wales slate workers (15) was of the form:

$$\text{x-ray category} = A \times \text{years worked} + 0.021 \text{ Age} - 0.85 \text{ SD } 0.87$$

where A varied from 0.224 for underground miners to zero for general and office workers; one practical implication is illustrated in fig. 8.13. The corresponding relationship for breathlessness is given in fig. 8.14. In this study x-ray category, unlike chronic cough and phlegm, showed no significant association with smoking. The proportion of quartz in the respirable dust was in the range 11–32%. Amongst U.K. foundry men exposed to mixed dust containing on average 10–15% quartz, the relationship to

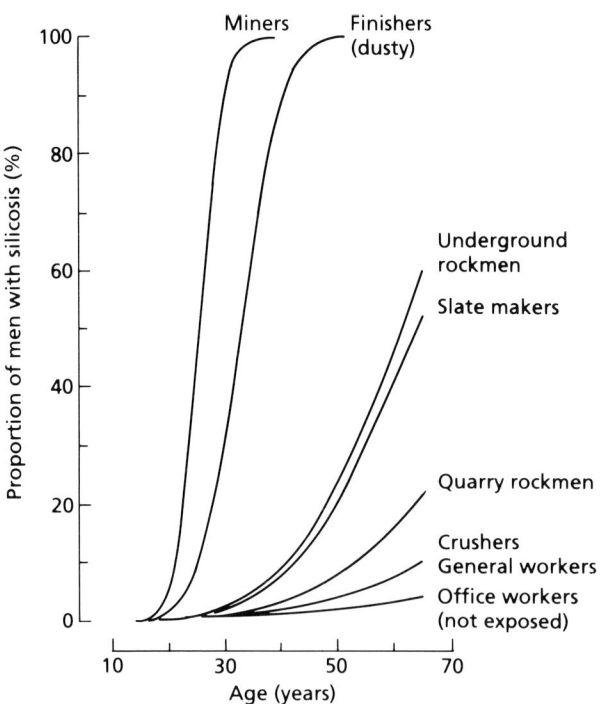

Fig. 8.13. Estimated proportion of slate workers with simple silicosis (x-ray category ⩾2) by occupation and age, if employment started at age 15. (By courtesy of J.R. Glover and colleagues (15); the results were analysed by Oldham.)

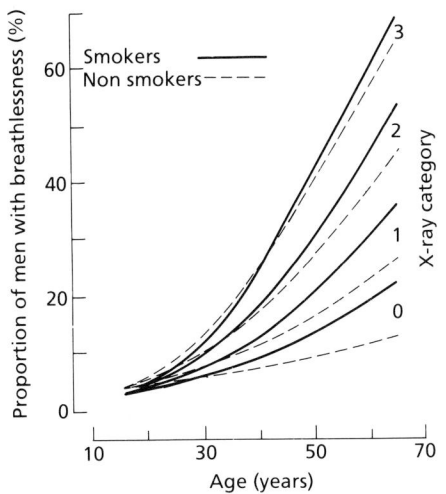

Fig. 8.14. Estimated prevalence of breathlessness (grade 2 or more) in slate workers, by age, smoking habit and category of simple silicosis at age 65, after working in the industry from age 15. (By courtesy of J.R. Glover and colleagues (15); the results were analysed by Oldham.)

gression and conglomeration can occur after exposure has ceased (figs. 8.8 and 8.12). Suggestions that susceptibility may differ between families or between ethnic groups do not appear to be based on hard evidence; the occupational exposure and the possible coexistence of tuberculosis, which may differ between groups, need to be taken into account in future studies. There does not appear to be any association with immunological status, which does not contribute even when abnormal (22), however, rheumatoid arthritis predisposes (page 150). Progression is influenced by the presence of haematite, coal, iron and other substances (fig. 8.2); this is discussed under the biological action of silica above. The interactions between coal and quartz dust in their effects on lung tissue are complex and merit further investigation.

Preventing silicosis

The potentially devastating nature of silicosis and the absence of specific treatment place a great responsibility on those concerned with prevention. This is primarily by recognizing the hazard and practising good occupational hygiene, including substitution by safer materials and removal of dust at source. Some examples of substitution are given in table 8.3 and methods of dust suppression are described in chapter 3. Dust control measures should be directed to keeping the concentration of silica in the inspired air below the threshold limit values (table 8.4). The effectiveness of control should

exposure was fairly similar but the prevalence was less (27). This is shown in fig. 8.15.

Progression of silicosis occurs by an increase in profusion of small opacities, enlargement in the size of opacities, (p or q opacities become r) and conglomeration leading to massive lesions. These changes are most likely if the onset is at a relatively young age and the exposure continues subsequently (e.g. fig. 8.7, page 153), but pro-

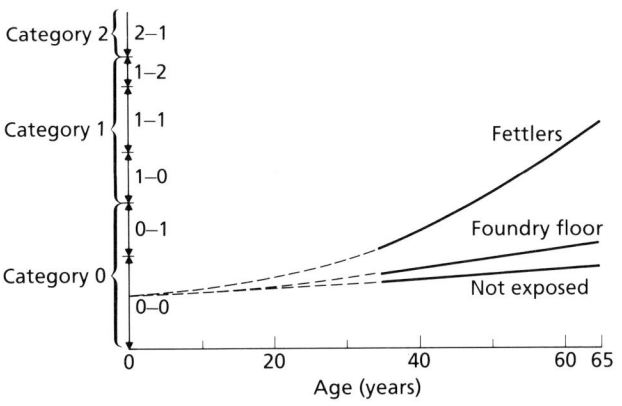

Fig. 8.15. Average category of simple pneumoconiosis (ILO 1958) in foundry workers by age and occupation. For purposes of calculation the categories were converted into a numerical score. (Data of T.A. Lloyd Davies (27); the results were analysed by Oldham.)

Table 8.3. Examples of substitution of quartz by other substances in industry (see also Table 8.1)

Industry	Process or substance	Initial use	Replacement
Metallurgy	Grinding, polishing	Sandstone, quartz abrasives	Carborundum, other abrasives
Coalmining	Dusting roadways	Shale dust	Gypsum, etc. (page 167)
Potteries	Biscuit firing	Powdered flint (36)	Calcined alumina
Foundries	Pattern making, parting powder	Sand and clay, quartz dust	Resins, etc. (page 368), zircon and other dusts
Ceramics	As body and for glazes	Flint, sand, china clay, feldspar	Wollastonite, synthetic calcium metasilicate

Table 8.4. Exposure limits for dusts which may contain SiO_2 and related compounds

Substance	Respirable dust (mg m^{-3})	Total dust (mg m^{-3})
Silicon tetra hydride (silane)*	7	—
Non-siliceous dust <1% quartz*†	5.0	10
Talc (also mica)*	1.0	10
Diatomaceous earth (natural)*	1.5	—
Amorphous silica	1.0	6.0
Quartz and fused silica	0.1	0.3
Cristobalite and tridymite	0.05	0.15

* Time weighted average over 8h shift.

† For respirable mixed dust the TLV is given by: 10/(% respirable quartz + 2) mg m^{-3}.

be monitored by regular dust sampling (chapter 2). Where this shows the presence of some airborne silica within the hygiene standard, the dust monitoring should be supplemented by biological monitoring which, in this instance, should be by serial chest radiography; the interval between x-rays should normally be 5 years but shorter in high risk situations. The films should be read both clinically and epidemiologically to provide information on individuals and on the group (chapter 5). There is no strong case for also undertaking screening by assessment of lung function (except to obtain 'base-line' values) since the respiratory impairment appears not to precede the radiological abnormality (15). However, a lung function assessment should be carried out on persons with radiological silicosis (category 1 or above) as part of the clinical evaluation. In addition, where sufficient dust suppression is unrealistic, clean air may be supplied to the operatives,

either in cabins or personally by one of the methods described in chapter 3. Any respirators should be appropriate in design and fitting, should be worn regularly and be regularly serviced. The casual use of such equipment (e.g. 37) is inexcusable. Proper care and attention, including observance of the threshold limit value should lead to further reductions in prevalence of silicosis but, given the nature of man's environment, occasional new cases are almost certain to occur. These would be prevented if prior to using any crushed mineral for the first time the silica content of the dust was ascertained.

References

1 Allison AC., Effects of silica and asbestos on cells in culture. *Inhaled Particles III* 1971:437–42. Walton WH (ed). Woking: Unwin.

2 Bailey WC, Brown M, Buechner HA, Weill H, Ichinose H, Ziskind M. Silico-mycobacterial disease in sandblasters. *Am Rev Respir Dis* 1974;**110**:115–25.

3 Bar-Ziv J, Goldberg GM. Simple siliceous pneumoconiosis in Negev Bedouins. *Arch Environm Hlth* 1974;**29**:121–6.

4 Becklake MR, Du Preez L, Lutz W. Lung function in silicosis of the Witwaterstrand goldminer. *Am Rev Tuberc Pulm Dis* 1958; **77**: 400–12.

5 Bendz G, Lindqvist I. (Eds). *Biochemistry of Silicon and Related Problems*. Nobel Symposium 40. New York: Plenum Press, 1978.

6 Caplan A. Pneumoconiosis on the Kolar gold field. In: Institution of Mining Engineers. *Silicosis Pneumoconiosis and Dust Suppression in Mines: Proceedings of a Conference held in London, April 1947*. London. 1947:33–67.

7 Chatgidakis CB. Silicosis in South African white gold miners. *Med Proc* 1963;**9**:383–92.

8 Christman JW, Emerson RJ, Graham WGB, Davis GS. Mineral dust and cell recovery from the bronchoalveolar lavage of healthy Vermont granite workers. *Am Rev Respir Dis* 1985; **132**:393–9.

9 Clark TC, Harrington VA, Asta J, Morgan WKC, Sargent EN. Respiratory effects of exposure to dust in taconite mining and processing. *Am Rev Respir Dis* 1980;**121**:959–66.

10 Cooper WC, Jacobson G. A 21-year radiographic follow-up of workers in the diatomite industry. *J Occup Med* 1977;**19**:563–6.

11 Corrin B, King E. Pathogenesis of experimental pulmonary alveolar proteinosis. *Thorax* 1970;**25**:230–6.

12 Costello JF, Moriarty DC, Branthwaite MA, Turner-Warwick M, Corrin B. Diagnosis and management of alveolar proteinosis: the role of electron microscopy. *Thorax* 1975;**30**:121–32.

13 Dutra FR. Diatomaceous earth pneumoconiosis. *Arch Environm Hlth* 1965;**11**:613–9.

14 Friberg L, Ohman H. Silicosis hazards in enamelling. A medical, technical and experimental study. *Br J Industr Med* 1957;**14**:85–91.

15 Glover JR, Bevan C, Cotes JE, Elwood PC, Hodges NG, Kell RL, Lowe CR, McDermott M, Oldham PD. Effects of exposure to slate dust in North Wales. *Br J Industr Med* 1980;**37**:152–62.

16 Graham WGB, O'Grady RV, Dubuc B. Pulmonary function loss in Vermont granite workers. *Am Rev Respir Dis* 1981;**123**:25–8.

17 Grundorfer W, Raber A. Progressive silicosis in granite workers. *Br J Industr Med* 1970; **27**: 110–20.

18 Gupta SP, Bajaj A, Jain AL, Vasudeva YL. Clinical and radiological studies in silicosis: based on a study of the disease amongst stone-cutters. *Ind J Med Res* 1972;**60**:1309–15.

19 Hale LW, Sheers G. Silicosis in West Country granite workers. *Br J Industr Med* 1963;**20**: 218–25.

20 Heppleston AG. The disposal of dust in the lungs of silicotic rats. *Am J Path* 1962;**40**: 493–506.

21 Heppleston AG. Silicotic fibrogenesis: a concept of pulmonary fibrosis. *Ann Occup Hyg* 1982;**26**:449–62.

22 Hughes JM, Jones RN, Gilson JC, Hammad YY, Samimi B, Hendrick DJ, Turner-Warwick M, Doll NJ, Weill H. Determinants of progression in sandblasters' silicosis. *Ann Occup Hyg* 1982;**26**:701–12.

23 Jain SM, Sepaha GC, Khare KC, Dubey VS. Silicosis in slate pencil workers: a clinico-radiologic study. *Chest* 1977;**71**:423–6.

24 Jones RN, Turner-Warwick M, Ziskind M, Weill H. High prevalence of antinuclear antibodies in sandblasters' silicosis. *Am Rev Respir Dis* 1976;**113**:393–5.

25 Jones RN, Weill H, Ziskind M. Pulmonary function in sandblasters' silicosis. *Bull Eur Physiopath Respir* 1975;**11**:589–95.

26 Kennedy MCS. Aluminium powder inhalations in the treatment of silicosis of pottery workers and pneumoconiosis of coalworkers. *Br J Industr Med* 1956;**13**:85–101.

27 Lloyd Davies TA. *Respiratory disease in foundary men. Report of a survey*. London: HMSO. 1971.

28 Lloyd Davies TA, Doig AT, Fox AJ, Greenberg M. A radiographic survey of monumental masonry workers in Aberdeen. *Br J Industr Med* 1973;**30**:227–31.

29 Lowrie DB. What goes wrong with the macrophage in silicosis? *Eur J Respir Dis* 1982; **63**:180–2.

30 Munizago J, Allison MJ, Gerszten E, Klurfeld DM. Pneumoconiosis in Chilean miners of the 16th century. *Bull NY Acad Med* 1975; **51**:1281–93.

31 Nagelschmidt G. The relation between lung dust and lung pathology in pneumoconiosis. *Br J Industr Med* 1960;**17**:247–59.

32 Oudiz J, Brown JW, Ayer HE, Samuels S. A report on silica exposure levels in United States foundries. *Am Ind Hyg Assoc J* 1983;**44**:374–6.

33 Palmer PE, Daynes G. Transkei silicosis. *S African Med J* 1967;**41**:1182–8.

34 Phibbs BP, Sundin RE, Mitchell RS. Silicosis in

Wyoming bentonite workers. *Am Rev Respir Dis* 1971;**103**:1–17.

35 Posner E. Pneumoconiosis in makers of artificial grinding wheels including a case of Caplan's syndrome. *Br J Industr Med* 1960; **17**: 109–13.

36 Posner E, Kennedy MCS. A further study of china biscuit placers in Stoke-on-Trent. *Br J Industr Med* 1967;**24**:133–42.

37 Samimi B, Weill H, Ziskind M. Respirable silica dust exposure of sandblasters and associated workers in steel fabrication yards. *Arch Environm Hlth* 1974;**29**:61–6.

38 Schuyler M, Ziskind M, Salvaggio J. Cell-mediated immunity in silicosis. *Am Rev Respir Dis* 1977;**116**:147–51.

39 Seaton A, Lamb D, Brown WR, Sclare G, Middleton WG. Pneumoconiosis of shale miners. *Thorax* 1981;**36**:412–8.

40 Seaton A, Ruckley VA, Addison J, Brown WR.

Silicosis in barium miners. *Thorax* 1986; **41**:591–5.

41 Sluis-Cremer GK, Hessel PA, Hnizdo E, Churchill AR. Relationship between silicosis and rheumatoid arthritis. *Thorax* 1986;**41**:596–601.

42 Snider DE, Jr. The relationship between tuberculosis and silicosis. *Am Rev Respir Dis* 1978;**118**:455–60.

43 Vitums VC, Edwards MJ, Niles NR, Borman JO, Lowry RD. Pulmonary fibrosis from amorphous silica dust: a product of silica vapour. *Arch Environm Hlth* 1977;**32**:62–8.

44 Warrell DA, Harrison BDW, Fawcett IW, Mohammed Y, Mohammed WS, Pope HM, Watkins BJ. Silicosis among grindstone cutters in the north of Nigeria. *Thorax* 1975;**30**:389–98.

45 Xipell JM, Ham KN, Price CG, Thomas DP. Acute silicolipoproteinosis. *Thorax* 1977; **32**: 104–11.

Chapter 9
Pneumoconiosis of Coalworkers and Related Occupations

Historical perspective
Coal mining
Tissue responses to coal dust
Chest illness, respiratory impairment and disablement in coal workers;
  does dust-related emphysema contribute?
Epidemiological studies
Safe conditions at work
Industrial Injuries Benefit

Historical perspective

Surface coal from outcrops and shallow drift mines has been used as fuel since the 9th century: deep mining became possible in the 18th century when mechanical pumps were developed which could be used to control flooding. Coal then replaced water as the source of energy which powered the first industrial revolution. In 1806 Laennec recognized a disease in the lungs of coalminers which he described as melanosis. A few years later Bayle reported that this form of phthisis gave rise to few symptoms and was compatible with life to an advanced age. Stratton in 1838 observed that anthrocosis could exist without any chest symptoms whatever. Subsequently, coalminers were observed to have a below average prevalence of tuberculosis and a trip down a mine was even recommended as a contribution to treatment! Meanwhile, in 1919 in the U.K., silicosis became a certifiable disease and the resulting scrutiny of applicants led to the recognition of much pulmonary abnormality amongst coalminers. Not long afterwards the advent of mechanization greatly increased the levels of dustiness.

In 1937, at the request of the Home Office to the Medical Research Council, Hart and Aslett investigated the respiratory health of South Wales coal miners; the ensuing report led in 1945 to the setting up of the MRC Pneumoconiosis Research Unit in South Wales. There followed a distinguished series of studies of individual cases in the laboratory, and of the distribution and effects of disease in coal mining communities. The latter were initiated by the MRC and expanded by the National Coal Board. Subsequently similar methods were applied in the U.S.A. The studies illuminated the nature and natural history of coalworkers' pneumoconiosis and laid the foundations for environmental monitoring and establishment of safe working conditions. In the process, the Pneumoconiosis Unit introduced new techniques and concepts which revolutionized occupational medicine, contributed to the formation of community medicine and helped to establish the double blind controlled trial as an accepted means for assessing the efficacy of any defined medical treatment. This work was done at a time when pneumoconiosis affected up to 70% of elderly miners in South Wales with a correspondingly high morbidity and mortality. Now, 30 years later, simple pneumoconiosis seldom occurs before age 45 years, morbidity from progressive massive fibrosis is infrequent and early death is largely a thing of the past. However, coalminers still incur more chest illness than most occupational groups: the reasons for this are considered below.

Coal mining

Formation and composition of coal

Coal is predominantly carbon which was formed by decomposition and compression of forest trees and related vegetation. Thus, although extracted by mining, coal is not strictly mineral since it is not of inorganic origin. The coal occurs in strata of varying thickness and purity, reflecting the length of time during which trees grew and were renewed and the nature, depth and duration of the subsequent covering with sedimentary deposits. The latter include sandstone from fragmented quartz, clay, shale from degradation of older quartz-bearing rock and limestone from the skeletons and shells of aquatic animals. The coal may rest on a bed of quartz or other mineral and this may have become intermingled with the coal as a result of movement of the earth's crust.

The first precursor of coal is peat which initially contains recognizable plant debris, also fungi, bacterial spores and other plant products. Dry peat contains a high proportion of organic substances, including amino acids, fats and carbohydrates; some of these may subsequently become oil or natural gas. The remainder may undergo progressive degradation with loss of molecules of oxygen and hydrogen. As a result the purest coal (anthracite) is approximately 92–94% carbon with a very low content of volatile substances. Bituminous coal contains up to 92% carbon, whilst in peat and lignite the carbon content is between 54% and 75% (table 9.1). A coal which is low in volatiles and high in carbon is said to be of high rank whereas a low rank coal is high in volatiles. In the past a high rank was associated with a high prevalence of pneumoconiosis. This was because the mining of high rank coal produced more airborne respir-

able dust and because the dust was cleared from the lung more slowly than in the case of bituminous coal. The association of pneumoconiosis with rank of coal is unrelated to the silica content which is relatively low in high rank coal (table 9.1); it is not related to the content of other minerals such as iron oxide, mica and clay. Silica is often present in high concentration in neighbouring strata and becomes airborne during the driving of roadways and in other types of 'stonework' underground.

Extraction

Coal seams were first exploited on a large scale in the U.K. but the U.S.A., Australia, South Africa, U.S.S.R. and Poland are now major exporters, much of their coal coming from big deposits in which the seams are 4–24m in height and large-scale extraction and opencast methods are used. In the older British coal mines, the majority of seams are 0.5–1.0m in thickness at a depth of 200–1000m. They are usually mined by the long wall and reverse face methods which are illustrated in fig. 9.1. The face is usually 150–300m in length. The coal is dislodged by undercutting, using cutting machines (engines) which are usually controlled by two men but may run automatically. The coal is then freed by controlled blasting (shot firing). Alternatively the engine may drive a toothed drum which

Table 9.1. Comparison of composition of lung and coalface dust for men with pneumoconiosis (data of Bergman & Casswell (3))

Coalface	South Wales		North-east England	Yorks.	East Midlands
Type of coal	Anthracite	Steam		Bituminous	
Rank of coal* (%)	92	90	88	86	83
No. of lungs	58	52	36	34	24
Dust retention† (dg/yr)	9.4	6.4	7.5	5.7	4.2
Dust composition†					
Coal (%)	83	76	74	50	38
Quartz (%)	2.2	3.8	4.6	9.7	12.4
Quartz (% of total mineral‡)	14	15	17	19	20

* % carbon in dry mineral-free coal.
† Significant correlation with rank of coal.
‡ % quartz in non-combustible residue.

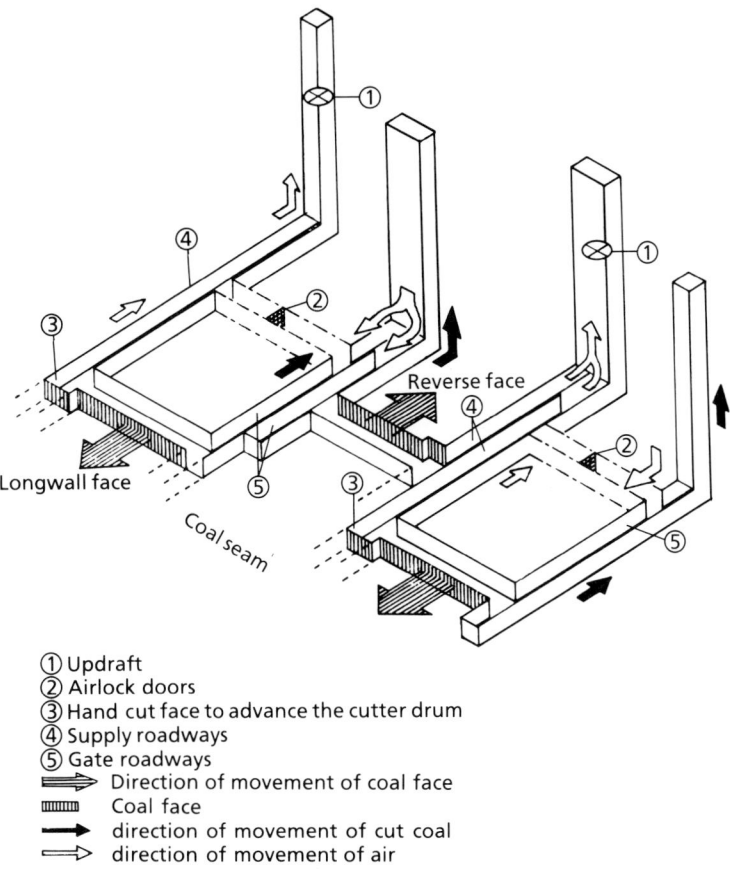

① Updraft
② Airlock doors
③ Hand cut face to advance the cutter drum
④ Supply roadways
⑤ Gate roadways
⟹ Direction of movement of coal face
▭ Coal face
➝ direction of movement of cut coal
⟹ direction of movement of air

Fig. 9.1. Layout of a coal mine: the long wall faces are advanced into the coal seam leaving reverse faces which can readily be mined automatically.

shears off the coal in chunks (fig. 9.2). Production at the coal face depends on the co-operation of many men working elsewhere, driving roadways, supporting the roof, providing ventilation and installing and maintaining conveyor belts and other haulage equipment used for bringing the coal to the surface. There is a risk of explosions from ignition of methane gas (fire damp) and when this occurs the flame may spread along underground roadways by igniting coal dust made airborne by the blast. This is prevented by scattering inert dust which, when it becomes airborne, prevents the formation of an explosive mixture; the dust formerly contained silica (table 8.3, page 162). Toxic gases, including oxides of nitrogen, are generated during shot

firing; because of this men are instructed not to return to areas of blasting until ventilation has carried these gases away. The occurrence of pockets of carbon dioxide (black damp) is another reason for maintaining the ventilation of the mine. However, the main health hazard is from coal dust.

Suppression of dust during mining

The first underground mines were not ventilated but they were often damp and the work was by hand so did not generate much dust. Conditions deteriorated with the advent of conveyors when the dust could obscure a man's lamp from the sight of the man working next to him. Compared

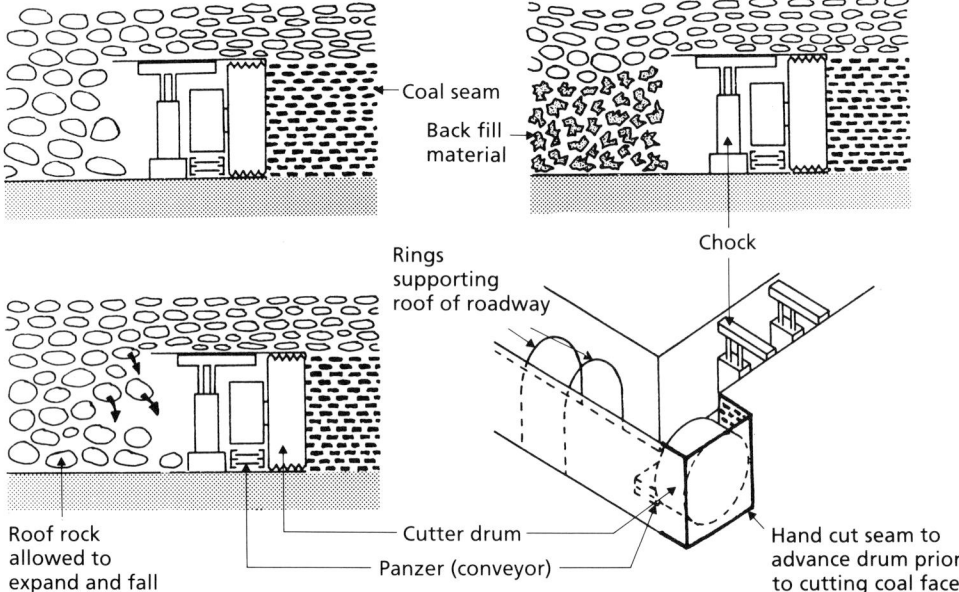

Fig. 9.2. Diagram showing coal cutting engine at the start of a traverse; the roof formed by the previous traverse is supported on mobile chocks with retractable cantilever arms. Roof rock exposed by earlier traverses is allowed to expand and fall or is supported by back fill.

with those days modern coal mines are clean places in which to work. Further reductions in dustiness could be achieved by using water jets or lasers to cut the coal; alternatively the dusty operations might be performed entirely automatically or be replaced by underground gasification (22).

The evolution of airborne dust is favoured by dry conditions so it is common practice to use water to suppress dust. The water is infused into the face under pressure prior to cutting and firing; it is also injected through the shafts of the drills used prior to inserting the explosive charges, and it is sprayed round the cutting teeth of the coal cutting and shearing machines. The quantity of dust is further reduced when the coal is obtained by shearing; compared with cutting and blasting this produces more chunks of coal and less dust, but more power is needed than with the older methods. Ventilation by local suction at the site of cutting is not yet practicable. Instead the face is ventilated by bulk flow of air which dilutes and carries away the dust. The resultant dust concentration, its

relation to pneumoconiosis and the recommended working conditions, including the use of respirators, are considered subsequently (page 194). Coal dust is also liberated in opencast operations, during sorting and size-grading of coal by screening, at points of loading and unloading conveyors wagons and ships, where the dustiest job is in the hold spreading the coal (coal trimming) and during the use of pulverized fuel in power stations, or in manufacture of smokeless fuel.

Other sources of carbon aerosol

Apart from its occurrence as coal, elemental carbon appears as graphite and in carbon black. Graphite is crystalline carbon; large crystals form sparkling black flakes, often in vertical lodes in quartz strata near coal deposits but the principal commercial form is small crystal or amorphous graphite. This is mined in many parts of the world, including Korea, Austria, U.S.S.R., China, Madagascar, Ceylon and Italy. The graphite is usually contaminated by quartz in concentrations of 0.2–11% and by other minerals. Artificial graphite is made by heating pitch and petroleum coke to 2500°C in an electric furnace whilst carbon black is a product of partial oxidation or thermal decomposition of hydrocarbons. Lamp black and soot are related products.

Elemental carbon withstands very high temperature, conducts electricity, has lubricating properties and is soluble in molten iron but not wettable by most alloys. In a finely divided form it adsorbs many chemical substances. These properties lead to a wide range of uses, such as generator brushes and electrodes, and in the production of steel where carbon is incorporated as a hardener. Graphite is used for crucibles and the lining of moulds in foundries and for electrotyping. Carbon fibres are used for the blades of jet engines and in a host of other applications including fume respirators (page 56). Carbon is an important constituent of pencils, carbon paper, black ink, many paints and proofing compounds, black rubber, gramophone records and other products.

Exposure to carbon aerosol may occur in the course of mining, manufacture, refining, or transportation of the raw materials, in manufacture of carbon black and use of the resulting products; one occupation which formerly carried a risk was that of cinema projectionist using a carbon arc projector. A small number of those who were exposed developed a condition indistinguishable from pneumoconiosis of coal workers (14).

Tissue responses to coal dust

Only the coal dust which reaches the alveoli contributes to the development of pneumoconiosis. To enter the alveoli the coal dust particles must traverse the airways where they are subject to removal by the processes described in chapter 4. These cleanse the air of all particles of aerodynamic diameter greater than 7µm and a proportion of those of smaller diameter (fig. 4.2, page 64). Some 94% of the remaining particles are subsequently exhaled but approximately 6% deposit on the respiratory epithelium of the acinus. The majority of these particles are in the size range 1–5µm; most are

ingested by macrophages and carried onto the ciliated epithelium whence they are removed via the mucociliary escalator. But some dust-laden macrophages are held up in the acinus or pass through its walls into lymphoid tissue around the respiratory bronchiole. Other particles are ingested by phagocytes in the epithelial lining of the respiratory bronchiole (fig. 9.3). The dust particles and macrophages accumulate in and around the respiratory bronchioles where they form the primary lesion of coalworkers' pneumoconiosis, the coal macule. This is best seen in lung tissue which has been inflated prior to fixation.

Preparation of lung tissue for histological examination

The lung should be fixed in an inflated condition by filling with a 10% aqueous formalin solution (4% formaldehyde) at a pressure of

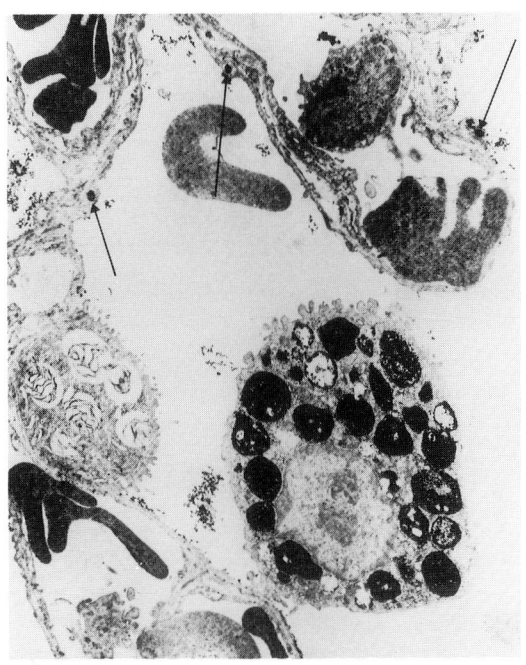

Fig. 9.3. Inert particles ingested by an alveolar macrophage and taken up by alveolar epithelium (indicated by arrows) in rat lung one day after intracheal injection of thorium particles. (By courtesy of B. Corrin, *Thorax* 1970;**25**:110.)

30cm of water through the trachea. Inflation can only be achieved if the lungs have been removed from the thorax without perforation of the visceral pleura, though small tears can be sealed with collodion. Large lung sections are prepared by the technique of Gough & Wentworth (16). The inflated lung is cut into slices 1cm thick; these are washed for 72h to remove the formalin, impregnated with 25% gelatine solution *in vacuo* at 60°C, frozen, partially thawed, then cut with a microtome into sections 1–2mm thick. The section is laid on a sheet of polished perspex, flooded with gelatine, covered with a filter paper, pressed to expel surplus fluid and allowed to dry, then peeled off the perspex (e.g. figs. 9.7, 9.10 and 9.15 below). The inflated lung is used as a source of tissue blocks for micros-

copy, both by conventional techniques and by mounting in 50 × 50mm transparencies for direct projection on to a screen.

The lung in simple pneumoconiosis

The primary lesion in pneumoconiosis of coalworkers is the coal macule. Macules occur throughout the lung but particularly in the upper and middle zones. Their profusion reflects the extent of dust retention. The macule has a diameter in the range 1–10mm and consists of dust particles, macrophages, reticulin tissue and fibroblasts accumulated round a second order respiratory bronchiole (fig. 9.4). There is relatively little fibrous tissue and macules are not discernible on palpation. The

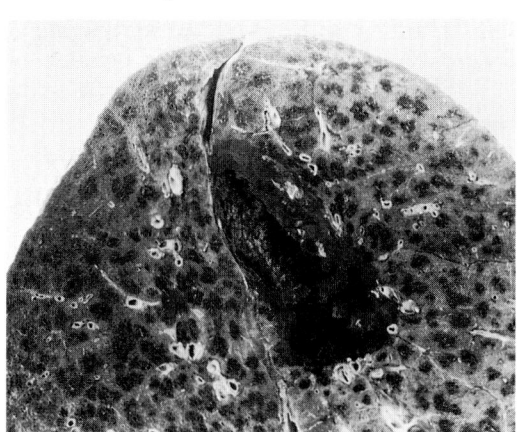

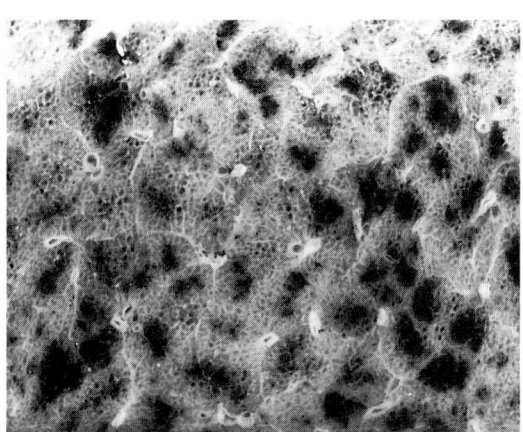

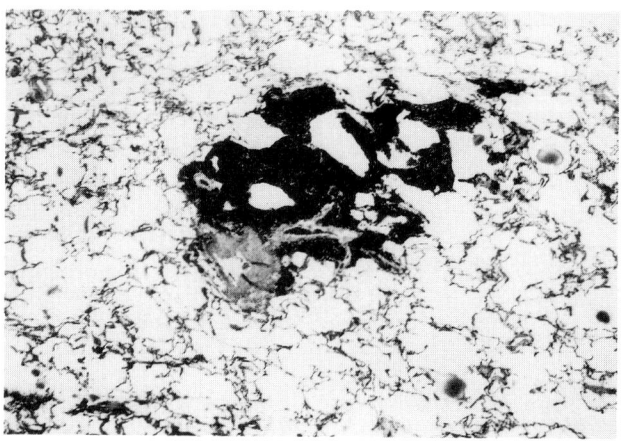

Fig. 9.4. *Top left*: Cut surface of inflated lung from a coal miner with pneumoconiosis showing coal macules and a PMF lesion (×0.5). *Top right*: Detail of macules showing normal alveolar structure (natural size). *Bottom left*: Coal macule forming round a respiratory bronchiole with intact alveoli (low power view). (By courtesy of T. Ashcroft.)

proportions of dust, cellular material and collagen vary widely depending on the type of inhaled dust; with high rank coal which is rich in carbon (table 9.1) the macules are largely acellular. By contrast, with low rank coal the macules contain less coal dust, are more cellular and may contain fibrous tissue, particularly if the quartz content of the dust exceeds about 8% (13, 40). These differences are reflected in the total dust content of the lung which varies from an average of 9–10g in category 0 to 20–40g in category 3, the higher figure in each case referring to high rank coal (40). Small macules enlarge slowly, compressing adjacent air spaces and engulfing capillaries which supply the affected alveoli. However, the process is usually self-limiting and the macules seldom have a diameter in excess of 3mm. Dust may be present in the adventitia of adjacent arterioles but obliteration of arterioles is infrequent. Dust accumulates around venules and along lymphatics, where it can form a lattice of dust tissue; it also occurs beneath the visceral pleura, in lymph nodes at the hilum and in the mediastinum. The lymphatic movement of dust is greater for silica than for carbon (6). Coal dust may also be present beneath the parietal pleura along the lines of the ribs but unlike asbestos does not cause pleural thickening. Changes in the centre of the coal macule lead to dilatation of the affected respiratory bronchiole (fig. 9.5).

This focal emphysema is due, at least in part, to the combined effects of atrophy of bronchiolar smooth muscle and increased rigidity of alveolar walls caused by dust; the changes reduce the resilience and increase the traction on the wall of the bronchiole during inspiration (18). The twin processes of dilatation and disruption occur together to merge into centrilobular emphysema in which loss of lung parenchyma is unequivocal. However, some of the destruction may be due to proteolytic enzymes or oxidants released from macrophages (page 383).

As macules enlarge more collagen is laid down and becomes discernible as grittiness when the lung is cut. These secondary nodules tend to protrude on the cut surface and they are palpable in the lung tissue (fig. 9.6). On large lung sections the nodules are either black throughout or black with pale centres depending on the coal and quartz content of the dust (table 9.2): they are of a circumscribed or stellate appearance and may show adjacent emphysema which is irregular in form. The collagen and reticulin fibres are usually arranged haphazardly in the nodules but extend outwards into the adjacent tissue to form a net. This is visible on the 50mm² section but not on a large lung section (fig. 9.6). The net is stained with coal dust and may contain expanded air spaces which gives the lung a cystic or honeycomb

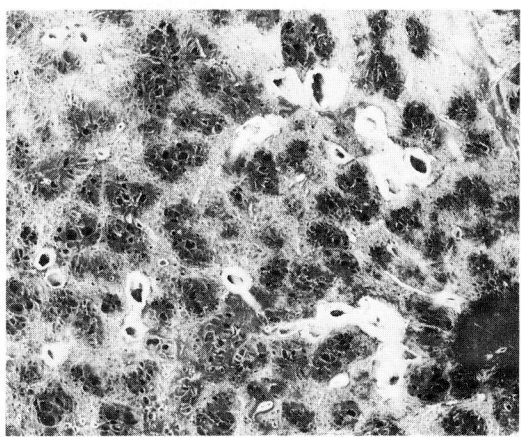 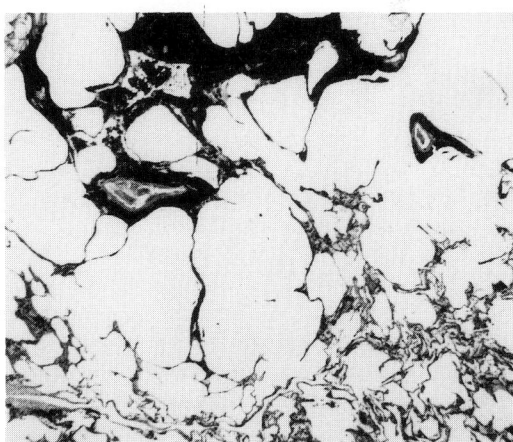

Fig. 9.5. *Left*: Cut surface of inflated lung showing focal emphysema in coal macules. *Right*: Coal macule with emphysema (magnification as in fig. 9.4). (By courtesy of T. Ashcroft.)

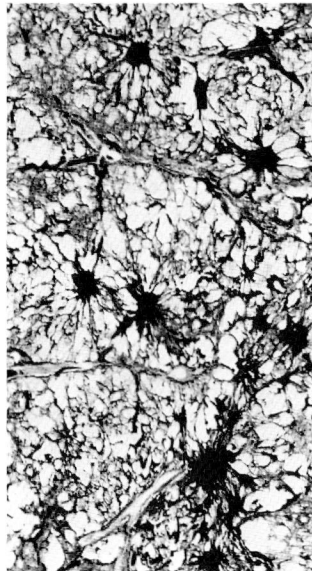 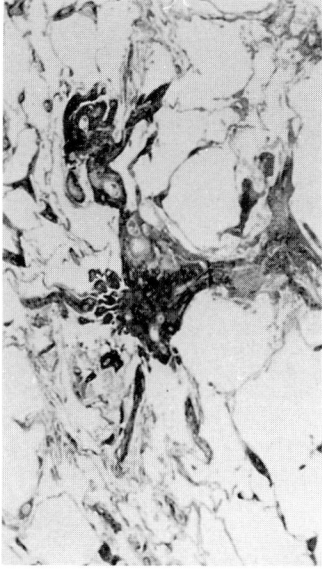

Fig. 9.6. *Above*: Stellate nodules in paper-mounted lung section and 50mm² transparency of the patient whose chest radiographs are shown in fig. 9.16 (left). *Below*: Paper-mounted section showing secondary nodules with emphysema from the lung of a man who worked on the coal face for 40 years (×0.8). He was asymptomatic. The chest radiography (right) was read as 2r. Death was from myocardial infarction. (By courtesy of J. E. M. Hutchinson.)

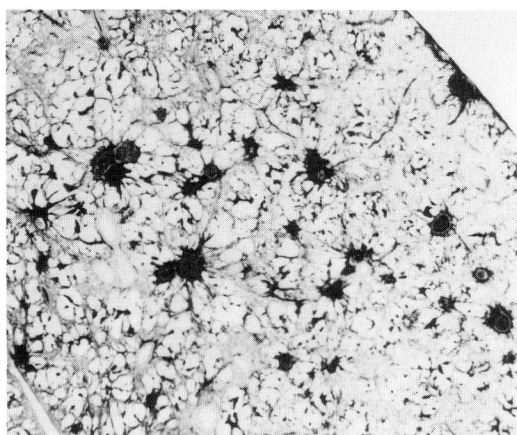 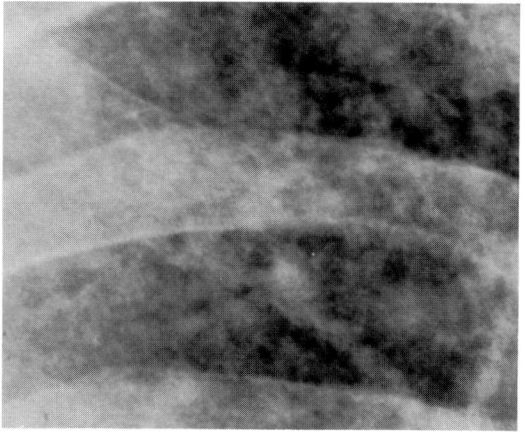

appearance. However, concentric whorls of fibrous tissue characteristic of silicosis may occur in the paler, more cellular lesions (13). The size of the dust foci influences the radiographic appearance, with the smallest foci (diameter 1–1.5mm) and the lattice type of dust distribution mainly giving rise to p-type opacities and the largest ones (diameter 2–10mm) to r-type opacities (40, figs. 9.7 and 9.8). The stellate secondary nodules resemble mixed dust fibrosis. Some features of these three types of simple pneumoconiosis are summarized in table 9.2.

In men at post-mortem the extent of emphysema in relation to dust foci is correlated positively with the quantity of coal dust in the lung and negatively with the silica content; it is more extensive than in non-miners (9,42) and is not dependent on the man being a smoker (29). Extensive emphysema is associated with irregular opacities on the chest radiograph (10, 28, fig. 9.9); they are of the s or t type and usually develop out of a background of round opacities of the p type which then become obscured (40). Thus emphysema is common in

Table 9.2. Comparison of features of simple pneumoconiosis due to silica, mixed dust and coal

	Silica	Mixed dust fibrosis	Coal
Description	Nodule	Medusa head*	Macule*
Dust content	Low	Intermediate	High
Proportion of silica	High	Intermediate	Low
Fibrous tissue	Concentric	Stellate	Very little
Emphysema	None	Irregular (if present)	Focal
Calcification	Yes	No	No
Relation to exposure	Yes	Yes	Yes
CXR small opacities	q–r	p–q and s	p–q
Age affects CXR reading	Yes	Yes	No
Incr. prevalence of TB	Yes	(Yes)	No
Usually affects lung function†	Yes	Yes	No
Progression after exposure ceased	Yes	Yes	No

* The stellate secondary nodule of coalworkers' pneumoconiosis resembles that of mixed dust fibrosis but the fibrosis is often less conspicuous than the emphysema: the circumscribed secondary nodule (infective nodule) resembles the coal macule but is often larger and contains collagen.

† After allowing for years of exposure and smoking.

late stage simple pneumoconiosis where it is an integral part of the disease process. However, its extent is usually small, less than 20% of the dustiest part of the lung (40). The associated respiratory impairment is considered on page 188.

Progressive massive fibrosis

Progressive massive fibrosis of the lung is a complication of simple pneumoconiosis. It is apparent during life as one or more large rounded opacities on the chest radiograph (fig. 9.10) and at post-mortem as a confluent lesion which is usually black in colour and often has a necrotic centre (fig. 9.4). Typically it is associated with breathing dust from high rank coal having a high carbon content and is due to progressive enlargement of a single coal macule. Less frequently PMF masses form by enlargement and fusion of adjacent nodular lesions of the fibrotic type and there is every gradation in between (13). PMF in association with a rheumatoid diathesis is discussed below. On the large lung section the typical PMF lesion appears as a black mass from which nearly all structural features have disappeared (fig. 9.10). The mass often engulfs bronchi and pulmonary arteries and extends across septa or from one lobe to another. Typically there is no clearly defined edge and no anatomical capsule of

fibrous tissue; instead the periphery of the lesion is made up of disorganized lung tissue, coal macules and secondary nodules, fibrous tissue and thrombosed pulmonary blood vessels. Endarteritis and thrombosis occur in adjacent pulmonary arteries. In some cases plasma cells are conspicuous. Except in the coalescent form of PMF, silicotic nodules are usually absent as is tuberculosis. The centre of the lesion has been shown by Wagner and colleagues to comprise mainly fibronectin which is a loosely stabilized insoluble protein based on the glycosaminoglycan series of acid mucopolysaccharides. The lesion also contains mineral dust and calcium phosphate (46). A PMF lesion which has ruptured into a bronchus may be empty or contain melanotic material diluted with fluid resembling blood plasma. Emphysema which occurs in association with progressive massive fibrosis may obscure the underlying simple pneumoconiosis; the emphysema may partly compensate for shrinkage of the inelastic PMF lesion. There may also be hypertrophy of the right ventricle and evidence elsewhere in the body of right ventricular overload.

Rheumatoid pneumoconiosis

The association of a nodular form of pneumoconiosis with rheumatoid arthritis or a rheuma-

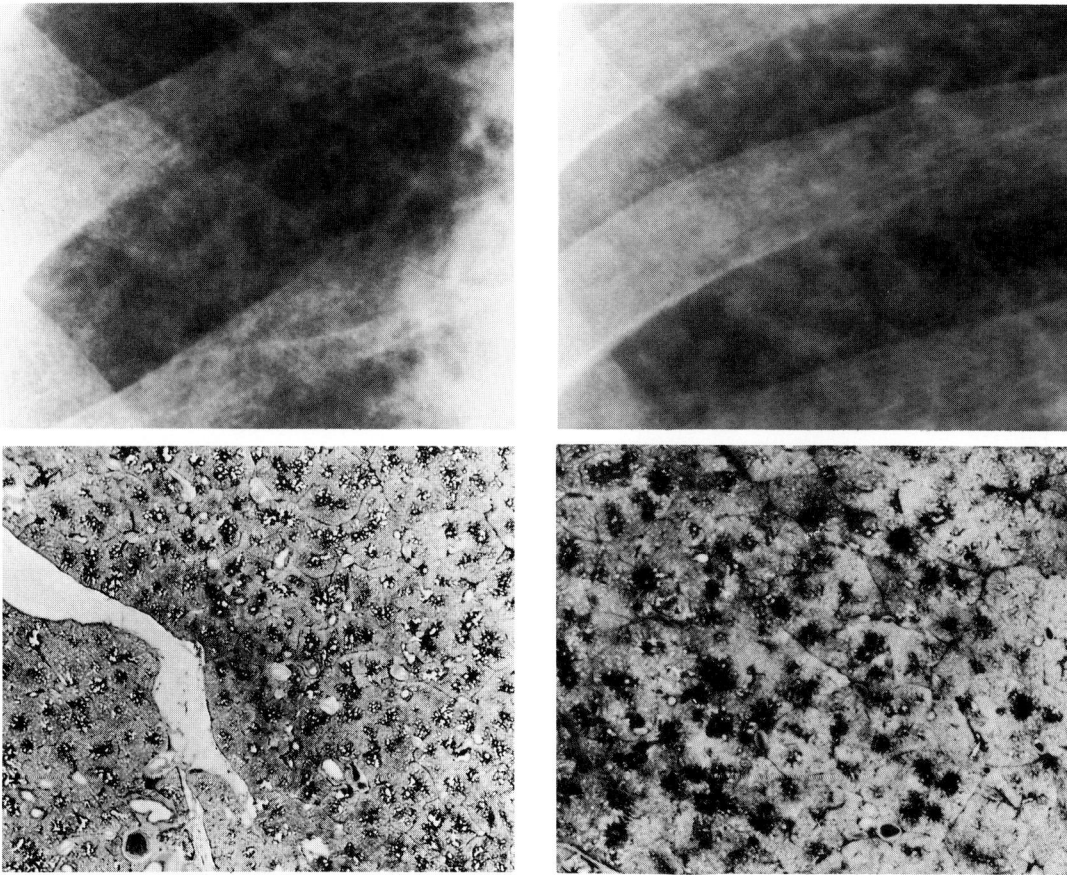

Fig. 9.7. Detail from chest radiograph shortly before death; comparison with lung pathology. Both these patients worked more than 30 years in the coal mines. They had normal ventilatory capacity; neither had any respiratory symptoms. Death was from myocardial infarction. *Left*: The chest radiograph was read as category 2p/q and the lung section showed dust macules with coal dust in the lung septa and focal emphysema. *Right*: The chest radiograph was read as category 3q and the lung section showed dust macules with no emphysema. (By courtesy of J. E. M. Hutchinson.)

toid diathesis constitutes Caplan's syndrome (page 184). At autopsy the lung contains some coal macules but usually fewer than in other forms of pneumoconiosis; it also contains characteristic nodular lesions formerly called infective nodules. These are usually of diameter 0.5–3cm palpable and often cavitated or calcified. The active zones of the nodules comprise macrophages containing coal dust, lymphocytes, polymorphonuclear leucocytes, numerous plasma cells (which may form a pallisade of rheumatoid cells) and occasionally giant cells.

These surround a central necrotic zone which in older lesions may calcify or cavitate. In some lesions there are alternating concentric zones of amorphous tissue and deposited dust (fig. 9.11) and these may shrink, leaving clefts which contain crystals of cholesterol. Arterioles and small pulmonary arteries in the vicinity of the lesions may exhibit endarteritis or thrombosis and the lesions themselves may coalesce to form larger massive lesions; typical PMF lesions may also occur concurrently.

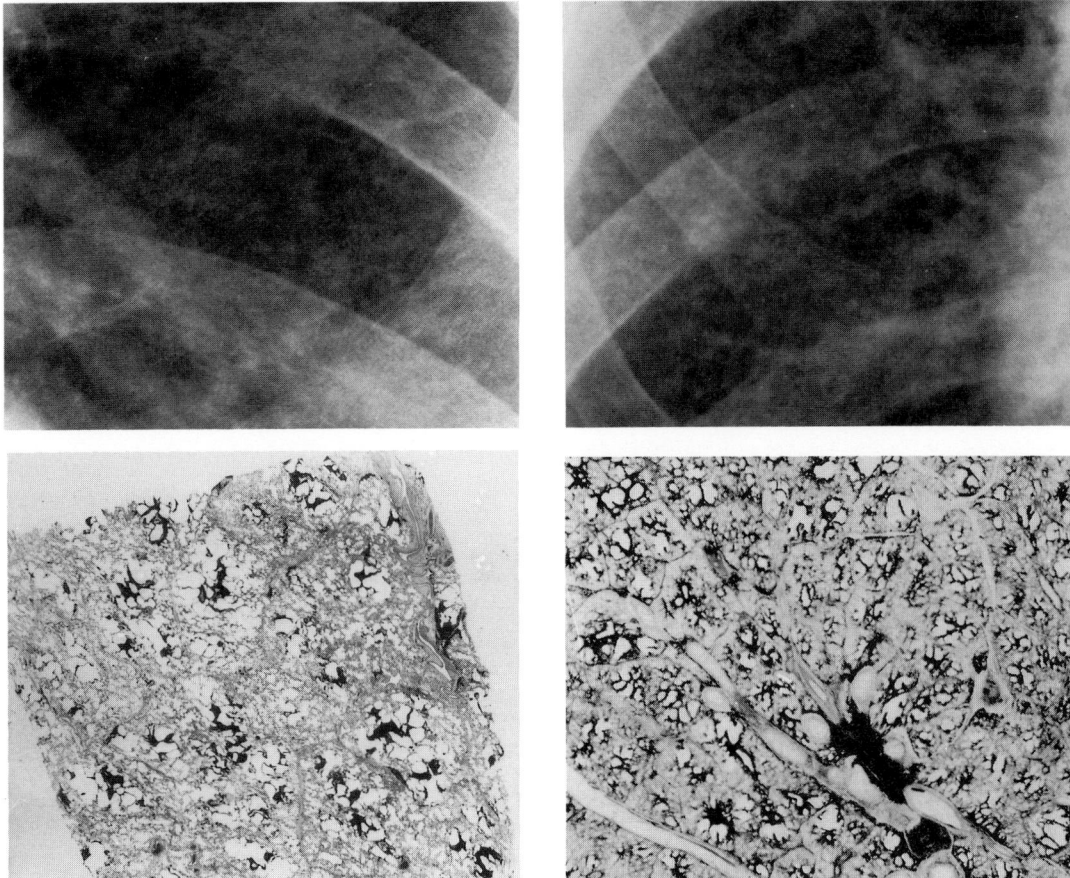

Fig. 9.8. Detail from chest radiograph shortly before death; comparison with lung pathology. *Left*: From a 68-year-old man who worked in the mines for 41 years doing a number of different jobs. He had no respiratory symptoms. Death was from ischaemic heart disease. The chest radiograph was read as category 2p. The lung transparency showed dust foci with emphysema. *Right*: From a 63-year-old man who had worked for 38 years in the mines. He smoked 25 cigarettes per day. Two years before death the FEV_1 was 1.08 l with a 20% improvement after salbutamol. Death was from right heart failure. The x-ray category was 3p/q and the paper section showed dust foci with extensive focal emphysema. Smoking probably contributed to the respiratory impairment. (By courtesy of A. E. Cockcroft.)

Aetiology of PMF and rheumatoid pneumoconiosis

Coal dust which enters the skin through a minor abrasion leaves a tattoo mark but no induration and the skin remains soft. The coal macule in the lung is similarly not scarred. However, the coal adsorbs protein including IgG and rheumatoid factor (IgM) which have been demonstrated in plasma cells adjacent to PMF lesions, in hilar lymph nodes and in the rheumatoid nodules of men with Caplan's syndrome. A raised serum titre of rheumatoid factor is a feature of Caplan's syndrome and, compared with other coal-miners, is commoner amongst men with PMF. The association led Payne to suggest that protein which is adsorbed onto coal dust is altered into a form which promotes rheumatoid activity; however, attempts to demonstrate this experimentally were unsuccessful (23). Moreover, in

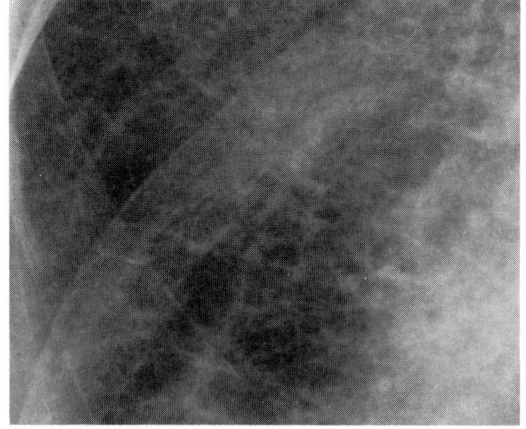

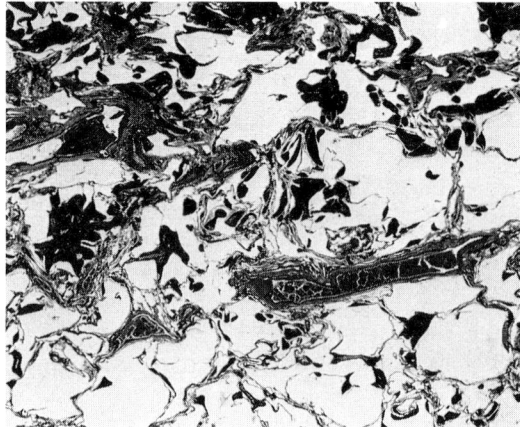

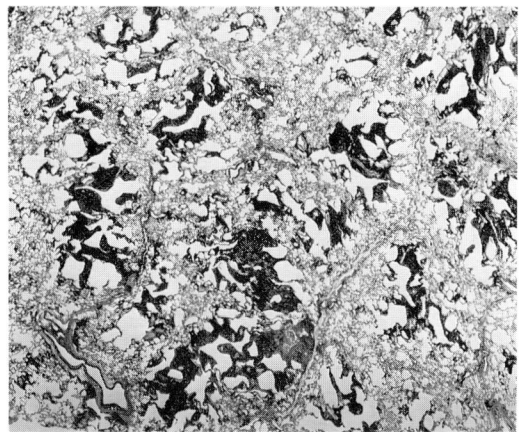

Fig. 9.9. Chest radiograph shortly before death showing irregular opacities (category 3t) associated with coal dust and marked emphysema on the lung transparency (left and above) in a 62-year-old man who worked as a coal miner for 46 years. He smoked 20 cigarettes per day up to age 59. At age 60 FEV$_1$ was 0.86 l and the transfer factor, which at age 49 had been normal, was now 45% of predicted. Death was from cardiorespiratory failure. Smoking may have contributed to the respiratory impairment.

some studies of men with PMF the prevalence of a raised rheumatoid titre was no greater than in men with simple pneumoconiosis (26). The serum titre of antinuclear factor is often increased in coalminers (45), particularly those from anthracite areas. Amongst men with PMF there is also an increased serum titre of lung reactive IgA antibodies against connective tissue collagen, elastin and reticulin (4). Thus pneumoconiosis is associated with increased antigenic activity in the body, but much of it is non-specific and there is, as yet, no good evidence for a causal mechanism.

The development of progressive massive fibrosis was formerly attributed to silica, tuberculosis or coal dust necrosis. The possible catalytic role of silica present with the coal was convincingly disproved by the observation that PMF could occur amongst workers exposed only to carbon black and artificial graphite which were completely free from silica (fig. 9.12). In addition the rank of coal does not influence the attack rate of PMF (44). The theory that PMF was a modified form of tuberculosis was similarly disproved by the realization that concurrent tuberculosis was present in only a minority of cases, even in an era when tuberculosis was relatively common. Treatment by antituberculosis chemotherapy (2) and reduction in the amount of active tuberculosis in the mining community were without effect on the long-term course of the disease. Similarly the possible role of viral and other infection was never convincingly demonstrated. There remains the possi-

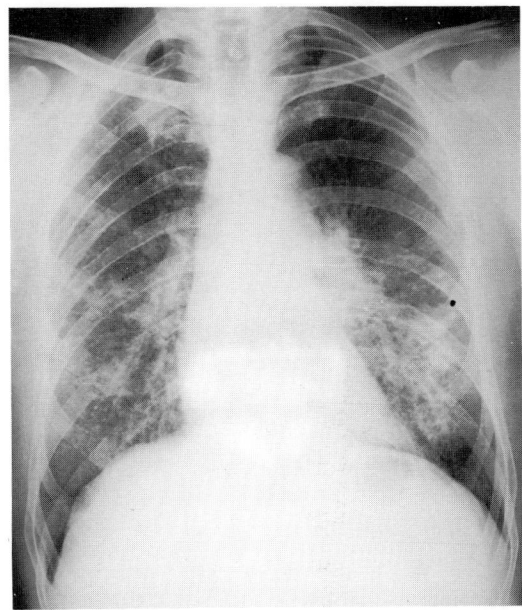

Fig. 9.10. Chest radiographs at ages 58 and 65 years in a coal miner who worked for 44 years in the mines. At the time of the former radiograph he had progressive massive fibrosis which progressed subsequently. He also had a positive sputum; this responded to antitubercular chemotherapy. Death was from respiratory failure (FEV_1 0.85l.) The large lung section (below) closely matched the radiograph taken 1 year before death. The extent of PMF and of emphysema are clearly shown. (By courtesy of J. E. M. Hutchinson.)

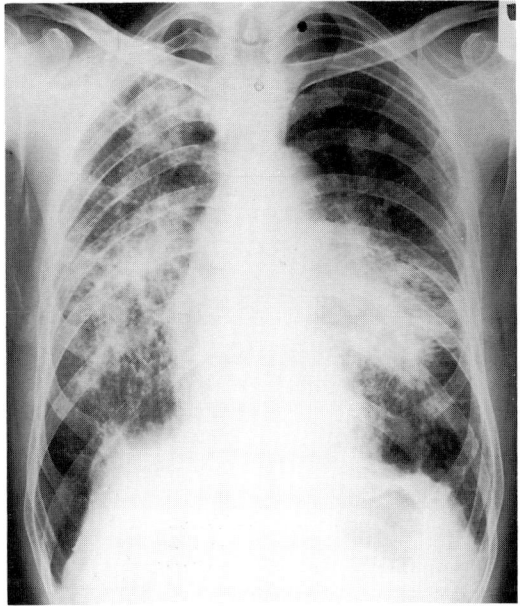

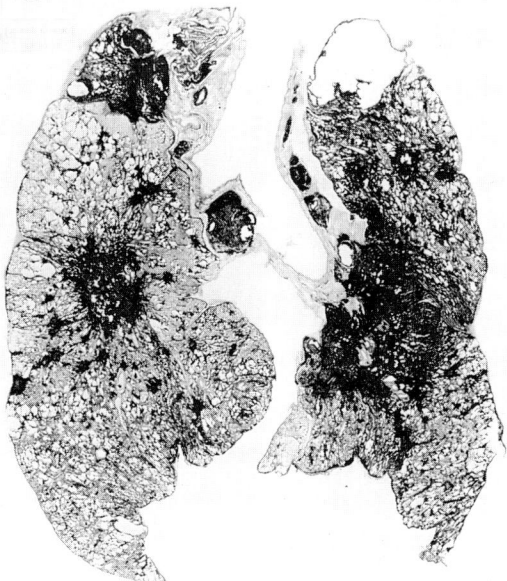

bility that PMF is due to obstruction of the lymphatic drainage of the lung. Either an enlarged gland erodes a bronchus or pulmonary artery (43) or the obstruction sets up a self-perpetuating local process of endarteritis, thrombosis and necrosis; whether or not PMF occurs in any individual coalminer is then a statistical phenomenon reflecting mainly the amount and distribution of dust in the lung. The evidence for this hypothesis is summarized in fig. 9.20 (page 193); the mechanism could still be immunological (see above).

Chest illness amongst coalworkers

Coal miners and others who breathe air contaminated with coal dust retain some dust in their lungs. The dust accumulates in small dust foci or macules which constitute simple pneumoconiosis of coal workers. With continuing exposure to a material concentration of dust the macules increase in number and become visible on the chest radiograph as multiple small round opacities. Simple pneumoconiosis is not associated with respiratory symptoms, does not shorten life and in the absence of chest radiography may not even be suspected. However, with passage of time following heavy dust exposure one or more macules enlarge or a number coalesce to form progressive massive fibrosis (PMF); the lesions progressively disrupt the normal function of the lung, give rise to respiratory symptoms and reduce life expectancy. This sequence constitutes classical pneumoconiosis of coal workers. In the absence of radiographic surveillance the condition presents with symptoms due to PMF and this presentation is described in detail below. In addition the inhalation of coal dust aggravates or may cause chronic bronchitis and emphysema, both of which occur unduly frequently in coalminers. However, the conditions are also caused by smoking and for men who have only worked in mines which meet the hygiene standard for airborne coal dust (page 194), smoking and not coal dust is the likely cause. The evaluation of respiratory symptoms in coal miners is critically dependent on the occupational history. This is sometimes difficult to interpret as coalminers often live and work in isolation from other people and in the past have developed their own idiom; a glossary of some coalmining terms is given in table 9.3.

Simple pneumoconiosis. A middle-aged or elderly coalminer who is referred because of multiple small round opacities on the postero-anterior chest radiograph is likely to have simple pneumoconiosis. The opacities appear first in the centre of the mid-zone of the right lung and extend both vertically to include the lower and upper zones and horizontally to fill the rib spaces from the hilum to the chest wall. The left lung is smaller and receives 15% less

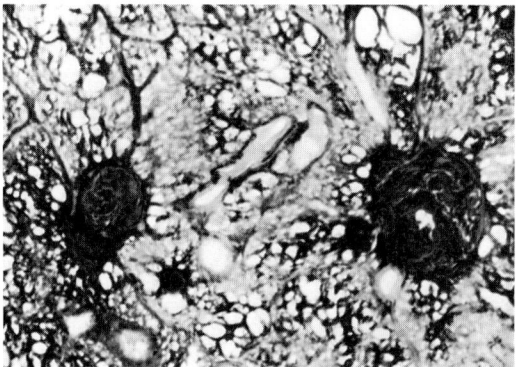

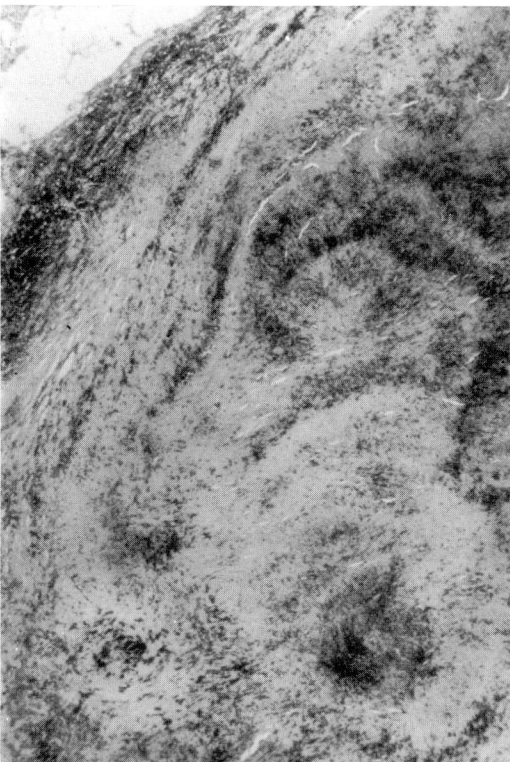

Fig. 9.11. Caplan's syndrome: Enlargement from paper-mounted lung section and histology showing concentric zones of coal dust, macrophages, collagen and clefts which contain cholesterol crystals. See also fig. 9.15 (page 184–5). (Histology by courtesy of R. M. E. Seal.)

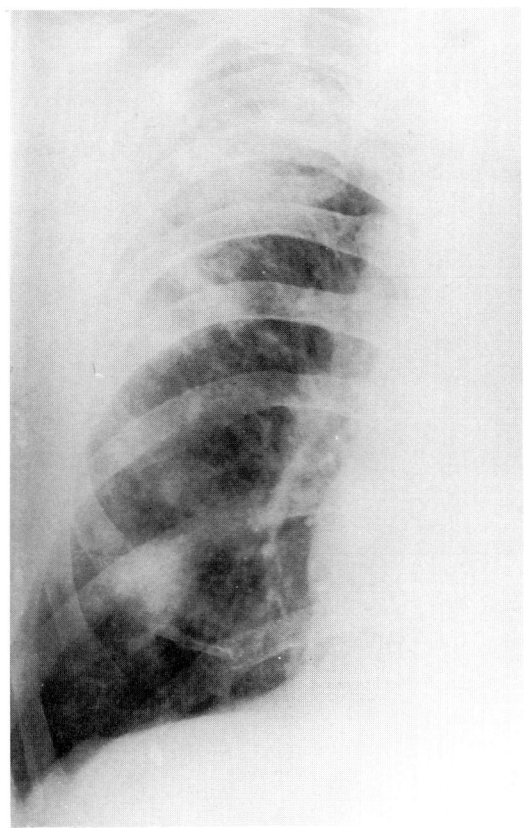

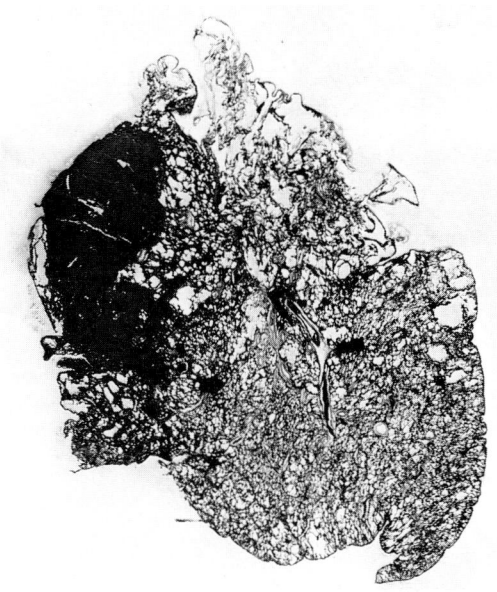

Fig. 9.12. Right chest radiograph 6 years before death and large lung section showing progressive massive fibrosis in a man who for 19 years was grinding carbon electrodes made from graphite. He never worked in a coal mine. Death at 70 was from congestive cardiac failure due to pneumoconiosis and chronic bronchitis. (By courtesy of J. E. M. Hutchinson and A. J. Watson (48).)

ventilation so is affected to a slightly lesser extent. The profusion of opacities may be graded on a 12-point scale from 0− to 3+ and the size as pinhead, micronodular or nodular (p, q or r) using the ILO international classification of chest radiographs (chapter 5). The profusion is correlated with the exposure to respirable coal dust; any detectable increase in profusion depends on continuation of exposure (unlike in silicosis) and takes place slowly over years, not months (30). Regression is rare and associated with development of emphysema. The size of the opacities usually remains relatively constant but the appearance of r opacities on a background of p opacities has been reported (36). The shape may progressively change from round to irregular; this is believed to indicate the development of stellate nodules which contain both coal dust and radiating strands of fibrous

tissue separated by emphysematous spaces. The patient is usually asymptomatic and the lung function normal unless chronic bronchitis or emphysema coexist. Emphysema is more common with p type simple pneumoconiosis than with the q and r types (page 188).

The diagnosis of simple pneumoconiosis is based on the characteristic radiographic features plus the occupational history and is seldom in doubt when the patient is asymptomatic and has normal lung function. Coexisting chronic bronchitis is diagnosed from the symptoms with or without chronic airflow obstruction (chapter 17). Emphysema is considered below (page 189). The differential diagnosis is given in table 9.4. There is no specific treatment for simple pneumoconiosis and in the absence of symptoms there is no indication for supportive therapy. However, simple pneumoconiosis is evidence of

Table 9.3.   Examples of terms used by coalminers

Description	South Wales	North England
Ground level	Pit top	Bank
Lift	Bon	Cage
Main tunnel	Lead-in	Mothergate
Supply tunnel	Supply heading	Tail gate
Foreman	Fireman	Deputy
Workmates	Butties	Marrows
Coal face worker	Collier	Filler
Men who dispose of stone rubble by backfilling	Packers	Buttmen
Men who build tunnels	Headers	Caunchmen
Men who maintain tunnels	Repairers	Back caunch men
Men who maintain railways	Road men	Waggon way men
Fault on coal face	Jump	Hitch
Work for a wage		Datal work
Work paid by results		Piece work
Food box/water container	Tommy box/jack	Bait/water bottle
Meal break	Snap time	Bait time
Earth and stone	Muck	Debris
Big hammer	Sledge	Mel
Hand pick	Mandril	Hand pick
Compressed air pick	Puncher/Jigger	Windy pick
Compressed air	Blast	Wind
Waggon	Dram	Tub
Train of waggons	Journey	Sets
Train attendant	Rider	Set lad
Wood used to brake waggons	Sprag	Dreg
Man controlling horses	Haulier man	Pit pony lad
Harness/shaft	Shaft/gun two pieces	Limbers/one piece

excessive exposure to coal dust which, if it is continued, may lead to progressive massive fibrosis; so the working conditions should be reviewed and the man's exposure to dust reduced (page 194). If the x-ray category is grade 2 or above the patient should ideally move from the coal-face to a non-dusty job in order to reduce the risk of his developing PMF; this may entail his leaving the coal mining industry. The further surveillance of such persons is considered subsequently. In addition there is a case for encouraging the affected miner to discontinue smoking since a small proportion will subsequently develop respiratory disablement from emphysema to which both the accumulated coal dust and tobacco fumes can contribute.

Progressive massive fibrosis. A coalminer with simple pneumoconiosis who gradually becomes unduly breathless on exertion and who is observed to have or to develop a rounded opacity on the chest radiograph probably has progressive massive fibrosis (PMF). Initially it cannot be distinguished radiographically from tuberculosis or bronchial carcinoma, though it is less likely to be either of these if bilateral. However, sputum examination for these two conditions should always be undertaken, especially when there is little or no evidence of simple pneumoconiosis in the rest of the lungs. If previous films are available the massive fibrosis sometimes appears to develop by coalescence of 'simple' shadows over the course of several years (figs. 9.13 and 9.14). But this is not always so and the diagnostic uncertainty has caused the initial shadows of PMF to be dubbed 'ambiguous' or Category A. Category A shadows are

Table 9.4. Differential diagnosis of simple pneumoconiosis of coalworkers

Condition	Distinguishing feature	Details
Inert dust pneumoconiosis	Occupational history	Page 229
Silicosis	Occupational history, radiographic appearance	Chapter 8 and table 9.2
Miliary tuberculosis	Short history, ill health, sputum sometimes positive	—
Sarcoidosis	Commonly involves mediastinum and other tissues; Kveim test often positive	Page 238
Coalworkers' cystic lung	Radiographic appearance	Text and table 15.5*
Extrinsic allergic alveolitis	History, fine râles, abnormal lung function, precipitating antibodies	Table 15.5*
Cryptogenic fibrosing alveolitis	Mainly lower zone irregular opacities	Table 15.5*
Asbestosis	Occupational history	Chapter 10 and table 15.5*
Fungal infection (e.g. histoplasmosis)	Geographical distribution, ill health, evidence for sensitization	Chapter 13
Schistosomiasis	Geographical distribution, positive complement fixation test	—

* page 331

usually asymptomatic, and never produce any recognizable physical signs.

During the course of a number of years the Category A shadows usually enlarge slowly and become kidney shaped. They are re-classified as Category B when this enlargement has reached the point at which the sum of the maximal diameters of all (usually two) A shadows added together exceeds 5cm, and further re-classified as Category C when the total area of all massive opacities exceeds one-third of the area of the right lung on a P-A chest radiograph (fig. 9.10). Progression entails not only enlargement of the initial apical shadows but also development of new shadows in the apices of the lower lobes and sometimes widespread throughout the lung. It is usually an extremely slow process taking 10, 15 or 20 years but occasionally a reactive individual is seen in whom the process 'gallops' in the course of a few years. A characteristic feature of the radiography of PMF is that as the lesions age they contract and appear to migrate towards the hilum. This contraction of part of the lung is accompanied by over-inflation of the peripheral parts of the lung in which emphysema, often bullous, can be seen to develop. The mediastinum and diaphragm are often distorted by the contracture, and the trachea and major bronchi become twisted and displaced. At this stage the patient is very severely disabled by breathlessness, but before contracture develops it is often surprising how little complaint accompanies widespread radiological abnormality.

The presenting symptom of PMF is nearly always breathlessness on exertion. This is barely perceptible to start with but over a period of many years increases until it becomes incapacitating. The breathlessness reflects increased work done in ventilating the lungs and an increase in the volume of air required to sustain a given level of activity. It is initially absent at rest; any complaint of sighing or 'inability to get air into the chest' is evidence for anxiety, not

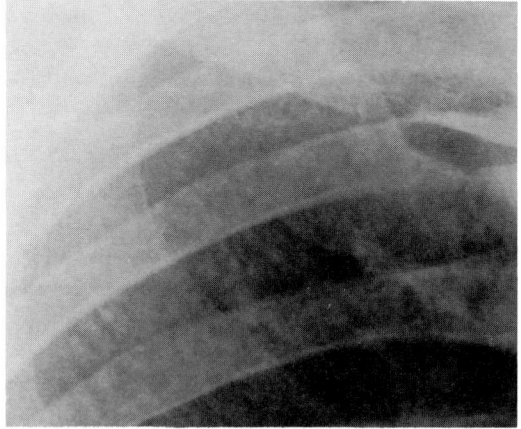 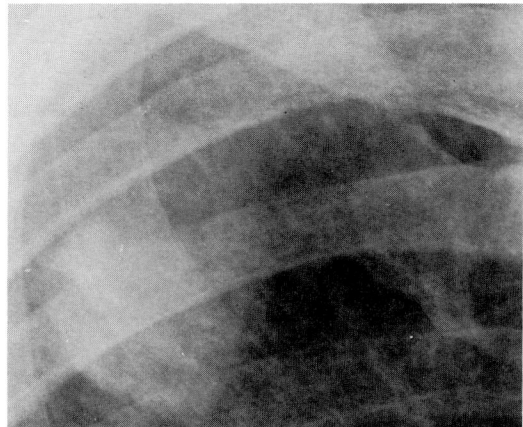

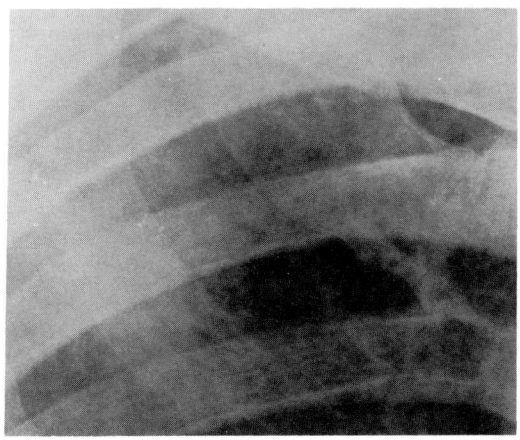

Fig. 9.13. Chest radiographs spanning a 22-year period showing the right upper zone of a 63-year-old man who for 38 years from the age of 14 worked as a collier. He was a non-smoker, had no respiratory or other symptoms and only left the industry because the pit closed. The films show the development of an A shadow on a background of simple pneumoconiosis (category 3p/q).

chest disease. Subsequent to the onset of breathlessness the patient may develop a productive cough, but a productive cough which precedes a history of breathlessness is not typical of pneumoconiosis. The sputum resembles that of other miners, its colour depending mainly on whether or not they are working. The sputum is frequently grey and may be streaked with coal dust or flecks of blood. The bleeding will usually stop without incident but occasionally it occurs a day or two before the rupture into a bronchus of the contents of a PMF lesion. Rupture occurs in massive lesions categories B and C and seldom in conglomerate nodular lesions. The sputum is ink black (melanoptysis) and has a foul taste and smell; the onset is often sudden without warning and the initial volume may be large,

exceeding half a litre. Thus the occurrence of melanoptysis can be alarming to all concerned. The viscid material is derived from central necrosis of a massive lesion and is usually bacteriologically sterile but stimulates the bronchial glands to produce mucus and often obstructs airways to adjacent parts of the lung; these then become infected. The cavity left by the melanoptysis is visible radiographically as a translucent centre to the PMF lesion, with or without a fluid level (fig. 9.14). Afterwards the cavity usually refills and is then no longer discernible on the chest radiograph; but melanoptysis may recur. Fortunately melanoptysis only occurs in a small proportion of patients with PMF. A more common complication is bullous emphysema (fig. 9.10); this is often basal in

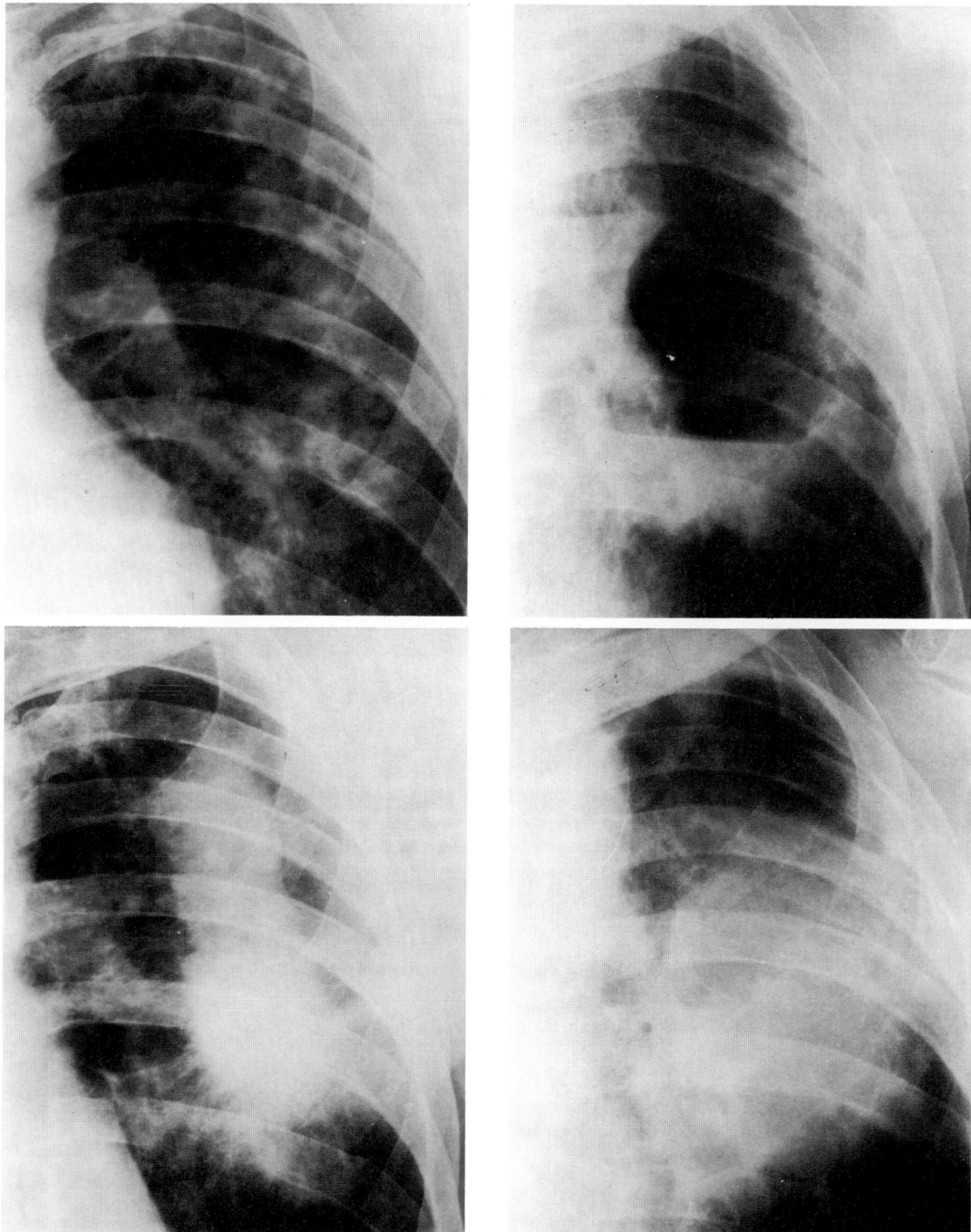

Fig. 9.14. Chest radiographs spanning 31 years showing the left upper zone of a man whose working life was spent as a collier. He developed a nodular type of simple pneumoconiosis, then progressive massive fibrosis (bottom left) which cavitated and refilled (right) on two separate occasions over a 2-year period.

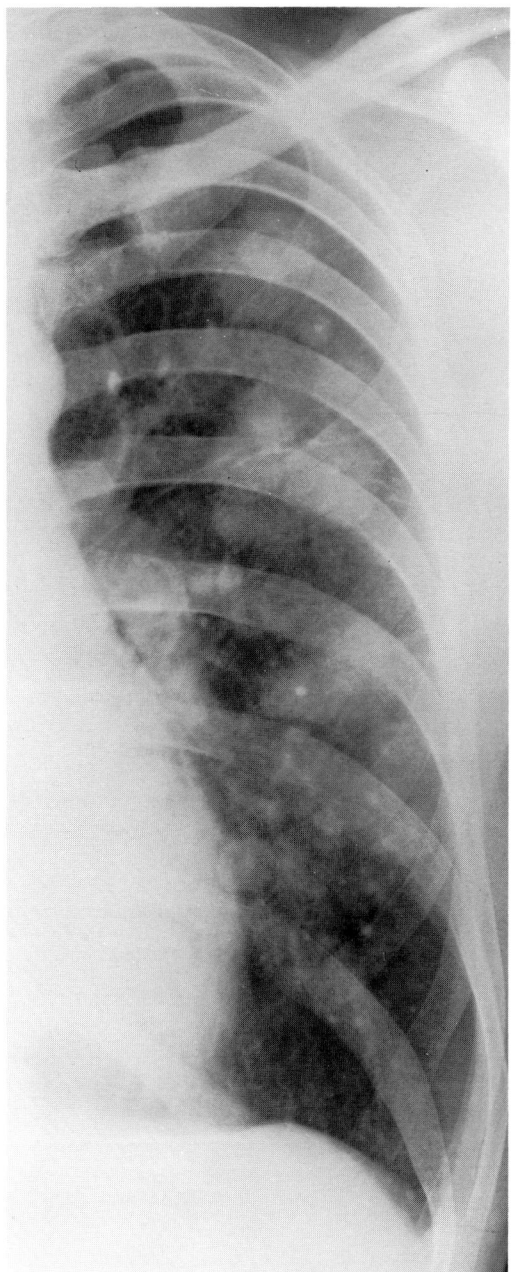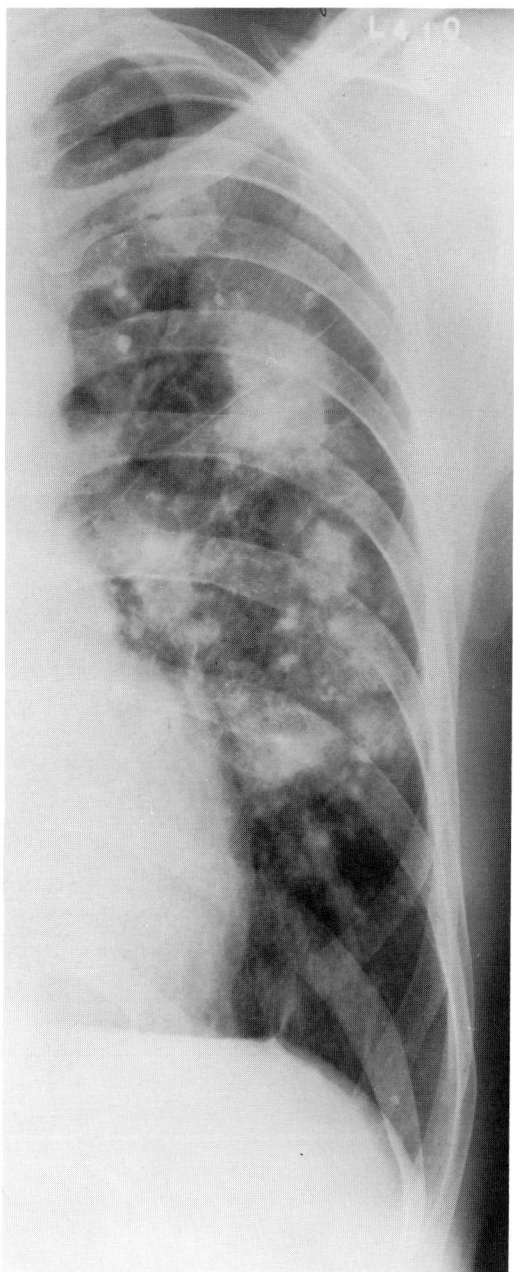

Fig. 9.15. Chest radiographs spanning a 15-year period, photograph of the hands, and paper-mounted lung section of a coal miner with rheumatoid pneumoconiosis. He was working as a labourer near the coal face for 12 years until age 30 when he developed rheumatoid arthritis; there was no family history. The chest radiograph showed 'finger print' opacities typical of Caplan's syndrome. Over the next 6 years the patient became progressively more disabled from arthritis; he also developed breathlessness on exertion and the radiographic lesions coalesced to resemble non-rheumatoid progressive massive fibrosis. The FEV_1 was

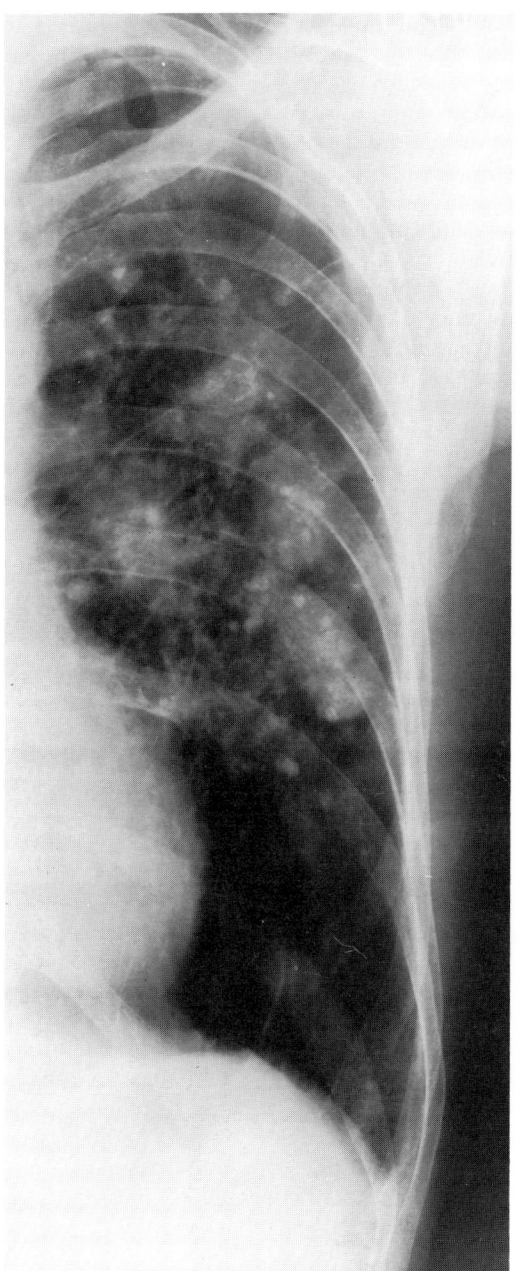

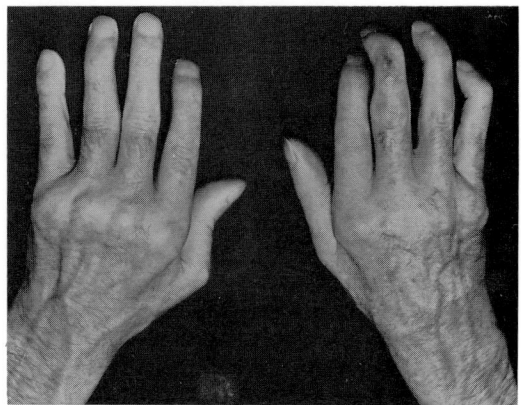

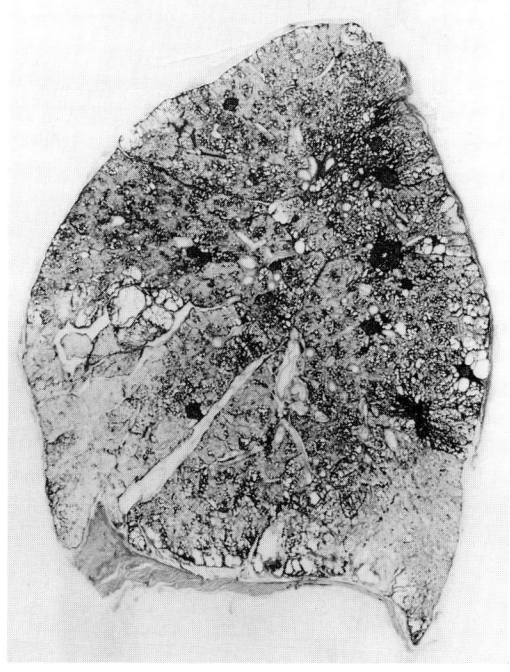

now 2 l (59% predicted) and the total lung capacity was reduced (80% predicted). Subsequently, the massive lesions diminished in size (burnt out Caplan's syndrome) but the patient became more breathless with features of emphysema (FEV_1 1.3 l, 38% predicted, transfer factor 3.7 SI units, 41% predicted) and he died in respiratory failure at age 48 years. At post-mortem the PMF lesions were shrunken with concentric zones containing dust, fibrous tissues and clefts. There was extensive emphysema. (Large lung section by courtesy of J. C. Wagner.)

distribution. The emphysema is a response to shrinkage and distortion of the lung by PMF; the patient usually has severe respiratory impairment and may develop episodes of acute breathlessness if pneumothorax follows rupture of a bulla. But the pneumothorax is often localized by pleural adhesions and may be inconspicuous radiographically.

Some coalminers develop a variant of PMF (Caplan's syndrome) in which multiple nodules of diameter 0.5–5cm appear on the chest radiograph, often over a period of weeks, not years (fig. 9.15); the lesions may come in batches and the radiological opacities may have a slight resemblance to finger marks on the film (but *not* to whorled prints, such as those used by police for identification). There is usually little or no simple pneumoconiosis (category 0 or 1), few respiratory symptoms and little respiratory impairment (11) but the patient has an inherited susceptibility to rheumatoid arthritis which may develop at the time of or subsequent to the lung lesions. Other members of the family often suffer from rheumatoid disease, and the Rose–Waaler red cell agglutination titre and the latex agglutination titre are increased. The syndrome was described by Caplan in 1953 (5) and bears his name; it is alternatively called rheumatoid pneumoconiosis. Rheumatoid nodules also occur on the forearms or on the Achilles tendon and the arthritis is frequently disabling, leading to the man giving up work as a miner. Respiratory complications include haemoptysis, which may be associated with cavitation of one of the lesions, acute pleurisy with constitutional upset, pneumothorax and progression to the massive form of PMF; this may subsequently regress (fig. 9.15). The principal differential diagnosis is multiple metastases. Diagnosis may present difficulty if there is no discernible simple pneumoconiosis or arthritis but, unlike the patient with metastases, the patient with Caplan's syndrome is usually asymptomatic, and the serum tests for rheumatoid factor are positive.

Advanced PMF is associated with breathlessness on mild exertion or at rest, chronic bronchitis with recurrent chest illness, right ventricular hypertrophy, and episodes of right heart failure. The patient loses weight and haemoptysis is not uncommon, especially with rheumatoid pneumoconiosis. Tuberculosis is an infrequent complication but infection by opportunist mycobacteria such as M. kansasii or M. avium is relatively common. The clinical physical signs are predominantly those associated with emphysema. When there is extensive upper lobe fibrosis breath sounds high in each axilla are often bronchial in type, and are sometimes amphoric overlying a cavity which has free communication with a bronchus. In these instances vocal resonance has the expected increase in these areas. The signs do not include fine basal crepitations or clubbing of the fingers; only melanoptysis is characteristic of PMF itself. The findings on assessment of lung function are similarly not diagnostic. They include the features of airflow obstruction, a space occupying lesion and emphysema, and are described below. Other findings include a raised erythrocyte sedimentation rate, pulmonary hypertension and a reduced haemoglobin concentration; this is often due to haemodilution. The total haemoglobin may be increased secondary to hypoxaemia. The clinical condition may remain stable or deteriorate with increasing breathlessness at rest and episodes of acute infection which threaten life. However, death is usually due to hypoxic cardiac arrest and occurs peacefully. Formerly the condition was a cause of death in early middle age but now that PMF is mainly a disease of elderly coalminers the life expectancy is only slightly reduced.

There is no specific treatment which either cures or arrests PMF. It is less likely to advance if the sufferer moves to light work on the surface than if he continues heavy work underground, but only symptomatic treatment can be offered. This takes the same form as in other chronic lung diseases and includes bronchodilator and antibiotic drugs, postural drainage and controlled assisted coughing, exercise training, long-term oxygen and other remedies. These are described in chapter 19. Their application is more effective than the downhill course of the disease might lead one to expect; minor remissions are frequent and may be enhanced by active intervention and attention to details of the patient's environment. By these means an acceptable quality of life may be preserved into a late stage in the disease.

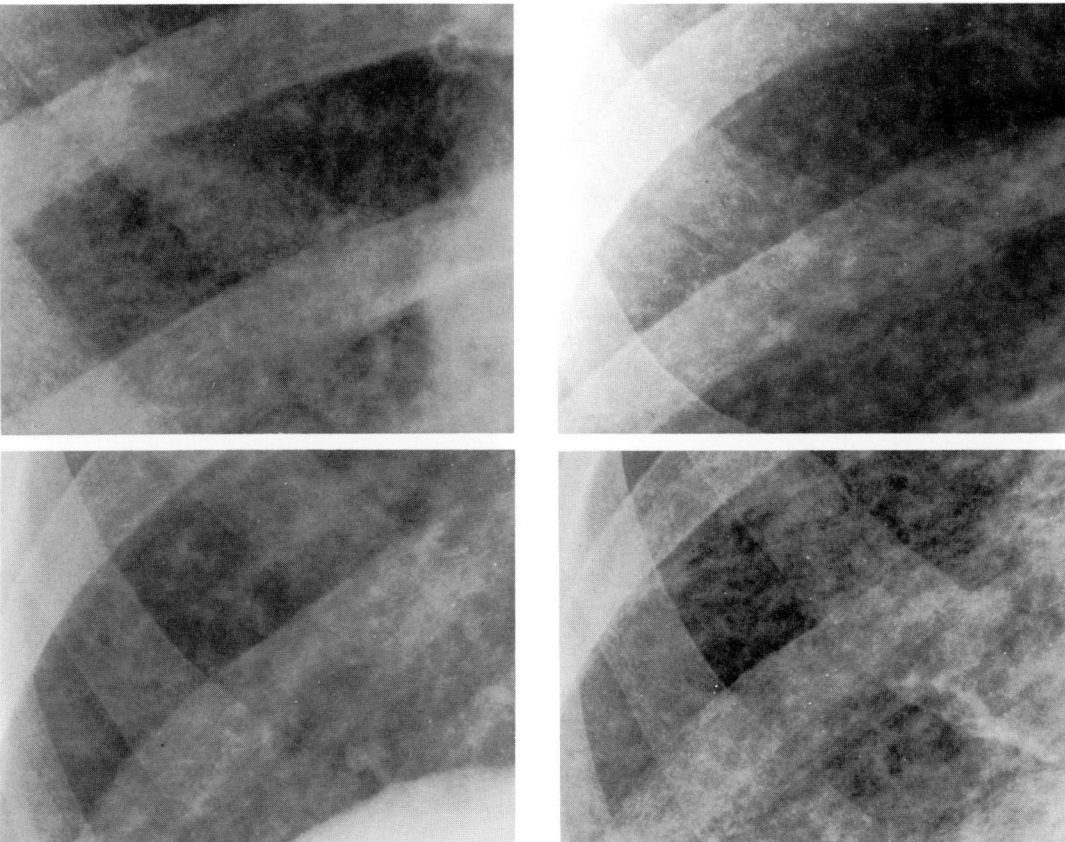

Fig. 9.16. Progression of irregular opacities. *Left:* Detail from chest radiographs at age 43 and age 56 of a man who worked as a collier for 34 years. He had formerly been a heavy smoker. On the second attendance, clinical examination revealed early finger clubbing, hyperinflation and some fine basal râles. There was moderate airflow obstruction (FEV$_1$ 1.8 l, 58% predicted) but a normal transfer factor. Death was from gastric carcinoma. The lung histology is illustrated in fig. 9.6. *Right:* Detail from chest radiographs at age 40 and age 55 in an asymptomatic collier (non-smoker). In both these patients the small opacities became more irregular; there was little change in their profusion.

Respiratory impairment in coalminers

Pneumoconiosis

The lung function of coalworkers with PMF was first investigated in depth by Gilson, Hugh-Jones, Meade & Oldham (15) in a classical study undertaken in 1949; this laid the foundations for much future work. These workers observed a reduction in ventilatory capacity and vital capacity, increase in residual volume, uneven distribution of lung ventilation, impairment of gas transfer (diffusing capacity) and increase in the ventilatory cost of standardized exercise. The total lung capacity measured by gas dilution was diminished by the presence of the PMF lesion. The mortality amongst these men was high and correlated with the respiratory impairment (38). A lesser degree of respiratory impairment was observed in men with simple pneumoconiosis; however, some of this was due to chronic bronchitis. Amongst the men with simple pneumoconiosis but no bronchitis, the initial lung function and the decline in lung function with age over a 22 year period were both within normal limits (12). Subsequent studies have largely confirmed these observations.

Effects of working in a coal mine

The development of a questionnaire for respiratory symptoms by Higgins, a spirometer for recording what is now called forced expiratory volume by Gaensler and others and an x-ray classification of pneumoconiosis made possible the large-scale investigation of respiratory health in coalminers and ex-miners. In a now classical study Rogan and colleagues (39) showed that after allowing for age and stature, the ventilatory function of working coalminers was impaired by smoking, by a history of bronchitis and by dust exposure, but not by the x-ray category of pneumoconiosis resulting from this exposure (table 9.5). Similar findings have since been reported from the U.S.A. (33) and studies of ex-coalminers are now in progress.

The reduction in forced expiratory volume is evidence for narrowing of lung airways. An increase in residual volume has also been reported (33) but these results contain ambiguities which make interpretation difficult. Detailed studies on small groups of subjects have also shown that, compared with control subjects, coalminers have a larger physiological

deadspace, increased alveolar-arterial tension difference for oxygen and larger shunt of mixed venous blood across the pulmonary capillary bed. However, many of the subjects for these studies were men with symptoms applying for industrial injuries benefit or smokers whose lungs may have been damaged on this account. Thus it is uncertain if the findings are due to working in mines: they do not seem to be related to category of pneumoconiosis which, in population studies, appears to have relatively little effect on lung function. An effect has also been looked for in selected men who were lifetime non-smokers and were free from respiratory symptoms. Amongst such men the occurrence of category 1 simple pneumoconiosis is associated with a significant reduction in elastic recoil pressure; in men with category 2 and 3, there is also evidence for narrowing of small lung airways, including an increased V-iso $\dot{v}$ and flow response to breathing helium; the closing volume is sometimes increased (24, 25).

Comparison of p and q type simple pneumoconiosis

The first evidence for a difference in lung function related to the size of small opacities came from Englert & De Coster who found the transfer factor to be reduced in the p type of simple pneumoconiosis. This has now been confirmed repeatedly (33). Several other differences between subjects with the p and q types of simple pneumoconiosis have been reported in individual studies but these have not been confirmed. The variability probably reflects differences in selection of subjects. The changes which may occur with p type opacities include an increase in lung distensibility (36), enlargement of the physiological deadspace, increased ventilation on exercise and a tendency for the pulmonary arterial pressure to be increased (33). In addition, the pattern of clearance of inhaled small particles suggests that the diameter of small airways is less in the p than the q type of simple pneumoconiosis, but the diameter of the peripheral air spaces is larger in the p type cases (17). These changes are consistent with the p type cases having more emphysema and this has been confirmed at post-mortem (28, 40).

Table 9.5. Multiple regression equation* describing the forced expiratory volume (FEV$_1$) of 3581 British coalminers. (Data of Rogan et al (39).)

Variable	Units	Mean	Regression coefficient
Dust exposure	gh m^{-3}	175	-0.6×10^{-3}
Smoking	cigs/day	13	-4.6×10^{-3}
Age	yr	47	-47×10^{-3}
Stature	m	1.70	3.1
Sitting height	m	0.90	0.86 (NS)
Body mass	kg	72	3.4×10^{-3}

NS = term not significant.

* Equation $y = ax_1 + bx_2 + \ldots -0.84 \pm 0.32$ l
The mathematical model allowed for interactions between exposure and either age or smoking but not between smoking and age (cf. page 117).

Irregular opacities

The 1971 ILO classification of small opacities on chest radiographs included irregular opacities; this prepared the way for study of the associated features. Amongst ex-miners with pneumoconiosis those with irregular opacities had a smaller total lung capacity and lower transfer factor than had the men with only rounded opacities; the slope of phase III of the single breath nitrogen test was reduced (10, 36). Independent of profusion of rounded opacities, working miners with irregular opacities who smoked had a lower forced expiratory volume and larger residual volume than smokers without irregular opacities (1). In a longitudinal study of men with simple pneumoconiosis, those with p type opacities were more likely to develop irregular opacities than men with q type opacities: some of these men showed an increased decline of transfer factor and K_{CO} with age (36). Thus irregular opacities are a relatively late feature; they commonly but not invariably occur on a basis of rounded opacities, may progress after exposure ceases, and are associated with impaired lung function; they are also associated with emphysema. It is important to know if these changes reflect a different disease or are part of simple pneumoconiosis.

Respiratory disablement in coal miners: does dust-related emphysema contribute?

Respiratory disablement and resulting breathlessness in a coal miner or ex-miner may be due to progressive massive fibrosis (category B or above) but this disease is now rare. Disablement is not a feature of classical simple pneumoconiosis. In the absence of PMF the breathlessness is usually due to airflow obstruction and negatively correlated with the FEV_1 (fig. 18.12, page 404). The obstruction is often caused or aggravated by smoking. It may be accompanied by chronic bronchitis which is aggravated by exposure to coal dust (chapter 17) whether or not the man has radiological pneumoconiosis. Airflow obstruction may also be due to late onset asthma or to emphysema which may be generalized as in non-miners (centriacinar or panacinar emphysema), secondary to progressive massive fibrosis (compensatory emphysema (27)) or localized in relation to the primary or secondary nodules of coalworkers' pneumoconiosis (focal emphysema or stellate nodule). Independent of airflow obstruction breathlessness may be due to fibrosing alveolitis, obesity, ischaemic heart disease or other medical condition which will often respond to the appropriate treatment. It may also occur as a consequence of anxiety or of voluntary overbreathing in association with a claim for industrial injuries benefit, but even in these cases there is usually an organic basis which is treatable. Outright malingering is fortunately very rare. Assessment and treatment of respiratory disablement are described in chapters 18 and 19.

Tobacco smoke causes airflow obstruction in several ways. Firstly, it stimulates irritant receptors in the bronchial epithelium; this initiates reflex contraction of bronchial smooth muscle (chapter 4). Secondly, it causes hyperplasia of mucous glands in the subepithelial layer of the bronchial wall: the enlarged glands encroach on the lumen and partially obstruct the bronchi. Thirdly, smoking causes destruction of lung tissue by mechanisms which are discussed in chapter 17. The destruction increases airflow resistance because it reduces the internal elastic forces within the lung which normally pull the (small) airways open by exerting traction on their walls. It results in emphysema of the centriacinar type which affects most smokers, including coalminers. In the latter the condition may resemble that in non-miners (fig. 17.3, page 382) or the air spaces may be outlined with coal dust but without coal nodules being present. As well as tobacco smoke the fumes from some explosives used for shot-firing formerly contained material concentrations of nitrogen oxides; these substances were a possible cause of emphysema in coal miners exposed to them (page 288).

Emphysema in coal workers is often present immediately adjacent to sites of accumulation of coal dust in the lung (figs. 9.7 and 9.8). In a coal macule the emphysema represents expansion of the affected respiratory bronchiole; it is, therefore, a centriacinar emphysema, also called focal emphysema. More emphysema occurs in association with secondary nodules (41); the emphysema is of irregular form or occurs in the angles between radiating strands of fibrous tissue (fig. 9.6). These forms of emphysema are more prevalent amongst miners than non-miners of similar age and smoking habit and are associated with an above average prevalence of dust macules (9); the emphysema is related directly to the lifetime's dust exposure and inversely to the silica exposure and silica content of the lung (40), (see also table 9.2). The emphysema is generally, but not universally (34), accepted as a consequence of coal dust in the lung and as a contributory cause of breathlessness on exertion.

Amongst non-smoking miners and miners with q-type round opacities any emphysema is usually of limited extent and not associated with functional impairment. Men with p-type opacities have rather more emphysema, the transfer factor is on average reduced and other aspects of lung function are also impaired (see above). In the absence of other factors the respiratory impairment is not material and the life expectancy is normal. The appearance of radiographic irregular opacities arising on a background of simple pneumoconiosis presages the development of widespread emphysema and fibrosis (page 172). The changes can be associated with respiratory impairment, disablement and premature death. Many of those affected were formerly smokers (e.g. figs. 9.8, right and 9.9) but disablement can also occur in non-smokers.

Where emphysema and pneumoconiosis are closely related, and death due to respiratory failure is preceded by features of dust emphysema or cystic lung rather than of chronic bronchitis, generalized emphysema or other lung disease, the dust-related emphysema must have been the main cause. It is important to know if such cases can be identified during life.

The miner with clinically significant emphysema presents with increasing breathlessness on exertion, and wheezing which is often nocturnal. The associated airflow obstruction can be partly reversed by bronchodilator drugs. In nonoccupational emphysema the static lung compliance and total lung capacity are usually increased. The chest radiograph often shows the typical features of centriacinar emphysema due to smoking, including increased transradiancy, hyperinflation and loss of peripheral blood vessels; the changes are most marked at the apices and in the upper parts of the lower lobes. In dust-emphysema the fibrous tissue between the emphysematous spaces prevents the increases in lung compliance so total lung capacity may be reduced. Such patients occasionally have clubbing of the fingers and end inspiratory râles may be heard on auscultation of the chest. The chest radiograph often reveals irregular opacities. These commonly arise on a background of p-type simple pneumoconiosis, either at the site of the round opacities or more often at the lung bases. However, unlike round opacities the irregular opacities become more numerous after withdrawal from exposure to coal dust and if initially basal they tend to extend progressively upwards into the middle zones of both lung fields (fig. 9.16). Irregular opacities are a feature of some older coal miners and when profuse are associated with breathlessness. In the late stage this condition resembles other end-stage chronic lung disease with breathlessness at rest, recurrent chest illness, polycythaemia, pulmonary hypertension and episodes of right ventricular failure. The radiographic picture may resemble that of cystic or honeycomb lung (fig. 9.9, page 176) or show the coarse irregular opacities of pulmonary congestion. Smoking appears to aggravate dust emphysema and contribute to the resulting disablement: however, the evidence is mainly anecdotal and there is need for more research.

The differential diagnosis of irregular opacities in a coalminer is between pneumoconiosis, emphysema due to smoking or other factors unrelated to coal dust exposure, fibrosing alveolitis, or other conditions; the features of some of them are summarized in table 15.5 (page 331). In a coalminer or ex-miner the following distinctions seem reasonable though they may need to be modified in the light of further research. Irregular opacities which develop gradually on a background of rounded opacities or have a similar distribution are evidence for a cystic type of emphysema with fibrosis arising from and forming part of classical simple pneumoconiosis, due to coal dust, not quartz. A coalminer with a low category of simple pneumoconiosis (0/1 to

1/2) and irregular opacities which extend upwards from the lung bases over a period of years probably has dust-related emphysema but may have fibrosing alveolitis. Irregular opacities which develop rapidly and, at an early stage, are accompanied by finger clubbing and râles are unlikely to be related to dust. Clinical and physiological emphysema not accompanied by irregular opacities is probably also unrelated to coal dust though this possibility cannot be excluded on the evidence at present available; some features of this type of emphysema are considered in chapter 17.

Epidemiological studies

Introduction

Mining coal mostly entails heavy work and, because there are few light jobs, men who become disabled leave the mines prematurely. The pressure to leave is increased at the present time of diminishing employment in the industry. Thus incomplete information is obtained by study of working coalminers and the information is least for PMF which may appear or progress after exposure to coal dust has ceased. In the 1950s these considerations led Cochrane to investigate coalworkers' pneumoconiosis in a whole community, choosing the Rhondda Fach valley in South Wales where coal mining was the only important occupation. The prevalence of pneumoconiosis was high and the movement of families in and out of the valley was probably less than in other areas. By this time, the Pneumoconiosis Unit had preliminary information on the relationship of simple pneumoconiosis in coal workers to the quantity of respired dust, based on x-rays read by a new ILO classification (1950) and measurements of dust concentration made at four pits. With the agreement of the National Union of Mineworkers, this work was taken over by the National Coal Board as the Pneumoconiosis Field Research scheme which now covers ten pits (formerly twenty-five) and is overseen at the Institute of Occupational Medicine in Edinburgh. Their results have shed unique light on the epidemiology of pneumoconiosis (e.g. 39). Comparable studies were subsequently set up in West Virginia,

U.S.A. (33) and in the Ruhr, West Germany. The National Coal Board's periodic examination scheme (1953–57) included all miners; it was unique in the extent, duration and standardization of the information collected and in its use to direct dust suppression economically. In the U.K. information on the amount of pneumoconiosis is also available from the Pneumoconiosis Medical Panels (chapter 1) but these data relate only to men who are accepted for compensation. Death certification is less biased, especially for cases selected prospectively, for example by inclusion in the Rhondda Fach study, but it is unreliable retrospectively as the recorded occupation is sometimes that to which the men moved after leaving coalmining; this leads to under-recording of coalmining as an occupation. In addition pneumoconiosis is sometimes given as a cause of death on meagre evidence.

Mortality

Mortality in coalworkers resembles that of other workers in heavy industry in being above the national average (standardized mortality ratio approximately 120 (8)). The overall rate is independent of whether or not the man has simple pneumoconiosis of the p, q or r types or category A of progressive massive fibrosis: it is increased in pneumoconiosis categories B and C and amongst miners who smoke, are bronchitic or have airflow obstruction (32). Mortality from lung cancer is reduced (e.g. SMR 66 for men in the Rhondda Fach followed for 20 years), whilst that from ischaemic heart disease is on average increased (SMR 111). The increased mortality from ischaemic heart disease is mainly amongst men without pneumoconiosis; in men with PMF category A it is apparently reduced, but why this should be is unclear (8). Due to progression of the PMF, men in category A resemble those with PMF categories B and C in having a material mortality from pneumoconiosis.

Prevalence

The prevalence of pneumoconiosis is highest for low categories and decreases progressively, through categories 2 and 3 of simple pneumoconiosis to PMF where the higher categories are now rare in working miners (fig. 9.17). The prevalence is related to cumulative dust exposure. This is a function of the prevailing level of dustiness and the duration of exposure; since the dust levels are now low, the duration of exposure and hence the age at which pneumoconiosis first appears is increasing steadily. The amount of dust inhaled is further reduced by wearing a respirator during periods of maximal dustiness and this practice is now on the increase (chapter 3). As a result of these changes simple pneumoconiosis, which in the 1950s was a condition of young men, now occurs mainly over the age of 50 years (fig. 9.18) and PMF, which was formerly killing men in middle life, now occurs in old age and seldom shortens life. This trend is also apparent in the returns of the Pneumoconiosis Medical Panels (fig. 9.19).

Relation to dust composition and other factors. In the U.K., the prevalence of pneumoconiosis was formerly highest amongst the anthracite miners of South Wales and lowest in the East Midlands coal fields (respectively high and low rank coal). This distribution is the opposite of what might have been expected if simple pneumoconiosis was usually due to silica and thus inversely related to rank of coal (table 9.1). It seems that the main cause of the regional differences in prevalence is the extent of exposure to coal dust. In South Wales boys formerly went onto the coal face straight from school at age 14 whereas elsewhere they did other mining jobs first and reached the face when they were on average 10 years older; in addition the anthracite mines, on account of the properties of the coal mineral, were formerly dustier than elsewhere. In Scottish coal mines

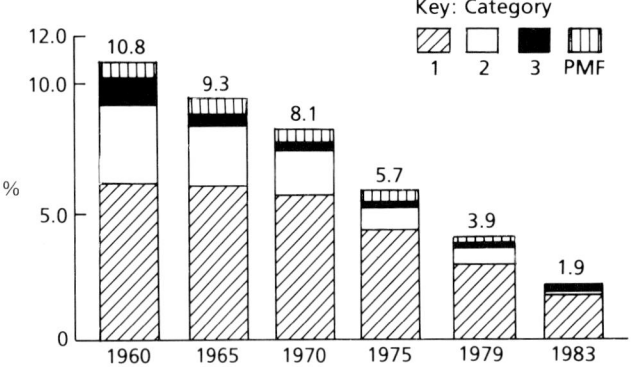

Fig. 9.17. Percentage prevalence of pneumoconiosis by radiological category in men under age 60 in forty-one British collieries surveyed at 5-yearly intervals. (By courtesy of the National Coal Board (37).)

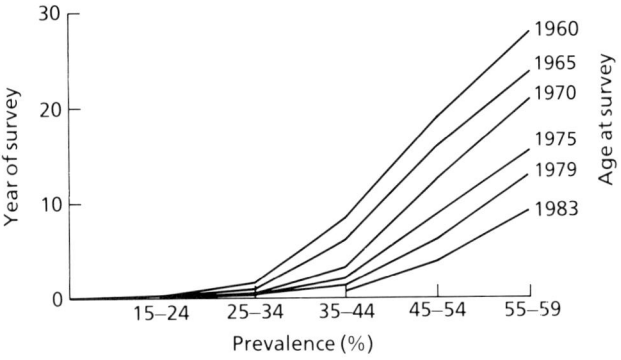

Fig. 9.18. Percentage prevalence of all categories of pneumoconiosis by age in forty-one British collieries surveyed over 23 years. (By courtesy of the National Coal Board (37).)

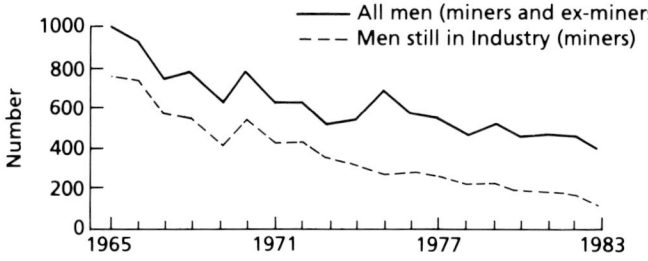

Fig. 9.19. Number of new cases of coal workers' pneumoconiosis diagnosed annually by Pneumoconiosis Medical Panels between 1965 and 1983. Amongst working coal miners the rate per thousand fell from 1.7 to 0.8. (By courtesy of the National Coal Board (37).)

the soot from miners' lamps was once a significant contributing factor (3). In the U.K. the quartz content of the dust does not influence the type of small opacities (p, q, r) but in Germany where the mine dust contains relatively more quartz a content of less than 15% predisposes to p type opacities. In the U.K. men who under present mining conditions show an increased rate of progression of simple pneumoconiosis have been exposed to a quartz content which is above the national average of 4.6% (19, 20). Increased retention of quartz is also associated with less emphysema (40); this might be expected from the pathology of silicosis (see e.g. table 9.2). High quartz contents may occur during driving the headings through rock; this predisposes to a nodular, silicotic type of disease. Independent of the dust composition the physical characteristics of the men, including their blood group, antibody profile or extent of pre-existing bronchitis do not influence the development of simple pneumoconiosis (35).

Progressive massive fibrosis. The development of progressive massive fibrosis was first investigated longitudinally in a representative complete population by Cochrane. Over an 8-year period up to 1962 he observed that the attack rate was related to category of simple pneumoconiosis (fig. 9.20) and was barely detectable below category 2 which he, therefore, proposed as a target threshold for prevention (7). Ten years later this hypothesis was largely confirmed by McLintock (31) but recently more than half the new cases of PMF are reported to have emerged from category 1 or less (44). Many of these cases appear to have been of the Caplan type but the difference may partly be an artefact due to a secular change in x-ray reading since compared with categories 2 and 3 the proportion

of men in category 1 is now higher than formerly. In the earlier studies, after allowing for x-ray category and hence exposure to coal dust, the attack rate was not influenced by age, energy expenditure at work, smoking, body type or current or previous tuberculosis. By contrast, progression of PMF lesions was faster in those who developed the condition relatively young and who continued to work at the coal face

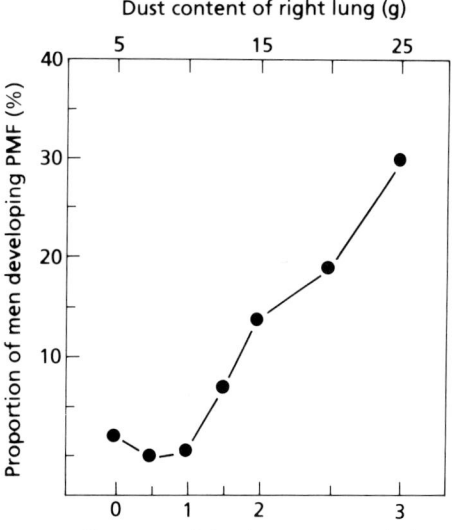

Fig. 9.20. Proportion of men developing progressive massive fibrosis in 8 years, in relation to initial category of simple pneumoconiosis amongst miners and ex-miners living in Rhondda Fach who were radiographed in 1950/51. Attacks in association with category 0 were diagnosed as tuberculosis. The original article should be consulted for details. (By courtesy of A. L. Cochrane (7).)

rather than taking a lighter job which usually entailed leaving the industry. It was not influenced by anti-tubercular chemotherapy (2). The relationship of antibody status to attack rate and progression does not appear to have been reported.

Safe conditions at work

In 1962 Cochrane recommended that the dust exposure over a working lifetime should be less than that which gave rise to category 2 simple pneumoconiosis. Estimates were made of the relevant levels of dust exposure and these were refined during the course of pneumoconiosis field research undertaken by the National Coal Board. The early estimates of dust concentration were made in terms of number of particles of respirable dust in the size range 1–5μm per ml of air sampled using a standard thermal precipitator. These were subsequently converted to mass concentration of particles of diameter 1–7μm expressed as mg m^{-3} obtained by gravimetric analysis using a standard elutriator (fig. 9.21). A mean concentration of 4.3mg m^{-3} corresponding to a maximal concentration in air leaving the coal face via the return airway of 8mg m^{-3} was initially accepted as a standard. This was estimated to give a 3.4% chance of a man developing category 2 over a working lifetime of 35 years. A probability of approximately 5% was obtained in practice. The current U.K.

standard for a long wall coal face is a maximum of 7mg m^{-3} in the return airway, corresponding to a mean concentration of 4mg m^{-3}. For underground roadways where there is a quartz hazard the maximal concentration is 3mg m^{-3} and for other localities 5mg m^{-3}. The corresponding U.S.A. standard is a mean concentration of 2mg m^{-3} obtained using a personal cyclone sample. This corresponds to a concentration of 3.2mg m^{-3} by the U.K. method of sampling. These and other standards and a strategy for dust sampling are discussed by Walton (47). Acceptable levels of dustiness are secured by dust suppression and additional protection is achieved by wearing a respirator at times of maximal dustiness (fig. 3.2, page 60). The health of the miners may be further protected by chest radiography performed every 5 years; this identifies men who are developing pneumoconiosis earlier than expected or whose disease is progressing unusually rapidly. These men should be withdrawn from further exposure to coal dust. If they are current smokers they should also be encouraged to discontinue smoking (page 180).

Industrial injuries benefit (see also page 8)

In the U.K. men with radiological pneumoconiosis category 2 or above are eligible for industrial injuries benefit; this is initially awarded at the nominal level of 10% and is increased when

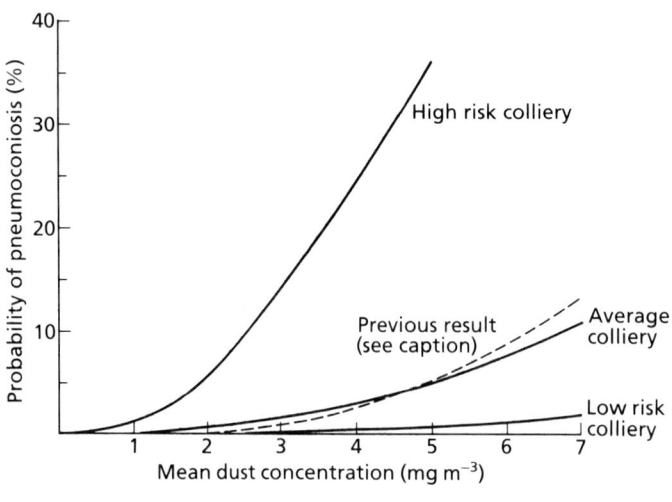

Fig. 9.21. Proportion of coal miners likely to develop simple pneumoconiosis category 2/1 or above, as a result of working for 35 years in different concentrations of respirable dust in ten collieries. The average result for eight collieries resembled that found previously (shown by interrupted line, 21); in two collieries the risk was very different. (By courtesy of J. E. Hurley and colleagues (19).)

there is PMF or respiratory disablement on account of pneumoconiosis. Additional benefit up to the level of that given for pneumoconiosis may be awarded for disablement from bronchitis or emphysema where these coexist (page 8).

As well as statutory benefits coalminers who are certified receive from the National Coal Board a lump sum payment; this replaces the right to claim under Common Law. The men and the dependants also receive a weekly supplementary income. Aspects of industrial injuries benefit in the U.S.A. and other countries are given in chapter 1.

References

1 Amandus HE, Lapp NL, Jacobson G, Reger RB. Significance of irregular small opacities in radiographs of coalminers in the USA. *Br J Industr Med* 1976;**33**:13–17.

2 Ball JD, Berry G, Clarke WG, Gilson JC, Thomas J, Exall C, Roberts M. A controlled trial of anti-tuberculosis chemotherapy in the early complicated pneumoconiosis of coalworkers. *Thorax* 1969;**24**:399–406.

3 Bergman I, Casswell C. Lung dust and lung iron contents of coal workers in different coalfields in Great Britain. *Br J Industr Med* 1972;**29**:160–8.

4 Burrell R, Flaherty DK, Schreiber JE. Immunological studies of experimental coal workers pneumoconiosis. *Inhaled Particles IV*, 1977; 519–29. Walton WH (ed.). Oxford: Pergamon Press.

5 Caplan A, Payne RB, Withey JL. A broader concept of Caplan's syndrome related to rheumatoid factors. *Thorax* 1962;**17**:205–12.

6 Chapman JS, Ruckley VA. Microanalyses of lesions and lymph nodes from coalminers' lungs. *Br J Industr Med* 1985;**42**:551–5.

7 Cochrane AL. The attack rate of progressive massive fibrosis. *Br J Industr Med* 1962; **19**:52–64.

8 Cochrane AL, Moore F, Moncrieff CB. Are coalminers with low risk factors for ischaemic heart disease at greater risk of developing progressive massive fibrosis? *Br J Industr Med* 1982; **39**:265–8. *See also* Atuhaire LK *et al Ibid.* 1985; **42**:741–5.

9 Cockroft A, Seal RME, Wagner JC, Lyons JP, Ryder R, Andersson N. Post-mortem study of emphysema in coal workers and non-coal workers. *Lancet* 1982;**ii**:600–3.

10 Cockcroft AE, Wagner JC, Seal RME, Lyons JP, Campbell MJ. Irregular opacities in coal-workers' pneumoconiosis—correlation with pulmonary function and pathology. *Ann Occup Hyg* 1982;**26**:767–87.

11 Constantinidis K, Musk AW, Jenkins JPR, Berry G. Pulmonary function in coal workers with Caplan's syndrome and non-rheumatoid complicated pneumoconiosis. *Thorax* 1978;**33**: 764–8.

12 Cotes JE. Serial data over 10–22 years for detailed lung function of working men. *Scand J Respir Dis* 1976;**57**:764–8.

13 Davis JMG, Chapman J, Collings P, Douglas AN, Fernie J, Lamb D, Ruckley VA. Variations in the histological patterns of the lesions of lung dust content. *Am Rev Respir Dis* 1983;**128**:118–24.

14 Gaensler EA, Cadigan JB, Sasahara AA, Fox EO, MacMahon HE. Graphite pneumoconiosis of electrotypers. *Am J Med* 1966;**41**:864–82.

15 Gilson JC, Hugh-Jones P. *Lung function in coal-workers' pneumoconiosis.* MRC Special Report Series No. 290.

16 Gough J, Wentworth JE. Thin sections of entire organs mounted on paper. In: *Recent Advances in Pathology*, 7th ed. Harrison CV (ed). London: Churchill, 1960:80–86.

17 Hankinson JL, Palmes ED, Lapp NL. Pulmonary airspace size in coalminers. *Am Rev Respir Dis* 1979;**119**:391–7.

18 Heppleston AG. The pathological anatomy of simple pneumoconiosis in coalworkers. *J Pathol Bact* 1953;**66**:235–46.

19 Hurley JF, Burns J, Copeland L, Dodgson J, Jacobsen M. Coalworkers' simple pneumoconiosis and exposure to dust at 10 British coal mines. *Br J Industr Med* 1982;**39**:120–7.

20 Jacobsen M, MacClaren WM. Unusual pulmonary observations and exposure to coalmine dust: a case-control study. *Ann Occup Hyg* 1982;**26**:753–65.

21 Jacobsen M, Rae S, Walton WH, Rogan JM. The relation between pneumoconiosis and dust-exposure in British coal mines. In: *Inhaled Particles III, Vol. II.* Walton W .H. (ed). Surrey: Unwin Brothers. 1971:903–17.

22 Jones ADW, Quinn JJ, Woolley KM. *Evaluation of coal winning technology.* Technical Change Centre, London. 1984.

23 Jones BM, Edwards JH, Wagner JC. Absorption of serum proteins by inorganic dusts. *Br J Industr Med* 1972;**29**:287–92.

24 Lapp NL, Block J, Boehlecke B, Lippmann M, Morgan WKC, Reger RB. Closing volume in coalminers. *Am Rev Respir Dis* 1976;**113**: 155–61.

25 Legg SJ, Cotes JE, Bevan C. Lung mechanics in relation to radiographic category of coalworkers' simple pneumoconiosis. *Br J Industr Med* 1983;**40**:28–33.

26 Lippmann M, Eckert HL, Hahon N, Morgan WKC. Circulating antinuclear and rheumatoid factors in coalminers. *Ann Intern Med 1973;* **79**:807–11.

27 Lyons JP, Campbell H. Relation between progressive massive fibrosis, emphysema and pulmonary dysfunction in coalworkers' pneumoconiosis. *Br J Industr Med* 1981;**38**:125–9.

28 Lyons JP, Ryder RC, Campbell H, Clarke WG, Gough J. Significance of irregular opacities in the radiology of coalworkers' pneumoconiosis. *Br J Industr Med* 1974;**31**:36–44.

29 Lyons JP, Ryder RC, Seal RME, Wagner JC. Emphysema in smoking and non-smoking coalworkers with pneumoconiosis. *Bull Europ Physiopath Respir* 1981;**17**:75–85.

30 Maclaren WM, Soutar CA. Progressive massive fibrosis and simple pneumoconiosis in ex-miners. *Br J Industr Med* 1985;**42**:734–40.

31 McLintock JS, Rae S, Jacobsen M. The attack rate of progressive massive fibrosis in British coalminers. *Inhaled Particles, III*, Vol. II. Walton W.H. (ed). Surrey: Unwin Brothers. 1971:933–52.

32 Miller BG, Jacobsen M. Dust exposure, pneumoconiosis and mortality of coal miners. *Br J Industr Med* 1985;**42**:723–33.

33 Morgan WKC, Lapp NL. Respiratory disease in coalminers. *Am Rev Respir Dis* 1976;**113**:531–59.

34 Morgan WKC. Coalworkers' pneumoconiosis. In: Morgan WKC, Seaton A. *Occupational Lung Diseases*, Philadelphia: Saunders. 1984:377–448.

35 Muir DCF, Burns J, Jacobsen M, Walton WH. Pneumoconiosis and chronic bronchitis. *Br Med J* 1977;**2**:424–7.

36 Musk AW, Cotes JE, Bevan C, Campbell MJ. Relationship between type of simple coalworkers' pneumoconiosis and lung function. A nine-year follow-up study of subjects with small rounded opacities. *Br J Industr Med* 1981;**38**:313–20.

37 National Coal Board Medical Service. *Annual Report*. 1983–4.

38 Oldham PD, Rossiter CE. Mortality in coalworkers' pneumoconiosis related to lung function: a prospective study. *Br J Industr Med* 1965;**22**:93–100.

39 Rogan JM, Attfield MD, Jacobsen M, Rae S, Walker DD, Walton WH. Role of dust in the working environment in development of chronic bronchitis in British coalminers. *Br J Industr Med* 1973;**30**:217–26.

40 Ruckley VA, Fernie JM, Chapman JS, Collings P, Davis JMG, Douglas AN, Lamb D, Seaton A. Comparison of radiographic appearances with associated pathology and lung dust content in a group of coalworkers. *Br J Industr Med* 1984;**41**:459–67.

41 Ruckley VA, Gauld SJ, Chapman JS, Davis JMG, Douglas AN, Fernie JM, Jacobsen M, Lamb D. Emphysema and dust exposure in a group of coal miners. *Am Rev Respir Dis* 1984:**129**:528–32.

42 Ryder R, Lyons JP, Campbell H, Gough J. Emphysema in coalworkers' pneumoconiosis. *Br Med J* 1970;iii:481–7.

43 Seal RME, Cockcroft A, Kung I, Wagner JC. Central lymph node changes and progressive massive fibrosis in coalworkers. *Thorax* 1986;**41**:531–7.

44 Shennan DH, Washington JS, Thomas DJ, Dick JA, Kaplan YS, Bennett JG. Factors predisposing to the development of progressive massive fibrosis in coalminers. *Br J Industr Med* 1981;**38**:321–6.

45 Soutar CA, Turner-Warwick M, Parkes WR. Circulating antinuclear antibody and rheumatoid factor in coal pneumoconiosis. *Br Med J* 1974;iii:145–7.

46 Wagner JC, Burns J, Munday DE, McGee Jo'D. Presence of fibronectin in pneumoconiotic lesions. *Thorax* 1982;**37**:54–6.

47 Walton WH. International Research Programmes in the Pneumoconioses—legislation, standards, medical aspects, etc. In: *Second Australian Pneumoconiosis Conference, Sydney Australia, 20–23 February 1978, Papers and Proceedings*. New South Wales: Joint Coal Board. paper A3.

48 Watson AJ, Black J, Doig AT, Nagelschmidt G. Pneumoconiosis in carbon electrode makers. *Br J Industr Med* 1959;**16**:274–85.

Chapter 10
Asbestos and Other Mineral Fibres

Asbestiform minerals

Asbestos from the Greek ασβεστός 'unquench-
able' is a fibrous silicate material which is tough
and fire-resistant. It occurs naturally in serpentine and amphibole mineral rock. The commonest form, chrysotile $(3MgO.2SiO_2.2H_2O)$, is a
sheet silicate (33). It was formed in fissures
amidst ultra-basic igneous rocks by the action of
great heat and water on magnesium oxide to
form layered scrolls of serpentine asbestos (fig.
10.1). The mineral does not contain quartz. It
occurs throughout the world but most comes
from opencast mines in the Quebec province of
Canada, the Ural mountains of the U.S.S.R. and
Southern Africa. Other sources include China,
Italy, Cyprus, U.S.A. and Western Australia.
Commercial production began in about 1880,
rose to a peak of about 6 million tonnes per
annum a hundred years later and is now diminishing. The fibre is usually liberated by wet
crushing and by hammer milling in a current of
air (69); the final product is a curved flexible
white fibre which is capable of splitting progressively into fibrils of exceedingly small diameter
(0.025μm, fig. 10.2). It has great tensile strength
and tolerates temperatures in excess of 600°C
but is alkaline, hence not very resistant to acids,
and vegetation will not grow in the waste.

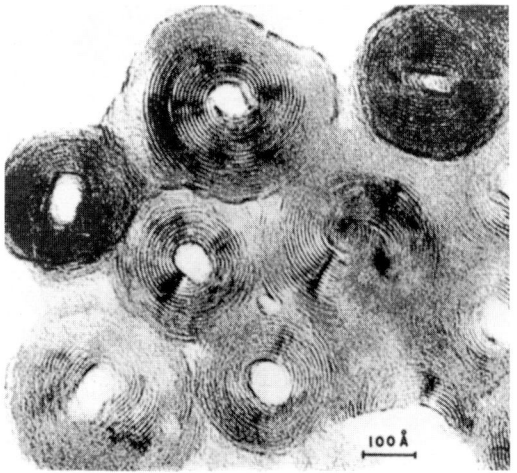

Fig. 10.1. Cross-section of a chrysotile fibre
showing the scroll-like structure of the
microfibrils. (Source Yada K. (1967) *Acta
Crystallographica* **23**:704–7.)

Fibrous amphibole asbestos is a chain silicate
with a straight lath-like structure; it has many
varieties including anthophyllite, a white,
somewhat brittle, heat resistant fibre which
occurs in a pure form in Finland, actinolite and
tremolite, which are not used commercially but
may be present as contaminants, and amosite, a

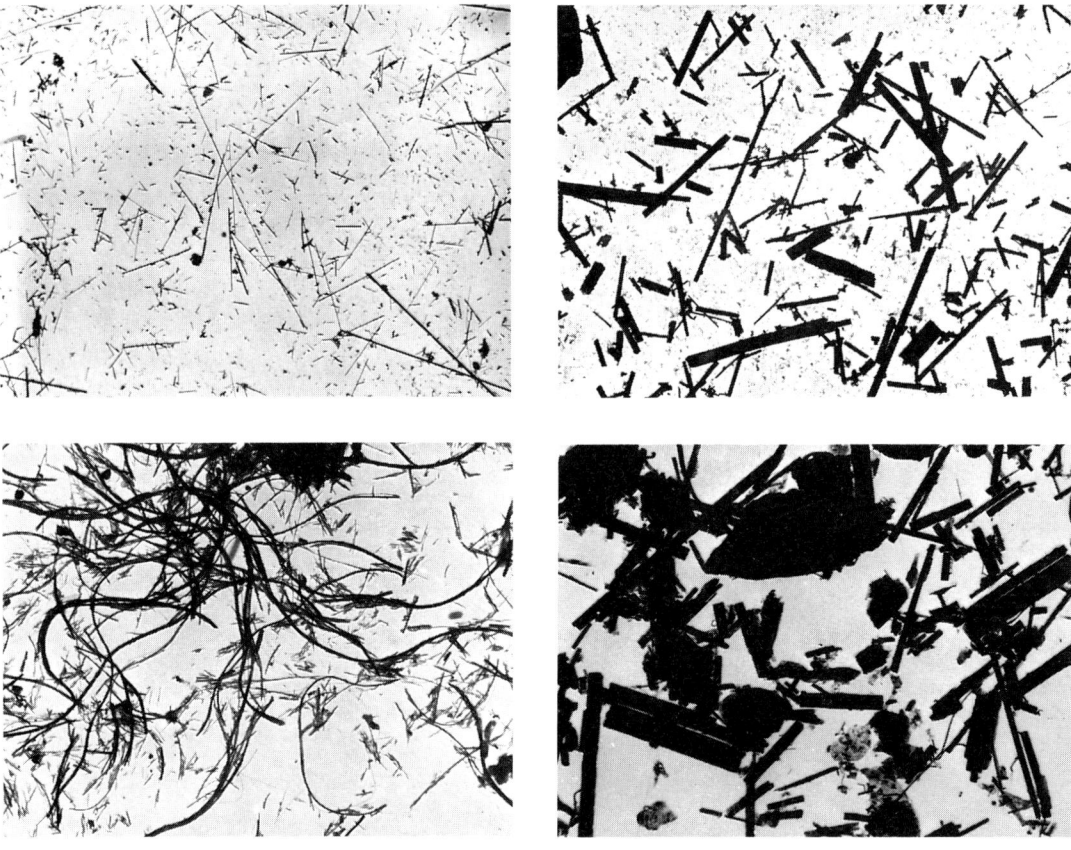

Fig. 10.2. Microscopic appearance of different types of asbestos (UICC standard samples). *Left*: crocidolite and chrysotile. *Right*: amosite and anthophyllite. (By courtesy of V. Timbrell.)

brown asbestos which is named after its origin in the asbestos mines of South Africa. However, the most important fibrous amphibole is crocidolite, the blue asbestos, which is mined in Southern Africa and at one time in Western Australia. Crocidolite from N. Western Cape Province in South Africa and from Wittenoom in Australia contains many exceedingly fine fibres (fig. 10.2). Until recently the production of amphiboles was rising relative to that of chrysotile and at the peak comprised some 3% of total world production. The deposits were formed by metamorphosis of pre-Cambrian sedimentary strata of banded iron-stone and the resulting fibres are straight, relatively long and thin, very tough and resistant to acid as well as heat.

Uses of asbestos

The main use in antiquity was for strengthening pottery and this application has continued in the form of asbestos cement which is used to make strong, inexpensive building materials such as boards, sheets, pipes, gutters, roofing-tiles and ventilation-ducts. The mixture contains between 12% and 15% of asbestos, which is now entirely chrysotile but was formerly a mixture of chrysotile and amphibole asbestos. Cement products account for some 70% of current world production of asbestos. Vinyl asbestos floor tiles may contain 20% of short fibre chrysotile and are another important application.

Table 10.1. Situations where there may be exposure to asbestos, subdivided by risk category

	High risk, full precautions essential	Low risk, good housekeeping necessary	Risk minimal in normal circumstances	Unacceptable risk, use discontinued
Production	Crushing, milling, packaging		Mining; transporting sealed bales	Transporting dusty consignments
Manufacture	Textiles; friction materials; preparing slurry in manufacture of other products	Cement products;* sheets, sections, tiles, pipes, conduits, etc.	Tarred felts;* mastics, underseals, adhesives	Millboard, paper fillers, battery boxes, insulation board
Use	Removal of old insulation	Building construction, roofing, flooring	Fitting brakes, etc.	Spraying pure fibre (mixed with silicate glue), lagging, packaging
Other	Demolition of structures containing asbestos; maintaining lagged equipment	Replacing brake linings	Using asbestos clothing,† mats, etc.	Sanding asbestos products

* After initial stages.
† If properly made and in good condition.

The second traditional use which has persisted was for fire-resistant cloth made from long-fibre chrysotile. This is used for protective clothing, e.g. for fire fighting, work in furnaces, military anti-flash jackets, fire-resistant blankets, conveyor belts and other products. However, at the time of its reintroduction in the 1880s asbestos was used mainly for thermal insulation, first of steam engines and then boilers, heating systems and other installations and appliances, including those on ships where the great durability and resistance to corrosion of crocidolite seemed to confer an obvious advantage. Asbestos mixed with cement was used as an adhesive cladding (limpet spray) for buildings. Asbestos reinforced bricks were used for lining furnaces. With few exceptions the use of asbestos for insulation is now being rapidly phased out in favour of safer materials. There is so far no fully satisfactory substitute for asbestos in friction materials, including clutch and brake linings, or for gaskets, packing for bearings and related products.

Occupations where asbestos may be a hazard

Mining and quarrying asbestos are relatively safe occupations; the risk starts with the processes of crushing and milling and continues through the intermediate stages of transportation and manufacture to the incorporation of asbestos in the final product. Under modern conditions the asbestos is usually quite safe but in the case of old buildings, ships, heating systems and other plant lagged with asbestos there is a risk during dismantling for repair work of any type and during demolition and subsequent disposal of the debris. These activities may result in the indirect exposure of persons in many occupations including fitters and electricians. Exposure leading to the development of mesothelioma has also occurred as a result of asbestos carried on clothing to the home, canteen or laundry, and airborne asbestos reaching people in the neighbourhood of a crocidolite milling plant or asbestos textile factory. Poorly

designed or fraying protective helmets and
clothing containing asbestos may also be a
hazard. Some occupations at risk are given in
table 10.1. Many of these are only of historical
interest and in the remainder the risk for new
entrants is now considered to be at an acceptable level. How this has come about is considered subsequently.

Diseases due to asbestos

That exposure to asbestos dust may lead to diffuse pulmonary fibrosis has been known since
early this century. The condition was given the
name 'asbestosis' by Cooke in 1927. Lung cancer
in asbestos workers was described by Wood &
Gloyne in 1934. Evidence for a causal association
was first provided epidemiologically by Doll in
1955 (see 60). The association of mesothelial
tumours of the pleura and peritoneum with
asbestos was noted in 1946 and epidemiological
evidence for the tumours being due to crocidolite
was obtained by Wagner and colleagues in 1960
(7: ref. 27). Other conditions which can be due to
asbestos are acute pleurisy, benign chronic
pleural disease including plaques, thickening
and calcification, and skin corns. Asbestos has
been charged with causing lung cancer in the
general population but this is almost certainly
incorrect (page 226). Previous very high exposures to asbestos appear to have caused carcinoma of the stomach, ovary, breast and larynx
(57). However, there is no good evidence for
moderately high exposures having these effects
(69, 76). The evidence for an association in the
case of non-Hodgkin's lymphoma of the gastro-
intestinal tract is also insubstantial (8). The
excess cancer risk appears to be virtually confined to the lungs, pleura and peritoneum of
persons who were exposed to amphibole, and to
a much lesser extent chrysotile, asbestos at a time
when the levels of pollution were not well controlled. The pathology of the asbestos-associated
diseases is described below (21, 61).

Benign asbestos pleural disease

Pleural plaques. Pleural plaques are circumscribed, raised areas of hyaline fibrous tissue
which, with the passage of time, may calcify (fig.
10.3). They are present in up to 40% of persons

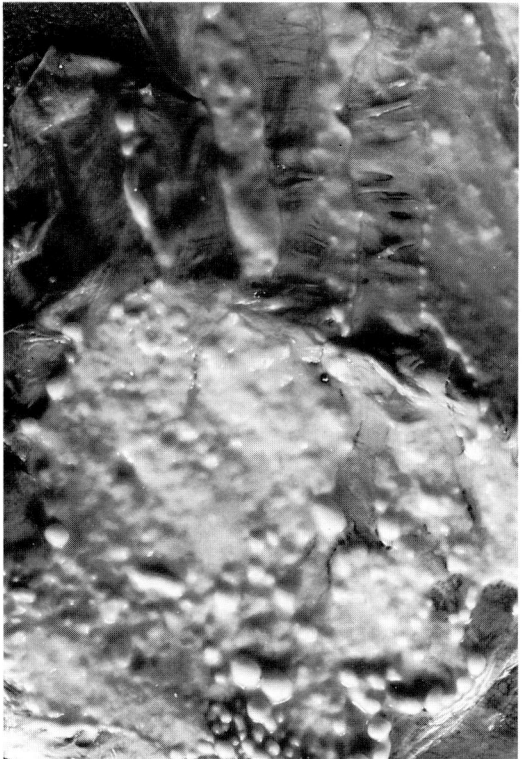

Fig. 10.3. Large pleural plaque which in places is
localized behind ribs, leaving the spaces between
clear. (By courtesy of T. Ashcroft.)

with a regular occupational or environmental
exposure to asbestos and also occur in places
where related minerals are present in the soil
(page 222). Away from sources of such fibres the
likelihood that plaques are due to asbestos
appears to be small (12). The proportion of persons affected is related more closely to the time
since first exposure to asbestos dust than to the
intensity of exposure. Smokers and ex-smokers
are more likely to develop visceral plaques than
are non-smokers (49, 82, 83) but it is not clear
whether this is true of the much commoner
parietal plaques.

Plaques in the parietal pleura usually occur
over ribs in the mid-zone and in the paravertebral sulci, or over the central part of the
diaphragm. The parietal pericardium on the left
side may also be affected. Large or calcified
plaques are easily identified radiographically

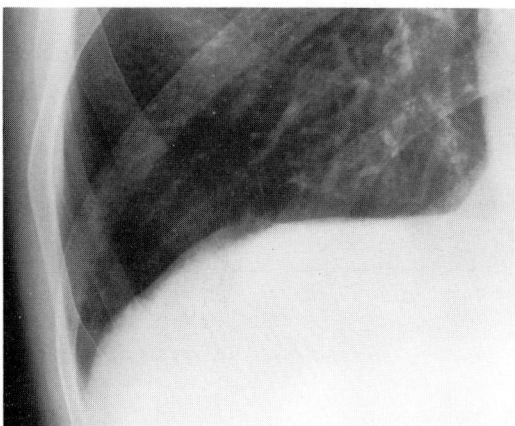 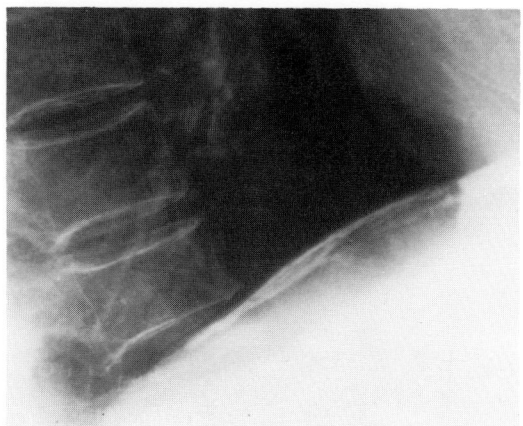

Fig. 10.4. Calcified diaphragmatic plaques more conspicuous on the lateral than postero-anterior chest radiograph. From a 59-year-old shipyard electrician (ex-smoker) who developed asthma following exposure to fumes in an electrical fire. He did not have asbestosis.

but small ones are not visible on standard chest films; they may be seen on lateral views (e.g. fig. 10.4) but even a heavily calcified plaque may be missed if the long axis is perpendicular to the plane of the film. Plaques are most readily seen edge-on as thickening beneath the lateral chest wall or as discrete, calcified lines or nodules; a calcified anterior plaque may resemble a holly leaf (fig. 10.5). More often the anterior plaque forms an irregular, soft opacity of waxy appearance which is sometimes confused with costal cartilage. Identification is greatly assisted by computer assisted tomography (CAT scans, 40, figs. 10.5 and 10.6).

Plaques in persons exposed to asbestos are now known to contain small asbestos fibres which appear to have migrated from the lung via the sub-pleural lymphatics of the chest wall; the process of migration is held up where the pleura overlies a rib and this may explain why plaques occur at such sites. Coalworkers may have coal dust deposited at the same site but without any reaction to it. Affected asbestos workers have a slightly increased risk of developing parenchymal changes compared with other asbestos workers (50). Plaques seldom give rise to symptoms and do not presage lung cancer or mesothelioma; however, the belief that they may do so is a cause of anxiety and of frustrated desire for compensation. The other complication is

restriction of lung expansion (13, 25, fig. 10.5). This is surprisingly uncommon and, except in association with diffuse pleural fibrosis or asbestosis, seldom gives rise to symptoms.

Benign pleural effusion. Pleural effusion in a person exposed to asbestos is usually evidence of a mesothelioma. However, this is not invariable and there are now many instances where the effusion has been innocent. In one series the average duration of exposure was 5.5 years and the interval between first exposure and presentation was 16.3 years (64). The condition is usually asymptomatic and detected by routine chest radiography. Alternatively the effusion presents with pleuritic pain which may be accompanied by fever, leucocytosis and low grade inflammation of the lung. The erythrocyte sedimentation rate is often increased. The visceral pleura is highly vascular and bleeding may occur into the effusion which is exudative in type. Pleural thickening is common either at the time or subsequently (fig. 10.6). In the series cited those effusions which resolved did so in an average of 4.3 months but one-third of patients experienced a recurrence during the subsequent 5 years; this was commonly contralateral. The condition may progress to diffuse fibrosis of the pleura.

Diffuse pleural fibrosis. This condition is present when the pleura is thickened to a width of

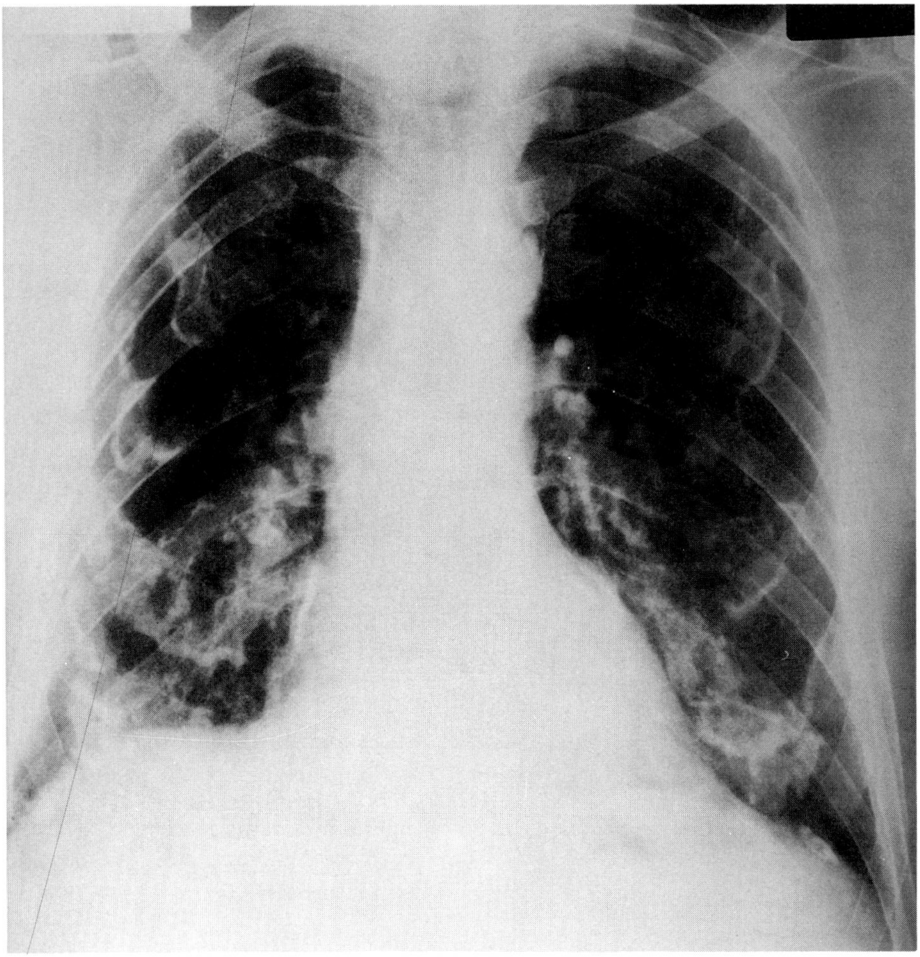

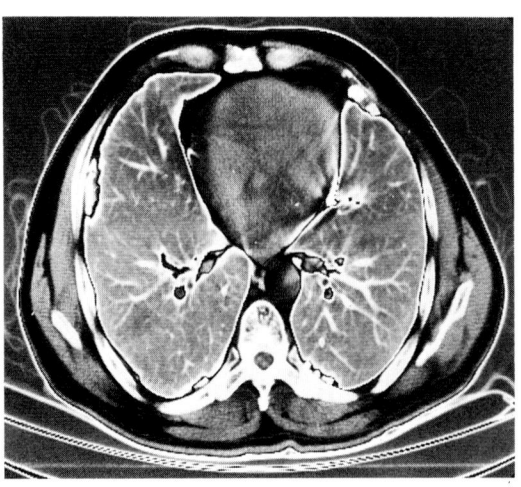

Fig. 10.5. Extensive plaques. Chest radiograph showing extensive calcified plaques diagnosed at routine radiography in a 60-year-old shipyard electrician. The CAT scan (below) showed the plaques indenting the lung in the paravertebral sulci and beneath some ribs. The patient had no respiratory symptoms but end inspiratory râles were present in the chest. Lung function assessment revealed a stiff lung but normal gas exchange (table 10.2).

at least 5mm over a length which is at least 25% of the chest wall on both sides or when both costophrenic angles are obliterated (page 89). It is then usually due to asbestos (2). Isolated filling of one costophrenic or cardiophrenic angle is commonly due to other causes. Diffuse pleural fibrosis may occur in isolation, with extensive pleural plaques (fig. 10.5), following benign pleural effusion (fig. 10.6), or in association with asbestosis. Except in the last of these conditions, there is no material involvement of lung tissue. However, the visceral pleura is inseparable from the lung itself, and at post-mortem is always found to be thickened to some extent in cases of asbestosis. In this condition the thickening often gives rise to an asymmetrical

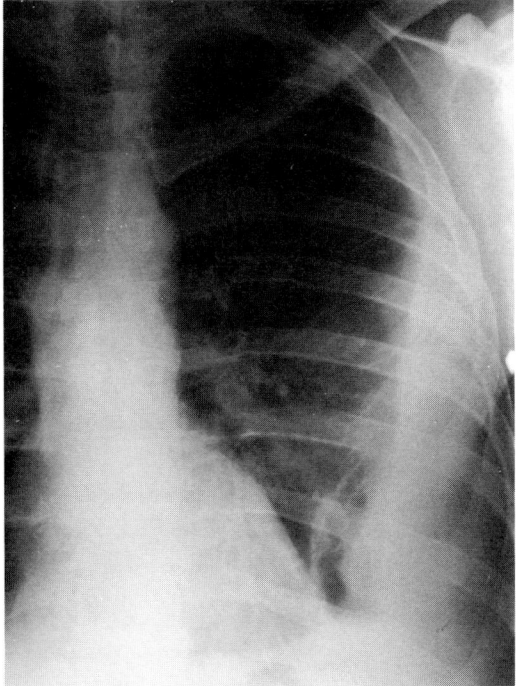

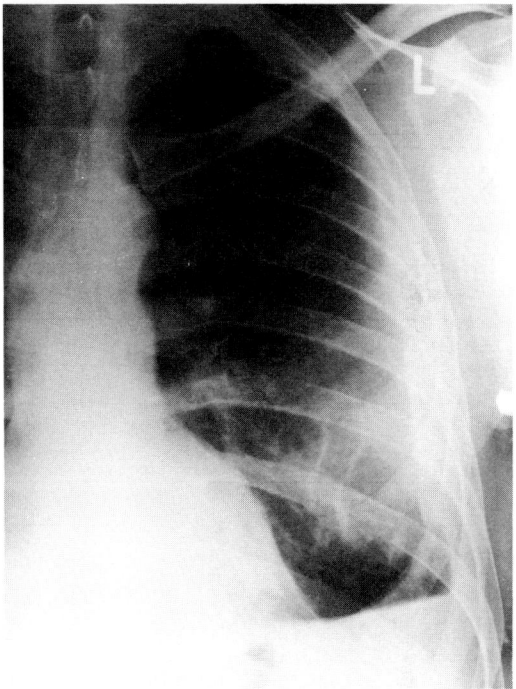

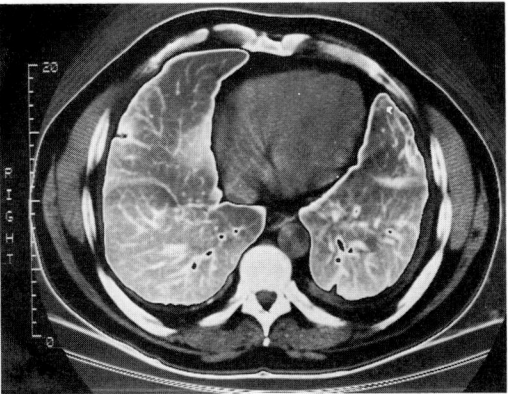

Fig. 10.6. Diffuse pleural thickening. Chest radiograph (top left) showing a loculated effusion in the left pleural space of a 36-year-old shipyard labourer who at one time was spraying asbestos; subsequently he developed pleural thickening. This is shown on the radiograph (right) and CAT scan (lower left). The scan also shows thickening of the right pleura with, posteriorly, a small patch of calcification which serves as a marker. By age 42 the patient was breathless on moderate exertion (grade 3), but had no cough despite being a heavy smoker up to that time. Some crepitations were heard at the lung bases. On assessment of lung function, the total lung capacity was reduced in association with a low compliance and moderately high recoil pressure but the transfer factor was relatively normal (table 10.2). The patient was considered not to have asbestosis.

Table 10.2.   Lung function in three men exposed to asbestos

| Details | Diffuse pleural disease | | Asbestosis (fig. 10.8) |
	Plaques (fig. 10.5)	Fibrosis (fig. 10.6)	
Age (a)	60	42	50
Height (m)	1.87	1.80	1.69
Weight (kg)	85	93	59
FEV_1 (l)	3.3 (3.5)*	1.9 (3.8)	1.2 (3.1)
FVC (l)	4.1 (4.8)	2.9 (4.8)	2.1 (4.1)
FEV%	81 (69)	64 (76)	57 (73)
TLC (l)	5.9 (7.7)	4.0 (7.1)	4.3 (6.1)
RV (l)	2.0 (2.6)	1.4 (2.1)	1.8 (2.0)
Cstat (l kPa^{-1})	1.7 (3.1)	1.1 (2.8)	1.0 (2.4)
P max (kPa)	5.0 (2.5)	3.5 (2.5)	5.1 (2.5)
Tl (mmol min^{-1} kPa^{-1})	8.6 (10.5)	7.6 (10.9)	3.4 (9.1)
K_{CO} (Tl/V_A)	1.6 (1.4)	1.9 (1.7)	0.9 (1.5)
$\dot{V}_E 45$ (l min^{-1})	33 (24)	34 (24)	42†(24)
Vt_{30} (l)*	1.0 (1.5)	1.0 (1.5)	0.8 (1.4)
SaO_2 (rest/ex.%)	96/96	NA	91/84

These patients all had a reduced total lung capacity associated with a low compliance and high recoil pressure. The low TLC contributed to reductions in exercise tidal volume (Vt_{30}) and in transfer factor; in asbestos pleural disease the latter effect was partly compensated for by an increase in K_{CO}. In all the patients the exercise ventilation was increased, mainly on account of an enlarged physiological deadspace. Exercise hypoxaemia occurred in the patient with asbestosis.
* Reference values are in parentheses: those for Vt_{30} are based on the predicted FVC. The upper limit for Pmax is 3.7 kPa.
† Extrapolated

haziness over the lower lung fields described as ground glass appearance, or to blurring of the cardiac outline giving the appearance of a shaggy heart. The lung function of two patients with diffuse pleural thickening is summarized in table 10.2. The principal change is restriction of lung expansion which reduces the tidal volume during exercise, increases the respiratory frequency and may give rise to breathlessness on exertion (chapter 18). In advanced cases all subdivisions of the total lung capacity are reduced starting with the inspiratory capacity and including the residual volume (48). Due to thickening of the visceral pleura the static compliance of the lung is usually reduced and the elastic recoil pressure increased (25). These changes reduce the forced expiratory volume and indices of forced expiratory flow; there may also be a reduced transfer factor, the computation of which is dependent upon total lung volume. When the lung is compressed from without, the alveolar surface area per unit volume is increased (the lung becomes denser) and this increases the K_{CO} (87). Consequently the transfer factor does not fall much (about 1 SI unit for each litre reduction in lung volume). A substantial fall in transfer factor in a patient with diffuse pleural thickening indicates disease of the lung parenchyma, even though the K_{CO} may be close to the reference value for a healthy person of the same age; the reference value is not applicable when the lung volume is reduced.

Diffuse pleural thickening seldom requires treatment; however, if breathlessness is a problem but the lung parenchyma appears normal the patient will sometimes benefit from surgical removal of the thickened pleura.

Asbestosis

General features. Asbestosis is a diffuse interstitial fibrosis of the lung; it occurs in persons who have had moderate or heavy exposure to

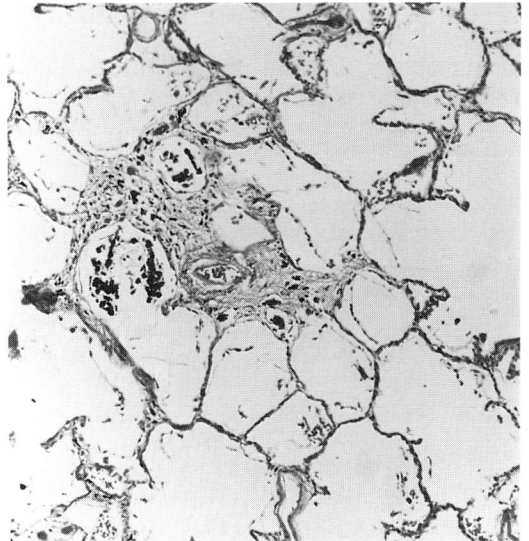

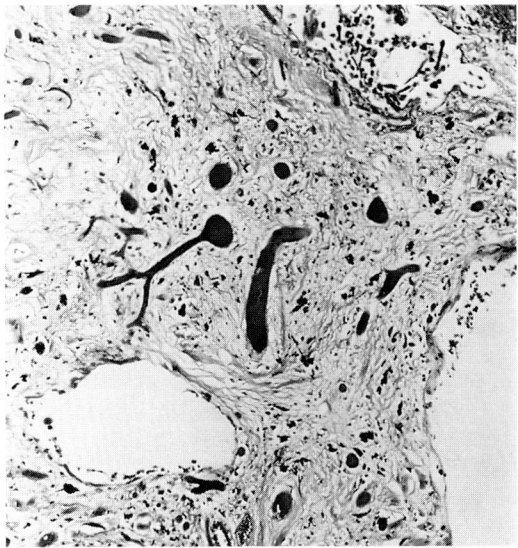

Fig. 10.7. Histology of asbestosis (low power view). Mild, moderate and severe fibrosis, the last showing cystic spaces between the strands of fibrous tissue, macroscopically appearing as honeycombing. Asbestos bodies and fibres are present in some alveoli. (By courtesy of T. Ashcroft.)

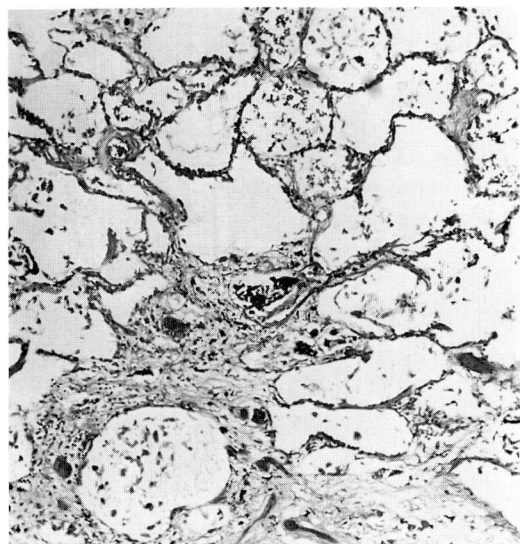

asbestos, usually some 12–20 years after first exposure. Smokers of more than 4 cigarettes per day are more at risk than non-smokers (65). The condition formerly presented with breathlessness on exertion but is now commonly detected as a result of a routine periodic radiographic examination of the chest. Sometimes the diagnosis is made a few months after an episode of pneumonia which may hasten the disease process; this initially takes the form of a focal pneu-

monitis with leucocytes, macrophages and fibroblasts accumulating round the inhaled dust fibres. The alveoli which open directly off respiratory bronchioles in the sub-pleural zone of the lung are affected first (fig. 10.7); they accumulate fibres which attract alveolar macrophages and stimulate the growth of alveolar type II cells; reticulin tissue is laid down and progresses to fibrous tissue (15, 7: ref. 62). This is grade 1 fibrosis; it is not unique to asbestosis as similar foci are seen in smokers not exposed to asbestos (21). In grade 2 the fibrosis extends into the adjacent alveolar ducts and alveoli but the lesions are discrete with normal lung between. In grade 3 the lesions become confluent. The lesions extend by enveloping the adjacent bron-chioles which are extensively damaged (86). The small pulmonary arteries are also narrowed or obliterated. Subsequently the fibrous tissue contracts and small cystic spaces up to 5mm diameter form between its strands (honeycomb lung, fig. 10.7). A similar mechanism may

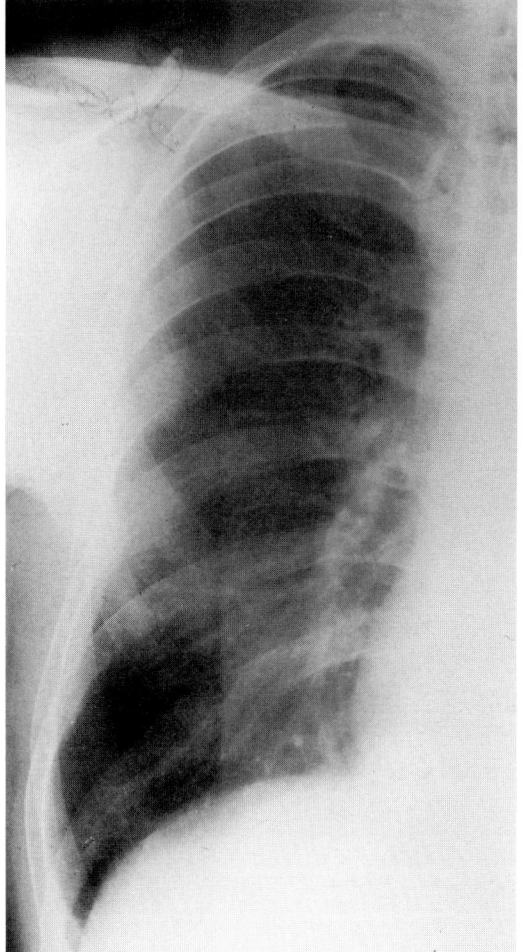 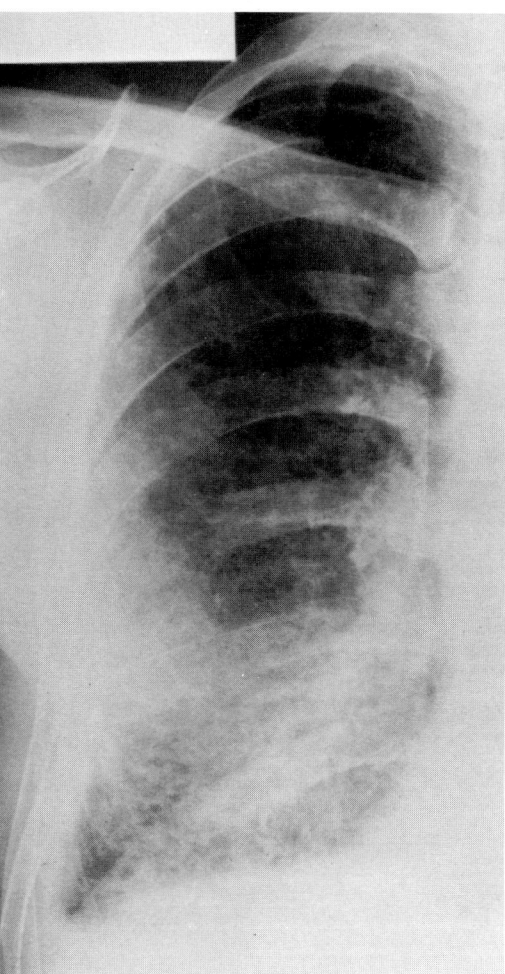

Fig. 10.8. Asbestosis. Chest radiographs at age 30 and 60 years of a man who for 21 years worked as a boiler coverer and insulator. The earlier film (left) was taken as a result of the father dying from asbestosis and lung cancer. A brother also died from these conditions. The patient's asbestosis was diagnosed at age 37. He subsequently developed a chronic productive cough with wheeze on most nights, and at age 60 was breathless on mild exertion (grade 4). He was cyanosed and had finger clubbing; râles and rhonchi were audible at the lung bases. The chest radiograph (right) showed some reduction in lung size associated with diffuse pleural thickening and irregular opacities in the lower half. The lung function results are given in table 10.2. As well as features typical of asbestosis the patient had irreversible airflow obstruction (a common complication). Despite this and the risk of lung cancer, demonstrated by the family history, the patient continued to smoke.

account for the rather uncommon development of cylindrical bronchiectasis. The honeycombing is categorized as grade 4 and is conspicuous on naked eye inspection. The distribution of asbestos fibres and resulting fibrous tissue is predominantly sub-pleural with the greatest amount at the lung bases (53); these are typically the site of small, irregular opacities on the chest radiograph (fig. 10.8). The middle zone, particularly on the right side, is also affected at an early stage but initially the changes are slight. Small rounded opacities may also occur, but only if the exposure has included other minerals (e.g. magnesia in makers and installers of lagging, rock dust in miners). In addition there may be other evidence for exposure, such as hyaline or calcified pleural plaques or diffuse fibrosis of the pleura. The radiographs can be categorized using the international classification (chapter 5). Breathlessness in patients with asbestosis is usually progressive, does not respond to bronchodilators and in severe cases is accompanied by hypoxaemia and cyanosis on exertion. There may be difficulty taking a deep breath or the patient may experience a dull ache in the chest when so doing: later there is cough which is dry or slightly productive of sputum. Fine râles (crackles) are usually heard on auscultation of the chest; typically these râles are high pitched clicks occurring with increasing frequency, in crescendo fashion, towards the end of inspiration and are not cleared by coughing. They occur in dependent parts of the lung, the axillary and posterior basal regions when the patient is erect and more extensively posteriorly when he is reclining. They usually disappear from the upper lung when the patient lies on one side. By contrast the crepitations of bronchiectasis are low pitched and occur at the start of inspiration. Those of heart failure and infection are of intermediate pitch and occur throughout inspiration. The pitch probably depends on the differential conduction of sounds by lung tissue. Crepitations occurring near the surface of the lung are high pitched, while if normal lung tissue intervenes between the source of sound and the stethoscope their pitch is lower (as in bronchiectasis). In population studies the prevalence of fine râles is positively correlated with the estimated exposure to

asbestos. Râles should be listened for with great care; they can be recorded on tape for subsequent reference. Clubbing of the fingers occurs in a small proportion of cases of advanced asbestosis. The condition is less common than formerly, possibly because with earlier diagnosis fewer patients develop a severe chest infection. The hyponychial angle may be measured (7: ref. 162) but it is not closely correlated with other indices of severity of the disease.

Lung function in asbestosis. The findings on assessment of lung function are typically those associated with diffuse fibrosis, i.e. restriction of expansion of the lung and a defect of gas transfer. However, since patients with asbestosis are usually smokers the features of chronic airflow limitation may coexist. The fibrosis reduces the lung compliance and increases the recoil pressure. These changes cause a reduction in vital capacity, usually without much change in residual volume. The forced expiratory volume is often reduced to a lesser extent so the FEV% is usually normal or raised. The increase in lung retractive force tends to expand the larger airways whilst the fibrous tissue diminishes the calibre of the bronchioles; these changes are reflected respectively in a normal or an increased forced expiratory flow at large lung volumes and decrease in flow rate at small volumes (37). The closing volume is usually increased.

The diffuse replacement of gas exchanging tissue by fibrous tissue leads to reductions in both the surface area of alveolar capillary membrane and the number of alveolar capillaries. These changes reduce the transfer factor and usually also the K_{CO} (transfer factor ÷ alveolar volume); the indices of transfer do not increase to the normal extent during exercise (chapter 18, ref. 8). The combination of a low transfer factor and an increase in oxygen uptake causes hypoxaemia (fig. 18.6, page 397); this stimulates the exercise ventilation which increases disproportionately. Ventilation is also increased by a change in the pattern of breathing. The reduction in lung distensibility makes the breathing shallower and more frequent, with a consequent increase in the proportion wasted in ventilating the anatomical deadspace. The wastage is accentuated by non-uniform distribution of the primary lesions which causes uneven ventilation of the lung and thus increases the physiological deadspace. Thus in asbestosis both the alveolar ventilation and the deadspace ventilation are excessive during exercise whilst the ventilatory capacity is usually reduced. These changes give rise to breathlessness on exertion (chapter 18). The lung function of a patient with asbestosis is given in table 10.2.

Diagnosis of asbestosis. Asbestosis is only one of many causes of diffuse fibrosis of the lung. It is diagnosed on the basis of the clinical, physiological and radiographic features described above. The features include fine basal râles at end inspiration, reduced lung distensibility and a low transfer factor. Clubbing of the fingers is no longer a useful criterion (see above). A history of recent pneumonia is relatively common. The cardinal feature is irregular, often linear, small radiographic opacities in both lower zones, sometimes more readily seen in oblique views than in the standard postero-anterior view of the chest. The diffuse fibrosis is likely to be due to asbestos if there is a history of significant exposure plus other suggestive features. The exposure should have entailed the handling of asbestos products for 2 or more years or a shorter period if the exposure was exceptionally heavy, for example spraying asbestos onto buildings (limpet spraying); the exposure should have occurred a minimum of 10 years previously. Shorter or proximity exposures rarely cause asbestosis. The information is elicited by taking a detailed occupational history (chapter 5). Other evidence of exposure

should be sought but this is no substitute for a good history. The chest radiograph may show pleural plaques but these often occur later in the disease. Asbestos bodies in any sputum which there may be or in fluid aspirated from the lung during bronchopulmonary lavage is evidence for exposure and a persistently negative result is against the diagnosis of asbestosis (75). An open biopsy specimen of lung tissue will exhibit evidence of diffuse fibrosis; the specimen should preferably be obtained from the lower part of the upper lobe or near the costophrenic angle. The specimen may contain asbestos bodies and fibres. An asbestos fibre content as assessed by phase contrast light microscopy in excess of one million fibres per gram of dry lung is strong supportive evidence for the diagnosis (table 10.3).

The differential diagnosis of asbestosis includes: (1) Extrinsic allergic alveolitis. This has its own characteristic history (page 327). The radiographic changes are predominantly in the upper half of the lung fields; they usually change over periods of months rather than years. Specific precipitating antibodies may be present in the serum. (2) Fibrosing alveolitis. The features may closely resemble asbestosis but the condition usually progresses over a few months or years and may respond to steroids. Sometimes there is conspicuous finger clubbing and a markedly reduced transfer factor but relatively normal lung mechanics. This is unlike asbestosis. If detailed, informed enquiry fails to reveal a history of adequate exposure at least 10 years previously the condition is not asbestosis. (3) Sarcoidosis: the differential diagnosis is dis-

Table 10.3. Asbestos fibre content of lung tissue analysed by light microscopy (21) (units: fibres per gram dry lung tissue)

Tissue	Circumstances	Mean count	Range ($\times 10^x$)
Lung	Healthy subjects (no industrial exposure)	30×10^3	0–0.1
Plaque	No asbestosis	4×10^3	0.5–15
Lung (mesothelioma cases)	No asbestosis	1×10^6	0.2–9
	Microscopic asbestosis	8×10^6	0.25–50
	Clinical asbestosis	40×10^6	1.0–400

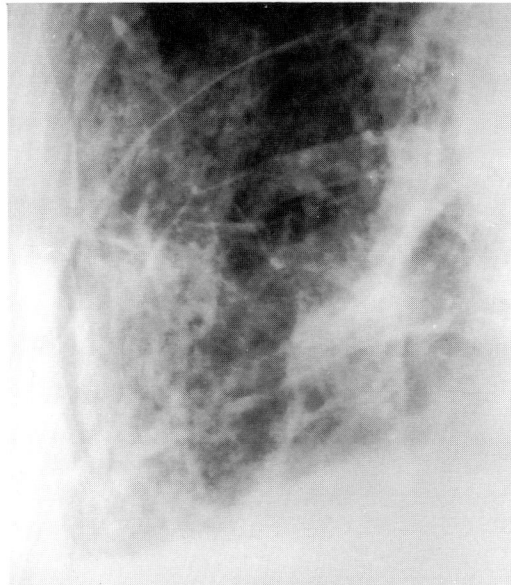

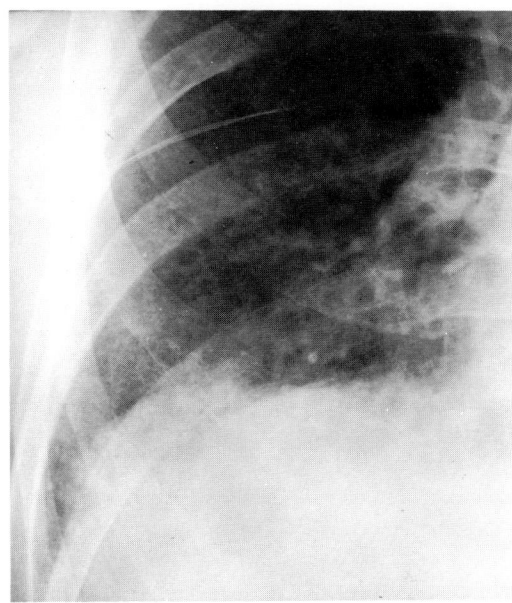

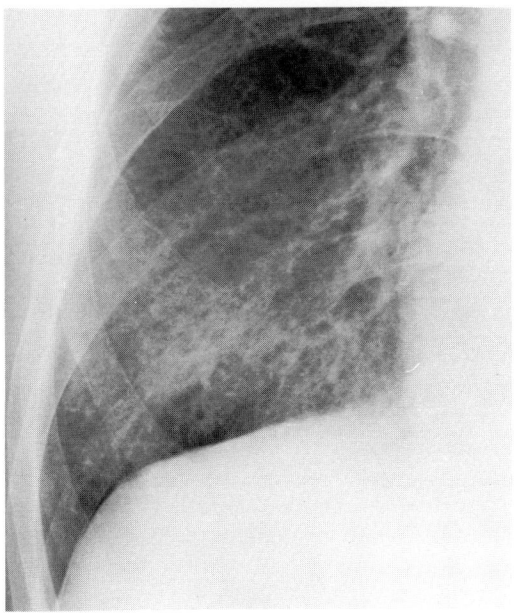

Fig. 10.9. Asbestosis? Chest radiographs showing detail from the right lower zone of three patients who were all referred on the same day with a diagnosis of asbestosis. *Top left* is from a 61-year-old shipyard electrician (a non-smoker) who had been intermittently exposed to asbestos. He was breathless on moderate exertion (grade 3) but did not have other symptoms; râles were present in the chest. The chest radiograph showed extensive pleural changes with plaque formation. There was a marked restrictive type of ventilatory defect and associated reduction in transfer factor. However, the K_{CO} was normal and there was no desaturation on exercise. The disease was considered to be mainly pleural. *Top right* is from a 59-year-old insulation worker who had few respiratory symptoms despite being a smoker. Ventilatory capacity, lung volumes and transfer factor were all within normal limits. However, he had clubbing of the fingers, basal crepitations, a high recoil pressure (4.5 kPa) and a fall in arterial oxygen saturation on exercise (97/89%). He was considered to have asbestosis. *Lower left* is from a 54-year-old coal miner who, after 21 years, temporarily left the mining industry to do 5 years' work for an insulation company. A previous chest radiograph at age 36 showed simple pneumoconiosis (Category 1p). He was breathless on moderate exertion (grade 3) but had no other respiratory symptoms despite smoking 20 cigarettes per day. The finger nails were curved (beaked) and there were some basal crepitations. The lung function (including compliance and recoil pressure) was within normal limits, and there was no desaturation on exercise. The differential diagnosis included early asbestosis and coal workers' cystic lung; the latter seemed to be the more likely but needed confirmation by lung biopsy. Asbestosis was diagnosed by default.

cussed on page 238. (4) Other rare types of diffuse fibrosis. (5) Cystic lung in an ex-coalminer (fig. 10.9). If the condition is very atypical the diagnosis is probably not asbestosis.

The lower limit of abnormality for diagnosis of asbestosis in an exposed person will be drawn at different levels depending on the circumstances. Adequate exposure is essential. Radio-

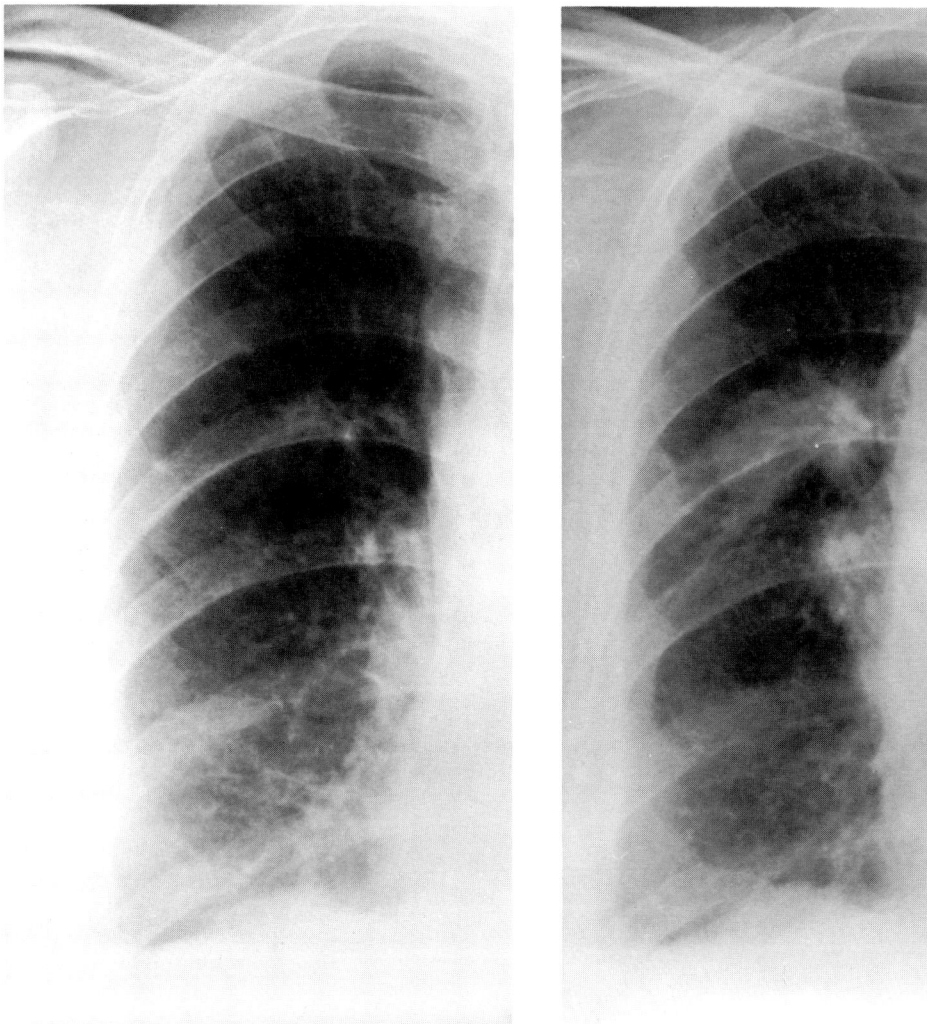

Fig. 10.10. Asbestos cancer. Chest radiographs showing pleural thickening (left) with subsequent lung cancer (right) in a 67-year-old plasterer. He smoked until age 48 (giving up to save money) and was symptom-free until age 60 when he became troubled by chronic cough and breathlessness. At assessment, he was overweight and had electrocardiographic evidence of myocardial ischaemia; a few crepitations were heard at the left base. There was no finger clubbing. The lung function showed a combined obstructive and restrictive ventilatory defect but normal transfer factor; the patient was diagnosed as having asbestos pleural disease with asbestosis confined to the periphery of the lung. Death was due to lung cancer. At post-mortem, there was a small cell anaplastic tumour of the right upper lobe main bronchus which had spread to the mediastinum. There was also asbestosis (fig. 10.11).

graphic abnormality is also essential except when there is an open lung biopsy and there should be some impairment of lung function, preferably both reduced distensibility and defective gas transfer; fine râles on auscultation of the chest are desirable but not essential.

The management of a patient with asbestosis is mainly symptomatic and is described in chapter 19. In addition special emphasis must be put on discontinuing smoking (see below) because there is synergism between smoking and asbestosis in the production of lung cancer. Care should be taken to treat all chest illnesses and the patient should preferably withdraw from exposure to asbestos on the grounds that both the severity and progression rate of asbestosis and the risk of lung cancer are all exposure-related.

Carcinoma of the lung

Lung cancer is primarily a disease of smokers but also occurs with excessive frequency following exposure to asbestos sufficient to cause at least mild asbestosis; the highest incidence is amongst those with exposure to both agents. The excess starts at about 15 years since first exposure and rises with exposure duration though it may fall off in those who live through to the age of 75 years or more. The asbestos content per gram of dry lung tissue as assessed by light microscopy is likely to exceed 1 million fibres (table 10.3). The tumour is usually squamous in type and occurs in a large airway, as do the small number of oat cell tumours. An intermediate proportion of tumours are adenocarcinomata arising at a bronchiolar bifurcation in the periphery of the lung. The tumour may present with any of the features of lung cancer including cough, haemoptysis, chest illness, weight loss, pain, endocrine disturbance or metastatic spread. It may also be detected during routine surveillance as a space occupying lesion on the chest radiograph; the presumptive diagnosis is then made relatively early as previous films are available for comparison (fig. 10.10). The diagnosis should be reviewed following examination of a biopsy specimen obtained at bronchoscopy or thoracotomy (fig. 10.11) or by cytological examination of the sputum; a bron-

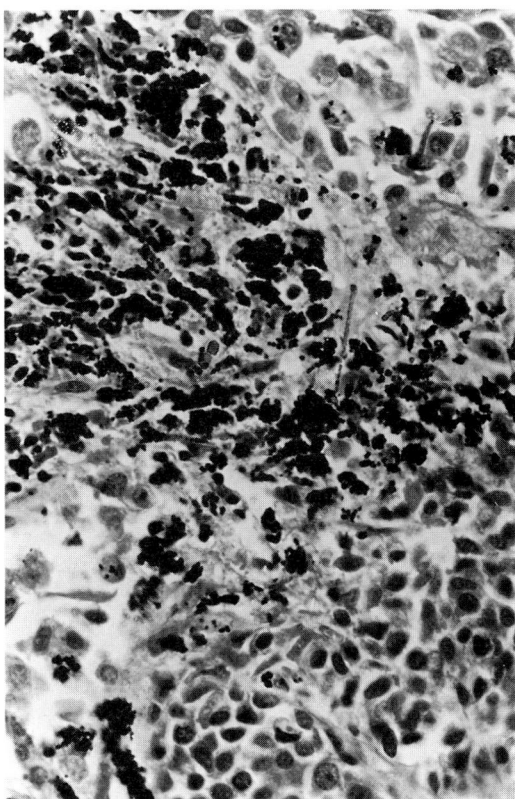

Fig. 10.11. Histological section from the lung of the patient with asbestos-related lung cancer described in fig. 10.10. The section shows tumour tissue (bottom right), interstitial fibrosis with asbestos bodies and fibres (also pigment) in the centre and macrophages in the alveolar space (top right). (High power view. By courtesy of T. Ashcroft.)

chial biopsy will seldom reveal histological evidence of asbestosis which is usually considered to be a necessary precondition if the disease is to be attributed to asbestos. Between 10% and 40% of persons dying with or from asbestosis also have lung cancer. It is, therefore, a very important terminal event in these patients. The treatment, as for any tumour of the lung, is by surgery, deep x-ray therapy or cytotoxic drugs; however, in an individual patient the choice may be limited because of extensive fibrosis. There is also need for appropriate support (page 215).

Mesothelioma

A patient who presents with pleural effusion or with continuous pain in the chest or shoulder and radiological thickening of the pleura may have developed a mesothelioma. Details of the condition have been reviewed by Elmes & Simpson (23). The thickening starts in the parietal pleura of the thoracic cage but may spread into the mediastinum, pericardium and visceral pleura of the lung (fig. 10.12). There is restriction of lung expansion and progressive shrinkage of the lung with accompanying

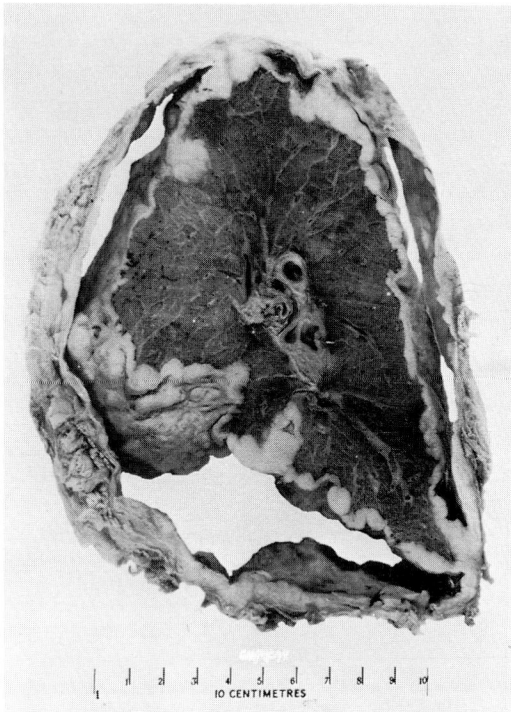

10 CENTIMETRES

Fig. 10.12. Mesothelioma enveloping and invading the right lung. The specimen was obtained at pleuropneumopericardectomy from a 47-year-old woman who presented with persistent right pleural effusion. She gave a history of having worked cutting blocks of asbestos fibre during her first year at work after leaving school 32 years previously. There was no subsequent exposure. Death occurred 18 months after the onset of symptoms. At postmortem, the tumour was of the mixed cell type. It had extended locally into abdomen and mediastinum and the related lymph nodes. (By courtesy of T. Ashcroft.)

breathlessness. Cough and haemoptysis are never features of mesothelioma. The breathlessness is aggravated by pleural effusion which is often haemorrhagic and may contain hyaluronic acid, white blood corpuscles and epithelial or mesenchymal cells which may be visibly neoplastic. The effusion, unlike that due to tuberculosis or viral infection, does not enlarge the hemithorax; it may be preceded by pneumothorax. The erythrocyte sedimentation rate is usually raised whilst clinical evidence of toxaemia including night sweats, weight loss and cachexia develop during the course of the illness. Half the cases die within 12 months; survival for more than 3 years should lead to a review of the diagnosis.

In 85% of the patients with mesothelioma there has been previous exposure to crocidolite, amosite or tremolite (i.e. to amphibole asbestos, 18, 77). Mesotheliomas are extremely rare in persons exposed only to chrysotile (e.g. 1). The exposure to amphibole is usually of occupational origin and of material intensity sufficient to cause a lung burden of asbestos in excess of 20,000 fibres per g dry lung as assessed by light microscopy (21, 84). The dosage seldom causes clinical asbestosis but this condition may be detected at autopsy. Occupational mesotheliomas exhibit a weak dose–response relationship (page 223) but not those due to exposure in childhood or to living near a source of atmospheric pollution by asbestos (76).

Mesothelial tumours also occur in the peritoneum, usually in persons with heavy past exposures and clinical asbestosis. Many cases are not diagnosed in life. The tumour causes ascites, constipation and obstruction to the bowel. Pain is not common and the ascitic fluid is glutinous so may not exhibit shifting dullness.

Types of mesothelioma. The tumours are usually of an epithelial type in that they contain glandular tubules, clefts lined with cuboidal cells and papillae (fig. 10.13); they are then difficult to distinguish from metastatic adenocarcinoma of the pleura arising from stomach, prostate or ovary. Special panels of pathologists have been set up in several countries to assist in diagnosis; their help is likely to be invaluable for the 10% of tumours which present diagnostic difficulty (21). The epithelial tumours are bulky,

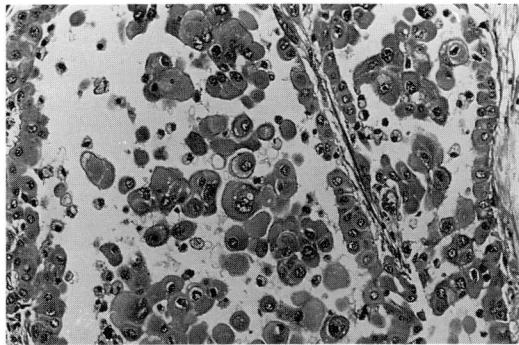 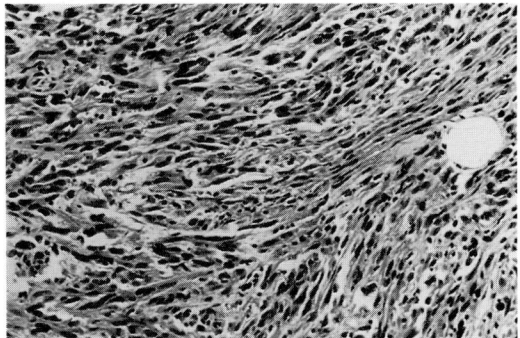

Fig. 10.13. *Left*: Histological section showing epithelial type of mesothelioma from the patient whose case is described in fig. 10.14. There are round or polygonal eosinophilic malignant cells with attempts at papillary formation. Other areas contained secretions which gave the characteristic staining reactions of hyaluronic acid. *Right*: Histology of connective tissue type of mesothelioma showing spindle-shaped cells with collagenous stroma, some mitosis and multinucleated cells. The patient was a 60-year-old plumber who from the age of 15 worked for 34 years in the shipyards. Five months before death he presented with breathlessness on exertion; this was associated with a right-sided pleural effusion. The subsequent aspiration led to the tumour spreading along the track of the needle. At post-mortem, the right lung was enveloped in and collapsed by the tumour. There were numerous peritoneal secondaries but the mediastinal glands were not involved. The left lung contained a few asbestos bodies and showed evidence of slight asbestosis. (High power view. By courtesy of T. Ashcroft.)

spread by direct extension and often give rise to large pleural effusions which may be bilateral; they may form metastases in regional lymph nodes. The prognosis is rather better than with other types of mesothelioma and the tumours occasionally respond to radiotherapy (41).

The connective tissue type of mesothelioma usually comprises sheets of round or spindle shaped cells resembling a fibrosarcoma; there may be areas of bone, cartilage or benign fibrosis and the tissue may be richly nucleated or acellular zones of hyaline material similar to benign fibrous plaques (fig. 10.13). These tumours spread locally in the chest wall, mediastinum and diaphragm but seldom give rise to effusions or regional or distant metastases. The survival is poor, rarely exceeding 3 years. Tumours containing mixed epithelial and connective cells also occur and have features of both parent cell types; they may give rise to large effusions, spread locally rather than via lymphatics or the bloodstream and have a poor prognosis. Thus the association between cell type (epithelioid or connective tissue) and morbid anatomical type (bulky encephaloid mass or scirrhous tumour) is

fairly loose. The cytology is not a reliable guide to clinical management.

Diagnosis of mesothelioma. In a person with a history of previous moderate or heavy exposure to crocidolite or mixed asbestos dust the risk of mesothelioma is in the range 3–8% (56). Diagnosis is then deceptively easy and care should be taken to exclude other tumours which may be more amenable to treatment (28). Alternatively the exposure may have been slight and incurred long ago; in these circumstances a comprehensive occupational history over the whole lifetime is essential. The tumour can often be visualized radiographically after inducing an artificial pneumothorax (fig. 10.14) or by computer assisted tomography (CAT scan). Diagnosis of a connective tissue or mixed cell tumour is usually made by histological examination of biopsy material: this should be obtained with circumspection as the tumour sometimes spreads along the incision or track of the biopsy needle. Histological diagnosis of an epithelial type tumour is more difficult on account of the large differential diagnosis; the biopsy specimen should comprise a minimum of 10g of tumour

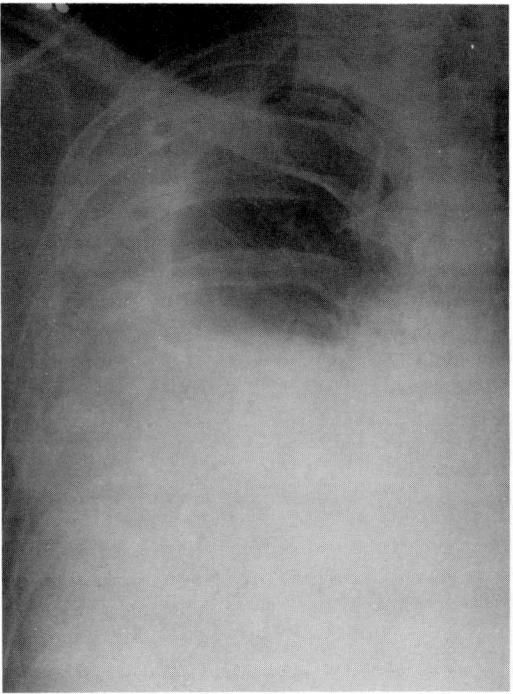 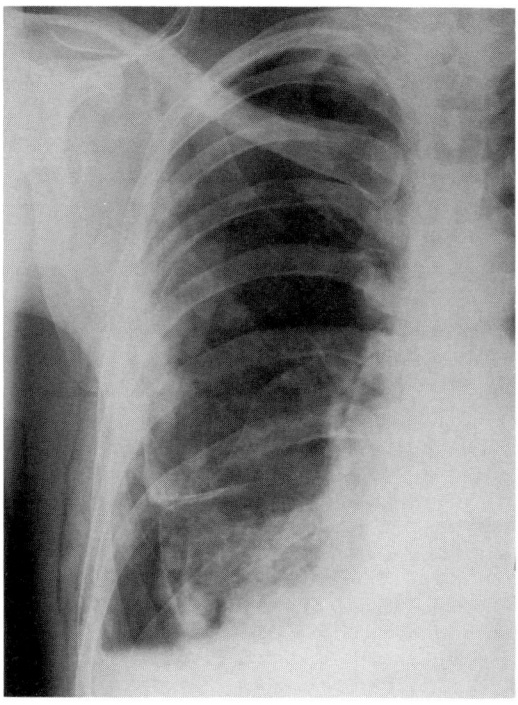

Fig. 10.14. Mesothelioma. Chest radiographs before and after aspiration of 7 l of pleural fluid and induction of partial pneumothorax to reveal mesothelioma. The patient was a plumber (non-smoker) who, when he was 16–17 years old, used asbestos for sealing joins in pipes. At age 41 he presented with a 6 weeks history of breathlessness due to the effusion and a transient, unproductive cough; there was never much chest pain despite the tumour subsequently infiltrating the chest wall. Persistence of the pleural effusion, despite numerous aspirations, was an indication for palliative pleurodesis and partial resection of the tumour; the lung then re-expanded temporarily. Deep x-ray therapy did not control the spread of the tumour and death occurred 8 months after presentation. The tumour was of the epithelial type (fig. 10.13). (By courtesy of S. J. Pearce.)

tissue. Tests for extracellular hyaluronic acid and its derivatives are helpful but not yet specific (4). Alternatively if there is an effusion, an epithelial type tumour may be diagnosed from the appearance of cells exfoliated from the tumour surface. Exfoliation occurs freely when the tumour is growing rapidly. The cells remain viable in the pleural fluid for up to 48h which gives time for a specialist centre to receive and comment on the specimen. However, interpretations may be difficult in the presence of a hae-mothorax as the blood may stimulate the mesothelial cells to divide and the clot may give the radiographic appearance of a tumour. Often the diagnosis follows a full post-mortem exam-ination and is made by a specialist panel of pathologists whose opinion may be supple-mented by an electron microscopic fibre analy-sis showing amphibole asbestos. Some cases certified at death as mesothelioma are not con-firmed when reviewed by the specialist panel, while in other cases the histological diagnosis is made too late for the condition to be entered on the formal death certificate (7: ref. 221).

Treatment of mesothelioma

There is at present no curative treatment so the possibility of an alternative diagnosis should be pursued energetically. The average time from the onset of symptoms to specialist referral has been reported as 3 months with death following on average 9 months later (23). The surgical procedures of pleuro-pneumonectomy with hemi-diaphragmectomy or stripping the pleura may help some patients with poorly differentiated epithelial tumours but the post-operative mortality is high (fig. 10.12, 16); BCG immunotherapy and cytotoxic chemotherapy have so far not influenced the prognosis though the latter given intrapleurally may prevent the reformation of effusions. However, the better policy is probably to aspirate those effusions which contribute to breathlessness. Pain should be relieved with drugs.

The relationship with the patient should strike a balance between early disclosure leading to sharing the travail of the terminal illness, and preservation of hope by emphasizing the real possibility that the diagnosis may be incorrect; thus preparing for the worst but hoping for the best. Achieving this balance is made difficult by the requirements for compensation, both statutory and arising from claims under Common Law. These aspects are best dealt with expeditiously during life when all information is available (chapter 1). In addition the relatives should be reassured that the condition is not infectious.

Experimental pathology

Deposition and clearance

Fibres are deposited in the respiratory tract by the processes of impaction, sedimentation and interception which are described in chapter 4. The processes are critically dependent on fibre size. Sedimentation is influenced by the aerodynamic diameter of the fibres and is not greatly influenced by fibre length. This has the effect that the maximal fibre diameter found in the lung is 3.5µm; the maximal length is determined by the geometry of the airways and is of the order of 200µm (73). Interception on the wall of the airway is influenced by the shape of the fibre; curved chrysotile fibres have a larger effective profile than the straight amphiboles and hence more often lodge on the bronchial or bronchiolar epithelium. Such fibres are eliminated from the lung via the mucociliary escalator. Thus relatively more amphibole than chrysotile fibres are deposited in the lung parenchyma; their greater fibrogenic and carcinogenic action in man (but not in some experimental studies) is consistent with this (30, 79, 81).

The mechanisms which protect against alveolar deposition are specific for fibres of different sizes; hence the size distribution of the respirable fibres in the environment greatly influences that in the lung (73). The environment may contain only relatively large respirable fibres which nearly all deposit in the airways, or very fine fibres of which a high proportion reach the lung parenchyma. In the asbestos industry 99% of airborne fibres have a length less than 5µm and deposition occurs mainly in the periphery of the lung (53). Clearance from the lung parenchyma is primarily by phagocytosis in alveolar macrophages (fig. 10.15, page 216). The macrophages migrate to the terminal bronchioles and onto the mucociliary escalator; few fibres migrate to pulmonary lymph nodes. Migration also occurs through the lung tissue, probably as a result of propulsion by the respiratory movements. Phagocytosis is effective for small fibres (<5µm) and occurs to a diminishing extent for longer fibres up to approximately 17µm (54); macrophages cannot ingest very long fibres (fig. 10.15). Migration to the periphery of the lung and out into the visceral pleura is a property of fibre dimensions; it occurs mainly for amphibole fibres of length less than 8µm (54); probably on account of their shape chrysotile fibres migrate more slowly and for the same reason fewer are retained in the lung. In addition chrysotile, but not the amphibole fibres, are cleared from the lung by disintegration; this occurs as a result of loss of magnesium by solution in lung tissue. Those which remain are mostly of small diameter and not visible by light microscopy (79). The majority of retained fibres are amphiboles and include all those of length greater than 20µm which have ever entered the respiratory bronchioles (fig. 10.15); their presence indicates the previous exposure to this form of asbestos. The size distribution of fibres retained in the lung relative to the environmental concentration is illustrated in fig. 10.16; the retention curve

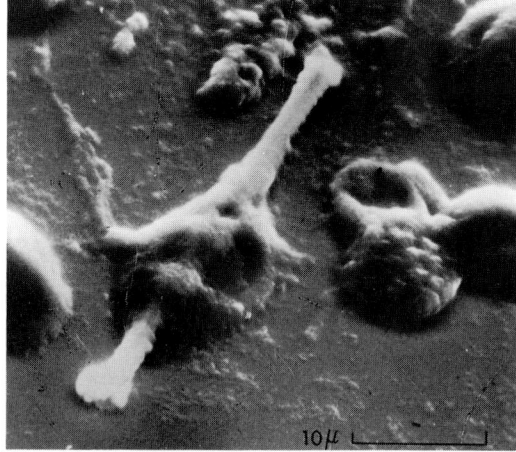

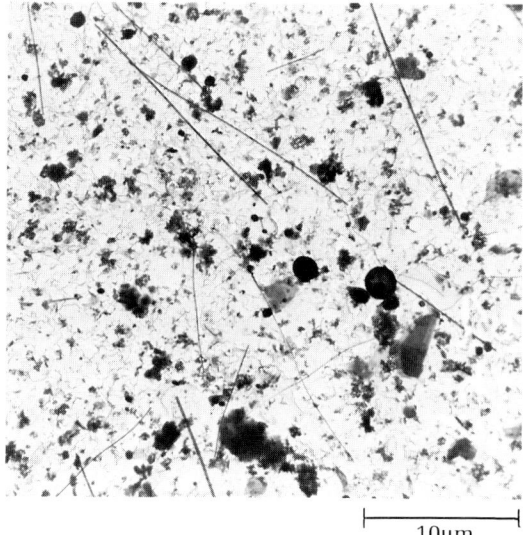

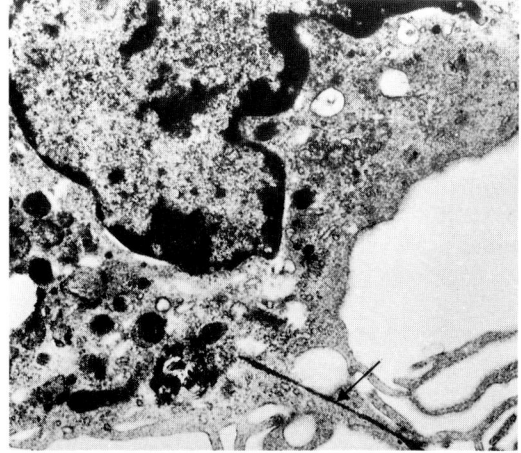

Fig. 10.15. *Top left*: Peritoneal macrophage attempting unsuccessfully to ingest a fibre 30μm in length. *Bottom left*: Amphibole asbestos fibre in lung tissue. (By courtesy of B. Corrin.) A high proportion of such fibres are more than 10μm in length. This is shown in top right which indicates the size of amphibole fibres obtained at post-mortem from the lung of an insulation worker. (By courtesy of A. Morgan & A. Holmes (52).)

differs from the deposition curve in containing fewer small fibres. The size distribution of the cleared fibres is illustrated in fig. 10.17. Clearance is impaired by smoking (47) and by interstitial fibrosis which reduces the size of communication channels in the lung; Timbrell has suggested that this permits local accumulation of fibres of mean length 10μm which may predispose to malignancy (73). The quantity of asbestos in lung tissue expressed in fibres per g dried lung (f/g) is the resultant of all these processes; the amount influences the type and extent of the subsequent disease (page 218).

Asbestos and other ferruginous bodies

The lungs and sputum of persons exposed to asbestos frequently contain asbestos bodies. Their core is usually a straight amphibole fibre of length 20-50μm. The core is coated with mucopolysaccharide containing iron which imparts a golden yellow colour; there may be knobs at the ends and the body may be segmented or in process of fragmentation (fig. 10.11). In persons with heavy exposure to asbestos the number of bodies is often of the order of 1 × 10⁶ per g dry lung tissue compared with up to

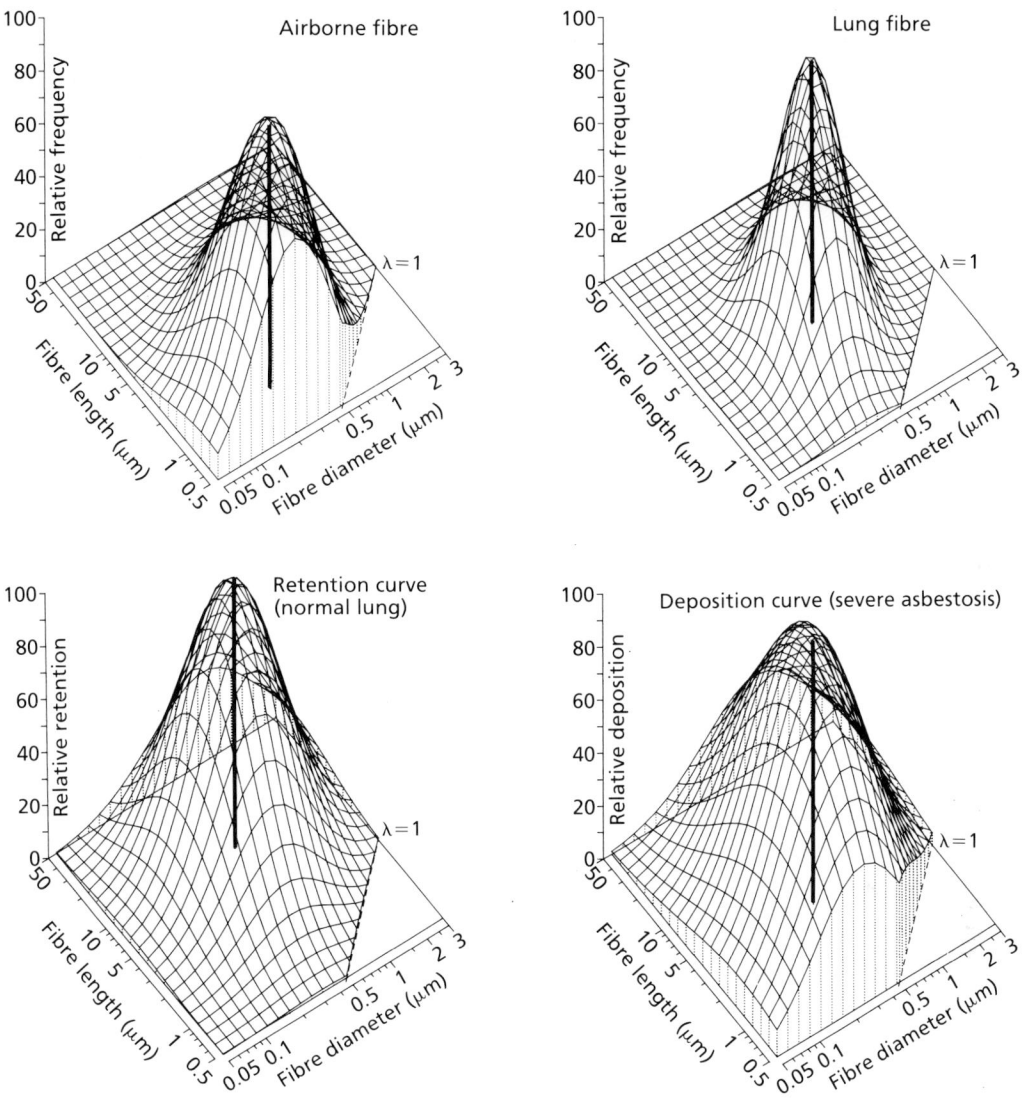

Fig. 10.16. Lung deposition and retention of airborne asbestos fibres. *Top.* Relative frequencies of the lengths and diameters of fibres in the air and in the lung parenchyma of a workman at the Pakkila anthophyllite mine studied by Timbrell. The commonest lengths were respectively 1.2µm and 4.0µm (corresponding widths 0.25µm and 0.37µm). Relative retention was calculated from these data, taking the fibre with the highest lung to air concentration ratio as 100. *Lower left.* Relative retention in a lung of normal structure after the clearance of small fibres by phagocytosis. Retention was greatest for fibres of length 10.1µm and diameter 0.48µm. *Lower right. Similar* information for the lung of a workman with severe asbestosis; this was effectively a deposition curve, as the diffuse fibrosis blocked the clearance but not the deposition of fibres. Compared with the normal lung there was a large excess of the small fibres which would normally have been removed by macrophages. There was no comparable excess of large fibres which, once deposited, inevitably remained in the lung (fig. 10.17). (By courtesy of V. Timbrell (73).)

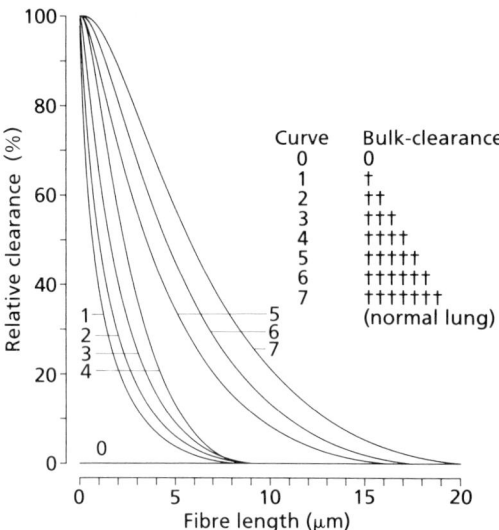

Fig. 10.17. Relative clearance of fibres deposited in lung parenchyma, analysed by fibre length and extent of bulk clearance from zero clearance in the presence of extensive interstitial fibrosis to the maximum which can occur in a healthy lung (curve 7). The curves were based on information of the type illustrated in fig. 10.16. (By courtesy of V. Timbrell (73).)

or not much more than 50/g in the general population (17). Intermediate numbers are found in industrial workers, especially those with some exposure to asbestos. Where the number is increased the bodies may be present in the sputum or the washings from bronchial lavage (75). Asbestos bodies are evidence for exposure to asbestos; their concentration in the lungs of routine autopsies on members of the general population has increased over the past 50 years, reflecting increased use of asbestos. However, in the absence of an identifiable exposure to asbestos the number of bodies present in the lungs of persons with bronchial and gastro-intestinal cancer is not apparently different from that in control subjects. This is part of the evidence that asbestos dust is not a significant hazard to the community in general. On rare occasions similar bodies are found to contain black carbon fibre, cosmetic talc and other material, hence their alternative name of ferruginous bodies. The contained material can usually be identified by light microscopy. This will also reveal uncoated

fibres which exceed the coated fibres by about 3:1. Under the electron microscope, which detects fibres of diameter less than 0.2μm, the ratio of uncoated to coated fibres is much higher.

Fibre type and disease

Retained asbestos fibres cause diffuse fibrosis of the lung. In animal experiments this response occurs with all types of asbestos, but in man, for the reasons discussed, chrysotile is less fibrogenic than the amphiboles. Thus in men with asbestosis coming to post-mortem, it is only the lung fibre counts for amphibole asbestos and not those for chrysotile which are correlated with the percentage disability (30, 79). Fibre length in the range 10–30μm appears to exert a maximal tissue response. In tissue culture the longer fibres appear to provide anchorage for fibroblasts and stimulate their growth. Fibres of length less than 5μm are not fibrogenic. However, Timbrell has recently shown that total fibre surface area per unit mass of lung tissue is the principal determinant of fibrogenicity (74). Fibre mass and number and fibre type, hence the cation content (iron or magnesium), do not contribute to the observed fibrogenicity after the effect of fibre surface area has been allowed for. This finding suggests that the fibrous reaction is due either to the mechanical action of the fibres or to the contained silica. Conditions which promote fibrosis predispose to bronchial carcinoma. This may be due to the fibrous tissue interfering with the normal processes of clearance and dispersion of fibres (73); the fibres remain concentrated at the site of impaction which, in the case of the amphiboles, is usually the bifurcation of a small bronchus. How asbestos predisposes to malignancy is not understood; some possible mechanisms are reviewed in chapter 12.

Mesothelial tumours arise in the parietal pleura of the lung more often than in the peritoneum and under experimental conditions may be produced by intrapleural administration of any type of asbestos. In man the disease is commonly due to crocidolite from North West Cape province of South Africa or Wittenoom in Australia. It can also be caused by amosite and possibly tremolite. Timbrell (72, 73) observed that the biologically active fibres are straight and slender, unlike chrysotile which is curved and unlike most amosite, anthophyllite and crocidolite from the Transvaal which occur as relatively broad fibres (fig. 10.2). The active fibres are more than 8μm long and have a diameter less than 0.25μm (70) but amongst such fibres the very thin ones (diameter <0.05μm) appear to be most active (73); these fibres are invisible by optical microscopy. They are capable of lancing individual cells but whether this is the cause of malignancy is not known. Glass fibres having these dimensions also give rise to tumours (70). The fibres reach the pleura or peritoneum by migration which in the lung may be impeded by lung fibrosis. This may explain why thoracic mesotheliomas are uncommon in persons with asbestosis. Conversely, children and persons who are lightly exposed only to crocidolite appear to be at increased risk. The reason is not known but the absence of significant fibrosis and, in the case of children, the small size of the lung will allow free movement of fibres within it. In the case of non-smokers the penetration of fibres into the bronchial tree may possibly also be enhanced by the small airways not being constricted by tobacco smoke (47, and chapter 17). Investigation of villagers in Anatolia where mesotheliomas occur naturally as a result of exposure to eronite, a fibrous zeolite, tends to confirm this hypothesis. The condition affects mainly adults who lived in the villages as children and not those who immigrated during adult life (6). Eronite also causes mesothelioma in mice (58).

Immunopathology

Much is known about the effects of asbestos upon lung macrophages but the information is not yet of practical use for prevention or management of disease. In the lung asbestos fibres become coated with surfactant or with IgG. The fibres activate complement and generate a chemotactic factor for polymorphonuclear leucocytes. They occasionally lyse red blood cells. Contact with macrophages sets in motion the process of ingestion with clustering of the surface proteins, depolarization of the outer membrane and contraction of macrophage

microfilaments. Reactive sites on the fibres combine with sialoglycoprotein from the lysosomal membrane. Fibres of length less than 5–10μm become enveloped within secondary lysosomes and exposed to their enzymes. An uncoated fibre may disrupt the lysosomal membrane and kill the cell (3). Coated fibres cause selective release into the surrounding medium of enzymes, including B galactosidase, B glucuronidase and N-acetyl BD glucosaminidase but not lactate dehydrogenase (20); this response differs from that to quartz which causes uncontrolled release of all the lysosomal enzymes and of oxidants which kill the cell. Macrophages which have engulfed fibres usually remain active and able to neutralize the fibrogenic and carcinogenic action of the contained asbestos. Fibres too long to be phagocytosed completely are potentially more harmful in these respects. In tissue culture asbestos fibres activate alveolar macrophages to cause proliferation of fibroblasts. In man the fibrogenic action may be associated with an increase in titre of rheumatoid factor and antinuclear antibody, especially IgM, but the change is not invariable or specific.

In the presence of asbestos fibres the rate of formation of fibrous tissue appears to be increased by infection which releases from blood serum a chemotactic factor for leucocytes. In addition a deficiency of T lymphocytes and of natural killer cell activity (page 76) may reduce the effectiveness of scavenging of potentially neoplastic cells. However, the evidence for these or other immunological mechanisms contributing to asbestosis and lung cancer is inconclusive (59). There is likewise no good evidence for increased susceptibility of persons in certain HLA antigen groups (19). Clearly more research is needed; it should preferably be undertaken using single varieties of asbestos, not mixtures (e.g. 44), and must take into account the dimensions of the fibres.

Epidemiology of asbestos-related diseases; establishing a dose-response relationship

Objectives and difficulties

In 1964 the first international conference on asbestos-related diseases was held in New York.

This meeting marked the start of a concerted international effort to understand and control what had become a man-made epidemic; the success of this venture owes much to the very different, but in retrospect complementary, contributions of Selikoff and Gilson. By about 1960 there was a clear need to discover the prevalence, attack rate, morbidity and mortality of diseases caused by asbestos and their relation to asbestos exposure. These questions proved difficult to answer for a number of reasons: they included the long latent period before the onset of positive features which were often difficult to define, the confounding effects of cigarette smoking, the tendency for exposure to involve more than one type of asbestos, the absence or recent establishment of dust sampling which initially was relatively unsophisticated (e.g. with respect to sensitivity, fibre type and submicroscopic fibres), the early practice in the U.S.A. of reporting total particle counts and not fibres only, the delay until 1968 in making an entry in the International Classification of Diseases for mesothelial tumours of pleura, the unreliability of diagnosis and the inexact certification of these and other asbestos-related diseases (28). In addition some organizations made it a practice to move employees between jobs on the basis of changes observed at periodic examination; since this might have removed from exposure the more susceptible individuals the results could not then be used for establishing a dose–response relationship.

The assault on these problems is still continuing (30). Some early developments included a quantitative method for describing finger clubbing (7: ref. 162), the first semi-automatic apparatus for measuring the transfer factor or diffusing capacity for the lung, extension of the ILO classification of chest radiographs to include irregular opacities and pleural diseases (chapter 5), development of improved methods for dust sampling, better appreciation of the significance of asbestos bodies, establishment of panels of assessors for chest radiographs and mesothelial tumours and international comparisons of scoring many of these variables. Less successful have been the attempts to equate figures for dust concentrations obtained at different times, the derivation of a factor for converting from millions of particles per cubic foot to fibres per ml and for unscrambling the effects of improvements in light microscopy, including the introduction of the eyepiece graticule, phase contrast illumination and membrane filters. In the case of fibres in the lung the prior removal of the tissue by potassium hydroxide digestion instead of by ashing improved the quality of the result (5, 53). On account of these and other differences the margin of uncertainty between laboratories counting asbestos fibres is by a factor of at least 2.5 and may be much higher (76). There is a similar uncertainty in converting from lung fibre counts by light microscopy to total counts, including submicroscopic particles where the conversion factor varies depending on the diameter of the fibres; typical factors are 100, 7 and 2.5 respectively for chrysotile, crocidolite and amosite (52). However, these uncertainties are small compared with those which obtained previously and have allowed very significant advances.

Prevalence

In almost all studies of persons exposed to asbestos the prevalence of clinical, physiological and radiographic features of asbestosis, and lung cancer has been significantly related to intensity of exposure; the association has been less readily demonstrated in the case for mesothelial tumours. The prevalence of pleural abnormality is related to the duration but not the intensity of exposure (table 10.5, page 221). For asbestosis and asbestos cancers there is a latent period of some 12–30 years and for mesotheliomas of 20–40 years before the condition develops. In addition there is a relationship to smoking; lung cancer and asbestosis but not mesothelial tumours occur only in or are commoner amongst smokers and ex-smokers than non-smokers. The effect of smoking is best described by a multiplicative model in which for a given exposure to asbestos the prevalence of bronchial cancer is relatively greater in smokers than in non-smokers; examples include persons formerly exposed to anthophyllite in Finland and members of the U.S. Insulation Workers Union. In these studies the risk for smokers compared with non-smokers were

Table 10.4. Relative contributions to mortality from lung cancer of smoking and of working with asbestos

	Mining			Manufacture
	Anthophyllite (51)	Chrysotile (46)		Mixed fibres (68: pages 473–90)
		(a)	(b)	
Non-smokers				
No asbestos exposure	1	1	1	1
Workers with asbestos	1.4	2	7	5.2
Smokers				
No exposure	12	6	12	10.9
With asbestos	17	8	25	53.2

(a) Moderate exposure or moderate smokers or both.
(b) Heavy exposure or heavy smokers or both.

increased respectively by factors of 1.4 and 5. (51, 68, pages 473–90). However, for chrysotile miners an additive model provides a better description of the findings (table 10.4). The evidence is reviewed by Rossiter and Berry (65) and by Saracci (66).

Any figure for prevalence needs to be interpreted in the light of the intensity and duration of exposure, the years since first exposure, age and the smoking history (10). Temporal factors also need to be taken into account, including improvements in industrial hygiene which have often been linked to legislation, the rising trend of mortality from smoking and, in the U.K., the exceptionally high concentrations of asbestos present in asbestos textile factories during the Second World War. The type of fibre is also important since a given environmental concentration of crocidolite is more fibrogenic than an equifibre dose of chrysotile (81). For mesothelio-

mas the fibre type and size is even more important; in man the tumours have not been reported after exposure to anthophyllite or in persons whose lungs contain only chrysotile (77). In most circumstances the tumours are probably due to exposure to crocidolite but may occur with amosite (30); the latter fibre in association with chrysotile is an important cause of mesotheliomas in North America. The role of fibre size is considered on page 218.

Results of prevalence studies amongst asbestos miners and millers in the province of Quebec based on a detailed study of 11,107 men born 1891–1920 are summarized in table 10.5 (46). This shows a wide range of prevalences of asbestos-related disease from zero for many indices in the lowest exposed groups to 34% for some indices in subjects who were heavily exposed. The prevalence is less for non-smokers than for smokers and is now declining (fig. 10.18).

Table 10.5. Relationship of respiratory abnormality to exposure amongst asbestos miners and millers. Where appropriate the results have been standardized for age, stature and years of exposure. (Data of McDonald et al, cited by Becklake (7).)

	Exposure category (m p ft^{-3} a^{-1})		
	<10	100–199	400–799
Prevalence of dyspnoea (%)*	7	23	30
Reduction in vital capacity (%)*	0	9	14
Reduction in transfer factor (%)*	0	6	9
Prevalence of radiol. abnormality (%)†			
Pleural changes	23	33	34
Irregular opacities (1/0 or above)	0	10	21

* Current workers.   † Current and ex-workers, 56–65 year age group.

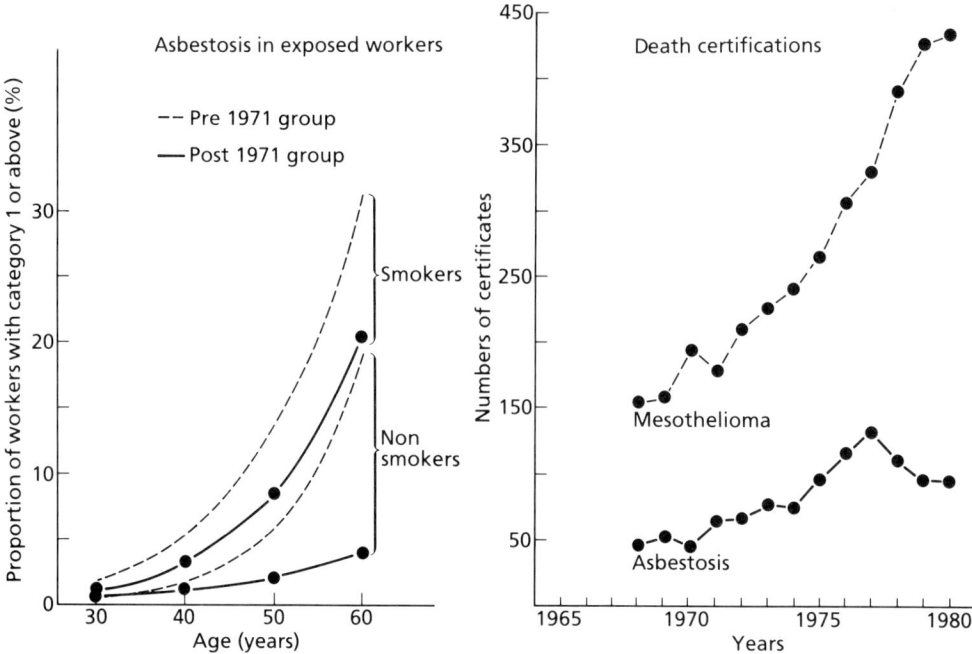

Fig. 10.18. Extent of asbestos related disease. *Left*: Estimated percentage of pneumoconiosis (category 1/0 or above) amongst U.K. asbestos workers having their first exposure pre and post 1971, analysed by age and smoking habits. *Right*: Number of deaths from mesothelioma and from asbestosis (alone or with other diseases including lung cancer but excluding mesothelioma) in England and Wales analysed by calendar year. (By courtesy of M. Jacobsen *et al* (36), the Health and Safety Executive and J. C. Gilson.)

Amongst marine insulation workers the prevalence of asbestosis after 20 years work was 12% and after 26 years was 19% (7: ref. 96). Amongst a sample of dockyard workers, of whom a proportion worked with asbestos, the overall prevalence of radiographic abnormality was 3%; the pleural changes exceeded the parenchymal ones by a ratio of 10:1 (7: ref. 75). Amongst those with plaques the risk of subsequently developing asbestosis was increased compared with dockyard workers without plaques (50). Thus asbestos-related pleural plaques are a warning sign but the association is weak; this is partly because other factors besides asbestos contribute to the formation of plaques. For example, calcified plaques are more common amongst workers in some Quebec asbestos mines than in other mines where there is comparable exposure to the same type of asbestos (27). Plaques are also common amongst persons exposed to anthophyllite, tremolite and zeolite respectively

in Finland, Austria, Bulgaria and Turkey amongst whom asbestosis and asbestos-related lung cancer are either uncommon or do not occur (6, 42, 51). In addition plaques in the general population do not have a serious connotation. Further research is required to elucidate these contradictions.

Mortality from lung cancer. The relationship between exposure and lung cancer is considered under environmental limits below. In summary there is a strong positive association at medium and high levels of exposure; the increased mortality is detectable some 16 years after first exposure and reaches its peak at about 30 years. The mortality is greatly influenced by the concurrent consumption of cigarettes. Some evidence is summarized in table 10.4 (page 221); this shows that the proportional increase in mortality between minimal and heavy exposure to asbestos is less than that between non- and heavy smoking. There is no positive evidence that lung cancer amongst members of the general population is due to asbestos. Persons who incur a small occupational exposure insufficient to cause clinically detectable asbestosis are theoretically at risk but the additional hazard over and above that due to smoking is too small to be detected by current methods (page 17 and below). In England and Wales the number of deaths per annum is approximately 100 (fig. 10.18).

Mortality from mesothelioma

Following the now classical study of Wagner and colleagues (page 200), mesothelial tumours of the pleura and peritoneum have been recorded with particular care in many countries. Some 85% are due to asbestos; the remainder, including most tumours in children, are of unknown origin. The prevalence of mesotheliomas is relatively high amongst asbestos workers and persons living in the vicinity of crocidolite asbestos mines in N.W. Cape province of South Africa. Cases have occurred in relation to mining crocidolite in Western Australia and a very few in relation to mining amosite (30). The great majority of mesotheliomas in adults have occurred amongst limpet sprayers, insulation workers and men working alongside them, in dockyards and insulation manufacturing plants. A few cases have occurred amongst wives and others who have regularly handled contaminated clothing. In England and Wales several thousand cases have been reported and new cases are occurring at a rate of approximately 500 per year (38, also fig. 10.18). In the U.S.A. the mortality in relation to the size of the population is a little lower. The tumours are due to exposure to crocidolite or amosite (18, 77). The latent period in adults from first exposure to the development of the tumour is usually in excess of 25 years. Thus cases are now occurring amongst workers who filled Service type gas mask filter canisters with well-crushed crocidolite asbestos during the Second World War. Amongst these women there is clear evidence for a dose–response relationship (39). No cases of mesothelioma have been reported amongst women who filled civilian gas mask canisters with chrysotile (1). Cases of mesothelioma are also occurring amongst naval dockyard workers who were spray insulating the undersides of decks and bulkheads with crocidolite in the late 1940s and early 1950s. A relationship of mesothelioma prevalence to exposure to asbestos was observed amongst asbestos textile workers using mixtures of chrysotile and crocidolite asbestos (56); the effective dose was less than that causing asbestosis or lung cancer but was usually material, being seldom less than 2 years' work in conditions of heavy exposure. However, an apparently slight exposure during childhood or in a relatively clean environment may also cause the disease.

Exposure limits

Bronchial cancer. The studies which have been reviewed demonstrate a clear association between mortality from lung cancer and exposure to asbestos. Additional evidence is provided by McDonald (45). However, for the reason given above, relatively few studies were suitable for establishing a dose–response relationship. The first estimates were obtained at the asbestos textile factory which was the site of Doll's initial study. In the U.K. this led to the establishment in 1969 of an exposure limit for the prevention of asbestosis of 2 chrysotile fibres per ml. However, the workers in the factory were subsequently found to have been exposed to crocidolite as well as chrysotile (79). The environmental conditions at the factory improved from 1933 onwards and for subjects recruited between 1933 and 1962 the risk of asbestos cancer, formerly 10:1 compared with the general population, was reduced to 1.6:1 (60). It will undoubtedly be much less for personnel who entered the factory recently on account of both lower fibre counts and the absence of crocidolite (see below). For comparison, in the Quebec study there was no excess mortality amongst men followed for more than 20 years whose estimated exposure did not exceed 2 fibres per ml (46).

Constructing a dose–response relationship for asbestosis entails extrapolation from higher concentrations which no longer obtain in practice (fig. 10.19). This is necessary if use is to be made of the epidemiological results. The process is

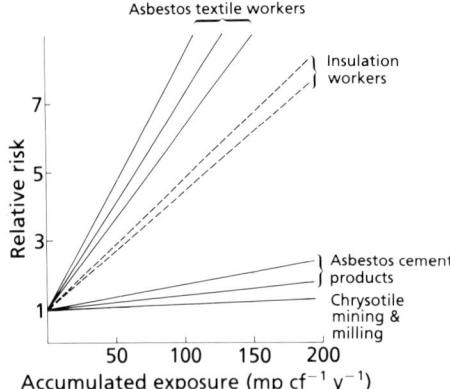

Fig. 10.19. Findings for eight cohorts of North American asbestos workers showing the relationship of lung cancer risk to exposure expressed as million particles per cubic foot per year (mp cf^{-1} y^{-1}, one mp cf^{-1} ≃ 6 fibres per ml. The data have been expressed in this form as not all the original relationships passed through the origin. The variation in slope between the groups is evidence that the accumulated exposure does not fully reflect the biological hazard. The distribution of fibre sizes, the type of asbestos, the smoking habits and, in the case of cement products, the cement itself, also affect the risk. (By courtesy of J. C. McDonald (45).)

Table 10.6. U.K. hygiene standard for asbestos (fibres ml^{-1})

	1973	1.1.83	1.8.84
Chrysotile	2	1	0.5
Amosite*	2	0.5	0.2
Crocidolite†	0.2	0.2	0.2

* Use banned from 1.6.84.   † Not imported since 1970.

insulation or for new products and amphibole asbestos no longer being imported into the country.

Mesothelioma. The relationship of mortality from mesothelioma to exposure to amphibole asbestos is inevitably approximate because the latent period is longer than that over which there are reliable estimates of exposure. Nevertheless, the association is so strong that in the U.K. it has led to a ban on the new use of crocidolite and to the supervised demolition by licensed operators of structures known to contain asbestos; however, some unsupervised demolition still occurs, particularly where the presence of asbestos is not recognized in advance.

Dust concentrations, sampling and analysis

Concentrations of asbestos fibres in respired gas have now been monitored for 50 years. Initially particle counts were made using an impinger, then samples were obtained using a Casella thermal precipitator (t.p.), later a long running t.p. was introduced and subsequently a membrane filter which was fed either from a fixed site (static sampling) or from a personal sampler. The counting was by light microscopy with visual scanning of whole fields and more recently of squares defined with an eyepiece graticule. Steel has estimated that by about 1974 these changes increased the sensitivity of counting by a factor of between 2 and 5 compared with the earlier methods (30: vol. 2, pages 85–7). The atmospheric concentration of fibres in any factory where the conditions have always exactly met the threshold limit value (now 0.5 fibre/ml) must have fallen proportionately. In

inevitably approximate. It leads to the conclusion that there is no level of exposure which is 100% safe, only levels at which the risk is very small. However, the linear model may be wrong or require modification (page 13), for example by allowing for variation in background mortality from other causes (43). The results are also compatible with the hypothesis of a threshold dose below which there is no excess risk. The average cigarette smoker accepts a 10% risk of developing lung cancer (or 50% if a heavy smoker) so a 1% excess risk for asbestos workers is possibly not unreasonable. Acheson and Gardner suggest that this corresponds to 3.30 chrysotile fibres per ml (76: pages 737–54). Thus the present U.K. exposure limit per ml of 0.5 fibres of chrysotile and 0.2 fibres of amphibole asbestos appears to provide an adequate margin of safety. This and earlier standards are given in table 10.6. In the U.K. the risk is further reduced by asbestos no longer being used for thermal addition fibre concentrations are now reported per ml and not particles/cu ft. The changeover was made possible by the decision to define a fibre as having a ratio of the maximal to the minimal dimension (aspect ratio) of at least 3:1 though a ratio of 5:1 might have been better (80). The conversion factor from the old to the new units depends on the ratio of fibres to particles which varies from 0.3 to 0.10 (80). The factor was also affected by the improvements in light microscopy. This now provides resolution down to a fibre diameter of 0.35μm or 0.2μm in exceptionally favourable circumstances. However, approximately two-thirds of airborne fibres and 95% of fibres from lung tissue are slimmer than this and not recorded by present routine methods. Fine fibres are counted by the laser technique of Timbrell (71). This entails aligning the fibres in a magnetic field and analysing with an electron microscope the light scattering patterns produced by a laser beam. The method accommodates all fibre sizes but not high fibre concentrations and has still to be shown to be useful in routine work.

Fibre composition is assessed by the method of Pooley (62); this uses the polycrystalline electron diffraction pattern obtained with a transmission electron microscope and x-ray analytical equipment. The method has provided the only reliable information on type, number and calculated mass of asbestos and other minerals in the lung and is likely to be used to an increasing extent in the future.

Present hazards from asbestos

Legislative framework

In the U.K. regulations for the surveillance of workers engaged in the manufacture of asbestos products, including periodic chest x-rays, were introduced in 1933; the regulations led to a great reduction in the number of new cases of asbestosis and lung cancer despite the regulations being relaxed during the Second World War (60). In 1969 the surveillance was extended to include users of asbestos, especially insulation workers. Concurrently hygiene standards for airborne asbestos dust were established and these were revised downwards in 1982 as a result of new

evidence on the biological effects of asbestos obtained in recent epidemiological studies. The standards were further revised in 1984, mainly to bring them in line with the best current practice (table 10.6, see also chapter 1). On the basis of the U.K. evidence the International Labour Organisation and many countries including initially the United States adopted similar standards and banned the use of crocidolite. The current practice in the U.K. is described below.

Control of asbestos exposure

The current exposure limit probably reduces the risk of asbestos-related cancer in smokers to less than one-tenth of the average due to smoking, with a correspondingly smaller risk for non-smokers. Indeed for persons only exposed within present limits the risk should now be barely detectable by present epidemiological methods and assuming a linear dose–response relationship (9, 11). In the U.K. by 1970 the importation of crocidolite was virtually discontinued, as was the use of asbestos for thermal insulation. Asbestos spraying was prohibited. By 1980 the use of asbestos fibreboard for building and the importation into the U.K. of amosite were largely discontinued. Other measures introduced by the Health and Safety Executive included the proper labelling of asbestos and asbestos waste and use of impermeable bags for transporting. Removal of asbestos required the use of water or exhaust ventilation and could only be done by approved contractors. The use of respirators and protective clothing whenever there was a risk of exposure to airborne fibres and the screening off of such processes from other workers became general.

The surveillance of persons exposed to asbestos is primarily by routine biennial chest radiography. This may be supplemented by the use of self-administered questionnaires and measurement of forced expiratory volume and vital capacity. The serial measurement of transfer factor is an additional safeguard against missing early abnormality but its use may not be cost-effective (7); for occupational surveys the measurement of ventilation during submaximal exercise is a more sensitive alternative (chapter 18, page 394).

Is there a risk from asbestos today?

Up to 1960 fibre counts in association with asbestos were commonly in the range 5–15/ml and counts of 50/ml were not exceptional. These high fibre concentrations led to an epidemic of asbestos-related diseases of all stages of severity and to increasing mortality from mesotheliomas and asbestos lung cancer. Due to the long latent period many persons who were exposed to these conditions in the past have still to develop clinical illness. This is reflected in the rising annual mortality rate for mesotheliomas (fig. 10.18).

However, the introduction of realistic hygiene standards in the late 1960s is now beginning to have an effect; this is shown by the change from an increase to relative constancy in the number of deaths from asbestosis per annum and the reversal of the upward trend is reinforced by a reduction in prevalence of early radiographic abnormality in persons first exposed subsequent to 1971 compared with those of similar age and smoking habit who were exposed previously (fig. 10.18). The epidemic is past its peak and is now on the decline, but this is not yet apparent to the general public who are rightly concerned by the present high mortality from asbestos-related disease. The evidence strongly suggests that under the conditions permitted by current regulations and practices there is no measurable hazard from inhaling asbestos fibres. The remaining unmeasurable risk is small compared with other hazards associated with daily living. The evidence is reviewed by Doll & Peto (ref. 10, page 22) and by Hughes & Weill (34). Many people are concerned that asbestos is present in most buildings and many machines and appliances (table 10.1). This is helpful when it leads to workers recognizing asbestos in old plant and to introduction of proper safety precautions, but destructive when the risk is exaggerated as by the ill-informed suggestion that single fibres kill. This aspect is considered in chapter 1. The tragedy is that on account of ignorance and neglect the situation arose in the first place. One consequence is that asbestos is now being replaced by substitutes which are often less suitable and for which the safe working conditions have not always been fully established. In this respect the careful scrutiny which has been undertaken of

persons exposed to man-made mineral fibres might serve as a model (page 228). Meanwhile at the personal level those who have been exposed to high concentrations in the past should avoid further exposure, abandon smoking and secure medical treatment for intercurrent chest illness. Routine surveillance should be as for those who are currently exposed (see control of asbestos exposure above).

Compensation

In the U.K., since 1948, certain diseases associated with exposure to asbestos in a prescribed occupation confer entitlement to disablement benefit or widow's death benefit. The compensation comes under the Industrial Injuries Scheme (chapter 1). The diseases include asbestosis, mesothelioma and, since 1985, diffuse bilateral pleural thickening sufficient to cause respiratory disablement. For exposures prior to 1948 benefit may be secured under the Pneumocrniosis, Byssinosis and Miscellaneous Diseases Benefit Scheme. Lung cancer confers entitlement if it is associated with asbestosis or diffuse bilateral pleural thickening; pleural plaques are not by themselves considered to be sufficiently reliable evidence of exposure. During the period 1965–80 the number of new cases of asbestosis accepted for compensation was fairly constant at about 140 per annum. The occurrence of asbestos-related disease may entitle the sufferer to sue his past employers for damages for negligence. The claimant then must show that on the balance of probabilities the disablement has resulted from the employer's negligence in failing to maintain safe working conditions. Thus only employment subsequent to the date of the relevant Act coming into force can be considered. The claim should be initiated within 3 years of the claimant being aware of the diagnosis (14).

Other mineral fibres

Talc

Talc is a mineral phyllosilicate ($Mg_3Si_4O_{10}$, OH_2) which is crushed and milled to produce an inert, lubricant powder with a wide range of

Table 10.7. Some uses of talc

Paint	Whiteners, fibres confer strength, prevent settling in tin	May be fibrogenic
Ceramic	Electrical insulators, ceramic tiles, refractory bricks, etc.	Firing to 1300°C may yield cristobalite which is fibrogenic
Filler	Putty, car and boat repairs, caulking, paper and fabrics, modelling compounds, rubber	Micronized talc for coating paper comprises mainly respirable particles
Parting agent	Roofing felt* rubber goods, confectionery†, salami, in shoe manufacture, etc.	
Polish	Rice (in U.S.A.)†, peanuts, pills, etc.	
Excipient	Pharmaceutical pills†, fertilizer, insecticides, cleaning powders (French chalk)	
Cosmetic	Face, talcum and other powders	Should not contain asbestos or quartz

* Now replaced by sand or other substance
† Talc should be of high purity

applications (31, 42, 63). The name is also given to any powdered mixture of associated minerals used to provide lubrication; the material may then contain crystalline or fibrous anthophyllite, tremolite, quartz or other mineral. These talc-like powders have been known to cause fibrosis and lung cancer or silicosis depending on their composition.

Phyllosilicate is a tri-octahedral sheet of brucite containing magnesium ions sandwiched between two sheets of silicate tetrahedra in multiple layers; these form stacks which are held together by weak Van der Waal's forces. The lubricant action is due to the application of slight force causing slippage parallel to the basal plane. The particles are flat, irregular flakes which are often very thin so when seen edge-on may be mistaken for fibres; usually only a small proportion is respirable. Some uses are listed in table 10.7.

Talc is mined in many parts of the world including Norway, U.S.A., France, China and Northern Italy where one mine provides 40% of the cosmetic talc used in the U.K. The miners and other users are subject to inert dust pneumoconiosis (chapter 13) which may be prevented by dust suppression to keep the concentration of respirable particles below the threshold limit value of 20 million particles per cu ft. The material itself is inactive in tissue culture and harmless to rats by mouth, by inhalation and on intraperitoneal injection. Studies of rubber workers exposed to non-fibrous talc have shown evidence for increased cough in those who are also smokers but few other positive features (24). By contrast, producers and users of fibrous talc may exhibit pleural calcification and features of asbestosis, including basal crepitation, clubbing of the fingers, radiological irregular opacities and impaired lung function (26). Thus proper preventive measures are needed including environmental dust monitoring, appropriate dust control and periodic examination of long-term employees. The type and source of the talc, including any additional constituents, should be recorded. In addition more information is needed about the contribution of various types of tremolite to the overall effects of asbestos including its role in producing pleural calcification (78) and lung cancer (22).

Wollastonite. Wollastonite is a fibrous monocalcium silicate ($CaSiO_3$) which has many of the attributes of asbestos; it is used for insulation in the form of mineral wool and wall board, for brake linings, fire blankets, exterior paints, etc.

(see e.g. table 8.3, page 162). It comes mainly from the U.S.A. but also Mexico and Finland. Persons exposed to the dust may have an increased prevalence of chronic bronchitis, radiographic evidence for mild pulmonary fibrosis, diffuse pleural thickening and physiological evidence for narrowing of small lung airways (35). The annual decline in peak expiratory flow is significantly correlated with the dust exposure (29). However, other studies have been largely negative (42). More information is needed.

Zeolite. Zeolite is a species of fibrous aluminium silicate which has recently been found to be of use as a molecular sieve, filler and, after calcining, as a lightweight aggregate. It is quarried from sedimentary volcanic deposits in U.S.A. and elsewhere and no harmful effects have been reported. However, the form eronite comprises long fibres of diameter mostly less than 0.25µm which have been found to be the cause of mesothelioma amongst the inhabitants of two villages in Anatolia and experimentally when inhaled by rats (page 219): Thus occupationally exposed persons may also be at risk. Since the latent period is of the order of 40 years there is a clear need for further scrutiny.

Man-made mineral fibres

For nearly 100 years fibrous materials have been manufactured from fusible slag or rock; since the 1930s fibres have also been made from glass. The fibres may penetrate the skin or mucous membranes but no clinical cases of lung fibrosis, cancer or mesothelioma have been reported (32). The manufactured products include glass fibre, rock wool and slag wool; they are used mainly as insulation but also for textiles, papers, filters, reinforcement for plastic and in construction. Many of these applications entail coating the fibres with oil or with resin which may occasionally give rise to occupational asthma (chapter 16). The fibres are amorphous silicates which melt at temperatures in the range 1000–1500°C. They are formed by centrifugation, blowing or drawing and the fibre diameter is usually controlled within fairly narrow limits. Subsequent processing does not reduce this further as, unlike asbestos, the fibres only

fracture transversely and not longitudinally. For most applications, including textiles and reinforcement, the fibre diameter is well above the respirable range; for insulation the mean diameter is usually 6µm with 8% of fibres being respirable (diameter <3µm). Fibres of diameter down to 1µm are used for filter papers, acoustic insulation and other applications; these fibres are all within the respirable range.

Evidence on the biological effects of man-made mineral fibres (MMMF) has recently been reviewed (85). Measurement of airborne concentrations of fibres shows that levels of dustiness are usually low, the fibres relatively large and most are cleared by the lung via the mucociliary escalator. The few fibres which are retained are encapsulated in ferro-protein, fragmented and probably clear from the lung more rapidly than amphibole asbestos. In studies using animals the delivery of MMMF to the respiratory tract has caused only minor changes in circumstances in which asbestos has caused fibrosis and cancer. The intraperitoneal injection of fibres of diameter less than 0.5µm causes mesothelioma (70). However, in epidemiological studies no mesothelioma has been reported amongst exposed persons. Thus, as in the case of asbestos, the risk in life is determined by the capacity of the fibres to penetrate and remain in the lining layers of the pleura and not their behaviour when they get there. At present there is no detectable risk to man of either mesothelioma or pulmonary fibrosis while the risk of lung cancer is very small, of the order of 1% (55). Long-term follow-up studies suggest that persons with an exposure in excess of 30 years may be at increased risk on this account but the evidence is inconclusive and more is needed (67).

MMMF is a much safer material than asbestos and should replace it whenever possible. However, very small fibres could still present a hazard, particularly if prepared in some new way which led to greater penetration and persistence in the lung. This is recognized in the hygiene standard (table 1.7, page 16). Scrutiny by animal inhalation should precede the use of such material. Meanwhile as with other materials the environmental conditions during manufacture are generally improving.

References

1 Acheson ED, Gardner MJ, Pippard EC. Crime LP. Mortality of two groups of women who manufactured gas masks from chrysotile and crocidolite asbestos: a 40-year follow-up. *Br J Industr Med* 1982;**39**:344–8.

2 Albelda SM, Epstein DM, Gefter WB, Miller WT. Pleural thickening: its significance and relationship to asbestos dust exposure. *Am Rev Respir Dis* 1982;**126**:621–4.

3 Allison AC. Pathogenic effects of inhaled particles and antigens. *Ann NY Acad Sci* 1974;**221**:299–308.

4 Arai H, Kang KY, Sato H, Satoh K, Nagai H, Motomiya M, Konno K. Significance of the quantification and demonstration of hyaluronic acid in tissue specimens for the diagnosis of pleural mesothelioma. *Am Rev Respir Dis* 1979;**120**:529–32.

5 Ashcroft T, Heppleston AG. The optical and electron microscopic determination of pulmonary asbestos fibre concentration and its relation to the human pathological reaction. *J Clin Path* 1973;**26**:224–34.

6 Baris YI, Artvinli M, Sahin AA. Environmental mesothelioma in Turkey. *Ann NY Acad Sci* 1979;**330**:423–32.

7 Becklake MR. Asbestos related diseases of the lung and other organs: their epidemiology and implications for clinical practice. *Am Rev Respir Dis* 1976;114:187–227.

8 Bengtsson NO, Hardell L, Eriksson M. Asbestos exposure and malignant lymphoma. *Lancet* 1982;**ii**:1463.

9 Berry G, Newhouse ML. Mortality of workers manufacturing friction materials using asbestos. *Br J Industr Med* 1983;**40**:1–7.

10 Berry G, Newhouse ML, Antonis P. Combined effect of asbestos and smoking on mortality from lung cancer and mesothelioma. *Br J Industr Med* 1985;**42**:12–18. See also Özesmi M. et al *Br J Industr Med* 1985;**42**:746–9.

11 British Occupational Hygiene Society. Report from the Committee on Asbestos. A study of the health experience in two UK asbestos factories. *Ann Occup Hyg* 1983;**27**:1–55.

12 British Thoracic and Tuberculosis Association: Medical Research Council Pneumoconiosis Unit. A survey of pleural thickening: its relation to asbestos exposure and previous pleural disease. *Environ Res* 1972;**5**:142–51.

13 Britton MG. Asbestos pleural disease. *Br J Dis Chest* 1982;**76**:1–10.

14 Britton MG, Hughes DTD, Phillips TJG. A guide to compensation for asbestos-related diseases. *Br Med J* 1981;**282**:2107–2111.

15 Brody AR, Hill LH, Adkins B Jr, O'Connor RW. Chrysotile asbestos inhalation in rats: deposition pattern and reaction of alveolar epithelium and pulmonary macrophages. *Am Rev Respir Dis* 1981;**123**:670–9.

16 Butchart EG, Ashcroft T, Barnsley WC, Holden MP. Pleuropneumonectomy in the management of diffuse malignant mesothelioma of the pleura. *Thorax* 1976;**31**:15–24.

17 Churg AM, Warnock ML. Asbestos and other ferruginous bodies: their formation and clinical significance. *Am J Path* 1981;**102**:447–56.

18 Churg A, Wiggs B, Depaoli L, Kampe B, Stevens B. Lung asbestos content in chrysotile workers with mesothelioma. *Am Rev Respir Dis* 1984;**130**:1042–5.

19 Darke C, Wagner MM, McMillan GH. HLA-A and B antigen frequencies in an asbestos-exposed population with normal and abnormal chest radiographs. *Tissue Antigens* 1979;**13**:228–32.

20 Davies P, Allison AC, Ackerman J, Butterfield A, Williams S. Asbestos induces selective release of lysosomal enzymes from mononuclear phagocytes. *Nature* 1974;**251**:423–5.

21 Davis JMG. The pathology of asbestos-related disease. *Thorax* 1984;**39**:801–8.

22 Davis JMG, Addison J, Bolton RE, Donaldson K, Jones AD, Miller BG. Inhalation studies on the effects of tremolite and brucite dust in rats. *Carcinogenesis* 1985;**6**:667–74.

23 Elmes PC, Simpson MJC. The clinical aspects of mesothelioma. *Quart J Med* 1976;**45**:427–49.

24 Fine LJ, Peters JM, Burgess WA, di Berardinis LJ. Studies of respiratory morbidity in rubber workers. Part IV: Respiratory morbidity in talc workers. *Arch Environm Hlth* 1976;**31**:195–200.

25 Fridriksson HV, Hedenström H, Hillerdal G, Malmberg P. Increased lung stiffness in persons with pleural plaques. *Eur J Respir Dis* 1981;**62**:412–24.

26 Gamble JF, Fellner V, Dimeo MJ. An epidemiological study of a group of talc workers. *Am Rev Respir Dis* 1979;**119**:741–53.

27 Gibbs GW. Etiology of pleural calcification: A study of Quebec chrysotile asbestos miners and millers. *Arch Environm Hlth* 1979;**34**:76–83.

28 Greenberg M, Lloyd Davies TA. Mesothelioma register, 1967–8. *Br J Industr Med* 1974;**31**:91–104.

29 Hanke W, Sepulveda M–J, Watson A, Jankovic J. Respiratory morbidity in wollastonite workers. *Br J Industr Med* 1984;**41**:474–9.

30 Health and Safety Executive. *Asbestos: Final Report of the Advisory Committee* Volume 1 and 2. London: HMSO. 1979.

31 Hildick-Smith GY. The biology of talc. *Br J Industr Med* 1976;**33**:217–29.

32 Hill JW. Man-made mineral fibres. *J Soc Occup Med* 1978;**28**:134–41.

33 Hodgson AA. Nature and paragenesis of asbestos minerals. *Phil Trans Roy Soc Lond* series A 1977;**286**:611–24.

34 Hughes JM, Weill H. Asbestos exposure—quantitative assessment of risk. *Am Rev Respir Dis* 1986;**133**:5–13.

35 Huuskonen MS, Tossavainen A, Koskinen H, Zitting A, Korhonen O, Nickels J, Korhonen K, Vaaranen V. Wollastonite exposure and lung fibrosis. *Environm Res* 1983;**30**:291–304.

36 Jacobsen M, Miller BG, Murdoch RM. *A study of a sample of chest radiographs from the Health and Safety Executive's survey of asbestos workers.* Edinburgh: Institute of Occupational Medicine: 1983.

37 Jodoin G, Gibbs GW, Macklem PT, McDonald JC, Becklake MR. Early effects of asbestos exposure on lung function. *Am Rev Respir Dis* 1971;**104**:525–35.

38 Jones B, Thomas P. Incidence of mesothelioma in Britain. *Lancet* 1986;**i**:1275.

39 Jones JSP, Pooley FD, Smith PG. Factory populations exposed to crocidolite asbestos—a continuing survey. *INSERM* 1976;**52**:117–20.

40 Kreel L. Computed tomography in mesothelioma. *Seminars in Oncology* 1981;**8**:302–12. *See also:* McLoud TC *et al.*, *Am J Roentgen* 1985;**144**:9–18.

41 Law MR, Hodson ME, Heard BE. Malignant mesothelioma of the pleura: relation between histological type and clinical behaviour. *Thorax* 1982;**37**:810–15.

42 Lemen R, Dement JM, (Eds) *Dusts and Disease.* Conference on occupational and environmental exposure to selected fibrous and particulate dusts and their extension into the environment. Illinois: Pathotox Publ Inc 1979.

43 Liddell FDK, Hanley JA. Relations between asbestos exposure and lung cancer SMRs in occupational cohort studies. *Br J Industr Med* 1985;**42**:389–96.

44 McDermott M, Bevan MM, Elmes PC, Allardice JT, Bradley AC. Lung function and radiographic change in chrysotile workers in Swaziland. *Br J Industr Med* 1982;**39**:338–43.

45 McDonald JC. Mineral fibres and cancer. *Annals Acad Med* 1984;**13**;No.2 suppl:345–52.

46 McDonald JC, Liddell FDK, Gibbs GW, Eyssen GE, McDonald AD. Dust exposure and mortality in chrysotile mining 1910–75. *Br J Industr Med* 1980;**37**:11–24.

47 McFadden D, Wright JL, Wiggs B, Churg A. Smoking inhibits asbestos clearance. *Am Rev Respir Dis* 1986;**133**:372–4.

48 McGavin CR, Sheers G. Diffuse pleural thickening in asbestos workers: disability and lung function abnormalities. *Thorax* 1984;**39**:604–7.

49 McMillan GHG, Pethybridge RJ, Sheers G. Effects of smoking on attack rates of pulmonary and pleural lesions related to exposure to asbestos dust. *Br J Industr Med* 1980;**37**:268–72.

50 McMillan GHG, Rossiter CE. Development of radiological and clinical evidence of parenchymal fibrosis in men with non-malignant asbestos-related pleural lesions. *Br J Industr Med* 1982;**39**:54–9.

51 Meurman LO, Kiviluoto R, Hakama M. Mortality and morbidity among the working population of anthophyllite asbestos miners in Finland. *Br J Industr Med* 1974;**31**:105–12.

52 Morgan A, Holmes A. Concentrations and characteristics of amphibole fibres in the lungs of workers exposed to crocidolite in the British gas-mask factories, and elsewhere, during the Second World War. *Br J Industr Med* 1982;**39**:62–9.

53 Morgan A, Holmes A. Distribution and characteristics of amphibole asbestos fibres measured with the light microscope in the left lung of an insulation worker. *Br J Industr Med* 1983;**40**:45–50.

54 Morgan A, Talbot RJ, Holmes A. Significance of fibre length in the clearance of asbestos fibres from the lung. *Br J Industr Med* 1978;**35**:146–53.

55 Morgan RW, Bratsberg JA. Mortality study of fibrous glass production workers. *Arch Environm Hlth* 1981;**36**:179–83.

56 Newhouse ML, Berry G. Predictions of mortality from mesothelial tumours in asbestos factory workers. *Br J Industr Med* 1976;**33**:147–51.

57 Newhouse ML, Berry G, Wagner JC. Mortality of factory workers in East London 1933–80. *Br J Industr Med* 1985;**42**:4–11.

58 Özesmi M, Patiroglu TE, Hillerdal G, Özesmi C. Peritoneal mesothelioma and malignant lymphoma in mice caused by fibrous zeolite. *Br J Industr Med* 1985;**42**:746–9.

59 Parkes WR. *Occupational Lung Disorders.* Butterworths. London. 1982.

60 Peto J, Doll R, Howard SV, Kinlen LJ, Lewinsohn HC. A mortality study among workers in an English asbestos factory. *Br J Industr Med* 1977;**34**:169–73.

61 Pneumoconiosis Committee of the College of American Pathologists. Asbestos associated diseases. *Arch Path Lab Med* 1982;**106**:541–96.

62 Pooley FD. The identification of asbestos dust with an electron microscope microprobe analyser. *Ann Occup Hyg* 1975;**18**:181–6.

63 Pooley FD, Rowlands N. Chemical and physical properties of British talc powders. *Inhaled Particles IV* 1977:639–46. Walton WH (ed): Oxford: Pergamon Press.

64 Robinson BWS, Musk AW. Benign asbestos pleural effusion: diagnosis and course. *Thorax* 1981;**36**:896–900. *See also*: Yoshimura H *et al.*, *Radiology* 1986;**158**:653–8.

65 Rossiter CE, Berry G. The interaction of asbestos exposure and smoking on respiratory health. *Bull Eur Physiopathol Respir* 1978;**14**:197–204.

66 Saracci R. Asbestos and lung cancer: an analysis of the epidemiological evidence on the asbestos-smoking interaction. *Int J Cancer* 1977;**20**:323–31.

67 Saracci R, Simonato L, Acheson ED, *et al.* Mortality and incidence of cancer of workers in the man made vitreous fibres producing industry: an international investigation at 13 European plants. *Br J Industr Med* 1984;**41**:425–36.

68 Selikoff IJ, Hammond EC. Health hazards of asbestos exposure. *Ann NY Acad Sci* 1979; **330**:1–814.

69 Shapiro HA: (ed). *Pneumoconiosis: Proceeding of the International Conference, Johannesburg 1969.* Capetown: OUP, 1970.

70 Stanton MF, Layard M, Tegeris A, Miller E, May M, Morgan E, Smith A. Relation of particle dimension to carcinogenicity in amphibole asbestoses and other fibrous minerals. *J Nat Cancer Inst* 1981;**67**:965–75.

71 Timbrell V. Alignment of respirable asbestos fibres by magnetic fields. *Ann Occup Hyg* 1975;**18**:299–311.

72 Timbrell V. Deposition and retention of fibres in the human lung. *Ann Occup Hyg* 1982;**26**:347–69.

73 Timbrell V. Fibres and carcinogenesis. *J Occup Hlth Soc Astr* 1983;**3:part 1**:3–13.

74 Timbrell V, Ashcroft T, Goldstein B, Heyworth F, Meurman L, Rendale REG, Reynolds JA, Shilkin KB, Whitaker D. Dose response relationships for asbestosis. *Ann Occup Hyg*: (Proc 6th International Symposium on Inhaled Particles 1985) in the press.

75 De Vuyst P, Jedwab J, Dumortier P, Vandermoten G, Vande Weyer R, Yernault JC. Asbestos bodies in bronchoalveolar lavage. *Am Rev Respir Dis* 1982;**126**:972–6.

76 Wagner JC (ed). *Biological effects of mineral fibres.* International Agency for Research on Cancer. WHO: Lyons: 1980.

77 Wagner JC, Berry G, Pooley FD. Mesotheliomas and asbestos type in asbestos textile workers: a study of lung contents. *Br Med J* 1982; **285**:603–6.

78 Wagner JC, Chamberlain M, Brown RC, Berry G, Pooley FD, Davies R, Griffiths DM. Biological effects of tremolite. *Br J Cancer* 1982; **45**:352–60.

79 Wagner JC, Pooley FD, Berry G, Seal RM, Munday DE, Morgan J, Clark NJ. A pathological and mineralogical study of asbestos-related deaths in the United Kingdom in 1977. *Ann Occup Hyg* 1982;**26**:423–31.

80 Walton WH. The nature, hazards and assessment of occupational exposure to airborne asbestos dust. A review. *Ann Occup Hyg* 1982;**25**:117–247.

81 Weill H, Rossiter CE, Waggenspack C, Jones RN, Ziskind MM. Differences in lung effects resulting from chrysotile and crocidolite exposure. *Inhaled Particles IV* 1977:789–98. Walton WH (ed): Woking: Unwin.

82 Weiss W, Levin R, Goodman L. Pleural plaques and cigarette smoking in asbestos workers. *J Occup Med* 1981;**23**:427–30.

83 Weiss W, Theodos PA. Pleuro-pulmonary disease among asbestos workers in relation to smoking and type of exposure. *J Occup Med* 1978;**20**:341–5.

84 Whitwell F, Scott J, Grimshaw M. Relationship between occupations and asbestos-fibre content of the lungs in patients with pleural mesothelioma, lung cancer and other diseases. *Thorax* 1977;**32**:377–86.

85 World Health Organization. *Biological effects of man-made mineral fibres.* EURO Reports and Studies 81. WHO: Copenhagen: 1983.

86 Wright JL, Churg A. Severe diffuse small airways abnormalities in long term chrysotile asbestos miners. *Br J Industr Med* 1985;**42**: 556–9.

87 Wright PH, Hanson A, Kreel L, Capel LH. Respiratory function changes after asbestos pleurisy. *Thorax* 1980;**35**:31–6. *See also* Bohlig H, *et al IARC Sci Publ* 1980;**2**:497–506.

Chapter 11
Beryllium Disease

Properties and uses of beryllium
Clinical features
Beryllium cancer
Epidemiology
Risk factors
Hygiene standards
Environmental control
Surveillance

Properties and uses of beryllium

Beryllium is a rare element which is a constituent of beryl ore. This is a beryllium aluminium silicate $Be_3Al_2(SiO_3)_6$ of which a variant is the gemstone emerald. Beryl is distributed widely throughout the world and is biologically inert. By contrast, beryllium metal and salts are highly reactive; they also have remarkable and commercially valuable physical and chemical properties which more than offset the high cost of safe manufacture.

Beryllium is refined from beryl or other ore in U.S.A., Japan, U.S.S.R. and other countries. The process entails crushing the ore which is then mixed with sodium silicofluoride and soda ash to make briquettes. These are heated in a kiln to 750°C, crushed, and leached with water to extract the beryllium hydroxide. The hydroxide may be reduced by further heating to form beryllium metal which is then poured into moulds. Beryllium oxide is obtained by calcining; the oxide is used for the manufacture of tubes and solid objects by the processes of slip casting and cold and hot pressing.

The metal has a high melting point and great tensile strength and elasticity but a low density so is ideal for the heat shields of space vehicles, rotor blades and other applications requiring tolerance of high temperatures together with a high strength-to-weight ratio. Beryllium is permeable to radiation and on this account is used for the windows of x-ray tubes and microwave equipment. Beryllium copper or nickel alloys are good electrical conductors which are very durable because the alloy is hard, has a high fatigue limit and is not easily corroded; it is also non-magnetic. Components made of these materials are widely used in engines and other electric devices including switches, springs, connectors and controls. Beryllium oxide is also very resistant to corrosion and is both a good thermal conductor and an electrical insulator. This combination of properties is used in beryllium oxide tubes and mouldings for mounting and insulating electrical components where there is need to disperse heat. The material also makes excellent crucibles and is used in nuclear reactors as a moderator to slow down and reflect neutrons without absorbing them. It has been tested as a rocket fuel. Beryllium silicates have phosphorescent properties.

Beryllium disease

A non-caseating, granulomatous disease of the lungs due to beryllium was first reported by Weber and Englehardt in 1933 and the illness achieved epidemic proportions in the U.S.A. towards the end of and after World War II. The epidemic was caused by beryllium silicates which were used as a phosphor in early fluorescent tubes for display screens and lighting; the illness affected persons who handled broken tubes as well as those who made them. Alternative phosphors were substituted in the late 1940s. The epidemic led Dr. Harriet Hardy to establish a beryllium case registry at the Massachusetts General Hospital in 1952. The registry

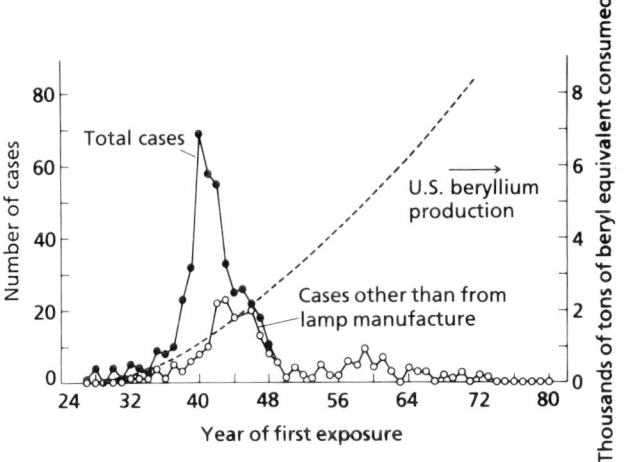

Fig. 11.1. Number of new cases of beryllium disease in the U.S.A. by year of first exposure compared with beryllium production. (By courtesy of M. Eisenbud and J. Lisson (5).)

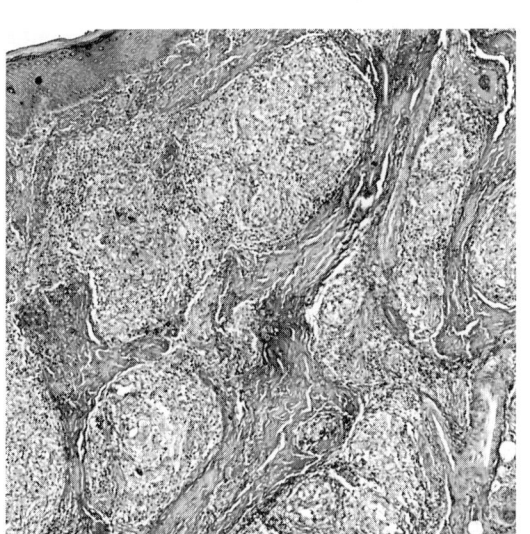

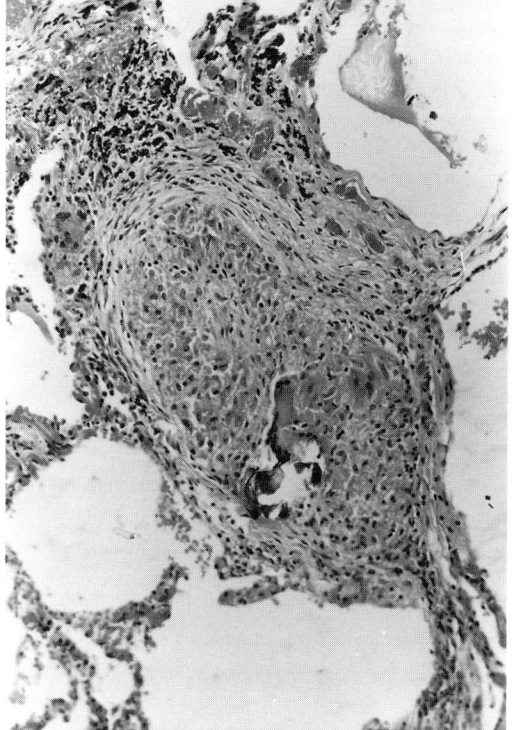

Fig. 11.2. Multiple non-caseating epithelioid granulomas due to beryllium. *Left*: from the dermis of the patient whose chest radiograph is illustrated in fig. 11.4. (By courtesy of W. Jones Williams.) *Right*: Chronic pulmonary granulomas from a 31-year-old female chemist who for 2 years from the age of 26 handled material containing beryllium in a fluorescent lamp factory (16). The lesion comprised epithelioid cells and multinucleated giant cells within a fibrous sheath. Lymphocytes, present in the upper left-hand part of the section, enveloped the lesion in the acute stage. The conchoid body (below centre) is formed from protein impregnated with calcium and is a non-specific feature. (By courtesy of I. Rannie and T. Ashcroft.)

is now maintained by the U.S. National Institute for Occupational Safety and Health at Cincinnati. The number of cases contained in the registry exceeds 888 but the incidence is now low (fig. 11.1). Fewer than forty cases have been reported in the U.K. However, recognition of the condition is important because the dramatic clinical features usually respond readily to treatment. Beryllium inactivates intracellular enzymes including plasma alkali phosphatase and phosphoglucomutase (1); it is a sensitizing agent and is carcinogenic to monkeys, rodents and rabbits (page 247). However, the mechanisms which underlie beryllium disease are not understood. Experimentally the condition provides a model for studying the action of intracellular enzymes. At the practical level it is a challenge to occupational hygienists whose largely successful efforts to achieve safe conditions have sometimes been hindered by the industrial secrecy which is associated with advanced technology (8, 9).

The *principal pathological feature* is the occurrence of non-caseating interstitial granulomas with follicles of epithelial cells and giant cells surrounded by lymphocytes and plasma cells (fig. 11.2). Reticulin in the granulomas may progress to fibrous tissue and the picture may then change to one of diffuse interstitial fibrosis with compensatory emphysema and bullae. The picture is similar to that of pulmonary sarcoidosis (12).

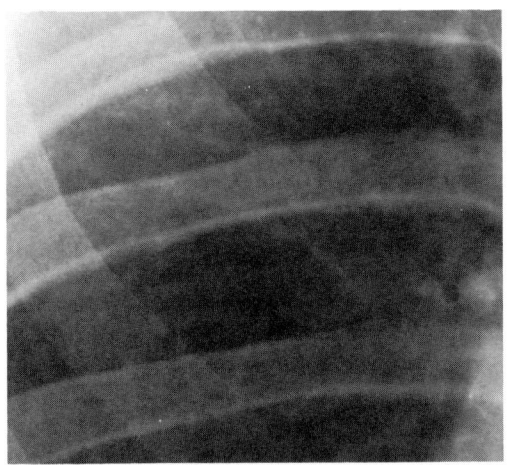

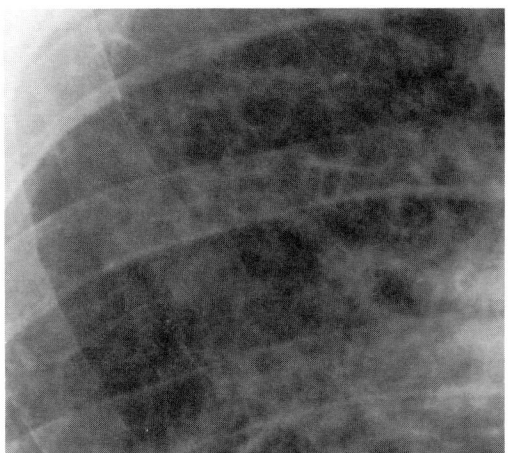

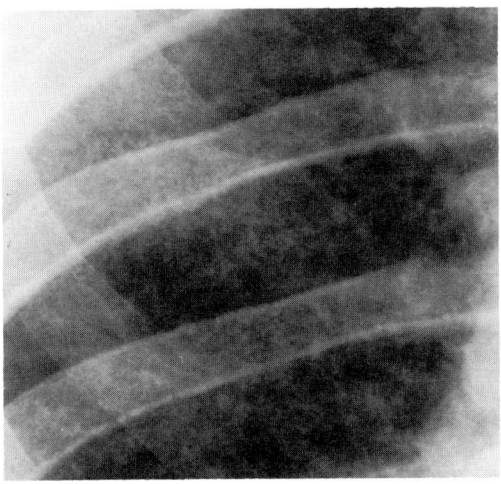

Fig. 11.3. Beryllium disease. Detail from chest radiographs at age 35, 37 and 56 years of a man who for 7 years worked with beryllium oxide. Apart from transient dermatitis he was in good health and the general atmospheric concentration of beryllium was within the hygiene standard (3). At the time of the first radiograph the patient was already in other employment; he was asymptomatic and extremely fit but a retrospective survey revealed early pneumoconiosis (category 1p, top left) and a reduced transfer factor (69% predicted); beryllium was detected in the urine. Two years later, after a small pneumothorax, the chest radiograph showed progression of the pneumoconiosis (category 2p). The lesion regressed in response to steroids (10mg/day); however, this dose did not prevent the subsequent development of diffuse interstitial fibrosis (right).

Clinical features

Exposure to beryllium metal and salts can cause reactions in several tissues or organs of the body but the parent ore, beryl, which is described above, seems to be biologically inert. The commonest abnormality is *contact dermatitis*, either immediate when it is probably due to chemical irritation by a water soluble beryllium salt, or after an interval when it may be due to sensitization of the skin (case 11.3). The lesion is an erythema or papulo-vesicular eruption and clears up on withdrawal from exposure. *Conjunctivitis* may occur as a splashburn or in association with dermatitis. *Implantation* of beryllium in the skin following a cut or abrasion may lead to chronic ulceration or the formation of a granuloma (fig. 11.2). Initially the lesion is at the site of implantation but secondary lesions develop elsewhere in the skin, lymph nodes and lung (13). The condition is prevented by careful cleaning of any injuries incurred during handling beryllium products; treatment is with steroid drugs supplemented where necessary by local excision.

Transient exposure to high atmospheric concentrations of beryllium causes *acute berylliosis*. This is a chemical, non-bacterial inflammation of the respiratory tract in response to water soluble beryllium salts or low-fired beryllium oxide (17); it can present as rhinitis, tracheitis or pneumonitis. Involvement of the lung results in dyspnoea, cyanosis, fever, râles on auscultation of the chest, and diffuse nodulation on the chest radiograph. In fulminating cases there is expectoration of blood-stained, frothy sputum and other features of pulmonary oedema. In the event of protracted illness loss of weight is common. The histological appearances are those of pulmonary and interstitial oedema and include an increased number of lymphocytes and plasma cells in the walls of alveoli, fibrin and red blood cells in the lumina and protein on the walls of alveoli giving the appearance of a hyaline membrane. During recovery the exudate is removed by phagocytic cells and the alveolar epithelium is repaired. The condition differs from chronic beryllium disease in that there are no pulmonary granulo-

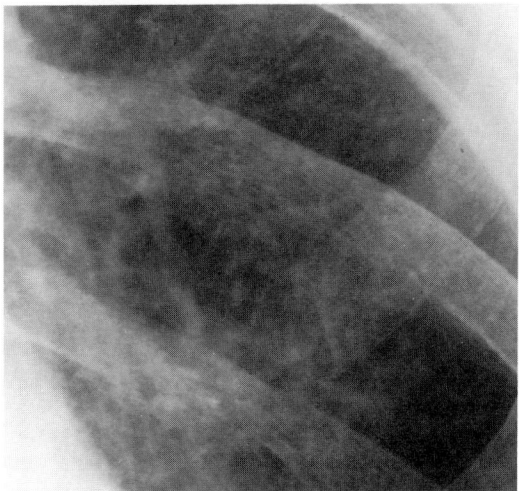 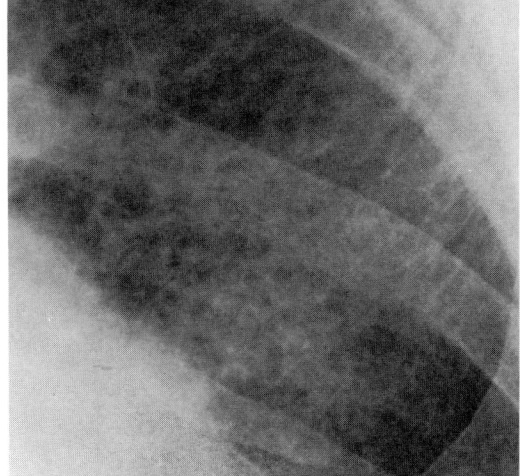

Fig. 11.4. Beryllium disease. Detail from chest radiographs of an engineer who at age 50 implanted beryllium in his finger whilst using a grinding wheel. At that time the chest radiograph (left) and the lung function were normal. A granuloma developed at the site of the injury, ulcerated, failed to respond to steroids and was treated by amputation. At age 56 a granuloma developed on the forearm (fig. 11.2) and was excised. Subsequently, despite steroid therapy, the patient became breathless on exertion (grade 2); at age 63 the total lung capacity and transfer factor were both reduced by approximately 15% and the ventilation on exercise was increased. The chest radiograph (right) showed small round and irregular opacities (3p/s). This early diffuse interstitial fibrosis subsequently progressed further.

mas or other evidence of sensitization to beryllium and in 90% of cases complete recovery
occurs following withdrawal from exposure.
The process of recovery is sometimes assisted by
medical treatment with oxygen and steroid
drugs. The use of steroids might also be
expected to reduce the small proportion of cases
who progress to chronic disease (19).

Chronic berylliosis. Inhalation of dust containing beryllium or its salts leads to the formation of chronic granulomas in the lungs and
other organs. The pulmonary condition can also
develop secondarily to contact dermatitis or
implantation granuloma (fig. 11.4). The onset is

usually insidious with breathlessness on exertion, dry cough and loss of weight or vague
symptoms including lassitude, anorexia, chest
pain, weakness and anxiety (fig. 11.5). Alternatively the patient may present with small
rounded opacities on the chest radiograph (fig.
11.3). Irregular opacities also occur either
initially or during the course of the disease. The
x-ray appearance may progress to one suggestive
of honeycomb lung (fig. 11.3). However, the
affected person can remain asymptomatic. On
physical examination, as well as tachypnoea,
there may be cyanosis, sometimes conspicuous
on exertion, mid- and late inspiratory râles at

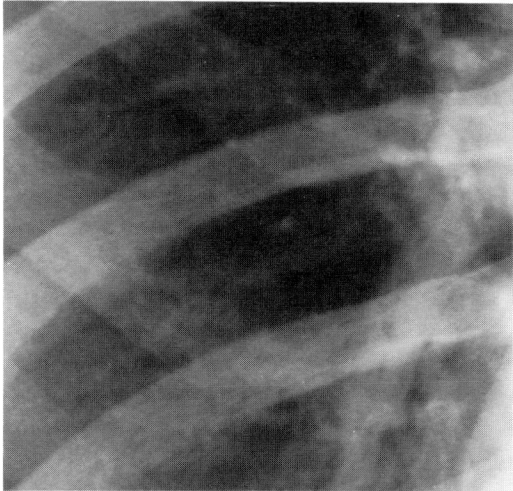

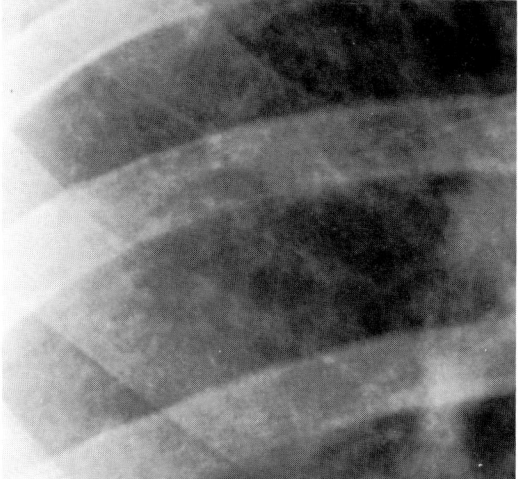

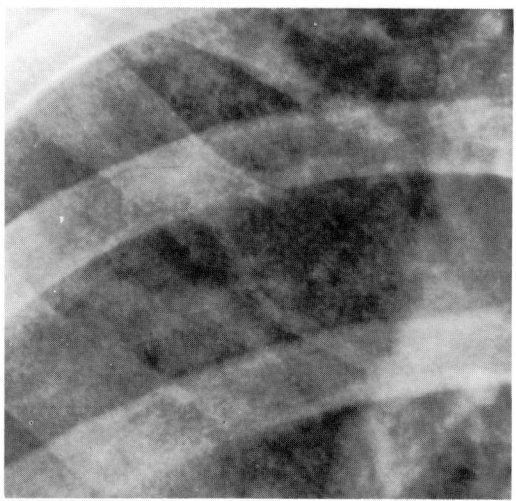

Fig. 11.5. Beryllium disease. Detail from chest
radiographs of a man who at age 26 spent a year
making beryllium copper alloy. At that time the
chest radiograph was normal (top left). At age 31 he
experienced symptoms suggestive of anxiety.
However, the transfer factor was reduced (49%
predicted), the exercise respiratory frequency was
greatly increase (Vt_{30} reduced) and the chest
radiograph showed simple pneumoconiosis
(category 3p). The condition responded to steroids
(60mg reducing to 15mg per day), but two further
reductions (one pre-meditated and one accidental)
led to severe exacerbations (fig. 11.6). The chest
radiograph during the second of these episodes at
age 35 and that at age 42 following successful
withdrawal of steroids are shown in the figure
(bottom left and top right respectively).

the lung bases and clubbing of the fingers. In the late stages there may be clinical or electrocardiographic evidence of pulmonary hypertension with or without congestive cardiac failure. The serum concentration of globulin is usually increased, there may be hypercalciuria and evidence of impaired liver function but the alkaline phosphatase is usually normal.

The findings on assessment of lung function are primarily those of defective gas transfer, with a low transfer factor and Kco, which on exercise give rise to hypoxaemia. This stimulates ventilation which is then high relative to the consumption of oxygen; hence $\dot{V}$E45 is increased. There is also rapid breathing (tachypnoea) which is probably due to stimulation of pulmonary J receptors (4); the depth of breathing, and hence the tidal volume at a minute volume of 30 l min^{-1} (Vt$_{30}$), are reduced relative to the vital capacity (chapter 18). Tachypnoea defined in this way is a feature of acute exacerbations associated with pulmonary granulomas (fig. 11.6); in the more chronic phase the tidal volume is consistent with the vital capacity which may itself be reduced. The static lung compliance may also be reduced and lung recoil pressure increased. These changes usually resolve with treatment but they may persist and are then associated with radiographic irregular opacities and features of interstitial fibrosis (fig. 11.3). In addition there is sometimes evidence for airflow obstruction which is probably secondary to distortion of the lung, and for emphysema which may be an expression of honeycomb lung.

Treatment requires withdrawal from exposure and use of prednisone or other corticosteroid drugs. Initially the drug should be given in sufficient dosage to control the symptoms and reduce the profusion of small round opacities on the chest radiograph. The irregular opacities do not respond to the same extent. Subsequently a maintenance dose should be given. This can sometimes be tailed off over a period of years leaving the subject asymptomatic. However, the time-course is years rather than months and very long-term supervision is essential to ensure that treatment is not stopped by omission.

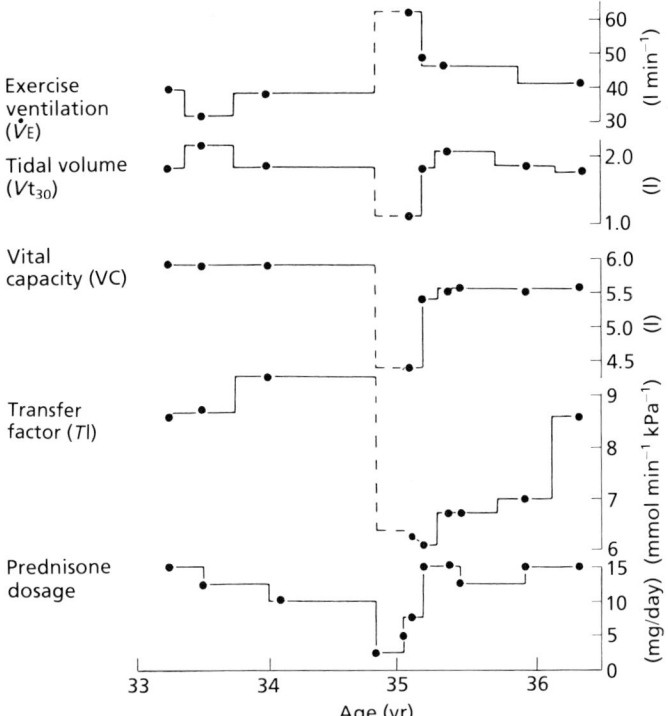

Fig. 11.6. Effect of a sudden reduction in steroid dosage upon the lung function of the patient whose case is illustrated in fig. 11.5. He became acutely breathless, hypoxaemic and tachypnoeic but recovered quickly when the dose of steroids was increased. (Source: Cotes J.E. *Lung Function* 4th edn. Blackwell Scientific Publications, Oxford: 1979: p. 424.)

Premature reduction of steroids leads to a return of the illness; this should be looked for by regular chest radiography and measurement of transfer factor and the ventilatory response to exercise. On no account should the steroids be withdrawn abruptly as this is liable to precipitate an acute exacerbation of the disease (fig. 11.6). In these circumstances the patient's life is at risk and the name chronic beryllium disease definitely a misnomer!

Differential diagnosis from sarcoidosis

A diagnosis of beryllium disease is usually based on the occurrence of appropriate changes in the lung of a person who has been exposed to beryllium, has one or more risk factors (see below) and does not have extra-pulmonary features of sarcoidosis; the latter include uveitis, enlarged lacrymal or salivary glands, isolated hilar gland enlargement, widespread superficial lymphadenopathy, erythema nodosum and bone erosion. In beryllium disease clubbing of the fingers may be present but is not invariable. In context to sarcoidosis basal râles are common and the Kveim test is negative. The tuberculin test is usually negative in both conditions. The presence of beryllium in the lesions is probably diagnostic (18) but not excretion of beryllium salts in the urine which is only evidence of exposure. This feature constitutes a rare cause of renal calculae. Changes in blood calcium are common to both conditions.

The difficulty of diagnosis has led to an extensive search for specific in-vitro tests for hypersensitivity using beryllium as the antigen. The results to date are incomplete; they suggest that despite high expectations the lymphocyte macrophage migration inhibition factor is not helpful and this appears also the case for the beryllium lymphocyte blast transformation test (20). Promising results have been obtained using a lymphocyte reactivity test (11) and the proportion of activated T cells found in bronchoalveolar lavage (6); the specificity and sensitivity of these procedures have still to be confirmed. Meanwhile in case of doubt the diagnosis may be established by histological and biochemical examination of not less than 10ml of tissue obtained by open lung biopsy.

Beryllium cancer

Malignant disease has been induced in animals by the administration of beryllium salts and cancer has developed in persons exposed to beryllium. In one instance the presence of beryllium was detected in the tumour but the association appears not to have been causal (7). In a follow-up study on persons exposed for more than 15 years an increased incidence of lung cancer which was on the borderline of statistical significance was observed by Mancuso (15) but in this study no allowance was made for the effects of smoking and the association with lung fibrosis, which is known to carry an increased cancer risk, was not reported. Thus the evidence remains ambiguous; the excess risk if present is probably small (10, 14).

Epidemiology

The risk of beryllium disease is largely confined to persons who work with beryllium oxide and salts and those who handle contaminated clothing. The neighbourhood cases are mostly of this type (17). The occurrence of acute beryllium disease is associated with an episode of high exposure to beryllium oxide or a soluble beryllium salt; sequelae are uncommon. The incidence may be obtained from the factory medical records and the prevalence may be obtained retrospectively by use of a questionnaire; in one study two men out of 130 developed episodes of acute beryllium pneumonitis over a 10 year period (3). The condition appears to be dose-related with a threshold below which no cases occur. Chronic beryllium disease was diagnosed on the basis of small opacities on the chest radiograph plus hypoxaemia at rest in eleven of 214 workers at a plant which was surveyed following the appearance of a clinical case (21). The peak environmental concentrations were up to 50 times the accepted peak limit value. Amongst workers in other factories the occurrence of clinical cases was also associated with poor environmental control (17). However, in a survey where a dose–response relationship was looked for none was observed (3). This may have been due to the clinical condition needing for its manifestation: (a) an adequate exposure, (b) development of sensitization, and (c) the presence of a trigger or risk factor. When the exposure is high enough the condition is probably dose-related with the other aspects not imposing much constraint but when the dose is near to the threshold the factors which influence sensitization and the presence of risk factors greatly influence the response.

Risk factors and subclinical disease

Subjects whose exposure to beryllium is minimal seldom develop significant disease. However, a few people are very susceptible, whilst some heavily exposed subjects remain healthy over many years. Susceptibility cannot yet be predicted and the cause is not understood. Its occurrence makes dose–response data difficult to interpret. Pregnancy is a common precursor in women; they should not be exposed to beryllium during the childbearing period. Cutaneous patch-testing with beryllium is liable to activate disease (24) and should not be performed in any circumstances. Withdrawal from exposure can precipitate disease in both man and animals (22, also figs. 11.3 and 11.5). Where aggravation does not occur a reduction in exposure leads to clinical improvement in mild cases (21). Infections, additional toxic exposures, surgery, and stress arising from a change in life-style can all contribute to appearance of active disease years after cessation of exposure. Assessment of their contributions will require further careful observation of exposed persons and better understanding of the underlying mechanisms of disease. There is need for more research both in the laboratory and by study of affected persons, including those who are asymptomatic.

Hygiene standards

The hygiene standard for personnel working with beryllium was established in 1944 by the U.S. Atomic Energy Commission (23). It comprised a threshold limit for regular daily exposure of $2\mu g$ m^{-3} as a time-weighted average and a ceiling for periods of 30min of $25\mu g$ m^{-3}. Also established was a general atmosphere threshold for air in the vicinity of a beryllium plant of $0.01\mu g$ m^{-3}. The ceiling was derived from experience of cases of acute disease. The factory threshold limit was an estimate based on the dose–response relationship for other toxic metals but reduced by a factor of 2 to allow for error (22). The adoption of these standards materially reduced the incidence of beryllium disease but cases continued to occur. Some were a result of recognized incidents or injuries leading to implantation. Others reflected long-term exposure to concentrations of beryllium which in several instances were above the threshold limit. Cases of chronic disease have also occurred amongst personnel whose occupational exposure appeared to comply with the hygiene standard (fig. 11.3, 3); in these instances the measurements were made using area and not personal samplers so may not have been representative of what was inhaled. However, lower concentrations are now readily attainable and are usually achieved in practice.

Environmental control

The risk to health of those who work with beryllium is reduced by enclosing the process in cabinets and by use of robots, remote controls and exhaust ventilation. The risk is then greatest when the automatic equipment breaks down or needs overhauling or cleaning. It can also be considerable amongst small-scale and intermittent users, including personnel undertaking development work and disposing of or reclaiming material from waste. In these circumstances there is a case for wet working and exhaust ventilation, and for using masks (chapter 3). The overalls worn during work should be prewashed before being laundered and not washed at home as this practice may liberate sufficient dust to cause disease, particularly in women of childbearing age (see below).

Surveillance of persons who are at risk

Women of childbearing age, persons with established chronic disease of the lungs, liver or kidneys, and those with a history of dermatitis should be excluded at pre-employment examination. The examination should include a full plate chest radiograph, spirometry and measurement of transfer factor; any abnormal result should lead to a critical review of the suitability for employment. Atopic status has been regarded as a contra-indication to employment but the evidence is not overwhelming. The chest radiograph and lung function results should be used as the starting points for long-term surveillance; this should include an annual chest radiograph. Compared with the radiograph, lung function tests and the ventilatory response to exercise appear to be less sensitive guides to the occurrence of exacerbations but are of greater use for their management when they occur; in the long term both types of information will contribute to understanding the condition. To this end the serum of exposed persons should be frozen for use when new sensitive tests become available; in relation to exacerbations measurements should be made of the ventilatory response to exercise. There are as yet no specific tests of susceptibility, nor any safe test of sensitization.

Acute berylliosis is prevented by eliminating high environmental concentrations of beryllium oxide; the records should be scrutinized regularly with this in mind. Beryllium implantation granuloma is prevented by exercising great caution when grinding beryllium compounds; exhaust ventilation, gloves, visors and protective clothing should be used and any injury cleaned very thoroughly. Chronic beryllium disease is prevented by consistently maintaining the mean environmental concentration at below the recommended level. The exposed person is at greatest risk at the time of a diminution in or withdrawal from exposure; a lesser risk persists thereafter. Thus surveillance should be continued after discontinuation of exposure and the worker's general practitioner should be advised to include chronic beryllium disease in the differential diagnosis of any future chest illness. Unfortunately there is, as yet, no acceptable way of diagnosing latent disease.

References

1 Aldridge WN. The toxicity of beryllium. *Lab Invest* 1966;**15**:176–80.

2 Cotes JE. *Lung Function. Assessment and Application in Medicine*: 4th edn. Oxford: Blackwell Scientific Publications: 1979.

3 Cotes JE, Gilson JC, McKerrow CB, Oldham PD. A long-term follow-up of workers exposed to beryllium. *Br J Industr Med* 1983;**40**:13–21.

4 Cotes JE, Johnson GR, McDonald A. Breathing frequency and tidal volume: relationship to breathlessness. In: Porter R (ed) *Ciba Foundation Hering-Breuer Centenary Symposium: Breathing*: London: Churchill: 1970:297–314.

5 Eisenbud M, Lisson J. Epidemiological aspects of beryllium-induced non-malignant lung disease: a 30-year update. *J Occup Med* 1983;**25**:196–202.

6 Epstein PE, Dauber JH, Rossman MD, Daniele RP. Bronchoalveolar lavage in a patient with chronic berylliosis: evidence for hypersensitivity pneumonitis. *Ann Intern Med* 1982;**97**:213–6.

7 Gold C. A primary mesothelioma involving the recto-vaginal septum and associated with beryllium. *J Path Bact* 1967;**93**:435–42.

8 Hardy HL. Beryllium poisoning—Lessons in control of man-made disease. *N Engl J Med* 1965;**273**:1188–99.

9 Hardy HL. *Challenging Man-made Disease; The Memoirs of Harriet L. Hardy MD*: New York: Praeger: 1983.

10 International Agency for Research on Cancer. Beryllium and cancer. *Lancet* 1981;**i**:399.

11 Jones JM, Amos HE. Contact sensitivity in vitro: activation of actively allergized lymphocytes by a beryllium complex. *Int Arch Allergy* 1974;**46**:161–71.

12 Jones Williams W. A histological study of the lungs in 52 cases of chronic beryllium disease. *Br J Industr Med* 1958;**15**:84–91.

13 Jones Williams W, Kilpatrick GS. Cutaneous and pulmonary manifestations of chronic beryllium disease. In: Iwai K, Hosoda Y (Eds): *Proceedings of the Sixth International Conference on Sarcoidosis*: Tokyo: University Press: 1974:141.

14 Kuschner M. The carcinogenicity of beryllium. *Environ Hlth Perspects* 1981;**40**:101–5.

15 Mancuso TF. Mortality study of beryllium industry workers' occupational lung cancer. *Environm Res* 1980;**21**:48–55.

16 McCallum RI, Rannie I, Verity C. Chronic pulmonary berylliosis in a female chemist. *Br J Industr Med* 1961;**18**:133–42.

17 Preuss OP. Epidemiology of beryllium disease—40 years experience of a major producer. *Arh Hig Rada Toksikol* 1979;**30**(suppl.): 349–53.

18 Prine JR, Brokeshoulder SF, McVean DE, Robinson FR. Demonstration of the presence of beryllium in pulmonary granulomas. *Am J Clin Pathol* 1966;**45**:448–54.

19 Rees PJ. Unusual course of beryllium lung disease. *Br J Dis Chest* 1979;**73**:192–4.

20 Reeves AL. Berylliosis as an auto-immune disorder. *Ann Clin Lab Sci* 1976;**6(3)**:256–62.

21 Sprince NL, Kanarek DJ, Weber AL, Chamberlin RI, Kazemi H. Reversible respiratory disease in beryllium workers. *Am Rev Respir Dis* 1978;**117**:1011–7.

22 Stokinger HE (Ed). *Beryllium. Its industrial hygiene aspects*. New York: Academic Press: 1966.

23 United States Environmental Protection Agency. *Beryllium and air pollution: an annotated bibliography*. North Carolina. Air Pollution Central Office: 1971 (Publication AP:83).

24 Waksman BH. The diagnosis of beryllium disease with special reference to the patch test. *Arch Industr Hlth* 1959;**19**:154–6.

Chapter 12
Occupational Lung Cancer

Background
Metal and mineral carcinogens
Radioactive gas
Organic chemical carcinogens

Background

Carcinogenesis

Cancer is a disordered overgrowth of cells which invade adjacent tissues and spread via lymphatics or blood vessels to other parts of the body. Tumours in the lung usually arise from epithelial or glandular tissue or occur as undifferentiated cells. The process of carcinogenesis is reviewed in many publications (3–9) and is usually, but not invariably, caused by a mutation in the genetic material deoxyribonucleic acid (DNA). The DNA is subdivided into approximately half a million genes per cell and of these only twenty-five appear capable of contributing to cancer. Thus the process of malignant transformation is specific to very few genes. These genes, now called oncogenes, have been identified in viruses and animal tissues and some have also been found in human tumours. They all have a normal counterpart called the proto-oncogene. Malignant transformation can be caused by infection with a virus which contains either or both an oncogene and oncogene activator (called a promoter) or is capable of translocating the genes into an order which promotes oncogene activity. Alternatively the proto-oncogene can be mutated by a chemical carcinogen, alpha particle, neutron, electromagnetic radiation or ultra-violet light. In addition to being caused by mutation a malignant transformation may be effected by an amplification in number of pre-existing oncogenes or by enhancement of their activity; the carcinogen croton oil may act in one of these ways.

Genes are templates for producing proteins. In the case of oncogenes the proteins either have different properties from those normally produced or they are produced in larger or smaller amounts. Nearly half the oncogenes act by adding phosphate groups to tyrosine or other amino acid. The amino acids are constituents of proteins which form part of the framework of cells (cyto-skeleton). One such protein is vinculin which in its normal form may control the multiplication of cells by causing them to adhere to adjacent surfaces. Another is a protein kinase which may by-pass the control on phosphorylation normally exercised by epidermal growth factor. Sis oncogene produces what is effectively normal platelet-derived growth factor, whilst the products of ras oncogenes may control the binding of guanine triphosphate and hence the cellular levels of cyclic AMP. Some oncogene products affect cell nuclei where they appear to regulate the formation of protein by certain genes. All these processes must by definition contribute to cell multiplication.

The process of tumour formation is usually initiated by a mutation which is effected by one of the agents listed. The cell is then primed but not yet capable of uncontrolled growth. This requires the presence of promoters, each of which is the product of a single oncogene. Thus two or more oncogenes are required to set off the process. A single oncogene rarely causes cancer. Once growth has started its progression is influenced by the local nutrition and other host factors. At any stage the process may be interrupted. The agent causing malignant transformation may also kill the cell. The products of the oncogenes may themselves kill the cell or be identified as foreign proteins which stimulate the production of antibodies. Cell death and phagocytosis may also occur for other reasons. Alternatively the cell or clump of cells may survive but not progress, or progression may only occur as a result of another intervention many years later. Very few mutations actually become tumours.

The process of carcinogenesis is multifactorial and influenced by many circumstances, both known and unknown. They lead to the risk being enhanced during childhood, in relation to pregnancy and in old age; in the latter event the tumour often progresses slowly. In the lung the process may be affected by the level of activity of enzymes such as aryl hydrocarbon hydroxylase, which metabolizes benzo(a)pyrene and other polycyclic aromatic hydrocarbons into a more mutagenic form. The immune system is actively involved in the defence process and may be stimulated by BCG or bacterial endotoxin (e.g. in cotton operatives; ref. 15, page 318) or impaired by viral or bacterial infections which may themselves initiate mutations. The blood concentrations of hormones, especially those which regulate metabolism and the reproductive system, influence all stages in tumour formation whilst in the lung some protection may be conferred by vitamins A and E. Dietary zinc and riboflavin may be protective in some circumstances and selenium compounds may also be anti-mutagenic.

The carcinogen may act on its own or require the presence of a co-carcinogen which is not itself mutagenic; alternatively the co-carcinogen may be inhibited by some other substance. Two or more carcinogens may act independently, when their effects are additive, or they may interact to cause more tumours than the sum of the two separately. Thus an active agent in tobacco smoke may act on its own as a carcinogen, it may interact with asbestos fibres or radon and daughter products to greatly increase the tumour prevalence, or under experimental conditions, it may act as a co-carcinogen. Sulphur dioxide is also a co-carcinogen for lung cancer in man. Mixed exposures to these and other substances occur during inhalation of the fumes from combustion of fossil fuels or emissions from coke ovens.

Testing for mutagens

Most carcinogens act by causing genetic mutation, both *in vivo* and during *in-vitro* tests which may, therefore, be used for screening. The Ames test and others like it assess the ability to cause mutations in bacteria; the most widely used is a subspecies of *Salmonella typhimurium* which cannot synthesize histidine except after treatment with mutagen. The suspected mutagen should not itself contain histidine. This requirement precludes the use of *S. typhimurium* for screening biological materials including blood, urine and faeces. However, other bacteria, including *E. coli*, and the fruit fly *Drosophila* can also be used. The tests are suitable for most substances but not metal carcinogens, of which only chromium compounds yield a positive result. Metal salts can be assessed by their ability to cause errors (infidelity) in the replication of DNA *in vitro*. The template is a DNA polymerase from avian myeloblastosis virus; this is incubated with two labelled deoxynucleoside triphosphates, one complementary and the other non-complementary. The degree to which the latter is incorporated is a measure of infidelity (8). The test is useful since one salt of a metal carcinogen may be active whilst another may be completely harmless. The speciation is also important. Single cell cultures of mammalian or human cells provide a test bed for raw chemicals and for substances which have undergone metabolic activation by prior incubation in a tissue preparation. This may convert the chemical into a more reactive mode. The reactive element can sometimes be identified and measured by chemical analysis, for example alkylating agents have been detected using 4-nitrobenzylpyridine. Cell transformation assays can depend on mutagenic transformation of hamster or mouse cells after exposure to metal salts, for example, or the enhancement of viral transformation of cells following treatment with chemicals. In man the extent of chromosome aberration and the occurrence of sister chromatid exchanges and of micronuclei have also been regarded as evidence of mutation. There is now a battery of tests for mutagens which may be applied to new substances or ones whose use is expanding as a result of technical change. However, with each additional test the likelihood of at least one positive result increases so a single positive result is now not considered to be a reliable guide to carcinogenicity (2).

Application of animal results to man

Tests of carcinogenicity in rodents or other mammals or birds form part of the assessment procedure for new substances and may yield positive results. In the U.S.A. under the Delaney amendment such results are considered in law to be evidence of carcinogenicity in man. However, tumour formation is often specific to one species and not transferable. A response which is relatively specific for man may be obtained by metabolic activation in human tissue of the substance to be tested, then applying the resultant complex to human cells in tissue culture. Evidence from studies on other mammalian tissues is not directly applicable to man and may be misleading.

Epidemiology: possible causes

The cumulative risk from lung cancer is high in the U.K. where on average it accounts for some 10% of deaths. It is lower by a factor of 10 in Nigeria with most other countries in between. Much of the mortality is from smoking and in the U.K. the risk is in the range 50% for heavy smokers to 1% for non-smokers. Some of the 1% is due to the non-smokers breathing exhalations of smokers. These figures indicate the great importance of tobacco smoke as a cause of lung cancer. They also contribute to the conclusion that some 85% of all cancers are of environmental origin (1)

although only about 5% are occupational. Thus, except with very potent carcinogens, the occupational component is likely to be smaller than that due to smoking. Proof that an occupational agent is contributing to the cancer prevalence usually depends on epidemiological evidence, since the results of in vitro and animal tests are not directly transferable to man. The requirements for establishing carcinogenicity have been reviewed by Doll and are summarized in table 12.1. In practice the evidence is often incomplete, of only moderate reliability and difficult to analyse on account of confounding factors. Ways of tackling these problems are considered in chapter 6. The main requirement is an unqualified association between tumour prevalence or mortality and the estimated exposure. Examples are given in tables 12.2 and 12.3. Dose–response relationships for asbestos and for radon and its daughter products, including the effects of smoking, are illustrated respectively on pages 224 and 256. In the case of asbestos the incidence of bronchial cancer seems to be proportional to the exposure, and current methods are unable to detect a threshold below which the risk is zero. This raises the fundamental question whether any dose is harmless and poses considerable problems in deciding what hygiene standard should be adopted (page 223).

Is there a threshold dose?

Completion of each stage in the formation of a tumour reflects a balance of probabilities. Thus the initial mutation, the incomplete repair, the production of an abnormal protein which confers malignant properties, the growth to tumour size and the subsequent progression are

Table 12.1. Requirements for establishing carcinogenicity from epidemiological evidence (1)

There should be a positive association between exposure and disease in groups of individuals with known exposures (case-control or cohort studies).

The association should not be explicable by bias in recording or detection or be due to confounding factors or to chance.

The disease prevalence should vary approximately with dose and time after exposure.

The observation should be made repeatedly in different circumstances.

Table 12.2. Lung cancer associated with occupations

Agent	Some occupations at risk
Arsenic	Mining, smelting Cu, Zn, Pb, manufacture, packaging and use of pesticides, page 246
Asbestos	Mining, manufacture of pipes, sheets, cloth, brake linings, etc., demolition of structures containing asbestos, page 199
Benzo(a)pyrene (B(a)P)	Coke plant workers, gas workers
Other polycyclic hydrocarbons	Steel production, asphalt workers, roofers
Bis(chloromethyl)ether (BCME) Chloromethyl methyl ether (CMME)	Chemical industry (alkylating agents)
Chromium	Chromate and steel production, chromium plating, tanning, Table 12.5
Mustard gas	Manufacture
Nickel	Refining, especially by nickel carbonyl process
Radon and daughter products	Mining uranium and other minerals
Tobacco smoke	Personal and general environmental hazard

all events which might or might not take place. Whether they do or not is determined by all the factors which have been discussed. Theoretically one molecule of carcinogen or one asbestos fibre might be sufficient. In practice the probability of a tumour arising in such circumstances is infinitely small. The agent must make contact with the cell during division, the mutation must confer malignant properties, the immune defences at the relevant site must be overwhelmed or deficient and the other requirements for tumour production must be met. The products of each stage are the survivors of the stage before and there must initially be many of them if the process is to be completed. These considerations are consistent with the practical experience that in experimental carcinogenesis there is always a dose below which no tumours occur. The duration and frequency of exposure are also important since mutation is more probable if exposure to the carcinogen is protracted than if the same dose is delivered all at once. Thus the threshold, though present, may be too low to be detected (see also page 13).

Table 12.3. Lung cancer: occupations where risk is not definite

Occupation	Suspected agent
Chemical producers and users	Benzoylchloride, chloroprene, Dimethylsulphate, di- and trichlorodibenzodiozan, hexachlorocyclohexane, epichlorohydrin, tritetrachlorocyclohexamin, vinylidine chloride (mixed exposure to vinyl chloride and acrylonitrile, page 256)
Machine users	Oil mist
Workers with: Beryllium	page 247
Cadmium	page 247
Lead	page 250

Metal and mineral carcinogens

Arsenic (As, atomic number 33, atomic mass 75)

Arsenic is a grey or black semi-metal which is widely distributed in the earth's crust: it occurs mainly as arsenic trioxide (As_4O_6) in arsenolite or combined with iron and sulphur in pyrites (FeSAs) and other minerals. The pentavalent form As_2O_5 also occurs. Arsenic is produced by smelting as was first described by Paracelsus in about 1520; arsenic is also a by-product of smelting copper, lead, gold and zinc. Principal producing countries are Sweden, Canada, West Germany, U.K. and U.S.S.R. The material is used as a preservative, pesticide, fungicide, defoliant, in glassware, industrial chemicals, pharmaceuticals, tanning, infra-red lenses and semi-conductors.

Arsenic enters the body by inhalation or ingestion of arsenic trioxide, pentoxide and organic compounds, of which the commonest is methylarsine (CH_3AsH_2). There are numerous more complex organic compounds both man-made and naturally occurring; many of the latter occur in crustacea and bottom-feeding fish. Ingested inorganic arsenic is taken up preferentially by red blood corpuscles and the skin; it is partially methylated in the liver to form methyl and dimethyl arsenic acids and is excreted mainly by the kidneys but also via the bile and in sweat. In man, following a single dose, the half time for excretion as trivalent inorganic arsenic is approximately 10h, and as methylated arsenic (formed *in vivo*), approximately 30h. Ingested pentavalent arsenic is excreted more slowly with an overall half time of 70h but with a small slow compartment having a half time of 38 days. Despite its slow excretion pentavalent arsenic appears to be less toxic than the trivalent form. With continued ingestion a near equilibrium is reached in about 5 days but in the long term the arsenic accumulates in the lungs, skin, hair and nails (17).

In high dosage arsenic affects most organs and tissues of the body; it impairs haematopoiesis, causes hyperkeratosis and skin pigmentation, affects the peripheral nervous system and may damage the liver, heart and blood vessels; however, the latter changes have occurred as a result of ingesting a large quantity of arsenic, not from chronic occupational exposure (17). The biological action of arsenic is mainly due to combination of trivalent inorganic arsenic with sulphydryl groups in proteins, especially mitochondrial enzymes, including DNA polymerase. Inactivation of this enzyme inhibits DNA synthesis and repair, so by this means arsenic acts at a relatively late stage in the sequence of changes leading to carcinogenesis (10). Exposure to arsenic is associated with an increased incidence of chromosomal aberration in peripheral blood lymphocytes. This change is consistent with the observed increase in prevalence of malignant disease in exposed persons; the tumours may affect the skin, lymphatic and haematopoeitic tissue, mouth, pharynx and lungs. Arsenic trioxide deposited in the nose can cause perforation of the nasal septum and inhaled arsenic has been incriminated as a cause of chronic bronchitis (chapter 17).

Lung cancer is associated with exposure to airborne arsenic during gold mining, smelting non-ferrous metals, in manufacture of chemicals including pesticides and fungicides, and during application of arsenicals as sheep dip and sprays to vines and other crops. There is a significant dose–response relationship (12, 13, 15, 17); it is independent of smoking and exposure to sulphur dioxide which were at one time thought to exert a synergistic effect (16). The exposure to arsenic may be relatively brief in relation to the working lifetime and the latent period has been reported as 37.6 years (11). Neighbourhood cases due to residence in the vicinity of a smelting plant or factory processing arsenic have been suspected but the evidence is not strong (14) and more research is needed.

The lung tumours associated with arsenic exposure are often made up of poorly differentiated epidermoid cells but other cell types also occur (16). The disease has not yet been reproduced in animals but may be in the future as a result of studies in which the arsenic is administered by inhalation rather than by ingestion. The tumours have usually followed prolonged exposure to high environmental concentrations; in one study of former copper smelters, for example, an estimated mean concentration of 50mg m^{-3} for 25 years was associated with a

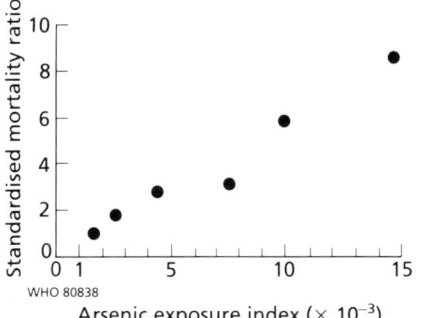

Fig. 12.1. Mortality from lung cancer in relation to estimated exposure to arsenic amongst 527 workers formerly employed in a copper smelting plant in U.S.A. For healthy subjects the standardized mortality ratio is 1.0 and the average arsenic exposure index is 1.25×10^{-3}. (Data of Pinto et al, 15.)

3-fold increase in incidence of lung cancer (fig 12.1, 15). In this study the environmental concentrations were estimated from the concentrations in urine. The risk of malignancy appears to be readily controllable by reducing the environmental concentration to within the hygiene standard; this is less for organic than for inorganic compounds of arsenic (table 12.4, below). Exposure during application of arsenical insecticides and fungicides to crops can be controlled by use of a respirator (chapter 3) and protective clothing. Monitoring the exposure is done by personal sampling or by analysis of urine, the normal concentration being in the range 10–50µg l^{-1} except after eating fish with a high content of organic arsenic compounds.

Table 12.4. Hygiene standards for atmospheric arsenic

	(mg m^{-3})
U.S.A.	0.2
U.S.S.R.	0.3
Japan	
Arsenic trioxide	0.5
Arsine	0.2
Sweden	0.05
U.K.	0.2

Such compounds should be excluded from the analysis by use of methods which are specific for dimethyl arsenic acid and inorganic arsenic. In surveys of persons occupationally exposed during smelting the average urinary concentration has been found to be in the range 50–800µg l^{-1} depending on the exposure (17).

Asbestos — see chapter 10

Beryllium

The distribution, processing and use of beryllium metal and its salts are reviewed in chapter 11. Many of these compounds cause lung cancer in rats and monkeys exposed by inhalation or intratracheal injection (18, 19). No tumours have been observed following exposure to the beryllium ore, bertrandite (20). The evidence from studies of man is summarized in chapter 11; so far it is suggestive but inconclusive. Thus beryllium should be considered as under suspicion of being carcinogenic to humans; it is not a confirmed carcinogen.

Cadmium (Cd, atomic number 48, atomic mass 112)

Cadmium sulphide is a constituent of most zinc ores and cadmium is liberated as a vapour in the early stages of smelting. It is a tin-white metal and takes a good polish. Cadmium is alloyed with lead, tin and bismuth in Wood's metal which has the remarkably low melting point of 68°C. Cadmium is widely used in electroplating as it is very resistant to corrosion. Other uses are as a stabilizer for plastics, in cadmium pigments and phosphors, the negative electrode of nickel–cadmium batteries, high-temperature alloys for bearings, solder for aluminium, fusible links and cores, neutron shields and control rods for nuclear reactors, fungicides and lubricants. Cadmium sulphide is the principal phosphor in many instruments and cathode ray tube screens. Many of these applications result in the liberation of cadmium oxide fume which may then be inhaled. The fume is also liberated during heating plated articles, for example cutting cadmium-plated bolts with an oxyacetylene torch.

Cadmium salts are biologically active. In common with zinc salts they can induce the formation of the metal binding protein, metallothionein; they also modify the metabolism of nucleic acids to reduce the fidelity of synthesis of DNA and enhance or inhibit the production of RNA. Chromosomal abnormalities have been reported in some studies of persons with a high body burden of cadmium and the balance of evidence suggests that some cadmium compounds are weakly mutagenic (24). Parenteral administration of cadmium compounds to rats causes local tumour formation and testicular atrophy (23). Lung cancers have been produced in rats following prolonged inhalation of cadmium chloride (26) but on account of species differences (speciation) this response cannot be extrapolated to man.

Cadmium vapour is highly toxic; acute occupational exposure causes pneumonitis and nephritis. The pneumonitis is usually reversible but may lead to diffuse interstitial fibrosis (27). The nephritis can progress to renal failure; it may have long-term sequelae (22). In one incident death from renal failure occurred following inhaling fumes generated by cutting five bolts. Cadmium has also been incriminated as a cause of occupational emphysema. The positive evidence relates to a previous era when the cadmium concentrations were probably 2 orders of magnitude higher than at present. Recent evidence has proved to be ambiguous. Thus in a follow-up study of 3025 nickel–cadmium battery workers the mortality from diseases of the respiratory tract other than lung cancer was not increased. The increased lung cancer mortality was in men exposed for more than 6 years and followed up for more than 29 years; these men were concurrently exposed to nickel and other substances so the cause of the increase, which was confined to workers exposed before 1940, has still to be established (25). Amongst nearly 7000 male cadmium workers born before 1940 and followed to age 85 years there were no excess deaths from prostatic cancer, cardiovascular disease or renal disease. The lung cancer mortality was above average but not related to exposure. However, there was a significant excess mortality from chronic bronchitis which was correlated with the duration and intensity of exposure. This finding may possibly reflect an increased prevalence of emphysema (cf. page 384) but in the absence of post-mortem information the suggestion remains speculative (21). If cadmium is a carcinogen it is a very weak one.

Chromium (Cr, atomic number 24, atomic mass 52)

Chromium is a hard steel-grey metal which occurs as chromite ($FeO.Cr_2O_3$), crocoisite, or chrome ochre ($PbO.PbCrO_4$) in ultra-basic igneous rock; the principal sources are the U.S.S.R., South Africa, Albania, Turkey, Zimbabwe, the Philippines, Finland and India. Chromium is produced by reduction of the ore with aluminium in an electric furnace or by electrolysis of a chromium-containing solution. The latter is obtained by heating the crushed ore with lime and potassium or sodium carbonate to form the corresponding chromate; this in turn is treated with SO_2 to form the sulphate salt, or with sulphuric acid to form dichromate or chromic acid depending on circumstances. The main uses of chromium are in ferrochromium alloys for making steel (see nickel below), in refractory materials for iron and steel processing, in glass-making and the manufacture of chemicals when the element may be in the trivalent or hexavalent form; some of the chemicals are listed in table 12.5.

Elemental chromium may enter the body by inhalation or ingestion but appears to be biologically inert. Inhaled trivalent chromium is also inert unless contaminated with hexavalent compounds. Its innocence is due solely to an inability to penetrate biological membranes in solution; on this account trivalent chromium compounds ((Cr(III)) in the concentrations normally experienced by man are neither mutagenic to bacteria nor carcinogenic to experimental animals. Very high concentrations may lead to ingestion by phagocytosis but the relevance of this observation is unclear. By contrast the soluble hexavalent chromate or dichromate ions readily cross all membranes in most but not all cell species; the transfer is effected by the sulphate system (39). Some sparingly soluble hexavalent chromates including strontium chromate and some zinc chromates behave in the same

Table 12.5. Oxidation state (valency), solubility (s) and principal uses of some chromium compounds

Barium chromate	$BaCrO_4$	(VI)	Pyrotechnics; high temperature batteries
Calcium chromate	$CaCrO_4$	(VI) s	Corrosion inhibitor
Chromic acetate	$Cr(OOCCH_3)_3$	(III) s	Printing and dyeing textiles
Chromic chloride	$CrCl_3$	(III) s	Mordant for alizarin dyes, chromium plating
Chromic oxide	Cr_2O_3	(III)	Green pigment
Chromium potassium sulphate	$CrK(SO_4)_2$	(III) s	Mordant for dyes
Chromium trioxide	CrO_3	(VI) s	Chromium plating
Cobalt–chromium alloy		(O)	Cutting tools, high temperature valves, turbine blades, pumps for corrosive liquids, etc.
Ferrochromium		(O)	Heat-resisting steel
Lead chromate	$PbCrO_4$	(VI)	Yellow pigment
Potassium chromate	K_2CrO_4	(VI) s	Mordant for dyes
Sodium chromate	Na_2CrO_4	(VI) s	Leather tanning, wood preservation, corrosion inhibition, pigment manufacture
Sodium dichromate	$Na_2Cr_2O_7$	(VI) s	Manufacture of other chromium compounds
Zinc potassium chromate	$Zn_2CrO_4(OH)_2$	(VI)	Corrosion inhibiting paint

way but the lead chromates are inert, presumably because the intracellular concentration does not reach the critical level (35). Once inside the cell the ions are reduced to trichromate; the rate of conversion varies between animal species and between different tissues. The trichromate forms stable compounds with nucleic acids, proteins and other compounds which contribute to the replication and repair of DNA. These changes lead to most inhaled hexavalent chromium(VI) compounds being both mutagenic and carcinogenic. The half life for the inhaled chromium is approximately 40 days (34). Of all metals the hexavalent chromium compounds best illustrate the hypothesis that carcinogenesis entails mutagenic mutation of somatic cells as a result of direct interaction with DNA. The evidence is reviewed elsewhere (33, 35, 39).

In man chromium compounds may cause acute toxic damage to the skin, gastro-intestinal tract, kidneys and respiratory tract; the nasal septum may perforate and chronic bronchitis has been reported amongst chromium electroplaters and welders using chromium alloy electrodes (29, 30). Sensitization may occur giving rise to dermatitis or occupational asthma (chapter 16). The excretion in the urine of β-glucuronidase and protein may be increased.

Peripheral blood lymphocytes may exhibit chromosomal aberrations and sputum cytology may show changes in the lining cells suggestive of pre-tumourous dysplasia (33).

Increased mortality from lung cancer, but not other cancers, has been reported in workers in chromium and chromate manufacturing plants since the 1930s. Dose–response relationships between exposure and death from lung cancer have been reported by Mancuso (36) and by Hayes and others (32) with a 2–4-fold increase in lung cancer mortality overall. In three U.K. factories manufacturing lead chromate pigment ((Cr(VI)) an increased mortality from lung cancer was observed amongst persons in high and medium exposure groups but not amongst those with 'low' exposure (28, 31). Amongst workers in fifty-four Yorkshire chromium plating plants the mortality from lung cancer amongst male and female process workers was approximately twice that in control subjects matched for age, sex and smoking habits (38). The excess was significant for persons who had been platers for more than 1 year when the mean period between first exposure and death was 13.6 years. For workers producing chromium ferro-alloys an increased mortality from lung cancer has been reported from the U.S.S.R. (37) but not from Sweden where the ambient concentrations for Cr(III) and Cr(VI) were respectively in the range zero to 2.5mg m^{-3} and 0.25mg m^{-3} (29). These and other studies provide clear evidence that the production of chromate compounds and the processes of chromium plating carry an increased risk of lung cancer. There is insufficient evidence as to whether or not welders of stainless steel also have an increased risk on this account.

Lead and lead compounds (Pb, atomic number 82, atomic weight 207.2)

Galena, a lead sulphide ore, is widely distributed in the earth's crust; when heated with lime the sulphur is liberated as sulphur dioxide and the lead which has a melting point of 327.5°C is run off into troughs, then purified by heating. Production is undertaken in most industrialized countries. Lead is soft, malleable and tough but is not ductile or tenacious. It has been used since ancient times for roofing, piping, shot etc., and in bronze which is an alloy containing 77% copper, 8% tin and 15% lead. It is alloyed with copper and zinc in brass, with tin in pewter (75% tin, 25% lead) and solder (usually 50% lead, 50% tin) and other fusible alloys. The proportional use of different lead-containing products differs widely from one country to another and is changing rapidly because of the introduction of safer and more convenient replacements. Its use in the U.S.A. in 1977 is given in table 12.6.

Lead has numerous biological effects of which the most frequent are on bone marrow, all

Table 12.6. Uses of lead metal in 1977 (42)

Storage batteries (including oxides, posts and grids)	57%
Antiknock additives for motor fuel	15%
Red lead (tetra-oxide) and white lead (monoxide) for paint, ceramics, oil refining	5%
Ammunition	4%
Solder	4%
Miscellaneous: pigment, weights, sheet, copper alloys caulking, cable covering, type metal, annealing, galvanizing, plating, etc.	15%

aspects of reproduction and post-natal mental development. Lead sub-acetate is carcinogenic to rodents and some chromosomal aberrations have been reported in experimental animals and man (42). An increased mortality from all malignant neoplasms including lung cancer has been observed amongst lead smelter workers but not battery plant workers (40, 41, 43); the smelter workers were also exposed to other substances including SO_2 and arsenic, so the excess cancer incidence cannot be attributed to lead. The risk of bronchial cancer appears to be very slight and is unimportant when compared with the many other manifestations of lead poisoning.

Nickel (Ni, atomic number 28, atomic weight 58.7)

Nickel from Kupfer-nickel (bedevilled copper) was first extracted from ore which resembled copper in Westphalia in 1751. It occurs principally as pentlandite, an iron nickel sulphide $(FeN_2)_9S_8$, which is mined mixed with copper ore in Sudbury, Ontario, the U.S.S.R. and other countries. It is also mined as garnierite, a magnesium nickel silicate which occurs mixed with cobalt ore in New Caledonia and elsewhere. Extraction of nickel from pentlandite is initially by flotation, roasting and smelting which leads to the separation of the iron as ferro-silicate slag. In the Orford process the residual matter containing 80% nickel and copper is fused with sodium sulphide and the mixture separates into two layers of which the lower is mainly nickel sulphide. This is ground, washed and sintered to oxide which is reduced to metal by heating with coal or hydrogen. The latter is the first step in the Mond process in which the impure nickel powder is reacted with carbon monoxide to produce nickel carbonyl gas, $Ni(CO)_4$; this is then decomposed by heat to produce pure finely divided nickel. The Mond process is carried out at Clydach near Swansea in South Wales using as raw material nickel matte (which also contains copper and sulphur) or nickel oxide from Canada. The metal is also obtained by electrolysis of nickel sulphate solution.

Nickel metal is used as an alloying additive to steel. A 3–5% addition greatly increases the tensile strength whilst the further addition of chromium confers hardness and resistance to fatigue and impact. Stainless steel may contain 18% nickel and 8% chromium but this alloy cannot be hardened and tempered. Nickel compounds are used for electro-plating, in batteries and as hydrogenation catalysts in the manufacture of edible oils, refining of petroleum, production of organic chemicals and purification of vehicle exhausts: these and other uses are given in table 12.7.

Table 12.7.   Uses of some nickel compounds

Nickel oxide	Stainless and alloy steels
Nickel carbonyl	Nickel powder manufacture, vapour plating of Ni, semi-conductors
Nickel sulphate	Electroplating (also other Ni salts)
Nickel carbonate	Hydrogenation catalysts, thermistors, ferrites
Nickel hydroxide	Nickel–cadmium batteries
Nickel fluoride	Battery electrodes

In experimental studies nickel compounds are readily phagocytosed, especially when in the form of negatively charged crystalline particles. Inside the cell the material dissolves to liberate nickel ions which bind to DNA phosphate; the activity of DNA and RNA polymerases is then impaired and this affects the fidelity of DNA replication. The changes induce strand breakages and DNA protein cross-links which can result in malignant transformation (36, 49). Carcinogenicity has been demonstrated in animals following inhalation or tracheal injection of metallic nickel, nickel subsulphide and other compounds (35). Some of these substances are also carcinogenic in man, but in the case of powdered metallic nickel no excess mortality was observed amongst persons exposed to a concentration of 0.5–0.9mg Ni m^{-3} over a 25 year period (44).

Cancer of the nasal sinuses and lungs due to exposure to nickel compounds was first reported in 1932 at the refinery in Clydach; by 1971 some 252 workmen had been affected but the relevant exposure appeared to have taken place prior to 1930. For nasal cancer the latent period was in excess of 15 years and the risk persisted thereafter more or less unchanged, but for lung cancer the risk decreased with time from last exposure (45). The refinery used the Mond process so the nasal tumours may have been caused by nickel carbonyl gas but this has not been confirmed. Elsewhere nickel sinter and ore containing nickel sulphide and oxide have been responsible for lung cancer amongst the workforce. In New Caledonia where the ore contains nickel oxide an increased cancer mortality has also been observed in people living in the vicinity of the refinery (47, 48).

The carcinogenic action of nickel can be inhibited by manganese but this is not of practical importance as with sensible attention to hygiene measures the risk of nickel carcinogenesis is now very small. The hygiene standard is given in table 1.7 (page 16).

Other effects of nickel carbonyl. Nickel carbonyl is a highly toxic gas. It appears to cause respiratory tract cancer (see above) and may cause occupational asthma (chapter 16), acute toxicity or chemical pneumonitis. The symptoms of toxicity are nausea, vomiting and severe headache but recovery is usually rapid except when there is pneumonitis. However, even in the absence of pneumonitis the condition may generate fear of subsequent lung damage which is sometimes hard to dispel. Thus careful assessment should be combined with reassurance. The pneumonitis comes on after an interval of a few hours up to several days; it presents with cough, chest pain and tightness, breathlessness and haemoptysis. There is often extreme weakness. Physical examination of the chest may reveal reduced expansion, impaired percussion and coarse crepitations and there may be radiographic features of pulmonary oedema or consolidation. The severity of the episode is related to the exposure which can be estimated from the urinary nickel concentration during the 3 days after exposure to nickel carbonyl; an initial 8h urinary concentration of less than 100µg l^{-1} constitutes mild exposure and more than 500µg l^{-1} a severe exposure which may be fatal. More usually there is a slow recovery but the condition sometimes progresses to diffuse interstitial pulmonary fibrosis (46). Treatment is by bed rest, oxygen therapy, steroid drugs and, in severe cases, intermittent positive pressure ventilation and prophylactic antibiotics. Sodium diethyl dithiocarbamate may also be used.

Uranium and associated minerals

Uranium commonly occurs in mineral deposits as U238 which is completely harmless in this form. It may capture slow neutrons or decay by loss of α and β particles to form substances which are radioactive. Their effects are discussed below.

Radioactive gas

Ionizing radiation

Radiations from electrical discharges or from disintegration of radioactive substances commonly take one of three forms, all of which may induce ionization of air and cause death, mutation or malignant change in living cells.

α particles are helium nuclei consisting of four nucleons (two neutrons and two protons): each has an atomic weight of four and a positive charge of magnitude equal to that on two electrons. α particles are formed by step-wise disintegration of uranium, thorium, actinium and their decay products. They cause dense ionization along the traverse path which in tissue extends for a distance of approximately 50μm; in bronchial epithelium this is to the level of the basement membrane. α rays emitted by radon gas, thoron gas and their daughter products are the main cause of radiation-induced lung cancer in miners.

α particles exert their effect upon DNA molecules during the course of cell division. The risk of cancer is, therefore, a statistical one depending on the numbers of both mitoses and α particles. It also depends on the distribution with respect to time since a trickle of α particles over a long time will intercept more dividing cells than a flood over a short time, some of which will converge on the same cells. The high energy particles are particularly potent because they have a longer traverse path, hence come into contact with more cells. They also kill more cells and this increases the number of cell divi-sions which must take place before the repair is complete.

β particles are electrons or positrons which initially have a velocity approaching that of light; they are formed in the course of decay of uranium and other isotopes and have considerable penetrating ability equivalent to several millimetres of aluminium sheet. β particles contribute to the tissue damage associated with uranium but probably not much to the risk of lung cancer following inhalation of radioactive aerosol.

γ-rays are electromagnetic waves with a wave length of 10^{-6} to 10^{-11}cm; the shorter the wave length the greater the penetrating ability and potential for tissue damage. Their production in an electrical discharge tube was discovered by Röntgen in 1895 (x-rays) and their release during radioactive decay of uranium by Becquerel in 1896 (γ-rays). Gamma rays have a considerably higher energy than x-rays; they are the main cause of tissue damage following a thermonuclear explosion, their effects being spread throughout the body and not specific to the lungs.

Distribution of uranium

Uranium (atomic mass commonly 238, atomic number 92) was discovered by Klaproth in 1789 and named after the planet which was observed 8 years earlier. It occurs in pitchblende, uraninite (U_3O_8) which is a brown or black solid with a greasy lustre found in Canada and Zaire and in the ore carnotite, a vanadate of uranium and potassium which occurs in Bohemia, Utah, Colorado and Arizona in U.S.A. Mining or deep quarrying of uranium bearing ore is undertaken in these and other countries including South Africa, Australia and U.S.S.R. Uranium ore is present, intermingled with other minerals, in Cornwall, Saxony, Norway (Kongsberg) and elsewhere. It may then be a cause of cancer amongst miners exposed to some species of granite, iron ore and other minerals.

Decay of uranium

Natural uranium exists in the forms U238 (99.3%), U235 (0.7%) and U234 (0.005%), of

Table 12.8. Uranium and thorium decay chains

Uranium series

Substance		Nuclear symbol	Decay α/β	MeV	Half-life	
Uranium 1	U$_1$	$^{238}_{92}$U	α	4.27	4.5×10^9	yr
Uranium X$_1$	UX$_1$	$^{234}_{90}$Th	β	0.205	24.1	d
Uranium X$_2$	UX$_2$	$^{234}_{91}$Pa	β	2.25	1.18	min
Uranium II	U$_{II}$	$^{234}_{92}$U	α	4.85	2.48×10^5	yr
Ionium	I	$^{230}_{90}$Th	α	4.76	8.0×10^4	yr
Radium	Ra	$^{226}_{88}$Ra	α	4.86	1622	yr
Radon	Rn	$^{222}_{86}$Em	α	5.59	3.8	d
Radium A	RaA	$^{218}_{84}$Po	α	6.11	3.05	min
Radium B	RaB	$^{214}_{82}$Pb	β	1.02	26.8	min
Radium C	RaC*	$^{214}_{83}$Bi	β	3.18	19.7	min
Radium C'	RaC'	$^{214}_{84}$Po	α	7.83	1.64×10^{-4}	s
Radium D	RaD	$^{210}_{82}$Pb	β	0.064	19.4	yr
Radium E	RaE	$^{210}_{83}$Bi	β	1.16	5.01	d
Radium F	RaF	$^{210}_{84}$Po	α	5.40	138.401	d
Radium G	RaG	$^{206}_{82}$Pb	Stable	–		

Thorium series

Substance		Nuclear symbol	Decay α/β	MeV	Half-life	
Thorium	Th	$^{232}_{90}$Th	α	4.08	1.39×10^{10}	yr
Mesothorium 1	MsTh1	$^{228}_{88}$Ra	β	0.053	6.7	yr
Mesothorium 2	MsTh2	$^{228}_{89}$Ac	β	2.18	6.13	h
Radiothorium	RdTh	$^{228}_{90}$Th	α	5.52	1.91	yr
Thorium X	ThX	$^{224}_{88}$Ra	α	5.78	3.64	d
Thoron	Tn	$^{220}_{86}$Em	α	6.40	51.5	s
Thorium A	ThA	$^{216}_{84}$Po	α	6.90	0.16	s
Thorium B	ThB	$^{212}_{82}$Pb	β	0.58	10.6	h
Thorium C	ThC+	$^{212}_{83}$Bi	{ α / β	6.21 / 2.25	60.5	min
Thorium C'	ThC'	$^{212}_{84}$Po	α	8.95	3.04×10^{-7}	s
Thorium C''	ThC''	$^{208}_{81}$Tl	β	1.79	3.1	min
Thorium D	ThD	$^{208}_{82}$Pb	Stable	–		

* 0.04% of RaC undergoes α decay to RaC'' ($^{210}_{81}$Tl) thence via β decay to RaD.
+ 64% and 36% of ThC decay respectively via ThC' and ThC'' to ThD.
Glossary: Ac, actinium; Bi, bismuth; Em, emanation; Pb, lead; Pa, protoactinium; Po, polonium; Tl, tellurium.

which U235 undergoes fission on capture of a thermal or slow neutron. U238 may similarly be converted into U239, then plutonium 239 (atomic number 94) which disintegrates on further bombardment with neutrons. Uranium 238 naturally disintegrates in a step-wise manner by the loss of α and β particles; the steps have time constants ranging from 4.5×10^9 years for uranium 238 to 3.05min for polonium 218. Some of the intermediate stages are given in table 12.8.

Lung cancer from ionizing radiation

Lung cancer from ionizing radiation, for the reasons given above, is a natural hazard of mining in rock containing uranium or where there is contamination by radon. The disease was first described amongst the miners of Schneeberg in the Erzgebirge mountains by Paracelsus in 1531 and radium was found in the pitchblende of adjacent Jáchymov (Joachimsthal) in Bohemia by Marie Curie in 1898. Pulmonary malignancy is a hazard of all uranium mining and of mining other minerals which are contaminated by uranium or its breakdown products. Thus there is or has been a risk associated with mining fluorspar (calcium fluorite) in Newfoundland, haematite in Cumbria (fig. 12.2), tin in Cornwall and silver, lead and zinc in Sweden. The lung cancer is due mainly to inhaling dust comprising the daughter products of decay of radon gas (table 12.8). The incidence of

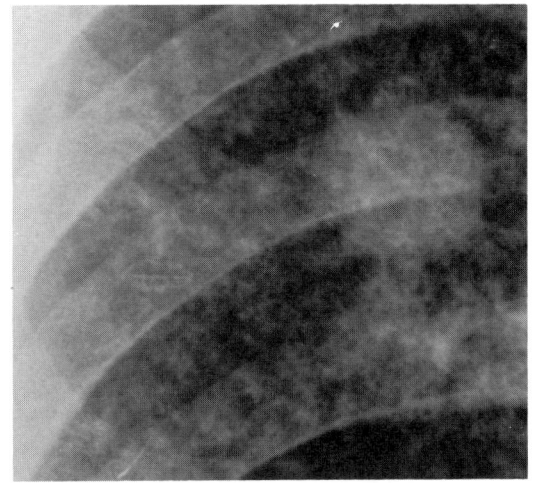

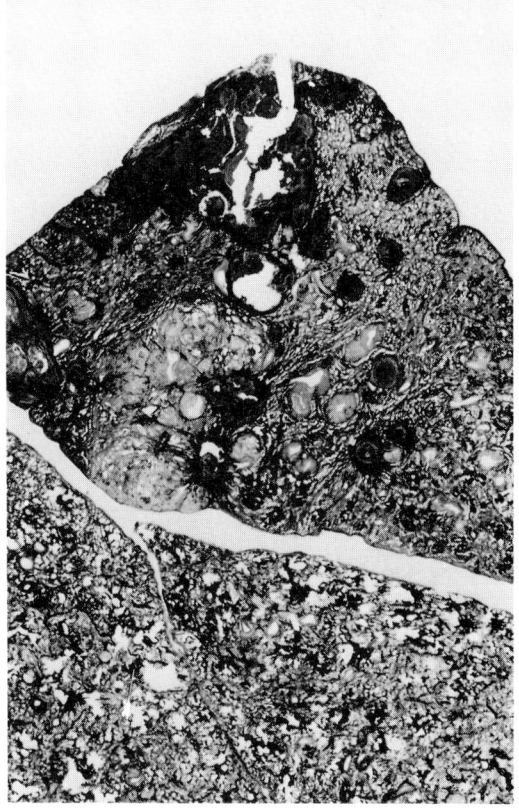

Fig. 12.2. Radiograph and paper-mounted lung section showing detail from the right lung of a 54-year-old Cumbrian iron ore miner who presented with breathlessness on exertion, having given up work on this account 12 years previously. He was diagnosed as having pneumoconiosis and tuberculosis but this was later revised to confluent silicosis. Subsequently he developed lung cancer and died at age 67 from the effects of metastases. At post-mortem there was a mass in the right upper lobe with further tumour tissue extending from the mediastinum. The tumour was present in the lung section (left of centre) and this also contained confluent and nodular silicosis. The lung was brown in colour on account of containing iron oxide. (By courtesy of J. E. M. Hutchinson.)

cancer varies over a wide range depending on the richness and distribution of the ore, the local conditions and the extent of surveillance and hygiene measures. Local pockets of rich ore and sites of accumulation of water containing radon from such pockets are particularly hazardous when combined with poor ventilation.

The tumours are in addition to those due to smoking and other causes; the excess incidence is most readily demonstrated at high levels of exposure and amongst such persons the predominant tumour type is the small cell anaplastic carcinoma (61). The average latent period for the development of these tumours has been reported as 15.9 years. Clinical disease is preceded by the appearance in the sputum of atypical cells and these may be assessed by the techniques of sputum cytology. Both smoking and mining exposure increase the probability of atypical cytology (50). Amongst twelve men whose cells were considered to be markedly atypical but not cancerous two developed the disease within 2 years. Cytology might supplement environmental and personal radiation monitoring as a means of protecting persons who are at risk. However, a positive result is usually evidence for irreparable damage and there does not appear to be evidence that cytology improves the prognosis of bronchial cancer.

The tumours are due to α particles emitted by 218Po and 214Po, of which the latter in particular have a very high energy level and an effective half-life from its precursor 214Pb of 33min. The polonium, formed by decay of radon gas, occurs as solid aerosol particles of diameter approximately 1μm. These can be adsorbed by droplet nuclei and smoke particles in the atmosphere and subsequently enlarge to form aggregates in the presence of water vapour. Inhaled aerosol particles behave in the manner described in chapter 4. The majority are exhaled: the remainder are deposited by sedimentation on the walls of airways throughout the lung, the distribution reflecting that of the respired gas. The aggregates are deposited preferentially by impaction at bronchial bifurcations near the hilum of the lung. This is also the site of deposition of aggregates containing tar from tobacco smoke. The tar includes benzo(a)pyrene and more radon daughter products which are possibly the main cause of lung cancer in cigarette smokers. In this event the effects of smoking and of occupational exposure to radon daughter products should be at the least additive, and an additive effect has indeed been observed in some studies (52, 60). However, the incorporation of polonium nuclei into aerosol aggregates is likely to be enhanced by smoking so this provides a mechanism for interaction whereby smoking might greatly increase the carcinogenic effect of occupational exposure to polonium. Interaction has been demonstrated by Doll from the data of Lundin, Lloyd & Smith (table 12.9, 51, 56): the extent of interaction appears to be related to the amount smoked (50, 55). The factors which may contribute have been analysed in detail by Martell (57) who points out that they also apply to the polonium aerosol present inside some granite houses and other domestic dwelling places (for example, in Aberdeen (58) and in parts of Sweden); this multiplier effect of smoking merits further investigation.

Thoron gas resembles radon in its decay via a series of α and β emitting substances. Of these 212Po has a very short half-life and emits exceptionally high energy particles (table 12.8). This species of polonium is a cause of lung cancer in workers processing thorium (59).

Environmental exposure and hygiene standards

Following the lead given by the U.S. Public Health Service the exposure to α particles is

Table 12.9.   Mortality amongst uranium miners from lung cancer (51)

	No. of deaths		Expected from model	
	Observed	Predicted	Additive	Multiplicative
Smokers	60	15.5	49.8	60.1
Non-smokers	2	0.5	12.2	1.9

expressed as the average environmental concentration per working month of duration 170h. The unit of concentration is 1.3×10^5 MeV of potential α energy per litre of respired air; this concentration when experienced for 1 month gives an exposure of 1 working level month (WLM). The equivalent in SI units, which are used by the International Commission on Radiological Protection, is 3.54×10^{-3} J h m^{-3}; however the conversion is approximate since the energy of an α particle depends on the element from which it is derived. The resulting dose of radiation received by the basal cells of the bronchial epithelium is approximately 3–10mGy (0.3–1.0 rad). Exposures in the range 120–4000 WLM increase the incidence of lung cancer (56). This is consistent with the dose of radiation needed to cause malignant change in tissue culture, which is approximately 800mGy, and the exposure of persons smoking one pack of cigarettes daily up to age 60 years which has been estimated as 380–970mGy (57). The risk associated with such an exposure is greater when it is accumulated over a relatively long time than when it is brief but intense. A dose–response relationship for Czechoslovak uranium miners followed for an average of 26 years is illustrated in fig. 12.3. This shows slight curvilinearity with a relative deficiency of cases amongst men with long exposures (54). A more linear relationship

is observed for Swedish iron miners amongst whom a significant excess of lung cancer is found at exposure levels above 25 WLM (60).

The exposure limit averaged over 12 months of mine work is 4 WLM with not more than 2 WLM over any 3 month period but the limit is now under review (53). The present level compares with an average level in some non-coal mines in the U.K. of 2.6 WLM and levels inside dwelling places of the order of 0.005 WLM (58). In a smoker an exposure of 2.6 WLM may be associated with a 10% excess risk of cancer (11% compared with an average of 10% from smoking alone) so on the basis of absolute risk there is a case for miners being recruited from amongst the non-smokers. If relative risk is the criterion some other protection is needed, especially as Radford and colleagues have evidence that an exposure of 4.8 WLM per year will lead to an excess death rate from lung cancer of approximately one in ten of the exposed population over a working lifetime (60).

Protection against ionizing radiation is by application of the principles of environmental hygiene described in chapter 3. The measures include diverting contaminated underground water courses, ventilating the mine, and erecting steel or concrete barriers to prevent the ingress of radon. If these measures are insufficient they may be supplemented by reducing the exposure through shortening the working week or imposing a ceiling on the life-time exposure; this is done by recording the cumulative exposure and only allowing the miner to continue at work up to a predetermined exposure limit.

Organic chemical carcinogens

Acrylonitrile

Acrylonitrile, formerly called cyanoethylene, has the formula $H_2C{=}CH{-}C{\equiv}N$. At room temperature it is a colourless liquid and may be formed from propane or by reaction of propylene vapour with ammonia and air in the presence of bismuth–iron catalyst. On account of its structure, acrylonitrile readily forms cross-linkages and this property is widely exploited; some of the resulting substances with their principal uses are given in table 12.10.

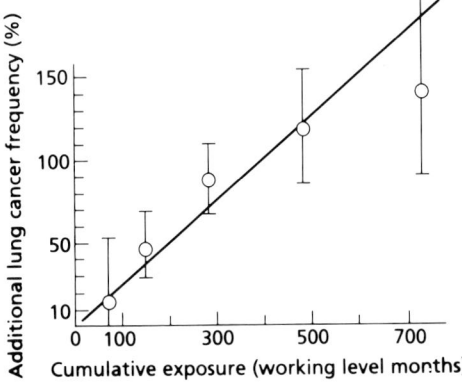

Fig. 12.3. Excess lung cancer mortality over 26 years in relation to cumulated exposure to radon amongst uranium miners in Czechoslovakia (Data of Kunz et al, 54. Reproduced from *Health Physics* 1979;**36**:699–706 by permission of the Health Physics Society.)

Table 12.10. Some uses of acrylonitrile

Acrylic and mod-acrylic fibres	Clothes, furnishings
Styrene-acrylonitrile resins	Instrument panels, drinking tumblers, kitchen hardware
Acrylonitrile-butadiene-styrene resins	Pipe fittings
Nitrile elastomers and latexes	Oil-resistant hoses, gaskets, belts, etc.
Adiponitrile	Intermediary in production of nylon
Nitrile resins: co-polymers with methyl acrylate and other substances	Beverage bottles
Mixed with carbon tetrachloride	Fumigant and pesticide for tobacco and in flour milling

Traces of free acrylonitrile are present in the derived materials and more may be liberated by heating in an atmosphere deficient in oxygen. The acrylonitrile may then break down to form cyanide and this substance is formed during its metabolism in the body. The cyanide is transformed to thiocyanate which is excreted in the urine.

Acrylonitrile is mutagenic when tested *in vitro* against bacteria. In animals it has been reported to cause foetal abnormalities and tumours in the gastro-intestinal tract, central nervous system and other tissues. Workers exposed to acrylonitrile in the early days of its manufacture and subsequently followed for 20 years showed an increased incidence of cancer of the lung and large intestine (62). Exposures within the hygiene standard (page 16) have no demonstrable ill-effects.

Acute poisoning may occur as a result of spillages, fires and other accidents. The harmful effects are due to breakdown of acrylonitrile to hydrocyanic acid (HCN) (page 274).

Benzo(a)pyrene, other polycyclic aromatic hydrocarbons and heterocyclic carcinogens

The polycyclic aromatic hydrocarbons (PAH) may be formed from most organic materials as a consequence of incomplete combustion. This liberates CH radicals which polymerize via nascent acetylene to form several series of compounds, many of which are carcinogenic (table 12.11). The temperature at a point of combustion is usually in the range 1000–1600°C whilst the more active products boil at temperatures in the region of 350°C so they form a carcinogenic

Table 12.11. Some polycyclic aromatic hydrocarbon and heterocyclic carcinogens

Benz(a)anthracene	$C_{18}H_{12}$	BP 400°C
Benzo(b)fluoranthene	$C_{20}H_{12}$	MP 168°C
Benzo(a)pyrene	$C_{20}H_{12}$	BP 475°C
Dibenzo(a,e)pyrene	$C_{24}H_{14}$	MP 241°C
Benz(c)acridine	$C_{17}H_{11}N$	MP 108°C
7H-Dibenzo(c,g)carbazole	$C_{20}H_{13}N$	MP 150°C

BP = Boiling point; MP = Melting point.

aerosol; prolonged inhalation may give rise to lung cancer.

In cell culture the polycyclic aromatic hydrocarbons and heterocyclic carcinogens become bound to cellular macromolecules and undergo hydrolysis with formation of toxic metabolites; of these some have been shown to be carcinogenic, for example cis-dehydrodiol derivatives of BA and β-hydroxymethyl B(a)P. The precise mechanism appears not to be known.

In rats and mice the compounds have been found to cause cancer of the lung following intravenous or intratracheal injections of doses of the order of 0.25mg. In one study rats exposed for 1h/day for 1 year to B(a)P aerosol at a concentration of 10mg m^{-3} developed lung cancer when the aerosol was fortified with SO_2 in the concentration 3.5ppm. Neither ingredient caused lung cancer in isolation (65).

In man an excess risk from lung cancer has been demonstrated amongst coal carbonizing process workers, especially those who formerly worked at the tops of retorts producing coal gas (63). The aerosol produced by heating crude oil, coal tar or pitch is also carcinogenic. Thus lung

Table 12.12.   Sources of benzo(a)pyrene aerosol and some estimates of concentration (64)

Industrial stack effluent	up to 2.7mg m^{-3}
Coal and pitch coking plants	0.3–35μg m^{-3}
⎧ Vapour from tar at 300°C	4.4%
⎨ Dose to workman	0.3–3mg h^{-1}
⎩ Laying tar (atmospheric concentration)	78μg m^{-3}
Gas works retort houses	1.4–4.8μg m^{-3}
Cigarette smoke	1.6μg/100 cigs.
Internal combustion engines	
Petrol exhaust	20μg m^{-3}
Diesel exhaust	3μg m^{-3}
Commercial garage	0.03μg m^{-3}
Combustion of all sorts	Variable
Urban air	0.002–2.2μg m^{-3}

Table 12.13.   Lung cancer in chloromethyl ether workers (67)

			Lung cancer cases	
Exposure	No. of men	SMR	Proportion of smokers (%)	Latent period (a)
Nil	981	1.1	94	—
Low	339	1.9	100	18.7
Intermediate	97	6.9*	80	17.8
High	29	30*	60	14.2

* $P<0.01$.

cancer from pitch used to bond carbon electrodes for refining aluminium has recently been reported (page 265). There does not appear to be evidence on the possible aggravating effect of tobacco smoke, or of a role for sulphur dioxide or other co-carcinogen. As well as forming aerosol the hydrocarbons adsorb onto particles of carbon liberated during combustion and the resulting soot may cause skin cancer, for example cancer of the scrotum of chimney sweeps. This was described by Percival Pott in 1775. Coal soot is more harmful than wood soot which contains relatively little of the principal carcinogen, benzo(a)pyrene (B(a)P). Bladder cancer may also occur (63). Some sources of airborne B(a)P are given in table 12.12.

Chloromethyl ethers (CME)

Bis(chloromethyl)ether (BCME, ClCH$_2$OCH$_2$Cl) is a potent human and animal carcinogen (66, 67). It can be produced by saturating a solution of paraformaldehyde in cold sulphuric acid with hydrogen chloride. The substance occurs as an impurity in chloromethyl methyl ether (CMME) in chemical plants in Philadelphia and elsewhere. CMME is used as an alkylating agent in the manufacture of anion exchange resins and other compounds. The Philadelphia plant began using chloromethyl ethers in 1948 and the mortality experience from lung cancer in relation to a semi-quantitative cumulative time-weighted index of exposure to airborne CME is given in table 12.13. The duration of exposure was the main variable whilst the intensity did not vary much between groups: overall there was a significant dose–response relationship which could not be explained by the effects of smoking. The predominant tumour was the small cell undifferentiated type. Similar observations have been made in the U.K. (66). The cancer is believed to be due solely to BCME but a minor contribution from CMME cannot be excluded on present evidence. The hygiene standards for these substances are given in table 1.7 (page 16).

Formaldehyde (H.CHO)

The gas is prepared by heating methanol vapour in air; it decomposes readily to form metaformaldehyde and is reformed by heating. Formaldehyde is used as the starting point for many chemical processes, for which purpose it is reacted with ammonia, phenol, urea and other substances. Some of the resulting compounds may dissociate to liberate formaldehyde; an example is urea formaldehyde used for wood glue, mouldings and cavity wall insulation.

Formaldehyde and a 40% solution in water (formalin) are widely used for disinfection of wool, skins and laboratory apparatus, fixing and preserving tissues, tanning leather and vulcanizing rubber. The substance is also used in the dye industry and as a feedstock for the synthesis of many drugs. Its potential to cause occupational asthma in a wide range of occupations is considered in chapter 16.

Squamous cell carcinoma of the nasal epithelium occurs in rats and mice after exposure to formaldehyde in the concentration range 5–14ppm (70). By contrast, post-mortem room staff and other persons occupationally exposed to formaldehyde do not have an increased incidence of malignancy (68, 69, 72) but this possibility should not be forgotten. In the U.S.A. there is disagreement as to whether formaldehyde should be regarded as a carcinogen which would lead to its use being severely curtailed or as a sensitizing agent to which empirical hygiene standards are applied (71). In the absence of further evidence the hygiene standard of 3 ppm (page 16) seems to provide an adequate margin of safety.

Mustard gas. Bis(2-chloroethyl)sulphide ($Cl.CH_2.CH_2–S.CH_2CH_2.Cl$)

Mustard gas is an oily liquid without colour or smell which solidifies at 13°C and boils at 216°C. It is soluble in fat and in organic solvents and sparingly soluble in water. The gas was used as a vesicant in the First World War and in Ethiopia in 1936. It was produced but not used during the Second World War. More recently there have been reports of its use in the Middle East and production continues in some countries. Thus the properties of mustard gas are still of practical importance. The substance also provides a model for biological studies of alkylating agents.

In low concentrations the gas is actively mutagenic in many test systems; it inhibits DNA synthesis in *E. coli* bacteria, induces mutations in *Drosophila* and causes chromosomal abnormalities in cell culture of mammalian lymphosarcoma and leukaemia tissue. A single 15min exposure to air saturated with mustard gas vapour is sufficient to cause lung cancer in mice. Lung cancer also occurs after intravenous injection (75).

In man there is evidence for an increased prevalence of lung cancer amongst soldiers who experienced mustard gas poisoning during the First World War and amongst workers engaged in the manufacture of mustard gas before and during the Second World War. The strongest evidence is from Japan where over the period 1952–67 amongst 495 former workers, thirty-three died of cancer of the respiratory tract compared with 0.9 expected. The conditions in the factory appear to have been bad, with the environmental concentrations attaining levels of the order of 70mg m^{-3} (77). American servicemen who were exposed to mustard gas in 1917–1918 and who were followed up in 1930–39 had an increased prevalence of chronic bronchitis and rather more deaths from lung cancer than men who developed influenza or were wounded (table 12.14). Amongst 1267 British mustard gas casualties the subsequent mortality from chronic bronchitis was increased (217 compared with twenty-one expected) but not that from lung cancer (74). A possible carcinogenic action might have been masked by a change in smoking habits since a significantly higher proportion of men had given up smoking by age 40 years in the exposed group compared

Table 12.14. Mortality from lung cancer in 1930–39 of U.S. servicemen exposed to mustard gas 1917–18 (73)

Category	Date	No.	Lung cancer	
			Observed	Expected
Mustard gas	1917–18	2718	39	26
Influenza	1918	1855	15	18
Wounded	1917–18	2578	30	26

with the control group of non-exposed men with chronic bronchitis (76). However, the carcinogenic effect of wartime exposure, if present, is not large. In this respect manufacture poses a more serious hazard.

Organic substances

Sensitizing agents. Diffuse pulmonary fibrosis is usually considered to carry an increased risk from lung cancer; however, this view was formed from observation of patients with fibrosing alveolitis and collagen diseases of the lung, not extrinsic allergic alveolitis. There is no evidence to suggest that farmers' lung, bird handlers' lung or similar conditions carry an increased risk of lung cancer.

Wood dust. Dust from hard woods used in the manufacture of furniture can cause adenocarcinoma of the nose and maxillary sinuses (page 65). The dust does not contribute to lung cancer (78) but terpenes and other products of heating coniferous wood may do so (79).

References

General

1 Doll R. Occupational cancer, problems in interpreting human evidence. *Ann Occup Hyg* 1984;**28**:291–305.
2 Doll R, Peto R. *The Causes of Cancer.* Oxford University Press: 1981.
3 Holmberg B, Ahlborg U. Symposium on biological tests in the evaluation of mutagenicity and carcinogenicity of air pollutants. *Environm Hlth Perspects* 1983;**47**:1–341.
4 Hunter T. Oncogenes and proto-oncogenes: how do they differ? *J Nat Cancer Inst* 1984;**73**:773–86.
5 Lucier GW, Hook GER. Proceedings of a workshop conference on the role of metals in carcinogenesis. *Environm Hlth Perspects* 1981;**40**: 1–252.
6 Saffiotti U, Wagoner JR (Eds). Occupational carcinogenesis. *Ann NY Acad Sci* 1976;**271**:1–516.
7 Sattaur O. Cancer genes—the enemy within. *New Scientist* 1984;**104**:12–16.
8 Sirover MA, Loeb LA. Infidelity of DNA synthesis in vitro: screening for potential metal mutagens or carcinogens. *Science* 1976;**194**:1434–6.

9 Sunderman FW. Mechanisms of metal carcinogenesis. *Biol Trace Element Research* 1979; **1**:63–86.

Arsenic

10 Brown CC, Chu KC. A new method for the analysis of cohort studies; implications of the multi-stage theory of carcinogenesis applied to occupational arsenic exposure. *Environm Hlth Perspects* 1983;**50**:293–308.
11 International agency for research on cancer: *Arsenic and arsenic compounds.* IARC monographs on the evaluation of the carcinogenic risk of chemicals to humans. 1980;**23**:39–141.
12 Lee AM, Fraumeni JF Jr. Arsenic and respiratory cancer in man: an occupational study. *J Nat Cancer Inst* 1969;**42**:1045–52.
13 Mabuchi K, Lilienfeld AM, Snell LM. Lung cancer amongst pesticide workers exposed to inorganic arsenicals. *Arch Environm Hlth* 1979;**34**:312–20.
14 Pershagen G. The carcinogenicity of arsenic. *Environm Hlth Perspects* 1981;**40**:93–100.
15 Pinto SS, Enterline PE, Henderson V, Varner MO. Mortality experience in relation to a measured arsenic trioxide exposure. *Environm Hlth Perspects* 1977;**19**:127–30.
16 Welch K, Higgins I, Oh M, Burchfiel C. Arsenic exposure, smoking and respiratory cancer in copper smelting workers. *Arch Environm Hlth* 1982;**37**:325–35.
17 World Health Organization. *Environmental Health Criteria 18. Arsenic.* Geneva: WHO: 1981.

Beryllium

18 Groth DH, Kommineni C, Mackay GR. Carcinogenicity of beryllium hydroxide and alloys. *Environm Res* 1980;**21**:63–84.
19 Vorwald AJ, Reeves AL, Urban ECJ. (1966) cited by Reeves AL. Beryllium carcinogenesis. In Schrauzer GN (Ed), *Conference on Inorganic and Nutritional Aspects of Cancer.* New York: Plenum Press. 1978:13–27.
20 Wagner WD, Groth DH, Holtz JL, Madden GE, Stokinger HE. Comparative chronic inhalation toxicity of beryllium ores, bentrandite and beryl with production of pulmonary tumours by beryl. *Toxic Appl Pharmacol* 1969; **15**:10–29.

Cadmium

21 Armstrong BG, Kazantzis G. The mortality of cadmium workers. *Lancet* 1983;**i**:1425–7.

22 Gompertz D, Fletcher JG, Perkins J, Smith NJ, Chettle DR, Mason H, Scott MC, Topping MD. Renal dysfunction in cadmium smelters: relation to in-vivo liver and kidney cadmium concentrations. *Lancet* 1983;**i**:1185–7.

23 International agency for research on cancer. *Cadmium and cadmium compounds*. IARC monographs on the evaluation of carcinogenic risk of chemicals to man. 1976;**11**:39–74.

24 Kazantzis G. Mutagenic and carcinogenic effects of cadmium. *Toxic Environm Chem* 1984;**8**:267–78.

25 Sorahan T, Waterhouse JAH. Mortality study of nickel–cadmium battery workers by the method of regression models in life tables. *Br J Industr Med* 1983;**40**:293–300.

26 Takenaka S, Oldiges H, Konig H, Hochrainer D, Oberdörster G. Carcinogenicity of cadmium chloride aerosols in W rats. *J Nat Cancer Inst* 1983;**70**:367–71.

27 Townshend RH. Acute cadmium pneumonitis: a 17 year follow-up. *Br J Industr Med* 1982; **39**:411–2.

Chromium

28 Alderson MR, Rattan NS, Bidstrup L. Health of workmen in the chromate-producing industry in Britain. *Br J Industr Med* 1981;**38**:117–24.

29 Axelsson G, Rylander R, Schmidt A. Mortality and incidence of tumours among ferro-chromium workers. *Br J Industr Med* 1980;**37**:121–7.

30 Bovet P, Lob M, Grandjean M. Spirometric alterations in workers in the chromium electroplating industry. *Int Arch Occup Environm Hlth* 1977;**40**:25–32.

31 Davies JM. Lung cancer mortality in workers in chromate pigment manufacture: an epidemiological survey. *J Oil Color Chem Assn* 1979;**62**:157–63.

32 Hayes RB, Lilienfeld AM, Snell LM. Mortality in chromium chemical production workers: a prospective study. *Int J Epidemiol* 1979; **8**:365–74.

33 International agency for research on cancer. *Chromium and chromium compounds*. IARC monographs on the evaluation of the carcinogenic risk of chemicals to humans. 1980;**23**:205–323.

34 Kalliomaki P-L, Lakomaa E, Kalliomaki K, Kiilunen M, Kivela R, Vaaranen V. Stainless steel manual metal arc welding fumes in rats. *Br J Industr Med* 1983;**40**:229–34.

35 Levy LS. Respiratory toxicology of nickel and chromium. In: Stern RM, Berlin A, Fletcher AC, Järvisalo J (eds). *Proceedings of International Conference on Health Hazards and Biological Effects of Welding Fumes and Gases*, Copenhagen, 18–21 February 1985. Amsterdam: Elsevier. 1986:267–84.

36 Mancuso TF. Consideration of chromium as an industrial carcinogen. In: Hutchinson TC (ed). *Proceedings of International Conference on Heavy Metals in the Environment*. Institute for environmental studies, Toronto. 1975:343–56.

37 Pokrovskaia LV, Shabynina NK. O kantserogennoi opasnosti na proizvodstve khromovykh ferrosplavov. (Carcinogenic hazards in the production of chromium ferro-alloys). *Gig Tr Prof Zabol* 1973;**17**:23–6.

38 Royle H. Toxicity of chromic acid in the chromium plating industry. *Environm Res* 1975;**10**:141–63.

39 Venitt S. Genetic toxicology of chromium and nickel compounds. In: Stern RM *et al.* 1986:249–66. (See Reference 35).

Lead

40 Cooper WC. Mortality in employees of lead battery plants and lead producing plants, 1947–1980. *Proc 21st International Congress of Occupational Health*, Dublin, Ireland, 11 September 1984. 1985.

41 Cooper WC, Gaffey WR. Mortality of lead workers. *J Occup Med* 1975;**17**:100–7.

42 International agency for research on cancer. *Lead and lead compounds*. IARC monographs on the evaluation of the carcinogenic risk of chemicals to humans. 1980;**23**:325–415.

43 Rencher AC, Carter MW, McKee DW. A retrospective epidemiological study of mortality at a large Western copper smelter. *J Occup Med* 1977;**19**:754–8.

Nickel

44 Cox JE, Doll R, Scott WA, Smith S. Mortality of nickel workers: experience of men working with metallic nickel. *Br J Industr Med* 1981;**38**:235–9.

45 Doll R, Matthews JD, Morgan LG. Cancer of the lung and nasal sinuses in nickel workers: a reassessment of the period of risk. *Br J Industr Med* 1977;**34**:102–5.

46 Jones Williams W. The pathology of the lungs in five nickel workers. *Br J Industr Med* 1958;**15**:235–42.

47 Lessard R, Reed D, Mahenx B, Lambert J. Lung cancer in New California, a nickel smelting island. *J Occup Med* 1978;**20**:815–7.

48 Pedersen E, Andersen A, Hogetbeit A. Second

study of the incidence and mortality of cancer of respiratory organs among workers at a nickel refinery. *Ann Clin Lab Sci* 1978;**8**:503–4.

49 Sunderman FW Jr. Recent research on nickel carcinogenesis. *Environ Hlth Perspects* 1981; **40**:131–41.

Ionizing radiation

50 Band P, Feldstein M, Saccomanno G, Watson L, King G. Potentiation of cigarette smoking and radiation. *Cancer* 1980;**45**:1273–7.

51 Doll R. The age distribution of cancer: implications for models of carcinogenesis. *J Roy Stat Soc A* 1971;**134**:133–55.

52 Edling C, Axelson O. Quantititive aspects of radon daughter exposure and lung cancer in underground miners. *Br J Industr Med* 1983;**40**:182–7.

53 International Commission on Radiological Protection. Radiation protection of workers in mines. ICRP publication 47. Oxford: Pergamon Press. 1986.

54 Kunz E, Sevc J, Placek J, Horacek J. Lung cancer in man in relation to different time distributions of radiation exposure. *Health Phys* 1979;**36**;699–706.

55 Larsson LG, Damber L. Interaction between underground mining and smoking in the causation of lung cancer: a study of non-uranium miners in Northern Sweden. *Cancer Detect Prevent* 1982;**5**:385–9.

56 Lundin FEJV, Lloyd JW, Smith EM, Archer VE, Holaday DA. Mortality of uranium miners in relation to radiation exposure, hard rock mining and cigarette smoking—1950 through September 1967. *Health Phys* 1969;**16**:571–8.

57 Martell EA. Alpha radiation dose at bronchial bifurcations of smokers from indoor exposure to radon progeny. *Proc Natl Acad Sci USA* 1983;**80**:1285–9.

58 National Radiological Protection Board. *Radon In British Mines*. London: HMSO. 1981. *Human exposure to radon decay products inside dwellings in the UK*. London: HMSO. 1983.

59 Polednak AP, Stehney AF, Lucas HF. Mortality among male workers at a thorium-processing plant. *Health Phys* 1983;**44:Suppl 1**:239–51.

60 Radford EP, Renard KGStC. Lung cancer in Swedish iron miners exposed to low doses of radon daughters. *New Engl J Med* 1984; 1485–94.

61 Saccomanno G, Archer VE, Auerbach O, Kuschner M, Saunders RP, Klein MG. Histologic types of lung cancer among uranium miners. *Cancer* 1971;**27**:515–23.

Organic chemical carcinogens

Acrylonitrile

62 O'Berg MT. Epidemiologic study of workers exposed to acrylonitrile. *J Occup Med* 1980;**22**:245–52.

B(a)P

63 Doll R, Vessey MP, Beasley RWR, Buckley AR, Fear EC, Fisher REW, Gammon EJ, Gunn W, Hughes GO, Lee K, Norman-Smith B. Mortality of gasworkers—final report of a prospective study. *Br J Industr Med* 1972;**29**:394–406.

64 International agency for research on cancer. *Certain polycyclic aromatic hydrocarbons and heterocyclic compounds*. IARC monographs on the evaluation of carcinogenic risk of chemicals to man. 1973;**3**:1–268.

65 Laskin S, Kuschner M, Drew RT. Studies in pulmonary carcinogenesis. In: Hanna MG, Nettesheim P, Gilbert JR (eds). *Inhalation Carcinogenesis*, US Atomic Energy Commission Symposium Series No. 18. 1970:321.

CME

66 McCallum RI, Woolley V, Petrie A. Lung cancer associated with chloromethyl methyl ether manufacture: an investigation at two factories in the United Kingdom. *Br J Industr Med* 1983;**40**:384–9.

67 Weiss W, Moser RL, Auerbach O. Lung cancer in chloromethyl ether workers. *Am Rev Respir Dis* 1979;**120**:1031–7.

Formaldehyde

68 Acheson ED, Barnes HR, Gardner MJ, Osmond C, Pannett B, Taylor CP. Formaldehyde process workers and lung cancer. *Lancet* 1984;**i**:1066–7.

69 Andersen SK, Jensen OM, Oliva D. Exposure to formaldehyde and lung cancer in Danish physicians. *Ugeskr Laeger* 1982;**144**:1571–3. (In Danish.)

70 Griesemer RA, (Chairman). Report of the federal panel on formaldehyde. *Environm Hlth Perspects* 1982;**43**:139–68.

71 Perera F, Petito C. Formaldehyde. A question of cancer policy? *Science* 1982;**216**:1285–91.

72 Walrath J, Fraumeni JF Jr. Mortality pattern among embalmers. *Int J Cancer* 1983;**31**: 407–11.

Mustard gas

73 Beebe GW. Lung cancer in World War I veterans: possible relation to mustard gas injury and 1918 influenza epidemic. *J Nat Cancer Inst* 1960;**25**:1231–52.

74 Case RAM, Lea AJ. Mustard gas poisoning, chronic bronchitis and lung cancer. An investigation into the possibility that poisoning by mustard gas in the 1914–18 war might be a factor in the production of neoplasia. *Br J Prev Soc Med* 1955;**9**:62–72.

75 International agency for research on cancer. *Mustard gas.* IARC monographs on the evaluation of carcinogenic risk of chemicals to man. 1975;**9**:181–92.

76 Norman JE. Lung cancer mortality in World War I veterans with mustard gas injury: 1919–1965. *J Nat Cancer Inst* 1975;**54**:311–17.

77 Wada S, Nishimoto Y, Miyanishi M, Kambe S, Miller RW. Mustard gas as a cause of respiratory neoplasia in man. *Lancet* 1968;**i**:1161–3.

Wood dust

78 Acheson ED, Pippard EC, Winter PD. The mortality of English furniture makers. *Scand J Work Environ Hlth* 1984;**10**:211–7.

79 Kauppinen TP, Partanen TJ, Nurminen MM, Nickels JI, Hernberg SG, Hakulinen TR, Pukkala EI, Savonen ET. Respiratory cancers and chemical exposures in the wood industry: a nested case-control study. *Br J Industr Med* 1986;**43**:84–90.

Chapter 13
Other Dusts, Gases and Vapours

Review of some ninety substances and classes of substances
in alphabetical order from acetyladelyde to zirconium.

Introduction

This chapter contains concise information about a number of solid, liquid and gaseous substances which can damage the lungs or impair the respiratory function of the blood. It is arranged alphabetically in order of principal substances but related compounds are included under many of the entries. Substances which may be lung carcinogens are given here by name and the page number in chapter 12 where they are described. Some substances which contribute to chronic bronchitis or emphysema are cross referenced to chapter 17. Substances which may give rise to extrinsic allergic alveolitis and occupational asthma are referred to respectively in chapters 15 and 16. Additional information about substances in this chapter may be obtained by consulting the selected references (page 303) or from the ILO Encyclopaedia of Occupational Health and Safety which is the source of some of the present material. The Encyclopaedia articles draw extensively on guidance notes, recommendations and reviews from the U.K. Health and Safety Executive and U.S. National Institute for Occupational Safety and Health. Permission to use the material is gratefully acknowledged.

Acetaldehyde (ethanal)

Acetaldehyde (CH_3CHO) is a colourless, flammable liquid with a pungent, fruity odour. It may be produced by any of a number of chemical reactions of which direct synthesis from carbon monoxide and hydrogen is possibly the most important. In turn acetaldehyde is used in the manufacture of acetic acid and other substances. The liquid boils at 20.8°C and the vapour is both irritant and narcotic. The respiratory effects include irritation of the nose, upper and lower respiratory tract and lung parenchyma where high concentrations cause pulmonary oedema. Death may occur from respiratory failure.

Acrolein (acrylic aldehyde)

Acrolein (CH_2CHCHO) is a yellow liquid with a pungent odour. It is produced by catalytic oxidation of propylene and is used as a starting point for manufacture of plastics, synthetic fibres, animal foodstuffs and other products. The aldehyde is a constituent of diesel fumes, cigarette smoke and fumes from melted fat. It is exceedingly irritant to the eyes and respiratory tract and causes lachrymation in low concentration. Higher concentrations damage the cilia of the respiratory tract. Leakage or spillage of acrolein has caused acute bronchoconstriction and pulmonary oedema; subsequent death or permanent lung damage have been reported. (See also diesel fumes.)

Acrylonitrile - chapter 12, page 256

Allyl chloride and related compounds

Allyl chloride (CH_2CHCH_2Cl) is a colourless liquid with a pungent odour which is used in production of epichlorohydrin for epoxy resin, glycerol and other substances. The vapour is a powerful irritant of the upper respiratory tract.

Aluminium

Aluminium is a silvery, ductile, non-magnetic metal. It is present in bauxite which contains up to 55% alumina (Al_2O_3) together with fluorine, silica, iron and other substances. The ore occurs in many parts of the world. Extraction is by open-cast mining followed by crushing and washing to remove clay and silica. Alumina is obtained by the Bayer process in which bauxite is digested under pressure with hot caustic soda, then calcined in a kiln. To produce the metal the alumina is dissolved in sodium aluminium fluoride (cryolite, Na_3AlF_3) and reduced in an electric furnace; the electrodes are graphite made from heating ground coke with pitch. The furnaces are known in the trade as pots. They operate at high temperature and the carbon electrodes are consumed in the process. This liberates toxic gases and fumes which are mostly contained in the pot except when the lid is removed for filling or for siphoning off the aluminium. The gases include hydrogen fluoride and oxides of carbon, nitrogen and sulphur. The particulates are mainly aluminium fluoride, alumina and pitch plus some quartz, nickel and vanadium. The process is associated with high temperatures, high noise levels and the risk of electric shock.

Aluminium powder is prepared in the form of flakes by stamping or grinding aluminium metal or foil and as granules which are made from molten metal. The flakes may be treated with animal, vegetable or mineral oil (stearine, spindle oil or paraffin) in order to prevent aggregation. Aluminium is used very extensively in the engineering, electrical and construction industries, commonly as an alloy with one of the other non-ferrous metals. Aluminium foil is used for packaging and aluminium powder for paints and pyrotechnics. Surface coatings are also applied by anodization. Aluminium is used in welding rods and there are many other applications.

In 1947 Shaver reported the occurrence of pulmonary fibrosis in men engaged in smelting bauxite. The disease was attributed to aluminium but is believed now to have been due to silica. Both bauxite and alumina appear to be inert and subsequent to 1947 miners and refi-

nery workers have not been recognized as having any occupational lung disease. However, excess lung cancer from pitch used to bond the carbon electrodes has been reported from some pot rooms by Gills and other workers. The cancer is probably due to benz(a)anthracene and benzo(a)pyrene (page 257). Pot room workers may have an increased prevalence of chest tightness but respiratory impairment is uncommon. Alumina administered as an aerosol to animals is without effect except when the cloud contains a high proportion of extremely small particles (diameter $<0.04\mu m$); this circumstance is rare commercially. Dust from alumina used for biscuit placing in potteries (page 265) and granular aluminium powder used in the experimental treatment of pneumoconiosis (page 158) have not been observed to damage the lungs.

Thus despite the large number of potentially harmful substances associated with the process, the expectation raised by Shaver's observations and the ever present risk of fluorosis, the production of aluminium appears to carry little risk. This is also true of the great majority of applications. However, aluminium fumes from welding and powder produced by stamping or flaking are known to cause pulmonary granulomas and diffuse fibrosis in man, and Corrin reproduced the condition in rats. Aluminium silicates are the principal constituent of clays and can cause simple pneumoconiosis (page 273). Aluminium powder may cause epileptiform convulsions or encephalopathy. Fumes liberated in the electrolytic reduction of alumina may also be harmful. Thus Field has observed occupational asthma in some pot room workers and a transient decline in lung function in susceptible individuals at times when the pots were open. Additional evidence is summarized by Simonsson and by Chan-Yeung and colleagues who also found that compared with control subjects the men who spent most of their time in the pot room had a reduced forced expiratory volume and more cough and wheeze. These findings suggest that whilst work with aluminium and its compounds does not normally damage the lung there are circumstances when it may be harmful. This possibility should be borne in mind when an aluminium worker presents with lung disease and a thorough exploration of the circumstances should be undertaken. Meanwhile persons exposed to dust or fume containing aluminium should adopt precautions appropriate for the level of risk which is involved.

Ammonia

Ammonia (NH_3) is a colourless, easily liquified gas with a sharp odour. It is present in decaying organic matter and is usually produced commercially by reaction of pure nitrogen with hydrogen at high temperature and pressure in the presence of a catalyst. Ammonia is used for manufacture of agricultural fertilizers, nitric acid, plastics, explosives and other substances; it is also used in dyeing, as a refrigerant and as an additive in furnaces. High atmospheric concentrations may occur from spillage or leakage during manufacture and as a result of traffic accidents during transit in tankers and railway waggons. The industrial leakages may be accompanied by carbon monoxide or hydrogen sulphide and carry a risk of explosion. The gas is highly soluble in body fluids and does not normally reach the lower respiratory tract. It irritates the eyes and upper respiratory tract where it stimulates irritant receptors and causes reflex changes in the pattern of breathing.

Higher concentrations cause airway narrowing with cough, retrosternal pain, haemoptysis, burning of the pharynx and larynx and pulmonary oedema. Death may occur acutely from laryngeal spasm or subsequently from secondary infection of the lung. In the event of recovery the patient may be left with bronchiectasis or narrowing of small lung airways. Treatment is by removal from exposure, neutralization of the caustic alkali with dilute citric acid solution as a douche and by inhalation, and administration of oxygen. Assistance to respiration may be needed and prophylactic chemotherapy is recommended.

Anthrax

B. anthracis is a spore-bearing bacterium which infects sheep, goats and other herbivora following the ingestion of contaminated fodder. The infection is a generalized septicaemia and is usually fatal. It is endemic in North and East Africa and much of Asia. Human infection is acquired from contact with infected animals or animal products including flesh, hide, hair, horn and bones. Infection may be acquired from blankets, brushes, clothes, dried meal or rugs made from these products. Infectivity is low but it persists for a long time because the spores are almost indestructable. In man the condition affects the skin, where it forms a papule which ulcerates, or the gastro-intestinal tract. Pulmonary anthrax is rare. It is due to inhaling anthrax spores from wool (hence wool sorters' disease), bone meal or other product. The pneumonia presents with fever, haemoptysis and pleurisy and if untreated progresses rapidly to septicaemia and death which may occur within 24–48h. Treatment is with anti-anthrax serum, penicillin and supportive measures. Prophylaxis entails (i) control of the disease in animals; this is achieved through vaccination, localization of outbreaks, proper disposal of carcases and disinfection of premises, (ii) fumigation of potentially infected wool and other products; this is done by immersion in 2% formaldehyde solution at 40°C followed by drying at 200°C, and (iii) protection of persons at risk; this is effected by vaccination and exhaust ventilation in the workplace. In conditions of high risk these measures should be supplemented by personal respiratory protection and prophylactic tetracycline.

Antimony

Antimony (atomic mass 121.8) is a silvery-white metal which readily burns to form antimony oxide (Sb_2O_3) and may be alloyed with lead, tin and other metals. It is contained in stibnite (SbS_3), valentinite (Sb_2O_3) and other ore; this is extracted by crushing, settling and flotation. The metal is produced through roasting and reduction by carbon under a flux of sodium carbonate or sulphate. Antimony is used in semi-conductors and in alloys as babbitt, pewter, white metal, Britannia metal and heavy metal. These are employed for bearing casings, printing-type, battery plates, cable sheathing, solder and other products.

Antimony trioxide, produced by oxidation of

References page 303

Table 13.1. Some antimony compounds

Stibine	(SbH_3)	From treating Sb with acid	Destroys red blood cells
Antimony trioxide	(Sb_2O_3)	Pigment, flame proofing compound	Suspected of causing lung cancer
Antimony pentoxide	(Sb_2O_5)	Pigment, for pharmaceuticals	Non-toxic
Antimony trichloride	$(SbCl_3)$	⎰Used to blue steel and	⎰Corrosive may cause
Antimony pentachloride	$(SbCl_5)$	⎱aluminium, as catalyst, etc.	⎱pulmonary oedema

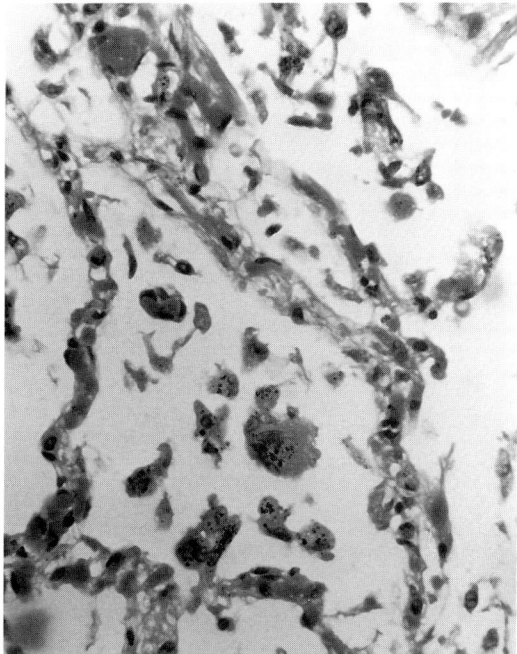

Fig. 13.1. Lung histology from a 55-year-old man who for 25 years was engaged in refining antimony sulphide. His respiratory health was excellent (no respiratory symptoms, FEV_1 124% of predicted) but routine chest radiography showed simple pneumoconiosis (category 2p). Death was from myocardial infarction. The section showed multinucleated cells containing bi-refringent particles (probably antimony sulphide). The structure of the lung was normal. (By courtesy of G. L. Leathart and T. Ashcroft.)

metal or ore, is purified by volatilization. The oxide is evolved as a very fine fume which is trapped by filtering the air from the furnaces through cloth bags. A small fraction of the antimony oxide dust inhaled by workers on this process is retained in the lungs and may even-

tually reach sufficient concentration to be visible as micronodulation on a chest radiograph. The condition is not accompanied by any material loss of function and there is no fibrosis of the lungs at post-mortem (fig. 13.1). Since antimony oxide is virtually insoluble in body fluid there are none of the symptoms associated with administration of soluble antimony compounds, which are very toxic (table 13.1). The possibility that antimony trioxide may cause lung cancer has not been confirmed.

Arsenic - chapter 12, page 246

Asbestos products - chapter 10

Barium

Barium (atomic mass 137.3) is a silvery-white metal which may ignite spontaneously in air and has few industrial uses. Some details of the salts are given in table 13.2. The principal sources are barytes $(BaSO_4)$ and wetherite $(BaCO_3)$ and the only hazard to the lungs is simple pneumoconiosis following prolonged inhalation of the dust (fig. 13.2). However, the dust has a high radio-opacity and is not fibrogenic so the radiographic lesions look more serious than they actually are. The lesions regress after cessation of exposure unless the condition is complicated by silicosis due to drilling through quartz or sandstone to secure access to the ore, contamination of the ore by siliceous rock or grinding with siliceous millstones. One such case is illustrated in fig. 8.4 (page 150).

Basalt

Basalt usually refers to marble which is a limestone (page 281). It also describes other rocks of

Table 13.2.   Some barium compounds

Barium sulphate	Filler in paper, etc., γ-ray-opaque glass and bricks, pigment, thixotropic mud in drilling oil wells, x-ray diagnosis	Causes simple pneumoconiosis
Barium carbonate	Bricks, tiles, glaze, rodenticide, etc.	Ditto: may cause abortion
Barium peroxide	Oxidizing and bleaching agent	Surface irritant
Barium hydroxide	Glass manufacture and other uses	
Barium chloride	Intermediary in manufacture of Cl_2. NaOH and other products; pigment; cardiac stimulant	⎱ Soluble salts, powerful muscle ⎰ stimulants and very toxic on ⎰ this account
Barium nitrate	Pyrotechnics, electronic ceramics	
Barium titanate	See titanium (page 297)	

similar appearance; many of these are siliceous (e.g. feldspar, page 146) and cause silicosis.

Benzo(a)pyrene and related substances –
chapter 12, page 259

Beryllium - chapter 11

Bismuth

Bismuth (atomic mass 209) is a hard, brittle metal which occurs as free metal in bismutite ($BiCO_3$) and in other ores. It is produced as a by-product of refining lead, copper and tin and is used in alloys which have a low melting point, for example Wood's metal; some alloys are used for welding. Bismuth is probably the least toxic of the heavy metals and does not damage the lung. It is capable of causing simple pneumoconiosis. Some bismuth compounds are given in table 13.3.

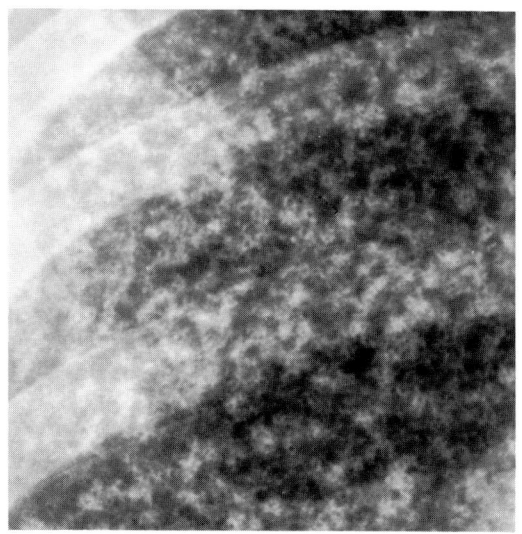

Fig. 13.2. Routine chest radiograph showing simple pneumoconiosis (category 3p/q) in a barytes worker whose job was to grind the ore. He was asymptomatic. (By courtesy of J. E. M. Hutchinson.)

Table 13.3.   Some bismuth compounds

Bismuth telluride	Semi-conductor	Causes simple pneumoconiosis
Bismuth oxide and other insoluble salts	Cosmetic	⎱ Rare cause of encephalopathy
Bismuth carbonate and other slightly soluble salts	Antacids, etc.	⎰
Bismuth butyl thiolamate	Anti-syphilitic	May cause nephrosis
Bismuth pentafluoride	Decomposes on heating	Fume causes pulmonary oedema

References page 308

Boron

Boron (atomic mass 108) is an insoluble brownish-black powder which is contained in borax ($Na_2B_4O_7.1OH_2O$) and other minerals. It is obtained by reduction of boron trioxide with magnesium or aluminium and is used as a degasifying agent in alloys and for shielding nuclear reactors. Boron forms borides with chromium (CrB_2), molybdenum (MO_2B_5), titanium (TiB_2), zirconium (ZrB_2) and other metals; these compounds are used for coating steel, in alloys, as catalysts and semi-conductors. Both ore and borides can cause simple pneumoconiosis. Details of some compounds of boron are given in table 13.4.

Bromomethane (methyl bromide)

Bromomethane (CH_3Br) is a colourless gas with a faint chloroform-like odour which is produced by reaction of methyl alcohol, sodium bromide and sulphuric acid. It is used as a refrigerant gas, in fire extinguishers, as an ingredient in manufacturing aniline dyes, and for killing plants, insects, fungi and rodents. The gas is highly toxic to most organs of the body, particularly the brain, liver and kidneys. Pulmonary congestion and oedema sometimes occur, either as a primary event or secondary to involvement of other organs. In low concentrations the nervous system is the principal target.

Brucellosis

Bacteria of the genus brucella cause infectious abortion and other illnesses in farm and related animals. The main species are *B. abortus* (cattle), *B. suis* (pigs) and *B. melitensis* (goats). The disease may affect persons coming in contact with infected animals, their discharges or infected premises. It also affects persons engaged in transport, food processing, workers with hair and hide, veterinary surgeons and laboratory staff engaged in analyses or producing vaccines and related products. Transmission occurs readily through an abrasion, the conjunctiva, mouth, gastro-intestinal tract or lungs. The pulmonary form is uncommon. It presents as an acute bronchitis which may progress to bronchopneumonia with fever and notable constitutional disturbance. More commonly the condition presents with malaise and unexplained fever; there may be glandular enlargement or septicaemia and the disease may subsequently localize in joints, intestines, meninges or genital organs. Following recovery the affected person may retain a hypersensitivity to *Brucella* antigen; this may lead to a hypersensitivity reaction occurring as a result of re-exposure. The site may be the skin, the bronchi or the joints.

Diagnosis of brucellosis is by blood culture and the presence of a high antibody titre in the serum; a positive intradermal skin test is not evidence for active disease. Treatment is by tetracycline plus supporting therapy and prophylaxis is by segregation and decontamination supplemented by immunization. In the U.K. the disease has nearly been eliminated by the slaughter of infected animals and the vaccination of those which are healthy. Veterinary surgeons are now at greatest risk. In the event of

Table 13.4. Some boron compounds

Boric anhydride	(B_2O_3)	Glass, enamel, glazes, in water forms boric acid	Skin irritant
Boron trifluoride	(BF_3)*†	Catalyst, flux for magnesium	Decompose to HF, HCl, HBr which may cause pulmonary oedema
Boron trichloride	(BCl_3)	Catalyst	
Boron tribromide	(BBr_3)	Radio-electronics	
Boron carbide	(B_4C)	Abrasive	Chronic bronchitis; lung fibrosis and emphysema in rats
Boron nitride	(BN)	Nuclear engineering	
Pentaborane (9)	(B_5H_9)	Fuel, chemicals	Toxic to all organs

* Gas: boiling point 100°C.
† Anti-cholinesterase.

an outbreak of infection, they may be protected by immunization with a purified antigen but the protection is relatively short-lived and re-vaccination may precipitate a hypersensitivity reaction. (References page 304.)

Cadmium - chapter 12, page 247

Carbon dioxide

Carbon dioxide (CO_2) is produced during the burning or fermentation of organic matter, calcination of limestone, reaction of sulphuric acid with dolomite and many other industrial processes. The gas may become dispersed in the atmosphere or it may be purified and compressed. It may also be absorbed by ethanolamine or alkali from which it is obtained as sodium carbonate. Some uses of CO_2 are given in table 13.5.

Table 13.5. Some uses of carbon dioxide

Gas	Liquid	Solid
Carbonating beverages	Firefighting	Refrigerant (Many applications)
Neutralizing alkalis	Inflating life-jackets, etc.	
Shielding for arc welding	Refrigerant	
Accelerating plant growth		

Carbon dioxide has a number of biological effects of which some are given in table 13.6. The gas is heavier than air so in a fermentation tank or other confined space the concentration is higher at the bottom than the top; in such circumstances a slip or fall may bring disaster.

The victim quickly loses consciousness, ceases to breathe and dies painlessly without sufficient warning of the danger. Any rescuer may suffer the same fate. The conditions which give rise to hypercarbia usually cause hypoxia but this only marginally affects the outcome.

Protection is provided by vigilance, exhaust ventilation and if necessary an airline respirator or breathing apparatus (page 56).

Carbon monoxide

Carbon monoxide (CO) is produced during the combustion of organic material which is incomplete on account of a relative deficiency of oxygen or because the temperature of the flame is reduced by local cooling. On a commercial scale the gas is produced by partial oxidation of natural gas or gasification of coal. It is used as a reducing agent in metallurgy, for organic synthesis and in the production of metal carbonyls, for example nickel carbonyl (page 250). Carbon monoxide is also a constituent of industrial gases used for fuel (water gas, blast furnace gas, producer gas, coal gas). In coal gas the concentration is in the range 5–15% and in the other gases 20–40%.

Exposure to carbon monoxide may occur in the vicinity of steel furnaces or other processes which either use carbon monoxide or involve combustion; in addition contamination of respired gas with carbon monoxide may occur from a nearby internal combustion or diesel engine, from naturally produced gas encountered during tunnelling, from welding fumes, explosions,

Table 13.6. Some effects of breathing carbon dioxide in air at sea level*

> 0.5%	Submarines	Alters acid–base balance	Tissue deposition of calcium increased (long-term)
1%	Confined spaces	Affects blood buffering	
5%	Breathing CO_2 in air	Dilates blood vessels, stimulates respiration	Headache, dyspnoea
8%			Confusion, tremor, papilloedema (if persistent)
10%	Silos, fermentation tanks; black damp in mines	Respiratory depression	Unconsciousness

* Under hyperbaric conditions the effects are increased proportionately.

tobacco smoke and other sources. When a fire occurs inside a building the carbon monoxide concentration usually exceeds 500ppm (0.05%). Poisoning may also occur following exposure to dichloromethane, which is used as a paint stripper, and related hydrocarbons; these substances liberate carbon monoxide during metabolism by the liver.

Carbon monoxide combines reversibly with haemoglobin for which its affinity is greater than that of oxygen by a factor of approximately 230. On this account an 8% saturation of haemoglobin with carbon monoxide occurs in equilibrium with an alveolar concentration of 50ppm (0.005%), whereas for oxygen the equivalent concentration is 1.2%. The corresponding concentrations to achieve 50% saturation are respectively 150ppm (0.015%) and 3.5%. Thus exposure to carbon monoxide decreases the capacity of the blood to transport oxygen from the lungs; it also displaces the oxyhaemoglobin dissociation curve to the left so for a given tissue oxygen tension more oxygen remains in the blood and less is released. In high concentration the utilization of oxygen is further deranged by the carbon monoxide combining with myoglobin and with the enzymes which contribute to oxidation of glucose.

In healthy non-smokers the alveolar carbon monoxide concentration is less than 10ppm. In smokers it is in the range 20–100ppm; the mean level is approximately 50ppm which is also the present hygiene standard for continuous exposure (page 16). At this level there is slight loss of visual acuity, impaired ability to learn skilled tasks, reduced capacity for heavy work and, in patients with ischaemic heart disease, aggravation of anginal pain.

In acute poisoning, if the saturation of haemoglobin with carbon monoxide is in the range 20–40%, the subject usually has symptoms of headache, giddiness and weakness; higher levels of carboxyhaemoglobin cause cerebral oedema. There may then be tachycardia and rapid breathing, a fall in blood pressure and sudden loss of consciousness. The patient is usually ashen grey and sweating but at postmortem the skin and mucous membranes may have a cherry-red appearance due to the presence of carboxyhaemoglobin. In chronic poisoning the subject may present with headache, irritability and dyspepsia and these changes may progress to loss of memory, personality change and muscle weakness. Similar features may present during recovery from severe acute poisoning associated with unconsciousness.

Carbon monoxide poisoning is often missed on account of the many conditions both acute and chronic which may present with similar features. The diagnosis is made by measurement of blood concentration of carboxyhaemoglobin or by analysis of alveolar gas collected after breathholding or a period of rebreathing. The equipment for the latter measurement is portable and relatively cheap; it should be available on all plant where there is a carbon monoxide hazard.

Persons with increased susceptibility to carbon monoxide poisoning include those at high altitude, heavy drinkers, pregnant women, children and patients with thyrotoxicosis, fever, anaemia and cerebral or cardiac atherosclerosis.

The rate of transfer of carbon monoxide between air and blood is determined by the tension difference between inspired and alveolar gas, the alveolar ventilation, the cardiac output and the prevailing tension of oxygen. Some of these variables are themselves affected by age and sex. The rate has been described mathematically by Joumard and his colleagues. Uptake is enhanced by exercise and by relative deficiency of oxygen such as occurs at altitude. Symptoms occur after a few breaths or up to an hour depending on circumstances. Elimination is also enhanced by activity; this may reduce the half-time from 210min which is normal for a resting man aged 30 years, to 100min or less depending on the intensity of the exercise. The half-time varies linearly with age and is less by about 10% in women compared with men. It is reduced to approximately 30min at rest by breathing 100% oxygen and to 8 or 5min by breathing oxygen at a pressure of 2 or 3atm in a compression chamber. This is the treatment of choice for acute carbon monoxide poisoning. Depending on circumstances the hyperbaric therapy may need to be supplemented by assisted ventilation and treatment of cardiac arrest or cerebral oedema.

Safe conditions are achieved by control of

References page 304

combustion, efficient use of chimneys, ensuring that pipes and burners are free from leaks, maintaining unobstructed exhaust ventilation and, where appropriate, by the catalytic oxidation of carbon monoxide to carbon dioxide. Particular care is needed in the use of fuel beds, gas manufacture, coke ovens, foundries, iron casting operations, manufacturing processes based on carbon monoxide and where internal combustion engines are used in confined spaces. Natural gas should be used for fuel instead of coal gas wherever this is practical.

Cement - see Limestone

Cerium

Cerium (atomic mass 140.1) is a rare earth present in cerite and other minerals including monazite which also contains the radioactive substance, thorium (described in chapter 12). Cerium dioxide is obtained by milling, flotation, electromagnetic separation and subsequent refining by electrolysis (see also Yttrium). The rare earths are radio-opaque, have anti-emetic and anti-coagulant properties, and can contribute to the regulation of glycolysis. They are used in deoxidants, catalysts, glass, polish for lenses, phosphors, ceramics, pyrotechnics and metal alloys. They are a cause of inert dust pneumoconiosis and of anaemia; they do not appear to induce a lung tissue reaction in man.

Chlorine

Chlorine (Cl_2) is a greenish-yellow gas with a pungent odour detectable at a concentration of 1ppm, though detection becomes impaired with continued exposure. It is produced by hydrolysis of sodium chloride in aqueous solution (brine); sodium hydroxide and hydrogen are produced concurrently as:

$$2\ NaCl + 2\ H_2O = Cl_2 + 2\ NaOH + H_2$$

The yield of sodium hydroxide is increased by use of mercury as an intermediary in the electrolytic process.

The gas is a powerful bleaching agent for textiles and paper, a disinfectant of water (including swimming pools) and a feedstock for many chemical processes; these include the production of metallic chlorides, solvents, refrigerants, pesticides and polymers. Exposure may occur in the course of any of these processes or during transportation of liquid chlorine by road or rail tanker. The risk of exposure is greatest during decanting and the transfer of gas in pipes from the container to the point of use. Rupture of a tanker may create a civil emergency.

Chlorine reacts with water on the surface of the eyes, nose, pharynx and respiratory tract to form hydrochloric acid and nascent oxygen. At a chlorine concentration of 5–30ppm these substances cause local irritation and stimulation of receptors which initiate reflex coughing, bronchoconstriction and pain felt behind the sternum. Higher concentrations cause tissue damage throughout the respiratory tract, including the lungs where the resulting pulmonary oedema may be fatal. The intense coughing may provoke vomiting which is often haemorrhagic and there is accompanying headache and acute anxiety. With overwhelming exposure, such as may follow a major spillage, death occurs rapidly from cardiac arrest. Treatment entails removal from further exposure and medication appropriate to the severity of the condition including bronchodilator or corticosteroid drugs, oxygen or intensive cardiac and respiratory support. For patients who survived the

Table 13.7. Some chlorine compounds which may cause pulmonary oedema

Substance	Formula	Use
Chlorine dioxide gas	ClO_2	As for chlorine
Sulphur chloride	S_2Cl_2	Vulcanizing of rubber, etc.
Thionyl chloride	$SOCl_2$	Chemical intermediary
Chlorsulphonic acid	$ClSO_2OH$	Chemical intermediary
Phosgene gas	$COCl_2$	See page 292

acute episode Weill and his colleagues found that recovery occurred within 3 weeks. There were no relapses. Chronic exposure to chlorine causes damage to the lung airways which is synergistic with that due to smoking; 5ppm exerts a material effect and 1ppm causes detectable airflow limitation in smokers. Some chlorine compounds which have similar toxic effects are given in table 13.7.

Leakage of chlorine gas or liquid is prevented by scrupulous observance of good industrial practices; these should extend throughout the industrial process as many accidents arise as a consequence of events which are themselves harmless. Leaks and faults in equipment should be looked for daily and any disconnection or repair preceded by purging the affected section. Major spillages should be avoided by good industrial design and emergency procedures drawn up to cope with any that do occur. Some of the relevant preventive measures are considered in chapter 3.

Chloromethyl ethers - chapter 12, page 259

Chromium - chapter 12, page 248

Clays (aluminium silicates)

Clay is malleable or plastic earth. The common variety is formed from the weathering of argillaceous rock and the principal constituent is hydrous aluminium silicate. This is called kaolinite after Kai-Ling, a hill in China where clay was first mined. Clay also contains a variable amount of quartz, from a trace up to 35%. For the manufacture of china the quartz content must be less than 5%. Fuller's earth gets its name from the property of absorbing oil and grease. The usual constituent is calcium montmorillonite which is an iron magnesium aluminium silicate. The material exhibits little change in volume when in contact with water and on this account in the U.S.A. is called low swelling bentonite. Bentonite, called in the U.S.A. high swelling bentonite, is sodium montmorillonite; it is formed by weathering of volcanic ash and is found in pure form at Fort Benton in Wyoming. Palygorskite (attapulgite) clays which are amphibole minerals are also used as Fuller's earth, particularly in the U.S.A.

Clay is extracted by quarrying or mining and the subsequent treatment, depending on the application, can include drying, calcining, crushing, grinding, sieving, bagging and loading. These processes can be very dusty. Clay is used in the manufacture of bricks, pottery, tiles and refractories, as a filler in paper, pharmaceuticals, other chemicals, cosmetics, rubber and plaster and for waterproofing dams and other structures. Fuller's earth is used mainly for refining and purifying oils and other liquids and for bonding foundry mouldings. It was formerly used for cleaning and thickening wool cloth. Bentonite has its main use as a lubricant and sealing agent in drilling oil wells. Synthetic crystalline aluminium silicate (mullite) which is a waste product of extracting potash from alunite clay has been used as cat litter.

The production of purified, finely divided kaolin creates much dust which can cause simple pneumoconiosis. This is a hazard of the manufacture of china clay as in Cornwall where in 1976 nearly 5% of workers were found to have category 2 or above. The presence of pneumoconiosis was associated with a reduction in vital capacity without much change in forced expiratory volume (FEV_1), residual volume or transfer factor. A cross-sectional study in the U.S.A. demonstrated respiratory impairment in men with progressive massive fibrosis. Exposure to kaolin appeared not to contribute to chronic bronchitis or wheeze but might have interacted with smoking to aggravate breathlessness on exertion. Thus kaolin pneumoconiosis causes a restrictive type of ventilatory defect but extensive fibrosis has not been reported. Fuller's earth pneumoconiosis is also very uncommon and similarly benign. No pneumoconiosis has been reported amongst workers with bentonite but the mineral is contaminated with cristobalite which can cause silicosis (page 145). Mullite used for cats' litter has been found to cause pulmonary granulomas with associated arthralgia and other features of a generalized constitutional disorder. The condition was thought by Musk and colleagues to have an immunological basis; it may progress to diffuse pulmonary fibrosis.

Coal dust - chapter 9

Cobalt

Cobalt (Co, atomic mass 58.9) is a hard, silver-grey, magnetic metal. It is obtained as a by-product of production of copper, nickel and zinc and is used in the manufacture of permanent magnets, high temperature alloys and sintered tungsten carbide cutting tools. Salts of cobalt are used as pigments in glass and pottery, as ink and as bleaching agents and catalysts.

Depending on circumstances the extraction and purification of cobalt may entail exposure to carbon monoxide, hydrogen disulphide, chlorine or arsenic as well as to cobalt fumes. Dust containing cobalt is released during the manufacture and grinding of tungsten carbide (hard metal) tools. Cobalt carbonyls have the additional hazard that they release carbon monoxide during decomposition. Radioactive cobalt (^{60}Co) is produced in nuclear reactors; it emits γ radiation (page 252).

Cobalt is an essential trace metal which is present in vitamin B12. It interferes with the action of decarboxylating and other enzymes including creatine phosphokinase and lactate dehydrogenase and has a number of biological effects; these include stimulating the production of red blood cells, damaging the islet cells of the pancreas and exerting a toxic effect upon the heart leading to cardiomyopathy which may be fatal.

Exposure to cobalt fumes can cause skin sensitization, occupational asthma (see refs.) and in high concentration, pulmonary oedema. Inhalation of dust from manufacture of hard metal may cause fibrosing alveolitis and this condition if not controlled may progress to diffuse interstitial fibrosis (see hard metal below).

Cotton dust - chapter 14

Cutting oils

Cutting oils are liquids used for cooling and lubricating metal during high speed cutting, grinding and turning. Formerly they were usually mineral oils or emulsions of mineral oil and water. Their use led to the formation of lipid aerosol (page 281). Now many cutting oils are

References page 304

synthetic liquids which contain no oil; instead they comprise a base liquid, usually water, plus additives which include antioxidants and other corrosion inhibitors, extreme pressure additives, antifoamers, colourants, germicides and deodorants. They may also be contaminated by bacteria and contain metal particles. Persons exposed to these liquids may develop occupational asthma from becoming sensitized to one or more of the constituents, for example, pine oil or colophony (chapter 16). The cutting oils may also contribute to chronic bronchitis (table 17.1, page 375).

Most recent studies of workers exposed to oil mists have shown little evidence of disease. This probably reflects awareness of the problem and application of preventive measures. These should not be relaxed because of the general risk and the particular effects of secondary bacterial infection of the oil. The latter may alter the chemical composition of the oil, introduce human pathogens into the lung or introduce normally saphrophytic *Pseudomonas* or *Klebsiella* which can become pathogenic in special circumstances, for example during treatment with immuno-suppressant drugs.

Cyanogen and related substances

Cyanogen ($(CN)_2$) is a pungent, colourless gas which in low concentration smells of almonds. It is produced from cyanide salts or from hydrocyanic acid (HCN). The latter may be produced by reaction of ammonia and methane with air or of coke oven gas with sodium carbonate; it is also formed by treating cyanide salts with acid or by the decomposition of formaldehyde or isocyanate. Some cyanide compounds are given in table 13.8.

Cyanides combine with cytochrome oxidase and related enzymes so that they are no longer able to transport oxygen. The cyanide ion also combines with that part of the blood haemoglobin (approximately 2%) which is normally in the form of methaemoglobin. In acute poisoning the blood oxygen tension remains high whilst the tissues become starved of oxygen. Hypoxia in the carotid body leads to hyperventilation. The patient is usually pale, giddy and confused, with a feeling of constriction in the chest. The

Table 13.8. Cyanogen and related compounds

		State at 20°C	Major uses
Cyanogen	(CN)$_2$	Gas	Fumigant
Cyanogen bromide	CNBr	Liquid	Pesticide, gold extraction, organic synthesis
Cyanogen chloride	CNCl	Gas	Fumigant, warning gas (irritant)
Hydrocyanic acid	HCN	Liquid	Manufacture of acrylonitrile (page 256), electroplating, rodenticide, insecticide
Sodium cyanide	NaCN	Crystalline	As for HCN, also hardening steel

breath smells of oil of bitter almonds. In addition the halogenated cyanide compounds (CNBr and CNCl) are highly irritant to the eyes and respiratory tract. In low concentration they cause lachrymation and in the concentration 10ppm may cause pulmonary oedema. The acute poisoning may progress to convulsions and death. Subacute cyanogen poisoning may be associated with headache, palpitations, nausea and vomiting whilst chronic exposure leads to muscular weakness and necrosis of the nasal mucosa which may progress to perforation of the nasal septum.

The diagnosis of subacute or chronic cyanogen poisoning depends on obtaining a history of exposure, but in the case of acute poisoning the clinical features may be sufficient indication. Diagnosis must be made early and even then may be to no avail. The patient should be removed from exposure and immediately treated with a nitrite drug, for example sodium nitrite by intravenous infusion; the dosage is 0.5mg given over 10min. The nitrite converts a proportion of the blood haemoglobin to methaemoglobin which then combines with cyanide ions in the blood to form cyanmethaemoglobin; the latter substance is chemically inert. The cyanide is subsequently detoxicated to cyanate by the enzyme rhodanase and this action is assisted by sodium thiosulphate which, given intravenously, provides a source of sulphur (CN^- + $S_2O_3^=$ → SCN^- + etc). If this treatment is ineffective or if the patient is comatose the cyanide should be inactivated with cobalt ethylene-diamine-tetraacetate (cobalt EDTA, Kelocyanor) in the dosage of 300 mg i.v. Assisted ventilation and intravenous noradrenaline and hydrocortisone may also be indicated.

Prevention of cyanogen poisoning is by practice of good occupational hygiene. This includes educating all those who may be at risk, labelling all products containing cyanides, achieving a high standard of personal and factory cleanliness and ensuring that the concentration of cyanide compounds in the respired gas is within the hygiene standard. Methods for achieving this are discussed in chapter 3. Where a respirator is used it should be fitted with a chemical cartridge for neutralizing toxic dust and hydrocyanic acid gas. Specialist publications should be consulted for details.

Diesel fumes

Compared with spark-ignition engines diesel engines have a higher thermodynamic efficiency and produce less carbon monoxide and hydrocarbon fumes. For these reasons they are more suitable for use in mines and confined spaces. There is an increased emission of oxides of nitrogen but this can be controlled by not overloading the engine, by ensuring that all parts are functioning optimally (including air filter, injection pump, nozzle, tuning and compression) and by arranging for partial re-use of the exhaust gases. The emission is greatest when the engine is cold and when it is overloaded. It can then contain smoke, odours and acrolein together with the substances mentioned above. The acrolein causes lachrymation and this together with the noise and smoke have given diesel fumes a bad reputation. The respiratory effects have been studied amongst personnel of bus depots, railway workers, miners of coal, salt and potash, and tunnel workers. In some instances an excess of respiratory symptoms has been observed but not impairment of lung function. Evidence for a dose–response relationship is inconclusive. There is no excess mortality from lung cancer. Further longitudinal studies are in progress but on present evidence diesel fumes do not constitute a material respiratory hazard.

Dimethyl sulphate

Dimethyl sulphate $(CH_3)_2SO_4$ is an oily liquid which is prepared by treating methyl alcohol with fuming sulphuric acid (oleum) and distilling *in vacuo*. It is widely used as a methylating agent in the chemical industry and as a solvent for separating mineral oils. In the presence of moisture the compound hydrolyses to sulphuric acid and methyl alcohol; the toxic effects are mainly due to the acid and resemble those of phosgene gas (page 292). The possible occurrence of bronchial carcinoma after long-term exposure has been suspected but not confirmed.

Dioxane

Dioxane $(OCH_2CH_2OCH_2CH_2)$ is a colourless, volatile liquid produced from ethylene glycol or other compounds. It is used extensively as a solvent for fats, dyes, paints, lacquers and organic substances, as a wetting agent in adhesives and for other applications in laboratories and elsewhere. In a concentration of 200ppm dioxane causes irritation of the eyes and respiratory tract. Higher concentrations may cause pulmonary oedema. However, the principal hazard is toxic injury to the liver and kidney following absorption through the skin.

Emulsifying oils - see cutting oils, page 274

Ethanol

Ethanol or ethyl alcohol (C_2H_5OH) is a colourless liquid which is a constituent of alcoholic beverages. It is the starting point for many processes in organic chemistry including some which lead to the production of plastics and synthetic rubber. It is also an additive for petrol and a solvent.

The principal toxic effects are upon the central nervous system, gastro-intestinal tract, liver

and heart. The lungs may be damaged as a result of being associated with other adverse factors. Alcoholics tend to be smokers and are exposed to tobacco smoke in bars and public houses. Some alcoholics have a diet deficient in vitamins and protein, live in cold or damp houses and suffer exposure to the elements; these features contribute to chronic bronchitis and impaired respiratory function. However, alcoholism is now a problem throughout industry; workers in the alcoholic beverage industry are at greatest risk. Much of the pulmonary abnormality is due to the circumstances of being an alcoholic. Occasionally the lung function may be impaired secondary to alcoholic cirrhosis of the liver. In addition the lungs may be affected by ethanol itself. Inhaled ethanol dilates the bronchi if they are constricted. In some subjects ethanol acts as a bronchoconstrictor whilst in others constriction occurs as a result of becoming sensitized to constituents of the beverage (chapter 16). Ethanol in high concentration reduces the respiratory responses to hypercapnia and hypoxia; in lower concentration it reduces the tone in the genio glossal muscle. This predisposes to obstruction to the airway during sleep, leading to sleep apnoea. Thus a high alcohol intake has a number of adverse consequences for the lungs as well as for other organs; they are an added reason for the occupational physician detecting and correcting the problem at an early stage.

Formaldehyde - chapter 12, page 259

Fumes from fires (fire-fighting)

Fire-fighting entails exposure to toxic gases which are generated by incomplete combustion, thermal degradation (pyrolysis) and vapourization. The gas mixture is critically dependent on the substrates present, the temperature which is achieved and the availability of oxygen. These variables are in turn influenced by the stage of the fire and the external circumstances. The combustion products may react chemically to produce additional toxic substances or they may interact biologically; the total tissue damage then exceeds that due to the components separately. Some substances to which fire-fighters may

Table 13.9. Toxic substances released by pyrolysis or partial combustion

Substance	Source	Page
Carbon dioxide	Product of combustion	270
Carbon monoxide	Incomplete combustion of substances containing carbon	270
Hydrogen chloride gas	Acrylonitrile, polyvinyl chloride	272
Phosgene (uncommon)		292
Hydrogen fluoride	Polytetrafluorethylene	—
Oxides of nitrogen	Veneers, wallpapers	285
Acrolein	Acrilan furnishing, polyethylene, polyurethane	265
Ammonia	Nylon	266
Formaldehyde	Polyethylene (see chapter 12)	259
Other aldehydes and vapours	Lacquers, chemicals	—
Isocyanates	Polyurethane foam	265
Hydrogen cyanide gas	Isocyanates, polyurethane foam, polyacrylonitrile	274
Sulphur dioxide	Sulphur compounds	294
Lipid aerosol	Burning fat	281

be exposed are listed in table 13.9. The table gives the page in the text where additional information may be found. The greatest hazards are carbon monoxide which causes tissue hypoxia and irritant gases; the latter damage the respiratory tract and may cause pulmonary oedema. The oedema is usually of late onset, occurring 12–24h after the fire.

Firemen who attend major fires often develop acute symptoms. These include pain in the eyes and beneath the sternum, cough, breathlessness on exertion, headache and nausea. There is bronchoconstriction leading to airflow limitation and uneven distribution of ventilation and perfusion leading to hypoxaemia. These changes are due to the irritant gases. Thermal injury to the respiratory tract is a rare and frequently fatal consequence of unconsciousness. Burns to the skin of the thorax can reduce vital capacity; the reduction is usually progressive over several days after which there is slow recovery.

The acute respiratory symptoms usually disappear within 24h; if they do not incipient pulmonary oedema should be suspected. The complication may be diagnosed early by a short period of observation in hospital and this is recommended for men who develop material acute symptoms during a fire; however, pulmonary oedema may occur in the absence of such symptoms and firemen need to be aware of this possibility. Appropriate treatment should be given as soon as practicable.

Following an acute episode recovery is usually complete but an enhanced annual decline of forced expiratory volume has been observed in some studies of working firemen; not all studies show this effect. In addition a small number of firemen have gone on to develop chronic bronchitis, persistent chronic airflow limitation or disease of the lung parenchyma; in some men toxic gases have been responsible but in others persistent smoking, and anxiety linked to a claim for compensation has contributed to the associated disablement.

Because of the high risk run by firemen new recruits are required to be intelligent, and well motivated, with good physique and normal pulmonary function; they should not give a history of respiratory symptoms, chest illness or atopy. Men so selected have an above average lung size; however, once in service and despite attempts at physical training they often put on weight and frequently do not have a high level of physical fitness. Thus long-term surveillance is essential.

Conventional hygiene measures cannot be used to protect firemen but correct technique may make the difference between life and death. When burning buildings are entered compressed air breathing apparatus must be worn. A respirator cannot provide protection against dangerous gases of unknown composition.

Haematite - see Iron

Hair spray

Hairdressers and beauticians use a wide range of substances including bleaches, dyes, permanent wave lotions, shampoos, depilatory creams or lotions and setting lacquers. These contain added colourants, perfumes, oils and excipients. They may be applied as pressurized aerosol, for which the propellant is usually a fluorochloro-hydrocarbon (freon), or as foam, liquid, cream or powder. Many of the substances are potentially harmful so there is risk of occupational disease.

The main health problem is skin sensitization and dermatitis which affect approximately 0.2% of hairdressers. An increased incidence of cancer of the urinary tract is also a possibility. Pulmonary complications include occupational asthma from sensitization to persulphate bleaching agents (page 368) and thesaurosis. This condition of diffuse pulmonary granulomatosis or hilar gland enlargement has been attributed in individual cases to inhalation of polyvinyl pyrrolidone, polyvinyl acetate and shellac. However, with respect to the last of these Parkes has suggested that the condition may be a lipid pneumonia due to oil used as a solvent. Some of the other reported cases were probably sarcoidosis. Epidemiological studies have so far not demonstrated an association with occupation but for many women hairdressers the period of exposure has been relatively short. In experimental studies a reduction in mucociliary transport and narrowing of small lung airways have been observed. Thus whilst the risk of hairdressers developing thesaurosis appears to have been over-estimated the possibility of respiratory symptoms being due to occupation should be borne in mind. Persons intending to set up a hairdressing salon should install open circuit exhaust ventilation despite the increase in overhead costs for heating which this entails.

Hard metal - see also Cobalt

Cemented or sintered metal carbides are

References page 305

extremely tough and hard and in consequence make excellent cutting tips for drills and other cutting tools. They are also used for armaments. The substances were developed in Germany in the 1930s and the disease associated with their production is known by the English translation of the German name, 'hart metale'. The main constituent is tungsten carbide produced from wolfram but other metal carbides may be added including titanium, tantalum and vanadium carbide. These substances are prepared by heating the powdered metal oxide with carbon in an atmosphere of hydrogen and the resulting carbide after sieving is mixed with powdered cobalt or other metal which serves as a binding agent. The mixture is milled, then the powder is separated off, mixed with wax, moulded and preheated in an atmosphere of hydrogen at 1000°C. The resulting pre-sintered blank is subsequently shaped, sintered at 1500°C in an atmosphere of hydrogen and ground wet with diamond or carborundum to give a cutting edge.

Workers producing hard metal are at risk of developing diffuse interstitial fibrosis though under modern conditions the incidence is low. The condition was formerly associated with exposure to respirable dust produced during milling the mixed ingredients but it has now been observed in the wet grinding stage. Here workers are exposed to aerosol containing ionized cobalt which is dissolved in the coolant fluid. The condition is believed to be due to the cobalt which is a sensitizing agent capable of causing dermatitis and occupational asthma in susceptible persons (page 273); however, its role in causing hard metal disease has not been confirmed. The condition may present as bronchoalveolitis with dry cough, breathlessness on exertion, loss of weight, râles on auscultation of the chest and irregular opacities on the chest radiograph. Histologically the features are typical of desquamating fibrosing alveolitis. They usually clear up completely on withdrawal from exposure but the sensitization persists so a short re-exposure causes rapid worsening of the condition. The illness can progress to diffuse interstitial fibrosis. A favourable outcome is assisted by treatment with corticosteroids and by the patient avoiding further exposure to cobalt.

Herbicides - see Paraquat

Indium

Indium (atomic mass 114.8) is a soft, malleable metal which is found in association with zinc mineral and is recovered commercially from the slag. The process may entail dissolution in acid and subsequent electroplating onto rods. The metal is resistant to corrosion and on this account it is used for coating other metals and glass, in alloys, bearings, motion picture screens, etc. The alloy with antimony and germanium is used in transistors and other electronic components.

Welding or soldering indium generates fumes which may acutely damage the lung parenchyma but the hazard appears to be small. In animal studies the main sites of tissue damage are the liver and kidneys.

Inert dust pneumoconiosis

The defence mechanisms against respirable particles depositing on the alveolar epithelium ensure that the great majority are removed during passage through the airways or are exhaled (chapter 4). The lung is subsequently cleansed of most deposited substances by their becoming dissolved, digested or phagocytosed and then eliminated. A few substances set up an acute toxic reaction (page 292), some initiate a specific response which is described in other chapters. Several merely accumulate in the lung where they cause a benign simple pneumoconiosis. The condition is diagnosed from the presence of simple pneumoconiosis on the chest radiograph (chapter 5) plus a history of occupational or environmental exposure. Substances which behave in this way are listed in table 13.10. In many instances the opacities disappear following removal from exposure (e.g. fig. 13.7, page 302).

Iron

Iron vapour and iron oxide are highly radio-opaque so dust inhaled into the lung readily causes siderosis which is simple pneumoconiosis due to iron (fig. 13.3). Exposure may occur during mining or quarrying haematite, limonite, magnetic pyrite or other ore containing iron. Other minerals or contaminants of the ore, including arsenic, may also cause symptoms. The ore may contain quartz when the condition merges into silicosis (sidero-silicosis, see fig. 13.4 and chapter 8). Cumbrian haematite mines are contaminated by radon gas from trace quantities of uranium and this is probably responsible for the raised prevalence of lung cancer (page 254).

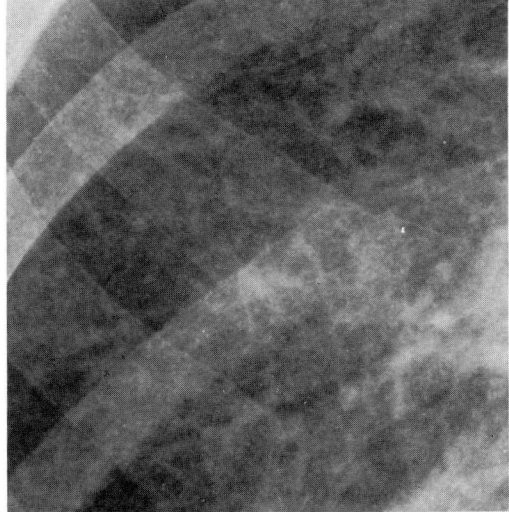

Table 13.10. Some causes of inert dust pneumoconiosis

Antimony	Iron (siderosis)
Barium (baritosis)	Manganese
Bismuth	Mica
Boron	Tin (stannosis)
Carbon*	Titanium
Cerium	Tungsten
China clay	Yttrium
Fuller's earth	Zirconium†

* May give rise to progressive massive fibrosis or be associated with emphysema (chapter 9).
† Granulomatous reaction occurs in animals.

Fig. 13.3. Detail from chest radiograph showing siderosis (category 3p) in a 61-year-old vehicle welder (ex-smoker). The patient presented with breathlessness on exertion due to moderate airflow limitation which was largely corrected by inhalation of salbutamol (FEV_1 1.49 l and 1.85 l, reference value 2.5 l).

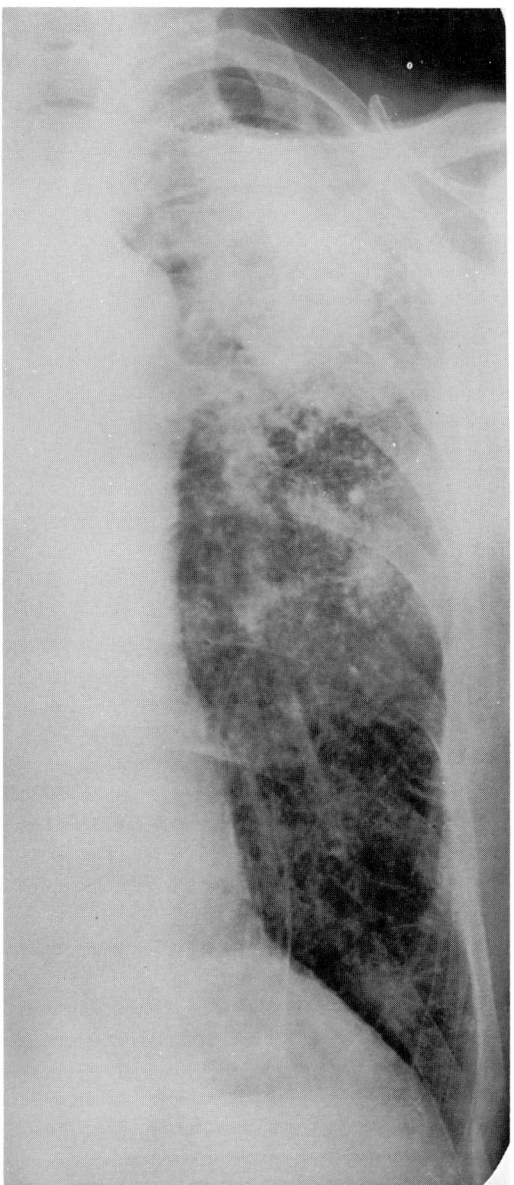

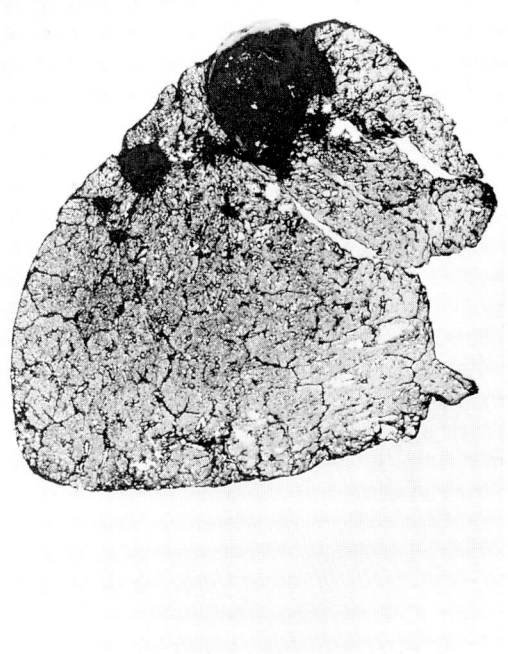

Fig. 13.4. Left chest radiograph and paper-mounted lung section showing confluent silicosis in a man who died at age 81 from carcinoma of the stomach. From age 24 to age 52 he had been a haematite miner and subsequently he developed respiratory insufficiency. Silicosis was diagnosed at age 69 and later was clearly visible on the large lung section. This was predominantly brown in colour due to the presence of iron oxide. (By courtesy of J. E. M. Hutchinson.)

Siderosis can occur from dust generated when processing the ore, using it as a pigment or for polishing, from scouring scaling or grinding ingots, boilers and other structures made of iron and from vapourization of iron during welding, cutting, gouging or cleaning iron objects with an oxyacetylene torch or electric arc. In most circumstances the condition is asymptomatic, the

References page 305

lung function is within normal limits and at post-mortem, whilst iron is present in the lung parenchyma, there is no tissue reaction. However, Sadoul observed that in the iron ore miners of Lorraine the siderosis was complicated by emphysema; there was then an increased physiological deadspace and hypoxaemia occurred on exercise. Siderosis in welders is considered on page 298. The quantity of iron, magnetite and other ferromagnetic material in the lung, including nickel, can be estimated by magneto-pneumography; the dust is magnetized in a powerful magnetic field which is then removed and the residual magnetism measured using a sensitive external magnetometer. The method is reviewed by Lippmann.

Lead - chapter 12, page 250

Limestone and lime

Limestone (calcite) is mainly calcium carbonate but may also contain magnesium carbonate (dolomite), clay or quartz. Of these substances only the quartz is harmful (chapter 8). Limestone is used in construction work, as a powder for preventing explosions in coal mines, and for production of cement, calcium oxide (CaO) and calcium hydroxide $Ca(OH)_2$. The stages in production are crushing, grinding, mixing with coal and other substances, calcining in a kiln which is usually operating continuously and melting the resulting clinker. The process liberates carbon dioxide from the calcium carbonate and carbon monoxide from incomplete combustion and these gases may cause respectively asphyxia and carbon monoxide poisoning (page 270). The calcium oxide (quick lime) may burn the conjunctivae and mucous membrane of the mouth or larynx; the burns are mainly due to heat liberated by reaction of aqueous secretions with anhydrous calcium oxide to form hydroxide. The intensity of the reaction usually protects the lower respiratory tract but chronic bronchitis and pneumonia have been reported. The limestone dust is soluble in body fluid and does not cause pneumoconiosis; however, when the dust contains more than 2% of quartz there is a risk of silicosis. This is the case for some pseudo-marbles (see Basalt, page 267) but not marble itself which is a limestone. The processing of gypsum which is crystalline calcium sulphate used for mortar and plaster board may carry a similar small risk from quartz contamination. Dust from lime or cement products to which asbestos has been added as reinforcement (e.g. asbestos cement) is a possible source of asbestosis (chapter 10).

Lipid aerosol

The respiratory defence mechanisms against inhaled fat particles appear to be relatively ineffective so if lipid aerosol is inhaled it may give rise to lipid pneumonia. This may occur in industry from inhalation of oil mist generated during spraying or by high-speed cutting or drilling, from water contaminated with oil, during firefighting, in catering operations, smoking oiled leaf tobacco, and other activities. Some of these are listed in table 13.11. For other effects of cutting oils see page 274.

Table 13.11. Some circumstances which may generate lipid aerosol

---

Spraying oil for rust preservation, lubrication or cutting
De-greasing with water jets
Aerosol formed during high speed rotation of spindles, drills, etc.
Vapour from cooling drop forgings, hot-rolled steel, dies, castings, etc.
Treatment of vegetable fibres (rope, sacking, etc.) and leather
Application of surface films
Spraying lipid-soluble chemicals in agriculture
Burning fat, e.g. for demonstrating fire extinguishers
Fighting oil fires
Heating oil for deep-frying
Smoking black-fat tobacco (rolled leaf softened with mineral oil)

Lipid pneumonia may be diffuse or localized depending on the nature of the exposure. Inhaled aerosol may cause lesions which are predominantly basal or widely distributed throughout the lung. Water contaminated with oil may cause massive lesions of part of the lung whilst the oil itself may cause localized granulomas. The clinical features reflect the type of exposure. Acute lipid pneumonia presents with cough, malaise, breathlessness and chest pain. The lung function is often materially impaired with reductions in vital capacity, transfer factor and arterial oxygen tension. The chest radiograph shows bilateral basal miliary nodules, or medium-sized opacities which are predominantly linear and may be mistaken for diffuse interstitial fibrosis. If the exposure is mild the radiographic features may develop insidiously without acute symptoms; subsequent progressively increasing breathlessness on exertion initially may be attributed to increasing age.

The lung at biopsy or post-mortem shows a spectrum of changes from acute pneumonia with fat-laden macrophages and giant cells through reticulin formation and accumulation of lymphocytes and plasma cells to endarteritis and the formation of granulomas, interstitial fibrosis, hyaline degeneration and necrosis. The fat droplets stain with Sudan IV, or in the case of most fats of vegetable or animal origin with osmium tetroxide.

The differential diagnosis of lipid pneumonia is extensive and whilst the condition may be recognized from the occupational history and clinical features it is easily missed. A good occupational history is essential. The diagnosis in an individual case may only be made at biopsy. The treatment is by removal from exposure and administration of corticosteroid drugs.

There is no clear evidence that oil mist is a lung carcinogen but the occurrence of skin warts and cancer, including scrotal cancer, from shale oil in cotton mill mule spinners and amongst users of neat cutting oils is well documented.

Lithium hydride

Lithium hydride (LiH) is a gas which is used for transporting hydrogen, as fuel and as a reducing agent. In low concentration the gas is an irritant and stimulates receptors in the respiratory tract to cause sneezing and coughing; in high concentration it causes pulmonary oedema. The hygiene standard is given in chapter 1.

Magnesium

Magnesium is the lightest of the structural metals and emits an intense light when it is burnt; these two properties determine its main uses. Production is usually by electrolysis of magnesium chloride or precipitation of carbonate from sea water, carnallite ore or chlorinated magnesium oxide. The metal fumes may give rise to metal fume fever (page 283) but do not damage the lungs. However, damage may occur

References page 305

in the event of fire (page 276) or from sulphur dioxide which is used to separate the metal from air during casting. Magnesium carbonate is used for thermal insulation in conjunction with asbestos; it may contribute to the small rounded opacities which are sometimes present on the chest radiographs of laggers.

Magnetite - see Iron

Manganese

Manganese is a major constituent of the earth's crust and is used extensively in the production of steel and steel alloys, welding rods, dry cell batteries and manganese chemicals which in turn have many uses. It is usually obtained from manganese dioxide which is mined in many parts of the world. The ore is sometimes contaminated with quartz which can give rise to silicosis. The manganese dust interacts with smoking to cause chronic bronchitis; the fumes may cause metal fume fever (see below) and the oxide may cause chemical pneumonitis as in the manufacture of high alloy steel. The manganese content of hair from exposed workers is reported to be increased. The principal chronic effect of manganese is upon the central nervous system where the symptoms resemble Parkinson's disease.

Man-made mineral fibres - chapter 10, page 228

Mercury

Mercury occurs naturally as sulphide in cinnabar ore which is mined in U.S.S.R., Spain, Algeria, China and other countries. The liquid metal is produced by heating or by reduction with iron or quick lime. It has a vast number of uses and is highly toxic so stringent precautions are necessary in its manufacture and use. Mercurial poisoning affects mainly the gastrointestinal tract, the kidneys and the central nervous system where the best known lesions are 'hatters shakes' and dementia from mercurial nitrate used for making felt, hence 'mad as a hatter'.

Mercury vapour enters the body via the respiratory tract. It is a cause of metal fume fever (q.v.)

and in high concentration causes chemical pneumonitis; this usually arises from an accident or from unintended misuse, for example, evaporating drops of mercury on a domestic stove. The vapour is invisible, odourless and tasteless and the first symptom is irritation of the pharynx and lungs some 4h after exposure. The irritation may progress to ulceration of the pharynx and to pneumonitis with pain, cough, dyspnoea and chest tightness. The victim may also have metal fume fever and signs of damage to the gastro-intestinal and central nervous systems. The pulmonary changes may progress to desquamation of alveolar lining cells, pulmonary oedema and death, either within the first few days or as a result of infection or interference with gas exchange. At this stage there is a hyaline membrane and cellular infiltration by lymphocytes. Recovery is assisted by energetic medical treatment of the pulmonary oedema supplemented by penicillamine and by intramuscular BAL (2,3-dimercaptopropanol). Subsequently the health is usually fully restored but the condition may progress to diffuse interstitial fibrosis.

Metal fume fever

The condition was originally called brass founders' ague. It occurs amongst workers exposed to fumes of zinc and other metals. Some are listed in table 13.12. The related conditions of polymer fume fever and cotton mill fever are considered respectively on pages 292 and 315.

Metal fume fever is due to fumes having a particle size in the range 0.05–0.5μm; these particles enter the acinus where many are deposited. The first symptom may be a dry, foul taste in the mouth; this is followed at 4–8h by pharyngeal or nasal irritation, cough, chest pain and generalized malaise with muscle pains, weakness, nausea, headache and anxiety. Fever

Table 13.12. Metals whose fumes may cause metal fume fever

Zinc	Aluminium	Manganese
Copper	Antimony	Mercury
Magnesium	Iron	Nickel
Cadmium		

may develop at about 12h preceded by rigors and followed after a few hours by deep sleep and profuse sweating. Polyuria and diarrhoea may occur and there is a polymorphonuclear leucocytosis. Recovery is usually complete within 24h but this is not invariable. The differential diagnosis includes influenza and acute cadmium poisoning which should be borne in mind as it is a much more serious condition (page 247).

Individuals differ in their susceptibility to metal fume fever and those who develop the condition usually acquire immunity; this is often short-lived and disappears during a few days away from work, for example, at the weekend. The condition may then reappear as Monday fever. Persons of above average susceptibility usually leave the industry and the remainder seldom develop symptoms; however, in shipyard welders an association with chronic wheeze has recently been observed. There is no specific treatment.

Metal, hard: see hard metal

Mica

Mica is an aluminium silicate containing potassium (muscovite), magnesium and iron (vermiculite), lithium and other combinations of minerals. The material is mined or quarried in India, South Africa, U.S.A. and other countries. Muscovite may be split into flat sheets which are transparent, tough, resistant to heat and do not conduct electricity. It formerly had many uses but is now being replaced by homogeneous synthetic materials. Mica powder is widely used in manufacture of electric cables, pneumatic tyres, welding electrodes, paints, dry lubricants, dielectric dressings, flameproof insulators and other products. Vermiculite expands on heating to form porous granules which provide excellent thermal insulation; the granules have replaced asbestos for many applications.

Mica dust can contribute to chronic bronchitis or cause simple pneumoconiosis in exposed persons but it appears not to be fibrogenic. However, the mineral is sometimes contaminated with other substances including tremolite which is fibrogenic and probably carcinogenic.

Thus the extraction and purification of mica is not always without risk.

Mustard gas - chapter 12, page 259

Mycotic infections of the lung

Fungal mycelia and spores are a relatively common cause of extrinsic allergic alveolitis; this condition is preceded by sensitization and in the active phase is characterized by the presence of appropriate antibodies in serum (chapter 15). Some fungal spores germinate and grow in the lung. The commonest is the *Aspergillus* species; this is present in most decaying vegetation and litter used by cattle and poultry. Thus, many people are exposed to *Aspergillus* species in the course of their occupation; however, illness on this account is uncommon and does not occur in the absence of predisposing factors. Three types of clinical picture are recorded. (i) In a lung previously damaged by tuberculosis, sarcoidosis or diffuse pulmonary fibrosis the fungus may grow to form a mycetoma in a cavity. The sputum may then contain mycelium and precipitins to the fungus are present in the blood. The chest radiograph shows a loculated lesion or a newly filled cavity, often with a crescent of air separating the mycetoma from the cavity wall; this contains granulation tissue which may bleed. Treatment is unsatisfactory and unnecessary in the absence of symptoms but significant haemoptysis may require surgical removal of the lesions. (ii) In atopic subjects sensitization to the spores may result in eosinophilic infiltration of the lung parenchyma and the production of viscid mucous plugs. The granulomas may be visible on the chest radiograph as patches of pneumonia in the upper zones; segmental or lobar collapse may occur where bronchi are obstructed by mucus. There may be fever associated with secondary infection. Prick tests for aspergillin produce an immediate positive reaction and precipitin tests are usually positive. These features occur mainly in asthmatics. In others allergic alveolitis may develop. Treatment is by corticosteroid drugs supplemented where appropriate by bronchodilators and antibiotics. (iii) Invasion of the lung parenchyma may rarely occur in the presence of an immuno-

logical deficiency state or where the patient is debilitated on account of severe disease. The condition is reviewed by Crofton & Douglas.

Coccidioidomycosis is an infection with *Coccidioides immitis* which normally grows in the soil in parts of Northern California, Southern U.S.A. and South America. The organism requires a dry climate and a light soil: it becomes airborne when the soil is disturbed by construction work, excavations or high wind causing a dust storm. Archaeologists, geologists and naturalists, service men and women and persons engaged in transporting or receiving materials from endemic areas are at risk. The condition presents as a low grade pneumonia, often 2–4 weeks after a storm. There is fever, usually with localizing symptoms and physical signs relating to the lung. The chest x-ray shows infiltrations, usually in the upper half of the lung fields, precipitating antibodies are present in the serum and the lung tissue contains fungal mycelium surrounded by granulomata. The attack rate following a storm has been assessed at 9% by Flynn and colleagues, with negroid and mongoloid people more at risk than those of Eurasian origin. In a proportion of cases the condition subsequently spreads via the blood stream to other organs or it may become chronic in the lung. Prevention and treatment are considered below.

Cryptococcus neoformans grows in droppings of pigeons and other birds. The human lung may occasionally become infected by spores inhaled during handling the birds or clearing away their excreta. However, this is uncommon except when the resistance to infection is reduced; the organism may then occasionally spread to other organs and tissues.

Histoplasmosis is due to infection with *Histoplasma capsulatum*. The fungus grows in infected soil or other media which is enriched with droppings (guano) from birds or bats; the latter species may become infected and then spread the disease. This exists in most countries between latitudes 45 degrees north and south of the equator, particularly in North and South America and in Africa. It is rare in Europe and then only following migration from an endemic area. The disease is prevalent amongst chicken farmers, in those clearing old silos contaminated

References page 305

with pigeon excreta, persons clearing city parks where there are starlings, maintenance engineers on bridges, vets, epidemiologists and spelaeologists. Infection, usually by inhaling the spores, is asymptomatic and confined to the lung. However, the condition may resemble pulmonary tuberculosis with fever, a primary complex in the lung, enlarged lymph nodes, multiple small discrete lesions and occasionally cavitation. Healed lesions may calcify. Dissemination of the infection may lead to enlargement of spleen and liver, anaemia and leukopenia. Addison's disease may occur from involvement of the suprarenals. The subject usually exhibits delayed skin hypersensitivity, complement fixing antibodies, precipitating antibodies and actively growing mycelium which may be cultured from the sputum.

Sporotrichum schenkii is a yeast which grows in soil in warm, damp places in the U.S.A. and elsewhere but not in Europe. Factory workers, greenhouse attendants, florists, horticulturists, workers in deep mines and laboratory technicians in endemic areas are at risk, but the condition is rare. Spores contaminate the sharp spines of plants or trees and may be carried into the subcutaneous tissue by inoculation if the skin is pierced. A granulomatous nodule may then form and ulcerate or the infection may spread along lymphatics. Pulmonary sporotrichosis occurs from inhaling the spores. The lesions are visible on the chest radiograph; they are usually asymptomatic and respond to treatment.

Prevention of pulmonary mycosis depends on disinfecting the spores, preventing them becoming airborne or providing personal respirators (chapter 3). Fungicides added to mine water were used to stop an epidemic amongst South African gold mines but in general the hygiene measures are seldom very effective. *Active treatment* is necessary only in a proportion of cases and should be carried out in hospital. It may take the form of intravenous or if appropriate intrathecal amphotericin B. The dosage is 0.5–1.0mg per kg body mass in 0.5 l glucose solution over 6h on alternate days for approximately 4 weeks. Heparin (10mg) can be added to reduce the risk of local venous thrombosis. Amphotericin has other disagreeable side-

effects which may need to be controlled with prednisolone. The antifungal drugs, nystatin and natamycin by inhalation may also be used; however, the chemotherapy seldom effects a complete cure.

Nickel - chapter 12

Nitriles

These substances contain a terminal cyano group and the general formula $R-C\equiv N$, where R is usually a hydrocarbon radical. They are highly reactive and used extensively in the manufacture of organic chemicals. On heating they decompose, liberating cyanogen fumes which are highly toxic (page 274). See also acrylonitrile (page 256).

Nitrogen oxides

Oxygen and nitrogen react to form a series of compounds having from one up to five oxygen atoms for every two atoms of nitrogen (table 13.13). The oxides are produced as by-products of a number of industrial processes and usually occur as a mixture. The exact composition of the mixture depends on local circumstances. The oxides may also be produced individually, for example nitrous oxide is formed by thermal decomposition of ammonium nitrate. This gas differs from the other oxides in being almost completely non-toxic; it is used extensively as a gaseous anaesthetic. Nitric oxide is a colourless gas with a sharp, sweet odour; it is generally regarded as non-toxic but in the presence of air oxidizes to nitrogen dioxide which in adequate concentration is highly toxic. Dinitrogen trioxide, dinitrogen tetraoxide and dinitrogen pentoxide normally occur only in low concentrations or for brief periods of time and are important mainly as steps in the formation of nitrogen dioxide (table 13.13).

Nitrogen dioxide is a dense, reddish-brown gas which becomes a liquid at below 21°C. It has an irritating odour which is a consequence of the gas reacting slowly with water on the nasal epithelium to form nitrous and nitric acids (e.g. $NO_2 + H_2O \rightarrow HNO_3$). Depending on the conditions of exposure nitric acid can cause damage

Table 13.13. Nitrogen oxides

N_2O	Nitrous oxide (nitrogen suboxide)	Inert, anaesthetic gas
NO	Nitric oxide	Oxidizable gas, apparently inert
N_2O_3	Dinitrogen trioxide	Traces present in mixtures ($N_2O_3 \rightleftharpoons NO + NO_2$)
NO_2	Nitrogen oxide (nitrogen dioxide)	Brown irritant gas (liquid at $<21°C$)
N_2O_4	Dinitrogen tetraoxide	Two forms in equilibrium ($2NO_2 \rightleftharpoons N_2O_4$)
N_2O_5	Dinitrogen pentoxide	White crystals which decompose at $> -10°C$
		$2N_2O_5 \rightarrow O_2 + 2N_2O_4 \rightleftharpoons 4NO_2 + O_2$

to any part of the respiratory tract. The biological action reflects the concentration of NO_2 and the solubility of the gas in an aqueous medium.

Sources. Nitrogen oxides are produced when nitric acid is used for oxidation in industrial processes, when organic nitro-compounds explode or burn, when air is heated to a high temperature and when inorganic nitrates decompose.

Nitric acid oxidation is used extensively in the chemical industry for the manufacture of acids and other substances including polyamine intermediates for synthetic fibres. In the explosives industry nitric oxide oxidation is used in manufacture of ethylene glycol dinitrate, nitroglycerin, trinitrotoluene (TNT) and other explosives. It is also used in the manufacture of dye stuffs and pharmaceuticals, in photo-engraving, for pickling engineering components and for engraving jewellery.

Organic nitrogen based explosives contain nitrogen dioxide radicals; for example, nitroglycerin and trinitrotoluene (TNT) each have three NO_2 radicals per molecule, as has cyclotrimethylene trinitramine (RDX). Thus TNT = $CH_3.C_6H_2.(NO_2)_3$ and RDX = $(CH_2N)_3(NO_2)_3$. The explosives are used for the primary blasting of rock or mineral *in situ* during mining, quarrying, tunnelling, trenching and construction work. Secondary blasting of dislodged material is also carried out. The hazard from fume is greatest when blasting is undertaken in confined spaces, for example coal mines (page 166). For this application there are now permitted explosives which have a relatively non-toxic fume.

Nitrogen oxides are formed by combustion in cigarettes, furnaces, internal combustion engines and during conflagrations involving organic nitro-compounds, for example soft furnishings, wall coverings and veneers. Firemen

are at risk on the latter account (page 276). Release from internal combustion engines is greater for diesel than for spark-ignition engines. The fume can be hazardous in coal mines since diesels are used in preference to petrol engines, the latter being unsuitable because of sparks and of carbon monoxide in the exhaust. The nitrogen oxide emission from diesels is influenced by the design and reduced by ensuring that fuel and air are well mixed prior to ignition.

Fixation of atmospheric nitrogen occurs when the temperature of air is increased. This happens during welding, burning or gouging metal with an oxyacetylene flame or electric arc. Other electrical discharges have a similar effect. Both the initial temperature and the subsequent cooling influence the composition of the resulting gas: a high initial temperature and rapid cooling by a mass of unheated metal favour the accumulation of NO_2. Under similar environmental conditions burning leads to a higher concentration than welding but in practice burning is seldom undertaken in confined spaces. Metal-inert gas electric arc welding has the additional effect of forming ozone which then oxidizes the lower nitrogen oxides (N_2O and NO) to dinitrogen pentoxide. This decomposes to form NO_2 (table 13.13). Nitrogen oxides also participate in other reactions which can lead to the formation of complex chemical substances. Petrochemical smog is the most abundant source but any process which results in the formation of nitrogen oxides and other gases can be the starting point.

Decomposition of inorganic nitrates occurs from chemicals present in soil or added as fertilizer or conditioning agent. The nitrate provides energy for bacteria which, at a moderately low pH, reduce it to nitrite; this converts to nitrous acid, then decomposes to liberate nitrogen oxides ($2HNO_2 \rightleftharpoons H_2O + NO + NO_2$); the nitric

References page 306

oxide subsequently oxidizes to NO_2. Nitrates are the main source of nitrogen oxides in the higher atmosphere where they are present in trace amounts. The same process is responsible for high concentrations of NO_2 occurring in silos; these are pits, troughs, barns or towers used for storing fresh grass which is then used as winter feed for cattle. The nitrogen oxides are formed soon after the fodder is put into the silo and are the cause of silo fillers' disease (see below).

Effects. Nitrogen dioxide in high concentration (100–500ppm) is highly toxic and has been responsible for a number of deaths amongst exposed persons. It is also toxic to experimental animals. The exposure can cause immediate bronchospasm and death from respiratory failure. More often there is initial mild irritation of the eyes and respiratory tract; after an interval of up to 30h this is followed by progressive pulmonary oedema which is frequently fatal. Methaemoglobinaemia may occur but is usually mild. The exposure also causes acute bronchiolitis. This becomes apparent following resolution of pulmonary oedema; it also occurs with somewhat lower concentrations of NO_2 insufficient to cause oedema. The bronchiolitis is associated with narrowing of the airways which develops acutely and persists on account of repair with fibrous tissue; this *bronchiolitis fibrosa obliterans* can be fatal but usually responds to early treatment. Recovery can be complete or the condition may persist as chronic bronchiolar fibrosis. In some cases apparent recovery is followed after a period of weeks by a second acute episode; this takes the form of pulmonary oedema, pneumonia or bacterial infection. It is a fairly common complication and probably due to the initial exposure impairing the pulmonary defence mechanisms. To detect the complication at an early stage the immediate treatment (page 292) should be followed by close surveillance for at least 3 months.

In animal studies nitrogen dioxide in the concentration range 2–30ppm has been used extensively to investigate the mechanisms of lung injury and repair. However, mammals respond in different ways and the results cannot be transferred uncritically to man. The initial lesion is in respiratory bronchioles where the epithelium becomes more permeable, the number of alveolar macrophages increases and changes occur in the structural proteins, both collagen and elastin. The collagen is depleted but at the same time the rate of collagen synthesis is increased so repair occurs despite continuing exposure. There is accompanying hypertrophy and hyperplasia of the bronchiolar epithelium and increased fibroblast activity; this can lead to bronchiolar stenosis. The depletion of elastin is probably due to enzymes contained in alveolar macrophages and persists for the period of exposure. It is the cause of the mild emphysema which has been observed in some studies; the best documented are hamsters heavily exposed to NO_2 at birth and the blotchy mouse which is unduly susceptible to emphysema on account of having genetically abnormal connective tissue.

In man a 2h exposure to nitrogen dioxide in concentration 5ppm causes an increase in airways resistance; this in turn increases the alveolar to arterial tension difference for oxygen and lowers the arterial oxygen tension. Exposure to lower concentrations of NO_2 can increase the bronchial hyperreactivity to acetylcholine. The increased bronchomotor tone has been attributed to stimulation of lung irritant receptors and to release of histamine from mast cells; however, narrowing of large airways is not a feature of the clinical condition so the relevance of these observations is unclear. During recovery from pulmonary oedema evidence has been obtained for narrowing of small airways but not for emphysema.

An association between childhood respiratory infection and nitrogen dioxide in fumes from domestic gas cookers has been suspected in a number of studies; these have been reviewed by Fischer and colleagues. Nitrogen dioxide has also been incriminated as a cause of chest illnesses and of respiratory impairment in populations exposed to polluted atmospheres. The evidence is not conclusive either way (see references).

Occupational aspects. The only confirmed hazard from nitrogen dioxide is acute pulmonary oedema or bronchiolitis which can be fatal but which should respond completely to prompt treatment. The condition is likely to develop up to 30h after the exposure. Thus prevention by adhering to the hygiene standard for NO_2, overnight observation of the victim following an apparently benign incident and provision of prompt effective treatment are mandatory. Workers on farms where silage is made (see below) are at special risk but any of the processes and activities listed above might in some circumstances result in an NO_2 concentration in excess of 50ppm. One such activity was shot-firing with Hydrox shells in coal mines. The resulting emission was incriminated by Kennedy as a cause of emphysema. However, his coalminer patients were apparently referred on account of symptoms and the study did not include a control group or take into account other aetiological factors, for example, smoking. In epidemiological studies of shipyard and dockyard welders no evidence for an increased prevalence of emphysema has been observed. Concentrations of nitrogen dioxide in the range 5–50ppm are unlikely to cause acute disease. Whether or not they contribute to chronic ill-health is not known but this possibility is the reason for the hygiene standard being set at a relatively low level (page 16).

Silofillers' disease. Nitrogen dioxide is produced by bacteria acting on ammonium salts in and applied to silage grass (see above). Production is maximal after 1 or 2 days and in the absence of ventilation can result in toxic concentrations. Since the gas is denser than air the NO_2 accumulates in hollows on the surface of the silage and in any holes or clefts. A worker not wearing appropriate protective equipment who steps into such a pocket is at great risk of pulmonary oedema. The risk is enhanced by the silo gas being deficient in oxygen and containing excess carbon dioxide. Both these circumstances stimulate breathing (via carotid chemoreceptors and central medullary receptors) so augment the exposure to NO_2. This shortens the latent period before onset of pulmonary oedema. The asphyxial gas mixture can also cause loss of consciousness or lead to the exposed person being unable to escape from the highly toxic environment.

Prevention entails educating those who work with silage and preventing access to others, particularly children. The risk is greatest for tower silos: these should have provision for loading and distributing the grass by mechanical means. The silo should also be fitted with a blower and this should be used for at least 30min to clear gas from the silo if an entry is to be made within a few days of filling. Subsequently the risk is less but if there is doubt an on-site gas analysis should be carried out. Alternatively entry should be made wearing a respirator (air line or appropriate chemical filter) and with a colleague at hand in case of difficulty.

Oil mist - see Cutting oils, page 274, Lipid aerosol, page 281

Organophosphates

A principal organophosphate is parathion $((C_2H_5O)_2\ PS.O.C_6H_4.NO_2)$. This substance is a brownish liquid formed from reactions between phosphorus trichloride, sulphur, sodium ethoxide and sodium p-nitrophenate. Parathion, malathion and related compounds are readily converted to the corresponding oxon; in this form they inhibit the cholinesterase group of enzymes. The compounds are used as insecticides and are similar to the active ingredient of nerve gas.

Symptoms are due to the uninhibited accumulation of acetyl choline at nerve endings and occur within a few seconds of exposure or up to 12h depending on dosage. Muscle weakness and visual, central nervous and gastrointestinal symptoms occur; there is sweating, salivation and bradycardia and in the chest, tightness followed by acute bronchoconstriction and pulmonary oedema; these features progress to respiratory failure. The condition often presents with faecal incontinence and diarrhoea and the diagnosis is confirmed by finding a reduced plasma or red cell concentration of cholinesterase. Treatment of the respiratory effects is by intravenous atropine sulphate in the dosage 2–4mg every 5–10min until atropinization occurs. In severe cases the atropine may be supplemented by 2-pyridinealdoxime methochloride (2-PAM) which reactivates cholinesterase.

Parathion poisoning may arise in the course of manufacture, distribution or use of the insecticide. Prevention is by isolation of the process, careful handling of the product, personal hygiene and use of protective clothing and respirators. Persons who may be exposed should not have any medical condition, including glaucoma, which might be aggravated by acetyl choline. Before exposure the red cell acetyl chlolinesterase concentration should be obtained on two or more days to obtain base-line values; these should agree to within 15%. Following exposure a reduction to less than 50% is an indication for withdrawal from exposure or active treatment depending on the clinical picture.

Ornithosis (psittacosis)

Infection by an organism of the group chlamydia is common amongst birds of the parrot family (psittacines), sometimes occurs in turkeys, other domestic poultry and sea birds and may affect most mammals. The disease can cause serious economic loss to those who breed or distribute birds and animals: the infection can spread to man. The infectivity is greatest for *Chlamydia psittaci* and progressively less for the other avian and mammalian strains of the organism. The avian illness may be latent, chronic with lethargy, loss of weight and reduced fertility or acute with discharge from the eyes and nose, bronchitis and diarrhoea. Amongst the perching birds sold as domestic pets the mortality is high and the dried secretions and excrement are highly infectious to man.

Persons at risk are those who may come in contact with infected birds or their droppings including breeders, distributors, turkey food processors, vets, laboratory workers and persons who care for birds in avaries or as pets. In addition the human disease is infectious and may be transmitted to people in contact with or caring for a primary case of ornithosis. However, in most instances the infection will be subclinical and only detectable by a positive complement fixation test performed using *Chlamydia* group antigen.

Clinical disease usually presents 7–14 days after exposure. There is a flu-like illness with fever which can be severe; it is then accompanied by rigors, conjunctivitis, photophobia, headache, nausea and other symptoms including vomiting, diarrhoea, myalgia, dry cough, chest pain, stupor and confusion. Usually the disease localizes in the lung when it may be seen on the chest x-ray as lobar or segmental consolidation. The physical signs in the chest seldom reflect the extent of the infection. Extrapulmonary manifestations include red spots due to cutaneous vasculitis, epistaxes, myocarditis and meningoencephalitis.

The diagnosis is made from the history, the presence of organisms in the sputum, blood or other fluid and the occurrence of a high serum antibody titre or a rising titre in specimens of serum taken 7–20 days apart. The antibodies overlap with those for *Chlamydia trachomatis* but the clinical features are quite different. The differential diagnosis includes typhoid fever, Legionnaires' disease and other infections. The early stages may be mistaken for extrinsic allergic alveolitis due to farmers' lung or bird fanciers' lung. The recovery phase when the symptoms have subsided but before the x-ray has cleared may be mistaken for a pulmonary neoplasm. Treatment with tetracycline or erythromycin should be given as soon as the diagnosis is suspected because the response is good, whilst the penalty for waiting for confirmation may be death.

Prevention depends on inspection and blood testing of birds prior to trans-shipment, use of medicated food during quarantine periods and, in the human cases, notification and adherence to isolation procedures.

Osmium

Osmium is a highly reactive metal which occurs combined with iridium as osmiridium usually in association with platinum ores. Production is by separating the osmiridium, distilling it with chlorine to form osmium tetrachloride and subsequent reduction. The metal is used as a catalyst in organic chemistry; the alloy with iridium is used for pen nibs, fine point bearings in compasses and watches and the tetraoxide (OsO_4) as a fixative in electron microscopy. The latter substance gives off a vapour which is extremely irritating to the eyes, nose and respiratory tract where it may cause pulmonary oedema. The vapour has a pronounced nauseating smell so there is never any doubt as to its presence.

Ozone

Ozone (O_3, atomic mass 48), is a highly active triatomic oxygen with two free radicals which confer strong oxidizing properties. It is formed when biatomic oxygen is exposed to radiation of wave length approximately 200nm; this occurs in the upper atmosphere and during exposure of air to x-ray sources, ultra-violet lamps, electric arcs, mercury vapour lamps, high energy linear accelerators and other electrical discharges. Ozone poisoning is a hazard of certain types of electric arc welding (page 298) and very high altitudes (page 130). To a lesser extent it may also occur with petrochemical smog. Ozone is stored dissolved in fluorocarbon liquid; it must be handled with care because of the risk from fire or explosive decomposition to biatomic oxygen. Heat, trauma, reducing agents and metals which might catalyse the reaction should be avoided. Ozone is used for disinfection, bleaching, thickening oil, producing azelaic acid and other chemical processes.

Ozone selectively oxidizes substances which contain double bonded carbon or sulphur linkages and on this account disrupts cellular function. It is formed in cells by ionizing radiation (page 252) and may contribute to the toxic effects of hyperbaric oxygen (page 138) and of paraquat (see below). Intracellular protection is provided by the enzyme superoxide dismutase.

Ozone in a concentration of 0.05ppm has a bracing smell resembling sea air. Symptoms begin to develop at approximately twice this concentration up to 5ppm which may cause pulmonary oedema. At intermediate concentrations there may be dryness of the throat, increased bronchial reactivity to histamine, airflow obstruction, dyspnoea and shallow breathing during exercise, headache and general malaise. Long-term exposure may accentuate the decline in lung function with age and contribute to the development of emphysema (page 383). On first exposure the threshold concentration for changes in lung function is in the range 0.2–0.4ppm for 2h. Tolerance develops during two or three daily exposures and may be the reason why residents of Los Angeles are less responsive than new arrivals. However, repeated exposure to low concentrations

(0.2ppm) does not reduce the response to higher ones (0.42 or 0.5ppm). The mechanism of adaptation is not known.

Protection against the harmful effects of ozone is by conforming to the guidelines for safe handling given above, using protective clothing during decanting the liquid from containers, and maintaining the air concentration within the hygiene standard (page 16) as described in chapter 3. Depending on circumstances the protection may entail enclosing the process, providing exhaust ventilation, having adequate ventilation and providing air-supplied respirators. For short periods, canister respirators with a catalytic ozone decomposing filter can be used. Limited prophylaxis is provided by ditocopherol and some disulphide compounds (cf. page 294). The risk of ozone poisoning is greatest for persons who are also exposed to other sources of free oxygen radicals including ionizing radiation, hyperbaric oxygen and peroxyacetyl nitrate which, like ozone, can occur in smog. Their effects are additive or in some instances multiplicative and provide a strong reason for taking into account the total environmental exposure of the subjects, particularly cosmonauts, persons engaging in high altitude flight and deep sea divers (chapter 7). Exposure to ozone does not aggravate the harmful effects of cigarette smoke or cause emphysema (page 383) and whilst it can be mutagenic, no evidence for malignancy has been reported in man.

Paraquat

Paraquat (1,1'-dimethyl-4,4' bipyridylium dichloride or disulphate) is a highly reactive compound which destroys chlorophyll by oxidation; it is absorbed onto and inactivated by soil. On account of these properties paraquat is used extensively as a contact weed killer which does not damage subsequent crops. Exposure may occur in manufacture or distribution, and during use by foresters, plantation or orchard workers and market gardeners; however, it usually occurs by accidental ingestion due to the liquid being mistaken for a beverage. Criminal administration also occurs. The solution is extremely toxic to all forms of life and may cause acute illness or death when inhaled,

References pages 306–7

ingested or absorbed through the skin. The local contact may cause ulceration of the skin, mouth or pharynx. Ingestion by mouth causes acute abdominal symptoms with pain, vomiting and diarrhoea. There may be acute pulmonary oedema, circulatory collapse and coma leading to early death. A less overwhelming dose may cause centrilobular necrosis of the liver, acute necrosis of renal tubules, toxic myocarditis and comparable changes in the lung which is the main target organ. The prospect of surviving the acute episode is strongly related to the plasma concentration of paraquat (fig. 13.5).

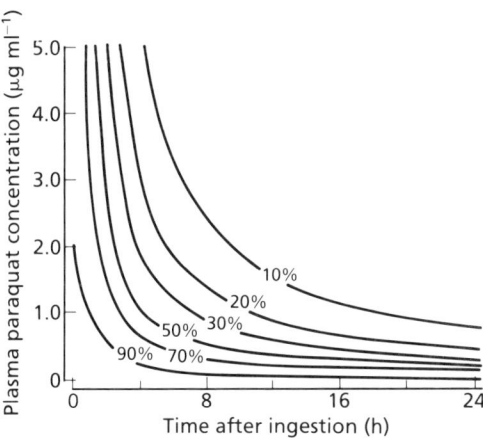

Fig. 13.5. Relationship of probability of survival after ingesting paraquat (expressed as percentage) to the plasma paraquat concentration. (By courtesy of T. B. Hart and colleagues (page 307).)

The effect of paraquat on the lungs is dose related and ranges from mild disease of the lung parenchyma to fulminating pulmonary oedema. Respiratory symptoms may develop immediately when exposure is by inhalation but this is uncommon. Breathlessness usually comes on after an interval of 2 or 3h up to 10 days; however, lung damage has occurred up to 14 days after a single dose whilst after repeated small exposures the onset may be delayed for weeks or months. In severe cases the alveolar epithelium disintegrates causing intra-alveolar oedema, haemorrhage and the formation of a hyaline membrane. Over the next few days mononuclear cells infiltrate the area and later transform to

fibroblasts which form collagen, both within and in the walls of alveoli. In less acute and subclinical cases the interstitial fibrosis occurs in discrete foci and here the pavement epithelium of the alveoli is replaced by cuboidal type II cells. Pulmonary arteries show hypertrophy of the muscle layer, thickening of the subepithelium and in some instances thrombosis with or without recanalization. The condition may progress to chronic fibrosis of the lung or it may resolve.

The changes in lung function are consistent with the pathology, ranging from gross derangement to a diminution in transfer factor without restriction of lung expansion: in the latter event the prospect for full recovery is excellent in the short term. There is need for longer follow-up to assess the eventual outcome.

Treatment of the acute episode is usually ineffective. The minimal lethal dose of paraquat is contained in only 10ml of the commercial preparation; this is a concentrated 20% solution (gramoxone or orthoparaquat) which is diluted on site. The diluted preparation (Weedol) comes in sachets, one of which constitutes a serious hazard. Following ingestion the chemical is rapidly absorbed from the gut, the peak plasma concentration being reached within 2h. Thereafter the concentration declines as the chemical is actively taken up by the lungs and other tissues and excreted by the kidneys; contact with the tissues causes local damage by release of superoxide. Thus after a potentially lethal dose the treatment must be given before absorption by the tissues has taken place. The options include giving Fuller's earth or bentonite by mouth to adsorb the chemical, perform whole gut lavage, achieve a forced diuresis or undertake haemodialysis or charcoal haemoperfusion. Before embarking on such heroic remedies the blood concentration should be ascertained to see if it approaches a dangerous level (fig. 13.5): treatment along these lines is too late if the clinical signs of acute poisoning are already present. A specific antidote such as the enzyme superoxide dismutase is needed but so far no satisfactory treatment formula has been evolved. Supportive treatment should be that for pulmonary oedema with sufficient additional oxygen to preserve cerebral function. Excess oxygen may add to the lung damage and is contraindicated. For less severe poisoning corticosteroid or cytotoxic drugs may be beneficial.

Prevention of paraquat poisoning is primarily by proper labelling and by education. The liquid should be kept in a safe place and not decanted into other containers. Care should be taken to avoid spillages, and this is helped by using a high viscosity preparation, including the incorporation of a distinctive colour and smell and emetic properties. Decontamination should be immediate. Protective clothing should be worn and spraying should not be done when high winds could cause drifting.

Phosgene

Phosgene ($COCl_2$) is a gas which is produced commercially by the combination of carbon monoxide with chlorine in the presence of activated charcoal catalyst. It is also formed from carbon tetrachloride and chlorinated hydrocarbons as a result of thermal degradation in a fire, or during welding, and from tetrachloroethylene which is used as a lubricant in the machining of high grade steel. The gas is used in the synthesis of many organic chemicals including isocyanates. During World War One it was used as a war gas. Phosgene is colourless and in low concentration has a smell of new-mown hay. In higher concentration the gas has a pungent smell and metallic taste, causes irritation or burning of the eyes and pharynx and a feeling of inability to take a deep breath which is probably of reflex origin (page 47). These symptoms disappear within 5min of the start of exposure, after which the gas can be inhaled deeply without immediate discomfort.

In the lung phosgene is hydrolysed to hydrochloric acid. The reaction occurs progressively over several hours and gives rise to symptoms after a latent period which is usually in the range 2–12h. Initially there is mild cough and breathlessness on exertion and these symptoms may progress to frank pulmonary oedema and death within 48h. If the victim survives this period the prognosis is reasonably good, but late deaths may occur from infection, lung abscess or vascular thrombosis. Survivors and persons exposed to lower concentrations are at increased

risk of developing chronic bronchitis. Treatment is as for exposure to chlorine (page 272); aspects of prophylaxis are discussed in chapter 3.

Polyfluorines

Polyfluorines are chains of -CF_2 units of high molecular weight; the most widely used is polytetrafluoroethylene (PTFE) formed by polymerization of tetrafluoroethylene (CF_2CF_2) which in turn is produced by pyrolysis of trifluoromethane (CHF_3) or related compound. PTFE is chemically inert, tolerates temperatures up to 260°C and has a slippery surface. On account of these properties it is used for surgical prostheses, for coating chemical vessels and non-stick pans, and in gaskets, gear wheels and bearings. The fume formed on heating to 315°C causes an influenza-like illness resembling metal fume fever. This has followed inhaling PTFE off cigarettes contaminated by unwashed fingers (Lawther, personal communication). Thus men should not smoke when the material is being processed. In a fire PTFE will liberate hydrogen fluoride gas which is highly irritating and corrosive; the effects resemble those of phosgene (see above).

Pulmonary oedema

Pulmonary oedema may develop following an exposure to a relatively high concentration of any irritant gas or aerosol. Many of the substances are discussed in this chapter: they are brought together in table 13.14. The oedema does not become manifest for at least 12h after exposure so any heavily exposed person should be kept under observation for 24h following the incident. The first evidence is then a fall in arterial oxygen tension in association with rhonchi from involvement of respiratory bronchioles. These features are followed by fine râles from alveolar oedema and fluffy shadows on the chest radiograph; the distribution is often predominantly perihilar giving rise to a 'bat wing' appearance. In other cases fine horizontal lines (Kerley B lines) appear in the costophrenic angles. The patient is breathless, anxious, restless, cyanosed and, with extensive oedema, coughs up frothy sputum.

References page 307

Table 13.14. Some fumes and vapours which can cause pulmonary oedema

Acetaldehyde (ethanal)	Nitrogen dioxide
Acid fumes	Nickel carbonyl
Acrolein (acrylic anhydride)	Osmium tetraoxide
Ammonia	Ozone
Antimony compounds (Table 13.1)	Organophosphates
Bismuth pentafluoride	Paraquat
Boron compounds (Table 13.4)	Phosgene
Bromomethane	Polytetra fluoro-ethylene
Cadmium vapour	Selenium dioxide
Chlorine and compounds (Table 13.7)	Sulphur dioxide and compounds (Table 13.15)
Cobalt vapour	Organo-tin compounds
Dimethyl sulphate	Titanium tetrachloride
Dioxane	Trimellitic anhydride
Fumes from fires	Vanadium compounds
Lithium hydride	Zinc chloride
Mercury fumes	Zirconium tetrachloride
Methyl isocyanate*	

Many of these substances also irritate the eyes and respiratory tract; they are either direct irritants or react with tissue fluid to form acidic or oxidizing radicals (see text).
* Also obliterative bronchiolitis as at Bhopal, India (Newman Taylor AJ, Jones B. *Ind J Med Res*, in press).

Following exposure the irritant substance should be removed or inactivated. The oedema should be treated with frusemide or other diuretic and oxygen in high dosage. Morphine is beneficial in allaying apprehension, reducing hyperventilation and suppressing the oedema. If there is hypercapnia the patient should be mechanically ventilated with oxygen via a cuffed endotracheal tube. Hypoxaemia which does not respond to this regimen is an indication for positive end expiratory pressure ventilation (PEEP). Antibacterial chemotherapy and steroid drugs are given respectively to prevent secondary infection and hasten the resolution of the inflammatory changes in the lung.

Quartz - chapter 8

Selenium

Selenium (atomic mass 78.9) is a red, crystalline substance resembling sulphur; it burns with a blue flame to form dioxide and also occurs in amorphous and grey hexagonal forms. The mineral is present in low concentration in rocks and soil. High concentrations, up to 15%, occur in the residues formed during refining copper from sulphide mineral and this is the only commercial source of selenium. The main uses are for rectifiers which convert alternating current into direct current and in photoelectric cells. It is also used for decolourizing green glass, making ruby glass, as an additive to stainless steel, in the rubber industry, as an insecticide and in photocopying. Selenium hexafluoride is used as a gaseous electric insulator. Hydrogen selenide has a particularly foul smell.

The mineral is harmless to man and in trace concentrations the salts are essential for life. The dioxide and other compounds cause local irritation or corrosion depending on their concentration; sites which are at risk are the skin, eyes, finger nails and gastro-intestinal and respiratory tracts. Inhalation leads to sneezing, rhinorrhoea, cough and chest tightness. The symptoms are transient but may be followed after a few hours by the onset of pulmonary oedema. Chronic exposure is associated with anosmia, an odour of garlic in the breath from dimethyl selenium, which is produced in the liver, and a metallic taste in the mouth. Protection is by appropriate environmental and personal measures. The hygiene standard for airborne selenium is given on page 16.

Sick building syndrome

In modern office buildings and factories the working environment is maintained at what is considered to be optimal levels of ventilation, temperature and illumination. These should promote good health. In practice, compared with workers in traditional buildings, the occupants often experience excess irritation of the eyes and respiratory tract, hypersensitivity reactions, headache, nausea and general malaise. This sick building syndrome does not have a unique cause. Its occurrence has led to a review of the many factors which may contribute, of which the most important may be organic solvents; however, the better documented factors should be considered first (table 13.15).

Silica - chapter 8

Sulphur

Sulphur (atomic mass 32.06) is a non-metallic element found in volcanic regions; it also occurs as metal sulphides, sulphates (e.g. gypsum) and hydrogen sulphide gas. Extraction is from sulphur deposits by using high pressure steam, from sulphides by heating or from refining copper, other metals and crude oil. The substance is a feedstock for the chemical industry and is used for matches, other incendiaries, the vulcanization of rubber, as a pesticide, fungicide etc.

Sulphur irritates and may corrode the eyes, skin and mucous membranes including the upper and lower respiratory tract. It is a cause of nasal catarrh, sinusitis and acute and chronic bronchitis with airflow obstruction. On chest radiography there may be irregular opacities associated with pulmonary congestion but without nodulation or other features of fibrosis. Sulphur forms numerous compounds; some of these are given in table 13.16.

Sulphur dioxide

Sulphur dioxide (SO_2) is obtained by combustion of sulphur, roasting of natural sulphides including iron pyrites or calcining of natural sulphates. It is used in the production of sulphuric acid, the manufacture of paper, as a bleaching and preserving agent and is the starting point for numerous organic syntheses. SO_2 is released into the atmosphere as a contaminant during these processes and also in the course of petroleum refining, combustion of coal rich in sulphur and other industrial activities. It is the most ubiquitous contaminant of the working environment and the principal toxic constituent of industrial air pollution. It was formerly the cause of much ill-health in Western Europe and U.S.A. and now affects the urban populations of many recently industrialized countries. SO_2 is highly irritant to human tissue because it reacts with water to form sulphurous acid on the surface of mucous membranes. The sulphurous acid may subsequently oxidize to sulphuric acid.

Acute poisoning with SO_2 may cause death directly from asphyxiation or laryngeal spasm or indirectly from irritation throughout the respiratory tract leading to pulmonary oedema which may itself be fatal. A less intense exposure causes reflex bronchoconstriction and impels the subject to seek fresh air. There may be sufficient absorption of SO_2 via the lungs and

Table 13.15.   Indoor air: factors which might affect health

Physical	Ventilation, temperature, humidity, ionization
Cigarette smoke (chapter 17)	
Combustion products	Nitrogen oxides, ozone (chapter 13)
Microorganisms	Infections, sensitizations (chapters 5 and 16)
Carcinogens	Radon gas, benzo(a)pyrene (chapter 12)
Volatile organic compounds (in adhesives, cleaning fluids, cosmetics, fuels, fumigants, glues, lubricants, paints, pesticides, propellants, solvents for plastics)	Examples: acetone, butane, chlordane, ethanol, formaldehyde, limonene, toluene, undecane, xylenes

References page 307

Table 13.16. Brief description of some sulphur-containing compounds

		B.P.*		
Carbon disulphide	CS_2	46°	Solvent: used in production of rayon, optical glass, etc.	Neurotoxic: may affect respiratory centre
Hydrogen sulphide	H_2S	−61°	Chemical feedstock, analytical reagent, disinfectant, constituent of sewer gas, by-product of many chemical processes	Acute irritant of eyes and respiratory tract, causes haemolysis, pulmonary oedema, blocks tissue enzymes, etc.
Sulphur dioxide	SO_2	−10°	(See text)	
Sulphur trioxide	SO_3	45°	Manufacture of sulphuric acid, oleum, dye-stuffs, explosives, etc.	Effects as for SO_2 but more pronounced
Sulphur hexafluoride	SF_6	(S)	Gaseous insulator	Inert unless decomposed by heat
Sulphur pentafluoride	S_2F_{10}	24°	Fluorinating agent	Hydrolyses to hydrogen fluoride and SO_2; more irritant to respiratory tract than phosgene (q.v.)
Sulphuryl fluoride	SO_2F_2	−55°	Insecticide and fumigant	May cause pulmonary oedema
Thionyl fluoride	SOF_2	−44°		

* BP = Boiling point °C.   (S) = sublimes.

gastro-intestinal tract to cause metabolic acidosis, interrupt metabolic processes, deplete the body stores of vitamins B and C and convert some haemoglobin to methaemoglobin.

Chronic exposure to SO_2 causes a dry burning sensation in the throat, nasal irritation, ulceration of the nasal septum, impaired sense of smell, destruction of dental enamel, tooth decay and irritation of moist areas of skin, for example in the axillae and round the scrotum. The exposure may initiate chronic bronchitis, aggravate chronic bronchitis associated with smoking or other atmospheric pollutant (chapter 17) or act as a co-carcinogen to nickel and radon daughter products in the formation of lung cancer (chapter 12). The hygiene standard for SO_2 is given on page 16.

The control of air pollution by SO_2 is along the lines discussed in chapter 3. Within buildings an acute emission may be neutralized with ammonia, either deliberately or by accident, as in the Smithfield Agricultural Show in 1952. The show was affected by a severe temperature inversion with build up of SO_2. This killed some of the prize-winning cattle whose stalls were immaculate but not others whose stalls were contaminated with ammonia from accumulated urine and faeces. Under exceptional circumstances temporary protection may be obtained by use of a respirator with appropriate chemical pre-filter (chapter 3). The management of personnel who are to some extent at risk includes the surveillance of respiratory health and discouraging smoking. Additional measures which, however, should not normally be necessary include monitoring the urinary acid and ammonia and regular use of a mouth-wash containing 10% sodium bicarbonate. Scrupulous personal hygiene should be encouraged. In the event of severe exposure the measures for resuscitation should be supplemented by application of sodium bicarbonate solution to burns on the skin, conjunctivae and mucous membranes.

Sulphuric acid

Sulphuric acid (H_2SO_4) is a strong acid and dehydrating agent. It is formed by hydration of sulphur trioxide which is obtained by oxidation of sulphur dioxide by air at high temperature in the presence of platinum or vanadium catalyst. Sulphuric acid is indispensable for a wide range of industrial processes in the chemical and metal refining industries, manufacture of fertilizers, dye stuffs, explosives, artificial fibres, extraction of titanium dioxide from ilmenite and of uranium from pitchblende, treatment of leather, wool and waste from scrap and many other applications. It is the acid used in lead/acid batteries. The acid readily vapourizes; the extra strong fuming variety (oleum) also emits sulphur trioxide.

The toxic effects are due to corrosion and affect particularly the skin, teeth and eyes. Inhalation of vapour in high concentration burns the nose and upper respiratory tract but low concentrations such as occur in manufacture of lead/acid batteries have no material pulmonary effects. The mechanism of adaptation is unclear. Safety is achieved by attention to the hygiene measures discussed in chapter 3. The hygiene standard is given on page 16.

Talc - chapter 10, page 226

Tantalum

Tantalum (atomic mass 181) is a hard, malleable, ductile metal which is very resistant to corrosion. It occurs in tantalite and columbite ore mixed with iron, manganese and niobium. Purification entails chemical extraction, reduction with molten sodium and heating in a vacuum or an atmosphere of argon or helium to prevent reaction with atmospheric gases. Its chief uses are in electrical capacitors for the chemical and electronics industries and for surgical sutures and plates. Tantalum is a component of hard metal but is not the cause of the interstitial pulmonary fibrosis which is probably due to cobalt (q.v.); tantalum itself appears to be inert.

Tellurium

Tellurium is a heavy element which occurs in conjunction with selenium in ore containing copper and is obtained as a by-product of copper

refining. It is used to improve the properties of steel, copper, tin and other metals, for vulcanizing rubber, as a pottery glaze and in selenium/tellurium rectifiers. The properties and medical effects of tellurium closely resemble those of selenium (q.v.).

Tin

Tin (atomic mass 119) is a soft, silvery-white metal which occurs in mineral deposits as the oxide (cassiterite, SnO_2) and the sulphide (stannite, Ca_2FeSnS_2 or tealite, $PbZnSnS_2$). The principal producers are in S.E. Asia, Malaysia, Thailand, Indonesia, China and Bolivia with lesser deposits in U.S.S.R., Zaire, Nigeria, Australia and Cornwall, U.K. Extraction of cassiterite is by dredging from the bed of the sea or river whilst the sulphide ores are quarried or mined; the latter is the usual method in Bolivia and in Cornwall. The metal is obtained by first concentrating the tin ore using physical methods, then smelting it with carbon, lime and quartz in a reverberatory furnace at 1200°C. Prior to this treatment the sulphide ore is roasted to remove arsenic and sulphur. The molten tin is moulded into blocks and subsequently purified by electrolysis or in other ways.

Tin was formerly used extensively as tin foil for wrappings, silvering mirrors and making collapsible tubes but plastics and aluminium are now used instead. Tin plating by dipping in a molten bath is used to confer resistance against corrosion on iron and steel utensils and containers. Molten tin is used in the float-process for making glass. Tin forms alloys with other metals and these substances have a wide range of uses. The alloys include tin–lead alloy used for soft solder, tin–copper alloy (speculum) used for reflecting surfaces and tin–niobium alloy used for electro-magnets. Other alloys of tin include phosphor bronze, brass, bronze, type metal and pewter. Tin oxide is used for the production of drill-glass, ceramics, porcelain and enamel. The chloride salt is used as a reducing agent and mordant in dye works. However, many of these uses are on the decline. The principal new uses are for organotin compounds in which tin or halogenated tin compounds are combined with hydrocarbons. These substances

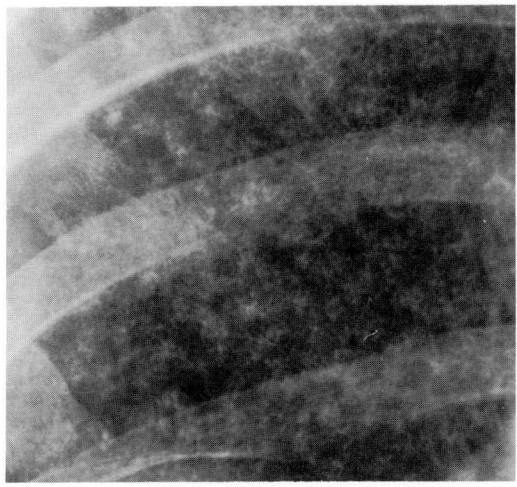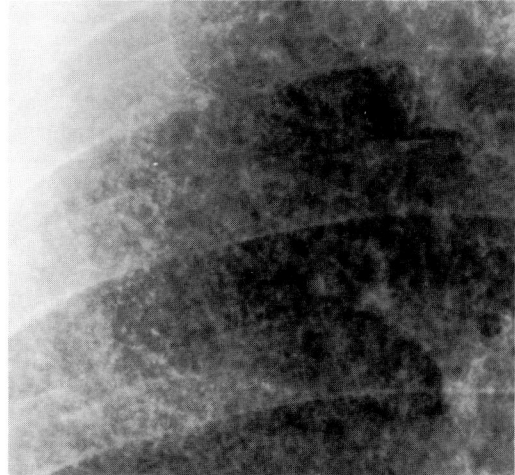

Fig. 13.6. Detail from routine chest radiographs of two men who processed tin oxide showing stannosis (categories 2p and 3p respectively). Both were asymptomatic. (By courtesy of M. McDermott.)

have a wide range of uses as stabilizers and catalysts in the plastics industry, as biocides and as intermediaries in the production of other compounds.

The mining and roasting of tin sulphide ore carries a risk from the associated exposures to quartz and sulphur dioxide. Tin oxide is very radio-opaque and on this account causes simple pneumoconiosis (stannosis) with numerous very fine dense opacities (fig. 13.6); these resemble those of baritosis (fig. 13.2, page 268); the condition is entirely benign but now rare. Tin mining can carry a risk of silicosis. Metallic tin powder is an irritant to the eyes and respiratory tract but illness on this account appears to be uncommon. Organotin compounds are powerful tissue irritants and in the respiratory tract cause local burns or pulmonary oedema. There is no excess risk from lung cancer. Thus the potential for serious injury exists but as normally used, tin appears to be quite harmless.

Titanium

Titanium (atomic mass 47.9) is a lustrous, white metal which is chemically active and flammable at room temperature. The parent ore usually contains iron oxide and extraction is by smelting to form titanium tetrachloride gas which is then condensed and reduced with the aid of magnesium. The metal is used for aircraft, rocket and marine construction, as an alloy in steel, for pyrotechnics, paint and other applications. Some titanium compounds are given in table 13.17.

Titanium, titanium oxide and the inert salts can cause simple pneumoconiosis. Titanium tetrachloride is a colourless liquid with a pungent smell; it hydrolyses in the presence of moisture to form hydrochloric acid and titanium hydroxide ($Ti(OH)_4$), both of which are irritant and caustic. Thus workers engaged on the chlorination and rectification stages of production as

Table 13.17.   Some titanium compounds

Barium titanate		Heavy duty capacitors	May cause
Titanium dioxide	TiO_2, white	Paint, ceramics,	simple
Titanium nitride	TiN, red	varnish, rubber	pneumoconiosis
Titanium carbide	TiC		
Titanium tetrachloride	$TiCl_4$	Mordant for dyeing, sky writing	Releases HCl, etc.

well as those who use the substance are at risk of sustaining damage to the eyes, skin and respiratory tract. Depending on the intensity and duration of exposure the latter effects may include tracheitis, acute and chronic bronchitis, pneumonitis and pulmonary oedema. These effects may be avoided by attention to the hygiene measures discussed in chapter 3. The hygiene standard is given on page 16. The personnel engaged in producing titanium dioxide are exposed not only to $TiCl_4$ but also to mist from sulphuric acid which is used to digest the ore and carbon monoxide which is formed during smelting.

Tungsten

Tungsten (atomic mass 184) is a tough metal which is used to harden steel, for high-speed cutting tools (hard metal, q.v.), as the filament in electric lamps, vacuum tubes and has other applications. It is produced from ores which are tungstates of iron (wolframite), calcium (scheelite) and magnesium. Production entails crushing and grinding the ore, concentrating the mineral by flotation, conferring magnetic properties by roasting, then undertaking magnetic separation; the pure oxide is reduced to metal powder, then converted into metal or heated with carbon to form tungsten carbide. The manufacture of hard metal is considered under this heading above. Tungsten is biologically inert and whilst it may give rise to simple pneumoconiosis this condition is now uncommon.

Uranium - chapter 12, page 252

Vanadium

Vanadium (atomic mass 50.9) is a light-grey, lustrous metal which greatly improves the tensile strength, elasticity and rust resistance of steel. It is used as a catalyst and the alloy with gallium is used for producing high magnetic fields. The substance occurs as vanadium sulphide in patronite found in Peru, lead–zinc vanadate in discloizite in South Africa and carnotite, a uranium ore, which is widely distributed. Vanadium also occurs in petroleum deposits on account of it being a constituent of

the blood of some marine fossils. It is, therefore, a constituent of soot and other residues from oil refineries, oil fired furnaces, gas turbines and other engines. The principal compound is vanadium pentoxide (V_2O_5) which comprises 50% of the soot from oil-fired furnaces; it is used as a catalyst, in metallurgy and for developing photographic plates. Ammonium metavanadate (NH_4VO_3) has similar uses to the pentoxide. Vanadium appears to be inert but in persons cleaning furnaces and jet engines the compounds may cause irritation throughout the respiratory tract from nose to alveoli. Depending on the concentration the effects range from the trivial to death. The respirable dust may cause wheeze and airflow obstruction. Recovery is usual and the subsequent occurrence of chronic bronchitis, whilst possible, has not been confirmed. Prevention is by the practice of good occupational hygiene supplemented by personal protection (chapter 3). The individual burden of vanadium may be assessed from the concentration in the urine.

Welding

A weld is a join effected by two surfaces being melted or pressed together; there is no intermediary as is the case with brazing, soldering or glueing. In metallurgy the heat is applied to the parts being joined by friction or electric current. Alternatively an oxygen flame or electric arc can be used to melt a rod of the same or related metal which then flows into the gap. A chemical flux may be incorporated in the rod to prevent oxidation at the surface of the metal and hence facilitate joining. Alternatively oxidation may be prevented by displacement of air with molten slag, inert gas (usually helium or argon) or reactive gas (usually carbon dioxide). Similar techniques are used for thermal cutting and for cleaning up metal surfaces prior to welding; an oxy gas flame is also used to supplement abrasion and chipping in the preparation of freshly cast ingots for processing. The tradesmen responsible are called respectively welders, cutters, burners and metal dressers (deseamers).

In gas welding the source of heat is a flame produced by combustion of oxygen and fuel gas which is commonly propane from a cylinder but

Table 13.18. Types of metal welding: many of the processes are also used for cutting

Type	Feature	Metal filler and flux	Type-specific hazards
Gas	Acetylene or other gas	Welding rod	Fire, explosion, products of combustion
Electric arc	Manual metal arc, gas shielded (CO_2,A,N_2,He)	Consumable electrode or separate rod (carbon or tungsten electrode)	Electrocution, u.v. light, ozone
Electron beam	In evacuated chamber		Radiation
Laser	For precision work	—	Burns
Metal spray*	Wire or powder sprayed through arc	—	See above
Plasma arc	Air, argon, hydrogen and other gases sprayed through arc (e.g. atomic hydrogen welding)	—	Radiation, noise
Resistance	Uses low voltage high current source and strong pressure (e.g. electro-slag, flash and spot welding)	—	Crush injury, noise
Spark erosion cutting (arc air gouging)	Discharge between electrode and electrolytic oil	—	Electrocution, fire, dermatitis, oil mist

* Need for prior sand blasting or pickling of parts to be welded.

may be hydrogen, town gas or acetylene; in low pressure gas welding the acetylene is generated on site by the addition of water to calcium carbide.

Arc welding is undertaken using an electric current flowing between an electrode and the pieces to be welded. The core of the electrode may be made of the metal to be joined (when it is consumed in the process) or of carbon or tungsten which are not consumed. If the electrode is non-consumable the weld metal is introduced mechanically or by hand as a separate consumable; however, for welding mild steel a stainless steel welding rod is sometimes used. In gas shielded arc welding the shielding gas can be nitrogen, argon, helium or carbon dioxide and the process is often largely automatic; the electrode may be any one of the types described and the process is known respectively as metal inert gas (MIG), metal active gas (MAG), carbon inert gas or tungsten inert gas (TIG) welding. When the weld is made manually the electrode is of the weld metal coated with a flux comprising cellulose, metal salts, silica, asbestos or other substances. The process is known as manual metal arc (MMA) or open arc welding. These

and other techniques for welding are listed in table 13.18.

The hazards of welding are partly type-specific and partly common to all types. Gas welding carries a risk of explosion and fire, arc welding of electrocution and ultra-violet radiation burns (e.g. arc-eye or eye-flash). With both forms of welding the intense heat, radiation and hot sparks may burn any exposed part. Fumes and toxic gases are generated during welding. Their nature depends on the metal or alloy being welded, the surface coating, the type of weld, the composition of flux and welding rod and the local environment. The medical conditions which may arise from these exposures are listed in table 13.19.

The hazards of welding are numerous but the evidence is fragmentary: it has recently been reviewed by WHO. The most prevalent condition is siderosis which is a benign simple pneumoconiosis due to iron oxide in the lung (fig. 13.3, page 279). The most frequent acute effect is metal fume fever which is experienced at some time by up to 30% of welders (page 283). The most significant condition is possibly ozone poisoning which is a hazard of argon shielded

Table 13.19.   Possible respiratory hazards associated with work as a welder

Weld metal and coating	Metal fume fever Inert dust pneumoconiosis Asthma Pneumonia Malignancy	Zinc (galvanized iron), etc. Iron (siderosis) Chromium, nickel (stainless steel) Manganese, cadmium (plating) Chromium, nickel, arsenic
Other coating	Polymer fume fever Asthma Pulmonary oedema	Tetrafluoroethylene resin Isocyanate, formaldehyde Phosgene (from degreasing solvents) Phosphine (from phosphate rust proofing)
Flux	Silicosis	
Thermal insulation	Asbestosis	From consumable electrodes, blankets, gloves
Inert gas shield	Asphyxiation	From carbon dioxide, etc.
Combustion	Carbon monoxide poisoning	From gas welding
	Lung disease from oxides of nitrogen	Gas and open arc welding and cutting
U.V. light	Ozone poisoning	Gas-shielded welding and arc-air gouging
Environment	Asbestosis, pleural plaques, mesothelioma	Working alongside laggers

electric arc welding, gouging or plasma cutting. The ozone is formed from molecular oxygen by the action of short wave length ultra-violet light (wavelength 1200–2000Å) at a distance of up to 1.2m from the arc. The rate of formation is related directly to the current used and inversely to the duration of welding. It is greatest for aluminium and its silicon alloy, when the ozone concentration 15cm from the arc can rise to 15ppm. In adverse circumstances concentrations of 2ppm can occur with mild and stainless steel but usually they are lower, and lower still in the breathing zone. (For ozone poisoning, see page 290.) Carbon monoxide and nitrogen dioxide are constituents of welding fumes but, whilst the latter in high concentration may cause pulmonary oedema or bronchiolitis, the evidence for either having a chronic deleterious effect is meagre (pages 270 and 285). Welders resemble other workers in heavy industry in having an increased prevalence of chronic bronchitis. In the U.K. the standardized mortality ratio for respiratory and cardiovascular disease in welding is a little above the national average. Thus there is proper cause for concern, and this has led to respiratory surveys of welders.

Persons welding mild steel have an above average prevalence of respiratory symptoms and when these occur the men may be off work for a longer time than other tradesmen. There are no symptoms associated with siderosis. On assessment of lung function the forced expiratory volume is on average within normal limits; however, it can be reduced as a result of heavy fume exposure, for example amongst men welding the double bottoms of ships. In young shipyard workers tests which reflect the calibre of small airways show evidence of abnormality; the changes are comparable to those due to smoking. There is evidence for synergism between these two ways of breathing polluted air; it leads to some welders giving up smoking. Welding mild steel is not incriminated as a cause of respiratory disablement or lung cancer. Welding stainless steel using a gas shielded electrode may possibly be associated with additional lung damage due to ozone and Stern has suggested that there is an increased risk from lung cancer due to chromium. As yet the evidence is inconclusive and further investigations are in progress. In dockyard welders there is a significant morbidity and mortality from asbestos-related

References page 307

diseases; this may be due to both dust from asbestos lagging and asbestos from the blanket or gloves used by the welder. Asbestos is no longer used as a coating for welding rods. In summary the harmful effect of welding as now practised is small and confined to a few occupations. The disease, welders' lung, does not seem to exist.

Protection against welding fumes requires good environmental hygiene including local exhaust ventilation. Particular attention should be given to aluminium and stainless steel welders, persons working in confined spaces, for example building the double bottoms of ships, those who are also exposed to asbestos and persons who by bad luck or incompetence consistently fail to get the benefit from exhaust ventilation. In addition the constituents of new surface coating materials and solvents should be scrutinized in case they may give rise to sensitizing agents or lung irritants. This possibility is a reason for enquiring about childhood or adult asthma at the pre-employment examination and appointing those affected to trades other than welding.

Wollastonite - chapter 10, page 227

Yttrium

Yttrium (atomic mass 88.9) is a rare earth resembling cerium from which it may be separated by its greater solubility in dilute mineral acids. For further details, see Cerium.

Zeolite - chapter 10, page 228

Zinc

Zinc (atomic mass 65.4) is a soft, silvery-white metal with a blue tinge. The metal is used as an alloy with a number of metals especially copper (q.v.). It rapidly acquires resistance to atmospheric corrosion by oxidation of the surface layer; this property is exploited to protect iron by plating with zinc to form galvanized iron and when zinc sheet is used for roofing, especially 'flashing'. The metal is also used as anode in many electrolytic processes; its use in manufacturing industry has largely been replaced by plastics. Other zinc compounds are given in table 13.20.

Zinc metal fumes are a potent cause of metal fume fever (q.v.). The salts are irritants and when inhaled cause nasal ulceration or damage to the respiratory tract. Pulmonary oedema can occur from spraying zinc metal or in exceptional circumstances as when a smoke generator containing zinc chloride is released in a confined space. The condition may then be fatal or progress to diffuse interstitial pulmonary fibrosis.

Zirconium

Zirconium (atomic mass 91) is an amorphous or grey-white, lustrous metal present in the gemstone, zircon ($ZrSiO_4$), some beach sands and in deposits of baddeleyite (ZrO_2). The minerals are widely distributed. In the U.S.A. zircon is sometimes used for sand-blasting as an alternative to quartz. The metal is highly reactive so is commonly produced by reduction of the chloride or iodide salt with liquid sodium in an atmosphere of argon or helium; it may also be produced electrothermically. The metal has a low absorption for neutrons and when alloyed with other metals is very resistant to corrosion so is used inside atomic reactors and for lining pumps and reaction vessels. For these applications the metal should be free of hafnium (atomic mass 178.4) which is in many ways very similar and

Table 13.20. Some zinc compounds

Zinc oxide	Pigment, filler, in pharmaceuticals, etc.	Inert
Zinc chloride	Dry battery cells, oil refining, etc.	
Zinc chromate	Pigment	Acute irritants
Zinc cyanide	Chemical reagent, pesticide	
Zinc phosphate	Rodenticide	

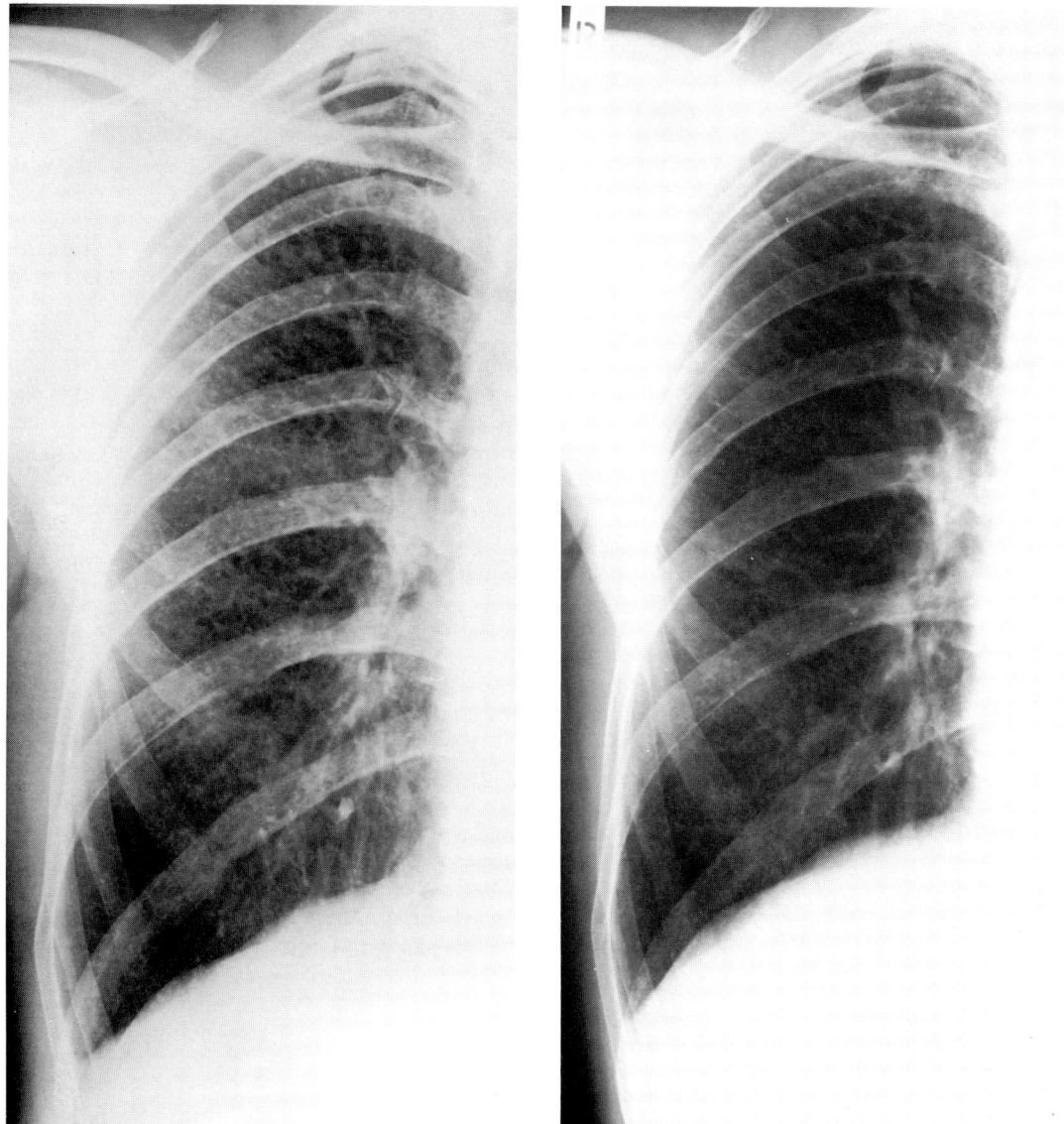

Fig. 13.7. Right chest radiograph at age 47 and 59 years in a man whose work from the age of 31 years entailed grinding zirconium silicate (zircon). He developed simple pneumoconiosis (category 3, left) following approximately 10 years of heavy dust exposure but had no respiratory symptoms and lung function was normal (FEV_1, FVC and Tl in range 94% to 110% predicted). Subsequently with adequate dust suppression the lesions regressed; the film at age 59 (right) was read as category 1/0. The patient remained asymptomatic despite smoking 25 cigarettes per day. (By courtesy of G. L. Leathart.)

occurs with it. Some information about zirconium compounds is given in table 13.21.

Inhalation of zirconium compounds in high concentration has been found to produce granu-lomas and diffuse interstitial pulmonary fibrosis in animals. McCallum & Leathart found simple pneumoconiosis in about half of a workforce who had had many years exposure to zirconium

Table 13.21. Some compounds of zirconium

Zircon (ZrSiO$_4$)	Refractories, ceramics, 'sand' blasting	Inert dust
Zirconium carbide	Refractories, cutting tools	
Zirconium diboride	Refractories, thermocouple jackets for furnaces	
Zirconium/columbium alloy	Superconductor used in magnets	
Sodium zirconium lactate	Body deodorant	May cause cutaneous granuloma
Zirconium dioxide	Jet and rocket engines, refractories	
Zirconium tetrachloride	Intermediary in production	May cause pulmonary oedema

silicate but there were no material symptoms and no respiratory impairment. The lesions can regress following withdrawal from exposure (fig. 13.7).

Further Reading

General

Hunter D. *The Diseases of Occupations*. London: English Universities Press: 7th edition: 1980.

International Labour Office: Encyclopaedia of Occupational Health and Safety: 3rd (revised) edition. Technical editor: Parmeggiani L. Geneva: ILO. 1983.

Klaasen CD, Amdur MO, Doull J (eds). *Casarett and Doull's Toxicology: The basic science of poisons*, 3rd edn. London: Macmillan. 1986.

Parkes WR. *Occupational lung disorders*. 2nd edition. London: Butterworths. 1982.

Aluminium

Andersen A, Dahlberg BE, Magnus K, Wannag A. Risk of cancer in the Norwegian aluminium industry. *Int J Cancer* 1982;**29**:295–8.

Chan-Yeung M, Wong R, Maclean L, Tan F, Schulzer M, Enarson D, Martin A, Dennis R, Grzybowski S. Epidemiologic health study of workers in an aluminium smelter in British Columbia. *Am Rev Respir Dis* 1983;**127**:465–9.

Chen W-J, Monnat RJ Jr, Chen M, Mottet NK. Aluminium induced pulmonary granulomatosis. *Human Path* 1978;**9**:705–11.

Corrin B. Aluminium pneumoconiosis II. Effect on the rat lung of intratracheal injections of stamped aluminium powders containing different lubricating agents and of a granular aluminium powder. *Br J Industr Med* 1963;**20**:268–76.

Field GB. Pulmonary function in aluminium smelters. *Thorax* 1984;**39**:743–51.

Gibbs GW, Horowitz I. Lung cancer mortality in aluminium reduction plant workers. *J Occup Med* 1979;**21**:347–53.

Maestrelli P, Marcer G, Clonfero E. Report of five cases of fluoride asthma. *Med Lav* 1981;**724**:306–12.

Simonsson BG, Sjoberg A, Rolf C, Haeger-Aronsen B. Acute and long-term airway hyperreactivity in aluminium salt exposed workers with nocturnal asthma. *Eur J Respir Dis* 1985;**66**:105–18.

Townsend MC, Enterline PE, Sussman NB, Bonney TB, Rippey LL. Pulmonary function in relation to total dust exposure at a bauxite refinery and alumina-based chemical products plant. *Am Rev Respir Dis* 1985;**132**:1174–80.

Ammonia

Cole TJ, Cotes JE, Johnson GR, Martin HDeV, Reed JW, Saunders MJ. Ventilation, cardiac frequency and pattern of breathing during exercise in men exposed to o-chlorobenzylidene malononitrile (CS) and ammonia gas in low concentrations. *Quart J Exp Physiol* 1977;**62**:341–51.

Ferguson WS, Koch WC, Webster LB, Gould JR. Human physiological response and adaption to ammonia. *J Occup Med* 1977;**19**:319–26.

Montague TJ, Macneil AR. Mass ammonia inhalation. *Chest* 1980;**77**:496–8.

Sobonya R. Fatal anhydrous ammonia inhalation. *Human Path* 1977;**8**:293–9.

Walton M. Industrial ammonia gassing. *Br J Industr Med* 1973;**30**:78–86.

Antimony

Cooper DA, Pendergrass EP, Vorwald AJ, Mayock RL, Brieger H. Pneumoconiosis among workers in an antimony industry. *Am J Roentg* 1968;**103**:495–508.

McCallum RI, Day MJ, Underhill J, Aird EGA. Measurement of antimony oxide dust in human lungs in vivo by x-ray spectrophotometry. In: *Inhaled Particles 3*. Walton WH (ed), London and Woking: Unwin. 1971:611–18.

Barium

Doig AT. Baritosis: a benign pneumoconiosis. *Thorax* 1976;**31**:30–39.

Brucellosis

McDevitt DG. Symptomatology of chronic brucellosis. *Br J Industr Med* 1973;**30**:385–9.

Sippel JE, El-Masry NA, Farid Z. Diagnosis of human brucellosis with ELISA. *Lancet* 1982;**ii**:19–21.

Carbon monoxide

Joumard R, Chiron M, Vidon R, Maurin M, Rouzioux J-M. Mathematical models of the uptake of carbon monoxide on haemoglobin at low carbon monoxide levels. *Environm Hlth Perspects* 1981;**41**:277–89.

Thomsen HK, Hjeldsen K. Threshold limit for carbon monoxide-induced myocardial damage *Arch Environm Hlth* 1974;**29**:73–8.

Cerium

Brochard P, Chamak B, Kine-Thouvenin A, Hadengue P, Philbert M. Pneumoconiose et cérium. *Archives des Maladies Professionnelles, de Médecine du Travail et de sécurité Sociale (Paris).* 1982;**43/4**:316–9.

Sinico M, Le Bouffant L, Paillas J, Fabre M, Trincard MD. Pneumoconiose due an cérium. Documents anatomopathologiques. *Archives des Maladies Professionelles, de Médecine du Travail et de sécurité Sociale (Paris).* 1982;**43/4**:249–52.

Chlorine

Hasan FM, Gehshan A, Fuleihan FJD. Resolution of pulmonary dysfunction following acute chlorine exposure. *Arch Environm Hlth* 1983;**38:2**:76–9.

Jones RN, Hughes JM, Glindmeyer H, Weill H. *et al.* Lung function after acute chlorine exposure. *Am Rev Respir Dis* 1986;**134**:1190–5. See also: *Am Rev Respir Dis* 1969;**99**:374–9.

Clays (aluminium silicates)

Kennedy T, Rawlings W Jr, Baser M, Tockman M. Pneumoconiosis in Georgia kaolin workers. *Am Rev Respir Dis* 1983;**127**:215–20.

McDermott M, McCarthy PE, Saunders MJ. Respiratory function and pneumoconiosis in Cornish china clay workers. In: *Proceedings of the VIth International Pneumoconiosis Conference, Bochum, 20–23 September 1983.*

Musk AW, Greville HW, Tribe AE. Pulmonary disease from occupational exposure to an artificial aluminium silicate used for cat litter. *Br J Industr Med* 1980;**37**:367–72.

Oldham PD. Pneumoconiosis in Cornish china clay workers. *Br J Industr Med* 1983;**40**:131–7.

Sakula A. Pneumoconiosis due to Fuller's Earth. *Thorax* 1961;**16**:176–9.

Cobalt

Roto P. Asthma, symptoms of chronic bronchitis and ventilatory capacity amongst cobalt and zinc production workers. *Scand J Work Environm Hlth* 1980;**6**: **Suppl.** 1–49.

Sjogren I, Hillerdal G, Andersson A, Zetterström O. Hard metal lung disease: importance of cobalt in coolants. *Thorax* 1980;**35**:653–9.

Cutting oils—see Lipid aerosol

Diesel fumes

Gamble JF, Jones WG. Respiratory effects of diesel exhaust in salt miners. *Am Rev Respir Dis* 1983;**128**:389–94.

Reger R, Hancock J, Hankinson J, Hearl F, Merchant J. Coal miners exposed to diesel exhaust emissions. *Ann Occup Hyg* 1982;**26**:799–815.

Schenker MB, Smith T, Munoz A, Woskie S, Speizer FE. Diesel exposure and mortality among railway workers: results of a pilot study. *Br J Industr Med* 1984;**41**:320–7.

Tollerud DJ, Weiss ST, Elting E, Speizer FE, Ferris B. The health effects of automobile exhaust VI. Relationship of respiratory symptoms and pulmonary function in tunnel and turnpike workers. *Arch Environm Hlth* 1983;**38**:334–40.

Weisenberger BL. Health effects of diesel emissions —an update. *J Soc Occup Med* 1984;**34**:90–2.

Ethanol

Breslin ABX, Hendrick DJ, Pepys J. Effect of disodium cromoglycate on asthmatic reactions to alcoholic beverages. *Clin Allergy* 1973; **3**:71–82.

Cotes JE, Field GB, Brown GJA, Read AE. Impairment of lung function after portacaval anastomosis. *Lancet* 1968;**i**:952–5.

Geppert EF, Boushey HA. An investigation of the mechanism of ethanol-induced bronchoconstriction. *Am Rev Respir Dis* 1978;**118**:135–9.

Krol RC, Knuth SL, Bartlett D (Jr). Selective reduction of genioglossal muscle activity by alcohol in normal human subjects. *Am Rev Respir Dis* 1984;**129**:247–50.

Michiels TM, Light RW, Mahutte CK. Naloxone reverses ethanol-induced depression of hypercapnic drive. *Am Rev Respir Dis* 1983; **128**:823–6.

Sparrow D, Rosner B, Cohen M, Weiss ST. Alcohol consumption and pulmonary function: a cross-sectional and longitudinal study. *Am Rev Respir Dis* 1983;**127**:735–8.

Firefighting

Brown A, Cotes JE, Mortimore IL, Reed JW. An exercise training programme for firemen. *Ergonomics* 1982;**25**:793–800.

Douglas DB, Douglas RB, Oakes D, Scott G. Pulmonary function of London firemen. *Br J Industr Med* 1985;**42**:55–8.

Genovesi MG, Tashkin DP, Chopra S, Morgan M, McElroy C. Transient hypoxaemia in firemen following inhalation of smoke. *Chest* 1977; **71**:441–4.

Loke J, Farmer W, Matthay RM, Putman CF, Walker–Smith GJ. Acute and chronic effects of fire fighting on pulmonary function. *Chest* 1980; **77**:369–73.

Sparrow D, Bossé R, Rosner B, Weiss ST. The effect of occupational exposure on pulmonary function. A longitudinal evaluation of fire fighters and non fire fighters. *Am Rev Respir Dis* 1982;**125**:319–22.

Unger KM, Snow RM, Mestas JM, Miller WC. Smoke inhalation in firemen. *Thorax* 1980; **35**:838–42.

Whitener DR, Whitener LM, Robertson KJ, Baxter CR, Pierce AK. Pulmonary function measurements in patients with thermal injury and smoke inhalation. *Am Rev Respir Dis* 1980;**122**:731–9.

Hairspray

Blainey AD, Ollier S, Davies RJ. Occupational asthma in a hairdressing salon. *Thorax* 1982; **37**:229.

Friedman M, Dougherty R, Nelson SR, White RP, Sackner MA, Wanner A. Acute effects of an aerosol hair spray on tracheal mucociliary transport. *Am Rev Respir Dis* 1977;**116**:281–6.

Parkes WR. *Occupational Lung Disorders*. 2nd edition. London: Butterworths: 1982:399–401.

Zuskin E, Bouhuys A. Acute airway responses to hair-spray preparations. *New Engl J Med* 1974; **290**:660–3.

Hard metal (see also Cobalt)

Bech AO, Kipling MD, Heather JC. Hard metal disease. *Br J Industr Med* 1962;**19**:239–52.

Coates EO, Watson JHL. Diffuse interstitial lung disease in tungsten carbide workers. *Ann Intern Med* 1971;**75**:709–16.

Iron (see also Welding)

Lippmann M. Magnetopneumography as a tool for measuring lung burden of industrial aerosols. In: Stern RM *et al. Proceedings of International Conference on Health Hazards and Biological Effects of Welding Fumes and Gases. Copenhagen.* Amsterdam: Elsevier: 1986:199–213.

Morgan WKC. Magnetite pneumoconiosis. *J Occup Med* 1978;**20**:762–3.

Sadoul P, Horsky P, Beigbeider R, Poncelet B, Pham QT. Siderosis of iron miners in Lorraine. *Archives des Maladies Professionnelles, de Médecine du Travail et de Sécurité Sociale (Paris)*: 1979;**40/1–2**: 15–23.

Kaolin

Altekruse EB, Chaudhary BA, Pearson MG, Morgan WKC. Kaolin dust concentrations and pneumoconiosis at a kaolin mine. *Thorax* 1984; **39**:436–41.

Kennedy T, Rawlings W Jr, Baser M, Tockman M. Pneumoconiosis in Georgia kaolin workers. *Am Rev Respir Dis* 1983;**127**:215–20.

Limestone

Doig AT. Disabling pneumoconiosis from limestone dust. *Br J Industr Med* 1955;**12**:206–16.

Davis SB, Nagelschmidt G. A report on the absence of pneumoconiosis among workers in pure limestone. *Br J Industr Med* 1956;**13**:6–8.

Lipid aerosol and emulsified oil mist (see also colophony, page 371)

Järvholm B, Bake B, Lavenius B, Thiringer G, Vokmann MD. Respiratory symptoms and lung function in oil mist exposed workers. *J Occup Med* 1982;**24**:473–9.

Miller GJ, Ashcroft MT, Beadnell HMSG, Wagner JC, Pepys J. The lipoid pneumonia of black fat tobacco smokers in Guyana. *Quart J Med* 1971;**40**:457–70.

Oldenburger D, Maurer WJ, Beltaos E, Magnin GE. Inhalation lipoid pneumonia from burning fats: a newly-recognized industrial hazard. *J Am Med Ass* 1972;**222**:1288–9.

Wagner JC, Adler DI, Fuller DN. Foreign body granulomata of the lung due to liquid paraffin. *Thorax* 1955;**10**:157–70.

Manganese

Morichau-Beauchant G. Pneumonies manganiques. *J Franc Med Chir Thorac* 1964;**18**:301–12.

Šarić M, Lučić-Palaić S. Possible synergism of exposure to airborne manganese and smoking habit in occurrence of respiratory symptoms. *Inhaled Particles IV*. Oxford: Pergamon Press: 1977:773–9.

Mercury

Hallee TJ. Diffuse lung disease caused by inhalation of mercury vapour. *Am Rev Respir Dis* 1969;**99**:430–6.

Milne J, Christophers A, de Silva P. Acute mercurial pneumonitis. *Br J Industr Med* 1970; **27**:334–8.

Mica

Davies D, Cotton R. Mica pneumoconiosis. *Br J Industr Med* 1983;**40**:22–7.

Mycotic infections

Baum GL, Donnerberg RL, Stewart D, Mulligan WJ, Putnam LR. Pulmonary sporotrichosis. *New Engl J Med* 1969;**280**:410–3.

Campbell CC. Histoplasmosis outbreaks: recommendation for mandatory treatment of known microfoci or *H. Capsulatum* in soils. *Chest* 1980;**77**:6–7.

Crofton J, Douglas A. *Respiratory Diseases*, 3rd edition. Oxford: Blackwell: 1981.

Di Salvo AF, Johnson WM. Histoplasmosis in South Carolina: support for the microfocus concept. *Am J Epidemiol* 1979;**109**:480–92.

Flynn NM, Hoeprich PD, Kawachi MM, Lee KK, Laurence RM, Goldstein E, Jordan GW, Kundargi RS, Wong GA. An unusual outbreak of windborne coccidioidomycosis. *New Engl J Med* 1979;**301**:358–61.

Mehta SK, Sandhu RS. Immunological significance of aspergillus fumigatus in cane-sugar mills. *Arch Environm Hlth* 1983;**38:1**:41–6.

Sorley DL, Levin ML, Warran JW, Flynn JPG, Gerstenblith J. Bat-associated histoplasmosis in Maryland bridge workers. *Am J Med* 1979; **67**:623–6.

Williams PL, Sable DL, Mendez P, Smyth LT. Symptomatic coccidioidomycosis following a severe natural dust storm. *Chest* 1979;**76**: 566–70.

Ornithosis

Anderson DC, Stoesz PA, Kaufmann AF. Psittacosis outbreak in employees of a turkey-processing plant. *Am J Epidemiol* 1978;**107**:140–8.

Anderson JP. Ornithosis in Somerset: Experience in the South Somerset Clinical Area 1964–71. *Post Grad Med J* 1973;**49**:533–4.

Andrews BE, Major R, Palmer SR. Ornithosis in poultry workers. *Lancet* 1981;**i**:632–4.

Byrom NP, Walls J, Mair HJ. Fulminant psittacosis. *Lancet* 1979;**i**:353–6.

Isaacs D. Psittacosis. *Br Med J* 1984;**289**:510–11.

Nitrogen oxides

Becklake MR, Goldman HI, Bosman AR, Freed CC. The long-term effects of exposure to nitrous fumes. *Amer Rev Tuberc* 1957;**76**:398–409.

Fischer P, Remijn B, Brunekreef B, Van Der Lende R, Schouten J, Quanjer P. Indoor air pollution and its effect on pulmonary function of adult non-smoking women: II. Associations between nitrogen dioxide and pulmonary function. *Internat J Epidemiol* 1985;**14(2)**:221–26.

Fleming GM, Chester EH, Montenegro HD. Dysfunction of small airways following pulmonary injury due to nitrogen dioxide. *Chest* 1979;**75**:720–1.

Freeman G, Stephens RJ, Crane SC, Furiosi NJ. Lesion of the lung in rats continuously exposed to two parts per million of nitrogen dioxide. *Arch Environm Hlth* 1968;**17**:181–92.

Horvath EP, do Pico GA, Barbee RA, Dickie HA. Nitrogen dioxide-induced pulmonary disease: five new cases and a review of the literature. *J Occup Med* 1978;**20**:103–10.

Kennedy MCS. Nitrous fumes and coal miners with emphysema. *Ann Occup Hyg* 1972;**15**:285–301.

Kleinerman J, Ip MP. Effects of nitrogen dioxide on elastin and collagen contents of lung. *Arch Environm Hlth* 1979;**34**:228–32.

Lam C, Kattan M, Collins A, Kleinerman J. Long-term sequelae of bronchiolitis induced by nitrogen dioxide in hamsters. *Am Rev Respir Dis* 1983;**128**:1020–23.

Last JA, Gerriets JE, Hyde DM. Synergistic effects on rat lungs of mixtures of oxidant air pollutants (ozone or nitrogen dioxide) and respirable aerosols. *Am Rev Respir Dis* 1983;**128**:539–44.

Morely R, Silk SJ. The industrial hazards from nitrous fumes. *Ann Occup Hyg* 1970; **13**:101–107.

Scott EG, Hunt WB. Silo-filler's disease. *Chest* 1973;**63**:701–706.

Von Nieding G, Wagner HM, Krekeler H, Löllgen H, Fries W, Beuthan A. Controlled studies of human exposure to single and combined action of NO$_2$, O$_3$ and SO$_2$. *Int Arch Occup Environ Hlth* 1979;**43**:195–210.

World Health Organisation. *Oxides of nitrogen. Environmental Health Criteria 4* 1977, Geneva: WHO.

Ozone

Adams WC, Savin WM, Christo AE. Detection of ozone toxicity during continuous exercise via the effective dose concept. *J Appl Physiol* 1981;**51**:415–22.

Dimeo MJ, Glenn MG, Hotlzman MJ, Sheller JR, Nadel JA, Boushey HA. Threshold concentration of ozone causing an increase in bronchial reactivity in humans and adaptation with repeated exposures. *Am Rev Respir Dis* 1981;**124**:245–8.

Dreschsler-Parks DM, Bedi JF, Horvath SM. Interaction of peroxyacetyl nitrate and ozone on pulmonary functions. *Am Rev Respir Dis* 1984;**130**:1033–7.

Gliner JA, Horvath SM, Folinsbee LJ. Pre-exposure to low ozone concentrations does not diminish the pulmonary function response on exposure to higher ozone concentrations. *Am Rev Respir Dis* 1983;**127**:51–5.

Lategola MT, Melton CE, Higgins EA. Pulmonary and symptom threshold effects of ozone in airline passengers and cockpit crew surrogates. *Aviat Space Environm Med* 1980;**51/9:Pt 1**:878–84.

Lunau FW. Ozone in arc welding. *Ann Occup Hyg* 1967;**10**:175–88.

Mihevic PM, Gliner JA, Horvath SM. Perception of effort and respiratory sensitivity during exposure to ozone. *Ergonomics* 1981;**24**:365–74.

Solic JJ, Hazucha MJ, Bromberg PA. The acute effects of 0.2ppm ozone in patients with chronic obstructive pulmonary disease. *Am Rev Respir Dis* 1982;**125**:664–9.

Paraquat

Cooke NJ, Flenley DC, Matthew H. Paraquat poisoning. *Quart J Med* 1973;**42**:683–92.

Fitzgerald GR, Barniville G, Gibney RTN, Fitzgerald MX. Clinical, radiological and pulmonary function assessment in 13 long-term survivors of paraquat poisoning. *Thorax* 1979;**34**:414.

George M, Hedworth-Whitty RB. Non-fatal lung disease due to nebulized paraquat. *Br Med J* 1980;**i**:902.

Hart TB, Nevitt A, Whitehead A. A new statistical approach to the prognostic significance of plasma paraquat concentrations. *Lancet* 1984;**ii**:1222–3.

Higenbottam T, Crome P, Parkinson C, Nunn J. Further clinical observations on the pulmonary effects of paraquat ingestion. *Thorax* 1979;**34**:161–5.

Levin PJ, Klaff LJ, Rose AG, Ferguson AD. Pulmonary effects of contact exposure to paraquat: a clinical and experimental study. *Thorax* 1979;**34**:150–60.

Phosgene

Diller WF. Medical phosgene problems and their possible solution. *J Occup Med* 1978;**20**:189–193.

Sick building syndrome

Gammage RB, Kaye SV (eds). Indoor air and human health. *Proceedings of the seventh life sciences symposium* Knoxville 29–31 October 1984. Chelsea, Michigan: Lewis: 1985.

Robertson AS, Burge PS, Hedge A, Sims J, Gill FS, Finnegan M, Pickering CAC, Dalton G. Comparison of health problems related to work and environmental measurements in two office buildings with different ventilation systems. *Br Med J* 1985;**291**:373–6.

Sulphur dioxide

Archer VE, Gillam JD. Chronic sulphur dioxide exposure in a smelter. ii. Indices of chest disease. *J Occup Med* 1978;**20**:88–95.

Charan NB, Myers CG, Lakshminarayan S, Spencer TM. Pulmonary injuries associated with acute sulfur dioxide inhalation. *Am Rev Respir Dis* 1979;**119**:555–60.

Dixon M, Jackson DM, Richards IM. Changes in the bronchial reactivity of dogs caused by exposure to sulphur dioxide. *J Physiol* 1983;**337**:89–99.

Federspiel CF, Layne JT, Auer C, Bruce J. Lung function among employees of a copper mine smelter: lack of effect of chronic sulfur dioxide exposure. *J Occup Med* 1980;**22**:438–44.

Ferris BG Jr, Puleo S, Chen HY. Mortality and morbidity in a pulp and a paper mill in the United States: a ten-year follow-up. *Br J Industr Med* 1979;**36**:127–34.

Tam WC, Cripps E, Douglas N, Sudlow MF. Protective effect of drugs on broncho-constriction induced by sulphur dioxide. *Thorax* 1982;**37**:671–6.

Sulphuric acid

Williams MK. Sickness absence and ventilatory capacity of workers exposed to sulphuric acid mist. *Br J Industr Med* 1970;**27**:61–6.

Tin

Cole CWD, Davies JVSA, Kipling MD, Ritchie GL. Stannosis in hearth tinners. *Br J Industr Med* 1964;**21**:235–41.

Vanadium

Knecht EA, Moorman WJ, Clark JC, Lynch DW, Lewis TR. Pulmonary effects of acute vanadium pentoxide inhalation in monkeys. *Am Rev Respir Dis* 1985;**132**:1181–5.

Kivuluotu M. Observations on the lungs of vanadium workers. *Br J Industr Med* 1980;**37**:363–6.

Lees REM. Changes in lung function after exposure to vanadium compounds in fuel-oil ash. *Br J Industr Med* 1980;**37**:253–6.

Welding—see also Ozone

Barhad B, Teculescu D, Craciun O. Respiratory symptoms, chronic bronchitis and ventilatory function in shipyard welders. *Int Arch Occ Environm Hlth* 1975;**36**:137–50.

Cotes JE, Feinmann EL, Male VJ, Rennie F. Respiratory health of shipyard workers. *Thorax* 1984;**39**:691 (abstract).

El-Gamal FM. Welding fumes as a cause of impaired lung function in shipyard workers. *PhD Thesis*. University of Newcastle upon Tyne. 1986.

Fawer RF, Gardner AW, Oakes D. Absences attributed to respiratory diseases in welders. *Br J Industr Med* 1982;**39**:149–52.

Hayden SP, Pincock AC, Hayden J, Tyler LE, Cross KW, Bishop JM. Respiratory symptoms and pulmonary function of welders in the engineering industry. *Thorax* 1984;**39**:442–7.

Hunnicutt TN Jr, Cracovaner DJ, Myles JT. Spirometric measurements in welders. *Arch Environm Hlth* 1964;**8**:661–9.

Jones JG, Warner CG. Chronic exposure to iron oxide, chromium oxide and nickel oxide fumes of metal dressers in a steel works. *Br J Industr Med* 1972;**29**:169–77.

Kalliomaki P-L, Lakomaa E, Kalliomaki K, Kiilunen M, Kivela R, Vaaranen V. Stainless steel manual arc welding fumes in rats. *Br J Industr Med* 1983;**40**:229–34.

McMillan GH. The health of welders in naval dockyards: the risk of asbestos-related diseases occurring in welders. *J Occup Med* 1983;**25**:727–30.

McMillan GH, Molyneux MK. The health of welders in naval dockyards: the work situation and sickness absence patterns. *J Soc Occup Med* 1981;**31**:43–60.

McMillan GH, Pethybridge RJ. The health of welders in naval dockyards: proportional mortality study of welders and two control groups. *J Soc Occup Med* 1983;**33**:75–84.

McMillan GH, Pethybridge RJ. A clinical, radiological and pulmonary function case-control study of 135 dockyard welders aged 45 years and over. *J Soc Occup Med* 1984;**34**:3–23.

Newhouse ML, Oakes D, Woolley AJ. Mortality of welders and other craftsmen at a shipyard in N. E. England. *Br J Industr Med* 1985;**42**:406–10.

Oxhöj H, Bake B, Wedel H, Wilhelmsen L. Effects of electric arc welding on ventilatory lung function. *Arch Environm Hlth* 1979;**34**:211–17.

Stern RM. Assessment of risk of lung cancer for welders. *Arch Environm Hlth* 1983;**38**:148–55.

Stern RM (Ed). *Proceedings of International Conference on Health Hazards and Biological Effects of Welding Fumes and Gases, Copenhagen*. Amsterdam: Elsevier. 1985.

Zirconium

Hadjimichael OC, Brubaker RE. Evaluation of an occupational respiratory exposure to a zirconium containing dust. *J Occup Med* 1981;**23**:543–7.

McCallum RI, Leathart GL. *Pneumoconiosis in zirconium process workers*. September 1975 XVIII International Congress on Occupational Health. Brighton. England.

Chapter 14
Byssinosis

Introduction

Byssinosis is probably the world's most prevalent occupational lung disease and the one which is least understood. This paradox arises from its frequently being of mild severity and depending for recognition on only one symptom complex which is not entirely specific; byssinosis merges into and is often difficult to distinguish from chronic bronchitis with airflow obstruction. There is no characteristic physical sign, lung function profile, radiographic feature or change at post-mortem and the causative agent is only known approximately. This is also the case for the prevalence and extent of morbidity and mortality which appear to vary widely depending on which vegetable fibre is responsible, the levels of dustiness and other factors. Thus there is a great need for more research.

The condition was first described in 1713 by Ramazzini in a classical account of which the following is a translation (40):

> We all know what a nuisance the maceration of hemp and flax can be in autumn when its offensive and highly injurious odour is perceptible from a considerable distance; likewise, those who card flax and hemp so that it can be spun and given to the weavers to make the fabric find it very irksome. For a foul and poisonous dust flies out from these materials, enters the mouth, then the throat and lungs, makes the workman cough incessantly, and by degrees brings on asthmatic troubles.

The term byssinosis from βνσσοζ for linen was introduced by Proust in 1870 (25) and modern research into the condition largely stems from Schilling, who initiated the first epidemiological surveys and inspired gifted collaborators including McKerrow, Bouhuys and many others. The condition occurs in workers with textile vegetable fibres including cotton, flax, sisal and soft hemp (cannabis sativa) but not jute or hard hemp. These same dusts may cause a febrile illness, particularly amongst new entrants to the industry but mill fever is unrelated to byssinosis and this is also the case for weavers' cough.

Processing cotton and flax

Cotton filament.

Cotton is produced by the plant species *Gossypium*. *G. herbaceum*, *G. barbadense* and other commercial varieties are cultivated in most countries within the limits 36 degrees north and south of the equator. The species is a perennial shrub but is often grown as an annual. It has alternate stalked and lobed leaves, large yellow to red flowers and a three or five lobed seed capsule which on ripening bursts open to liberate numerous black seeds enveloped in cotton filament. The filament is used for cotton textiles, the seed for its contained oil and as a source of vegetable protein; bark off the root was formerly used for its alleged medicinal properties. Both filament and seed are contained in the capsule or cotton boll (fig. 14.1). This was formerly picked by hand but is now either picked mecha-

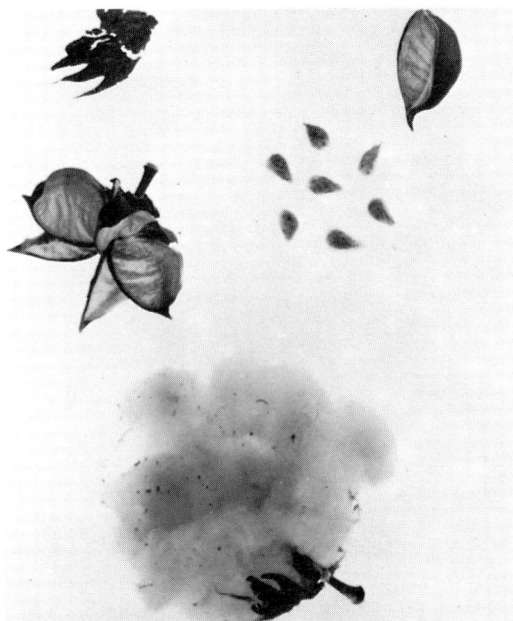

Fig. 14.1. Cotton boll showing the fibres (linters), small leaves at base (bracts), seed case (pericarp) and seeds. (By courtesy of M. McDermott.)

The cotton seed has its coating of fine cotton filament removed and is then dehulled prior to the seed kernels being baled for dispatch to the cotton oil seed mill.

The stages in the processing of raw cotton are described concisely in table 14.2 which should be consulted for details. In the table the relative dustiness of the different stages was that in 1960 when the greatest exposure to airborne dust was in the blowing room and in the vicinity of the scutcher and the carding engine. The debris from around these and other processes also contained many very small cotton fibres and dust from fragmented bracts which became airborne during cleaning up. By comparison with cotton bolls the processing of cotton seeds in oil and cake mills is relatively clean since the seeds are initially nearly free from bract and leaf debris

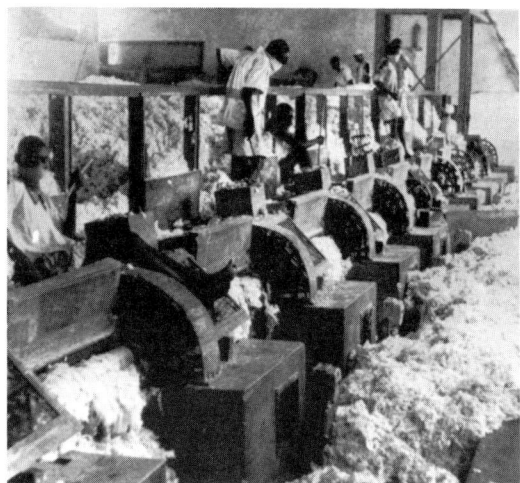

Fig. 14.2. Ginning cotton in Uganda. (By courtesy of J.C. Gilson (17).)

nically or the bolls are obtained by machine stripping; the latter process also harvests much plant debris, called trash. The yield from machine-picked cotton is given in table 14.1. This material immediately undergoes ginning (abbreviated from Middle English engyn) or raking to remove the seeds and much of the pericarp and other debris. This process was formerly very dusty (fig. 14.2) but is now usually clean (see below). After ginning the cotton filament plus some leaf debris and broken capsules (bracts) are baled for dispatch to the cotton mill.

Table 14.1. Material associated with 1kg of cotton lint (29)

Machine stripped (kg)		Machine picked (kg)	Composition of trash (%)			
Cotton seed	1.5	1.5				
Lint	1.0	1.0				
Trash	1.9	0.4	Pericarp	50	Stem	3
			Leaf	20 }*	Soil	1
			Bract	12		

* Poorly removed by ginning; thereafter represents 55% of trash.

Table 14.2. Processing raw cotton

Stages	Operative	Name given to waste cotton	Relative risk†
Harvesting the cotton bolls (seed heads)	Picker	—	—
Ginning (raking) to remove seeds	Ginner	Motes	+
Packing raw cotton into bale	Packer	—	+
Opening bale; removing debris by 'blowing' with compressed air	Blow room worker, Opener	Filter waste	+++
Scutching or beating to separate the fibres	Scutcher	Picker	++
Combing the cotton (carding) to form lap	Stripper/grinder, Card tenter, liner carder, carder, Lap carrier	Strip	+++
Drawing and doubling untwisted thread (sliver)	Draw frame tenter	Sweeps	+
Slubbing and roving (making the first twists)	Speed frame tenter	—	+
Winding and spinning	Ring spinner, winder, beamer	—	+
Weaving	Weaver		—*
Delintering cotton seeds (removing coating of fine fibres)		Linters	++
Garnetting (processing) waste cotton to make batting (for quilts and mattresses)			++

* Use of mechanical pickers is increasing the dustiness and hence the risk of byssinosis amongst spinners, winders and weavers.
† In 1960 (34) plus other information.

and the principal dusty process is the delintering (table 14.2). Dust is also formed during the process of dehulling. In the cotton-spinning mills the dustiness is now greatly reduced on account of application of the measures described on page 316; as a result the distribution of dust levels between processes is more uniform. However, one unintended consequence is that the cotton mill dust may contain one or more additives, for example machine oil, silicon spray, ethylene oxide and sorbitan monolaurate; it may also contain organic contaminants from the humidifier system (cf. page 340).

Flax fibre

Linum usitatissimum is an annual plant with small blue flowers, narrow stem and jointed leaves which grows some 2ft high in temperate climates; other varieties have longer stems including the New Zealand flax *Phormium tenax*. The stem contains long fibres which are used for making linen cloth. This is done in the U.S.S.R., Poland, Northern Ireland, the Netherlands and other countries but until recently the process was expensive; the industry is now experiencing a revival due to the introduction of new methods, including the use of defoliants. The seeds are a source of linseed oil and a feed for cattle. The processing of flax is similar to cotton after the initial stages; these differ due to the fibre being contained in the stalks and not the seed cases. The stalks are defoliated, then treated by wet rotting to soften and loosen the fibres. The rotting is carried out on the fields (dew retting), in tanks (wet retting), by alkalis (chemical retting) or by mechanical means (green retting). These processes are performed wet so are not dusty.

Clinical features of byssinosis

Symptoms

The characteristic feature of byssinosis is substernal unease which becomes worse on exertion when it is accompanied by inability to expand the lungs fully. The patient may describe the chest as being puffed up but the sensation differs from that of an attack of asthma

Table 14.3. Byssinosis questions to supplement MRC questionnaire of respiratory symptoms (38)

1. Do you cough on any particular day of the week?

2. Does your chest ever feel tight or your breathing become difficult?

   If yes: Only with colds?
         Apart from colds?
         If apart from colds, when?

3. Is your chest tight or your breathing difficult on any particular day of the week?

   If yes: Which day?
         Sometimes?
         Always?

4. Has your chest ever been tight or your breathing difficult on any particular day of the week?

Table 14.4. Grades of byssinosis (38)

Grade 0	No symptoms of byssinosis
Grade 1/2	Occasional chest tightness on the first day of the working week
Grade 1	Chest tightness on every first day of the working week
Grade 2	Chest tightness on the first and other days of the working week
Grade 3	Grade 2 symptoms accompanied by evidence of permanent incapacity from diminished effort tolerance and/or reduced ventilatory capacity

(which may coexist) and whilst it is also referred to as chest tightness this is an over-simplification (23). Initially the symptom develops over the first working day after a period away from exposure which may be the weekend or a holiday or a period of sickness. In western countries the return to work is usually on a Monday, hence Monday Tightness or Monday Sickness. In Islamic countries the first working day is usually a Saturday. As the condition advances the symptom appears on subsequent days as well. This sequence is usual though not invariable. It provides a way of grading byssinosis through answers to standard questions; these questions, which are intended primarily for use in epidemiological surveys, are listed in table 14.3 and the resulting grades are given in table 14.4. Grades 1/2 and 1 constitute classical byssinosis which is usually easily recognized if the right questions are asked but with grades 2 and 3 the subject may also have chronic bronchitis and be diagnosed as having this condition with or without asthma or emphysema. The diagnosis of byssinosis is then in doubt. However, cough and phlegm is more common in those with byssinosis than without (6) and its occurrence may follow a weekly cycle similar to that of the chest tightness and breathlessness; in these circumstances cough is probably an integral part of the disease (22). The bronchitis may also be a separate entity reflecting a high prevalence of smoking and exposure to environmental air pollution; it may be the sole abnormality or bronchitis and byssinosis may coexist. Asthma in cotton workers usually occurs separately and may be recognized as such by the patient. Bronchial hyperreactivity due to a viral infection or other cause can additionally confuse the clinical picture (37). To make the diagnosis then requires time and patience and may be difficult if the exposure to cotton ceased some time prior to the consultation.

Airflow obstruction

The symptom of chest tightness developing progressively over the first day back at work is usually accompanied by a reduction in forced expiratory volume (fig. 14.3) and peak expiratory flow; reductions in airflow conductance and forced expiratory flow ($\dot{V}_{50}$) have also been reported but the changes are not consistent (8, 16) and there is need for further work. Similar changes can occur when healthy subjects are challenged with aqueous extract of the dust but not all subjects respond. The fall in FEV_1 over the shift is usually regarded as evidence for byssinosis. However, symptomatic byssinosis may occur without it. The FEV_1 is the basis for a

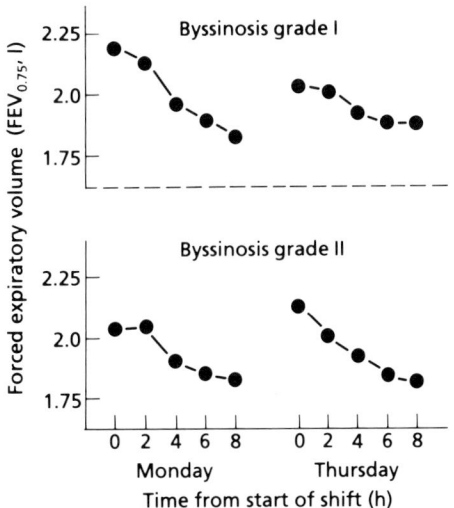

Fig. 14.3. Mean levels of $FEV_{0.75}$ over a working shift for cardroom workers with byssinosis grades I and II. In grade I the decline was most marked on Mondays but in grade II it occurred on other days as well. (By courtesy of M. McDermott (24).)

scale of functional impairment in byssinosis which is given in table 14.5. A reduction in FEV_1 over the first working shift in the week of more than 0.2 l or 5% is evidence for a definite acute effect of dust. The decline in FEV_1 over the shift is prevented or reversed by the use of a bronchodilator aerosol; in the early stages of work with cotton, recovery between shifts occurs spontaneously and it is usually only after some 10 years of employment that the FEV_1 may be conspicuously reduced compared with the reference value. The reduced ventilatory capacity is not diagnostic of byssinosis as it also occurs in association with non-specific respiratory symptoms (2).

Grade 3 byssinosis

Subjects with grade 1 byssinosis who remain in employment may experience an extension of their symptoms from the first day of the working week to other days (grade 2 byssinosis) and in addition may develop breathlessness on exertion due to persistent ventilatory impairment. This combination of features constitutes grade 3 byssinosis. There are no special findings on physical examination and the chest radiograph is usually normal but the subject may have persistent cough and phlegm sufficient to warrant the diagnosis of chronic bronchitis with airflow obstruction. At this stage the evidence for byssinosis may be elicited by careful enquiry into the clinical and occupational histories. The obstruction is only slightly ameliorated by bronchodilator therapy. The disease may progress to respiratory insufficiency and cor pulmonale. The treatment is that for these conditions and is described in chapter 19 (page 407). The evidence is conflicting as to whether or not byssinosis shortens life; most recent studies suggest that it does not (4, 14, 27) but in the period 1910–31 the mortality of Lancashire cotton mill strippers and grinders from respiratory and related diseases was materially increased (38). The recorded causes of death are probably not reliable but a high cotton dust exposure is likely to have been a material contributory factor. The mortality from lung cancer appears to be low amongst cotton operators; the mechanism is unknown (15) (cf. page 243).

Table 14.5. Classification of respiratory impairment in byssinosis (7)

Functional category	Change in FEV_1 over shift (l)	Reduction in FEV_1 (as % predicted)
F0	None (<0.05)	None (>80)
F1/2	Slight (0.06–0.2)	None
F1	Definite (>0.2)	None
F2		Slight – moderate (60 – 75%)
F3		Moderate – severe (<60%)

Post-mortem findings

At post-mortem the byssinotic lung looks completely normal; it even lacks the brown pigmentation which was implied by byssinosis previously having been called brown lung disease. On histological examination there is hyperplasia of mucous glands in the walls of the lobar bronchi, metaplasia of goblet cells and hypertrophy of bronchial smooth muscle. There is no significant involvement of the segmental bronchi and in this the appearances differ from those of typical chronic bronchitis associated with smoking. Emphysema may coexist but its prevalence is not greater than amongst other members of the local community and this is also the case for abnormality of the pulmonary blood vessels. Pulmonary hypertension is not common and there is no undue hypertrophy of the right or left ventricles of the heart. Giant cells may occur in the lung parenchyma, possibly in association with fragments of cotton, and so-called byssinotic bodies may be present but neither of these features is believed to be of any consequence; there are no changes suggestive of extrinsic allergic alveolitis (12). The increased capacity to secrete mucus is correlated with the cotton dust exposure during life but no similar association has been observed for emphysema or other post-mortem findings (33).

Mechanisms

The progressive airways obstruction over the first working day of the week may be due to any of several causes; these have recently been reviewed (19, 29). The simplest is that cotton dust stimulates irritant receptors in the airways (page 47) but this is unlikely since the response occurs at levels of dustiness which are below the

threshold for this effect. It might be due to 5-hydroxytryptamine or other bronchoconstrictor substances present in the dust but these substances are only present in very low concentration. At one time methyl piperonylate was thought to be responsible but its presence in the bracts has not been confirmed. An IgE-mediated hypersensitivity reaction such as occurs in asthma (page 346) is also unlikely since persons with byssinosis are usually non-atopic and cotton workers do not exhibit undue sensitivity to cotton-based antigens; however, amongst exposed persons those who are atopic exhibit a greater decline in FEV_1 than their non-atopic colleagues (20). On this account they often stay in the industry for only a short time and there is need for more studies of the contributory factors.

Most authors accept that the bronchoconstriction is mediated by intrinsic histamine which is released from mast cells in the lung; the mast cells usually degranulate nearly completely during the first day at work and regeneration is slow so in most workers no histamine is left for release on subsequent days. However, the regenerative ability of the mast cells probably increases as a result of stimulation since later in the disease the bronchoconstriction occurs on other days of the week besides Mondays. Breakdown products of histamine are excreted in the urine. The histamine release is prevented by prior administration of sodium cromoglycate which acts by stabilizing the membrane of the mast cell so that degranulation and release of mediator substances does not occur. Administration of histamine blocking agents (anti-histamines) may also prevent the onset of airways obstruction in some circumstances but the response is not invariable (36). This may partly reflect the proximity of the mast cells to the histamine receptor sites but other bronchoconstrictor substances may also contribute to the response.

The release of histamine may be due to a non-antigenic releasing agent present in the cotton (30). It may be due to bacterial endotoxins from bacteria associated with the cotton (31) or to an antigen–antibody reaction associated with a precipitating antibody present in the plasma (39). These hypotheses are the subject of intensive research (11). Of them the direct release hypothesis is the most widely held and is now buttressed by an elegant assay method using pig blood platelets (1). However the possible role of lipopolysaccharide endotoxin (LPS) from the walls of gram negative bacteria including *Enterobacter agglomerans* which grow on the surface of all textile vegetable plants is now attracting increasing attention (31, 35). The endotoxin may possibly explain all the features of byssinosis, including the bronchitis and the mill fever which may develop in the early stages of working in a cotton or flax mill. Thus LPS is chemotactic for polymorphonuclear leucocytes which are recruited into the airways and nose following exposure to cotton dust or extract. It also causes release of histamine in circumstances when release would occur with cotton dust extract, though whether the release is due to an effect on macrophages and blood platelets or on neutrophils or mast cells is still unclear. In acute studies a decline in FEV during a first day at work with cotton has been shown to be correlated with the LPS concentrations (35) whilst in epidemiological studies the extent of symptomatic byssinosis is correlated better with the amount of airborne gram negative bacteria and airborne LPS than the concentrations of airborne dust (10). However, following inhalation challenge with endotoxin the symptoms are not typical of byssinosis and bronchoconstriction is not invariable. In addition the bracts contain other bronchoconstrictor substances (9). Washed cotton also bronchoconstricts (32). Thus the endotoxin hypothesis remains unproven. Possibly different agents cause the symptoms, the acute decline in airway calibre over the working day and the long-term deterioration, and one or more agents may act as a trigger to allow another to exert a deleterious effect (19). There is clear need for more research and this would be helped by an animal model of byssinosis to supplement studies on men (29). Unfortunately a model presupposes that the disorder can be defined in objective terms; this appears not to be possible (page 309) so the advent of a model is still for the future.

Epidemiology: relationship to dust exposure

Amongst cotton operatives byssinotic symptoms are now uncommon with less than 4 years exposure and usually only occur after 10 or more years (28). Age and ethnic group do not influence susceptibility but men may be more susceptible than women (5). The prevalence in working populations is in the range 0–70% with an average in one report of 27% (28); the overall prevalence in a whole community including ex-employees, relatives and others appears never to have been assessed. A study of ex-flax workers has recently been reported (13).

The evidence for byssinosis being due to exposure to dust from cotton or other active

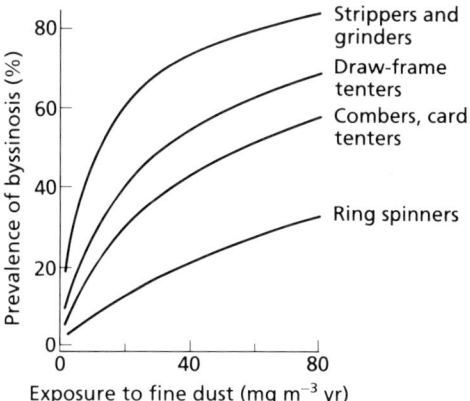

Fig. 14.4. Relationship of byssinosis prevalence (grade 0.5 or above) to estimated exposure to cotton dust for different occupational groups. After allowing for dust concentration at the time of survey, duration of exposure and smoking, there was a significant relationship to occupation. This could have been due to differences in the dust or to the previous exposures in the dustier occupation having been underestimated. (By courtesy of G. Berry *et al* (5).)

textile vegetable fibre is based on both observation of the acute changes (page 312) and the finding in epidemiological studies of a relationship between symptoms and exposure to cotton dust; the first of these was that conducted by Roach & Schilling (34). Subsequent studies (e.g. fig. 14.4) came to a similar conclusion (5, 21, 26). At the time of the earlier study there was a fairly consistent sequence of dustiness associated with the several stages of the industrial process; in the case of cotton this is given in table 14.2. The highest levels of dustiness in cotton mills were in the vicinity of the carding engines with peaks often occurring at the times when they were cleaned. Low levels were associated with spinning and weaving though there were systematic differences between mills depending on the quality of the cotton being processed; in general Lancashire (U.K.) used coarse cotton which was relatively dusty. Since 1960 the pattern has changed; dust concentrations are less predictable and the lower limit for development of byssinosis appears to have fallen. This is due to changes in the industry including replacement of hand picking of cotton bolls by machines which harvest more dirt and plant debris, the introduction of exhaust ventilation around the carding engines and a speeding up of the processes of spinning and weaving through the introduction of new machinery which also generates more dust. Due to these changes the dose–response relationships which were so conspicuous in the past are less apparent in recent studies but the conclusions which were drawn from the earlier ones are in the main still valid. In many surveys the prevalence of byssinosis has been found to be higher amongst smokers than non-smokers (5, 24) but this is not invariable (6) and there is no evidence for interaction between the effects of tobacco smoke and air-borne cotton fibres or debris similar to tobacco's interaction with asbestos (chapter 10).

The observation that byssinosis was associated with a reduction in forced expiratory volume on the first working shift of the week (page 313) was based initially on study of a small number of cotton operatives (24). It has since been observed in occupational surveys but the association is often weak; thus in one study (3) amongst forty-seven workers with byssinosis

only fourteen exhibited the change in FEV_1 whilst this feature was observed amongst twenty-six out of 120 operatives who did not have the typical symptom. Some of the discrepancy may have been due to occupationally-related cough not being classified as byssinosis (see above) and to some operatives being relatively insensitive to their airways obstruction. Evidence for the latter view comes from the findings that (1) workers who developed byssinosis during the survey had a significantly larger decline in FEV_1 over the first shift than those who did not and (2) amongst subjects with byssinosis grade 1/2 the decline in FEV_1 over the shift was significantly correlated with the environmental concentration of fine dust. The reduction reflected an approximately 50% increase in the annual decline of FEV_1 for cotton workers compared with persons in a mill processing man-made fibres. The decline was correlated with the duration of the employment, the dust exposure including working in proximity to the carding engine, bronchitic symptoms and whether or not the subject smoked. The changes extend beyond the period of employment into retirement (2). In future studies allowance should also be made for atopic status which additionally influences the decline in FEV_1 (20).

Safe conditions

The findings of Roach & Schilling which are summarized in table 14.2 provided the first reliable indication of what were likely to be safe conditions in the U.K.; these are now defined as a maximal average air-borne concentration of plant material and debris of less than 0.5mg m^{-3} less fly which is the larger particles excluded by a 2mm wire mesh gauze or appropriate elutriator. The U.S. standard for an 8h shift is 0.2mg m^{-3} as a time-weighted average obtained using a standard vertical elutriator with a cut-off at 15μm. In some cotton mills the attainment of safe conditions is ensured by totally enclosing the carding engines but this presents practical difficulties. In addition exhaust ventilation is in use round the engines and elsewhere in the factory; vacuum cleaning is undertaken extensively to reduce the accumulation of dust. The equipment in the model card room consists of a single bale opener, seeder and cotton card through which cotton is processed from bale to sliver. A laminar flow of re-circulated, cleaned and conditioned air moves through the room counter-currently to the flow of cotton. The effectiveness of the dust suppression is monitored by a large variety of gravimetric short-term and continuous air samplers (18) (see also chapter 2). Additional measures which may be applied include the use of steam or dust suppressant lubricants to moisten the cotton in the gin, where this procedure is more effective than when applied to the bale. Lint cleaners in the ginning line are also effective. The harvesting should preferably have been carried out using spindle pickers which generate less dust during the processing of the cotton than is the case for brush strippers.* Less dusty genetic variants of the commonly used textile plants have not yet been discovered but this is a strong possibility for the future. One likely development is of a variant with smooth-skinned (naked) seeds which avoid the need for delintering.

The hygiene measures are expensive, not least because cotton spinning is best undertaken in an atmosphere which is moist and very warm. The heat which is lost by exhaust ventilation is costly to replace. There is need to find out which remedies are cost-effective in any particular circumstances with respect to the equipment in the factory, the speed of use, the levels of ventilation and the type and dustiness of the cotton or other fibre. To achieve this the requisite environmental monitoring should be undertaken using personal samplers which are worn by employees on a random basis; this method effectively provides surveillance of all the operatives in the plant. The environmental monitoring should be combined with biological monitoring by periodic assessment of personnel and scrutiny of sickness absences and retirements on medical grounds with a view to confirming whether or not the environmental conditions are satisfactory.

* These terms are used in the U.S.A. In the U.K. they were formerly used to describe the men who cleaned the teeth of cards with a rapidly rotating brush.

Medical surveillance

The medical care of textile workers starts with the pre-employment examination when it is usual to recommend exclusion of persons with established respiratory disease or who are atopic or whose ventilatory capacity is below the normal range. These practices have much to recommend them but the exclusion of atopic subjects should perhaps be deferred pending the accumulation of more information (page 80). There is probably an equal case for excluding smokers though this is seldom done in practice.

The periodic examinations should include the questionnaire on symptoms (table 14.3) though the answers tend to be affected by the morale in the factory and the level of employment in the community, and may not be easy to interpret. The ventilatory capacity should be measured routinely and where appropriate the change in FEV_1 over a first day at work should be monitored. A watch should be kept on subjects whose change in FEV_1 over a first working day exceeds 0.2 l; this is functional capacity F1 (table 14.5). However, these figures need to be considered in the context of the local conditions including the prevalence of smoking and chronic bronchitis. In addition a reduction in the absolute level of forced expiratory volume of 0.25 l over a 5-year period should lead to a review of the case and a decline of 0.5 l to specific remedial action. Positive evidence for byssinosis occurring in an employee has serious implications for the medical health and economic viability of the mill so the condition must be prevented if possible.

Further Reading

Honeybourne D., Wales D.S., Watson A, Lee W.R., Saga B.F. (1982) *Byssinosis—causative agent and clinical aspects.* Shirley Institute Publications, Manchester.

National Research Council on Byssinosis (1982) Byssinosis: Clinical and Research issues, pp. 1–143. National Academy Press, Washington.

References

1 Ainsworth SK, Neuman RE, Harley RA. Histamine release from platelets for assay of byssinogenic substances in cotton mill dust and related materials. *Br J Industr Med* 1979;**36**:35–42.

2 Beck GJ, Schachter EN, Maunder LR. The rela-

tionship of respiratory symptoms and lung function loss in cotton textile workers. *Am Rev Respir Dis* 1984;**130**:6–11.

3 Berry G, McKerrow CB, Molyneux MKB, Rossiter CE, Tombleson JBL. A study of the acute and chronic changes in ventilatory capacity of workers in Lancashire cotton mills. *Br J Industr Med* 1973;**30**:25–36.

4 Berry G, Molyneux MKB. A mortality study of workers in Lancashire cotton mills. *Chest* 1981;**79:4(Suppl)**:11S–15S.

5 Berry G, Molyneux MKB, Tombleson JBL. Relationship between dust level and byssinosis and bronchitis in Lancashire cotton mills. *Br J Industr Med* 1974;**31**:18–27.

6 Bouhuys A, Barbero A, Schilling RSF, Van de Woestijne KP. Chronic respiratory disease in hemp workers. *Am J Med* 1969;**46**:526–37.

7 Bouhuys A, Gilson JC, Schilling RSF. Byssinosis in the textile industry. *Arch Environm Hlth* 1970;**21**:475–8.

8 Bouhuys A, Van de Woestijne KP. Respiratory mechanics and dust exposure in byssinosis. *J Clin Invest* 1970;**49**:106–118.

9 Buck MG, Wall JH, Schachter EN. Airway constrictor response to cotton bract extracts in the absence of endotoxin. *Br J Industr Med* 1986;**43**:220–6. *See also* Cloutier MM, Rohrbach MS. *Am Rev Respir Dis* 1986;**134**:1158–62.

10 Cinkotai FF, Whitaker CJ. Airborne bacteria and the prevalence of byssinotic symptoms in 21 cotton spinning mills in Lancashire. *Ann Occup Hyg* 1978;**21**:239–50.

11 Edwards J. Mechanisms of disease induction. *Chest* 1981;**79:4 (Suppl)**:38S–43S.

12 Edwards C, Macartney J, Rooke G, Ward F. The pathology of the lung in byssinotics. *Thorax* 1975;**30**:612–23.

13 Elwood JH, Elwood PC, Campbell MJ, Stanford CF, Chivers A, Hey I, Brewster L, Sweetnam PM. Respiratory disability in ex-flax workers. *Br J Industr Med* 1986;**43**:300–6.

14 Elwood PC, Thomas HF, Sweetnam PM, Elwood JH. Mortality of flax workers. *Br J Industr Med* 1982;**39**:18–22.

15 Enterline PE, Sykora JL, Keleti G, Lange JH. Endotoxins, cotton dust and cancer. *Lancet* 1985;**ii**:934–5.

16 Field GB, Owen P. Respiratory function in an Australian cotton mill. *Bull Europ Physiopathol Respir* 1979;**15**:455–68.

17 Gilson JC, Stott H, Hopwood BEC, Roach SA, McKerrow CB, Schilling RSF. Byssinosis: The acute effect on ventilatory capacity of dusts in cotton ginneries, cotton, sisal, and jute mills. *Br J Industr Med* 1962;**19**:9–18.

18 Hersh SP, Batra SK, Fornes RE. Review of cotton dust control technology studies at North Carolina State University. *Chest* 1981;**79:4(Suppl)**:101S–108S.

19 Honeybourne D, Wales DS, Watson A, Lee WR, Sagar BF. *Byssinosis—causative agent and clinical aspects.* Manchester: Shirley Institute Publications. 1982 ISSN 0306 5154:543.

20 Jones RN, Butcher BT, Hammad YY, Diem JE, Glindmeyer HW III, Lehrer SB, Hughes JM, Weill H. Interaction of atopy and exposure to cotton dust in the bronchoconstrictor response. *Br J Industr Med* 1980;**37**:141–6.

21 Jones RN, Diem JE, Glindmeyer H, Dharmarajan V, Hammad YY, Carr J, Weill H. Mill effect and dose-response relationships in byssinosis. *Br J Industr Med*, 1979;**36**:305–13.

22 Kamat SR, Kamat GR, Salpekar VY, Lobo E. Distinguishing byssinosis from chronic obstructive pulmonary disease. *Am Rev Respir Dis* 1981;**124**:31–40.

23 Lee WR. Clinical diagnosis of byssinosis. *Thorax* 1979;**34**:287–9.

24 McKerrow CB, McDermott M, Gilson JC, Schilling RSF. Respiratory function during the day in cotton workers: a study in byssinosis. *Br J Industr Med*, 1958;**15**:75–83.

25 Massoud A. The origin of the term byssinosis. *Br J Industr Med* 1964;**21**:162.

26 Merchant JA, Lumsden JC, Kilburn KH, O'Fallon WM, Ujda MD, Germino VH, Hamilton JD. Dose-response studies in cotton textile workers. *J Occup Med* 1973;**15**:222–30.

27 Merchant JA, Ortmeyer C. Mortality of employees of two cotton mills in North Carolina. *Chest* 1981;**79:4(Suppl)**:6S–11S.

28 Molyneux MKB, Tombleson JBL. An epidemiological study of respiratory symptoms in Lancashire mills, 1963–66. *Br J Industr Med* 1970;**27**:225–34.

29 National Research Council Committee on Byssinosis. *Byssinosis: Clinical and Research Issues.* National Academy Press: Washington. 1982:1–143. ISBN 0–309. 03276–8.

30 Nicholls PJ, Nicholls GR, Bouhuys A. Histamine release by compound 48/80 and textile dusts from lung tissue in vitro. In: Davies CN (ed) *Inhaled Particles and Vapours II*, London: Pergamon Press, 1966:69.

31 Pernis B, Vigliani EC, Cavagna C, Finulli M. The role of bacterial endotoxins in occupational diseases caused by inhaling vegetable dusts. *Br J Industr Med* 1961;**18**:120–9.

32 Petsonk EL, Olenchock SA, Castellan RM, Banks DE, Mull JC, Hankinson JL, Bragg KC, Perkins HH, Cocke JB. Human ventilatory response to washed and unwashed cottons from different growing areas. *Br J Industr Med* 1986;**43**:182–7.

33 Pratt PC, Vollmer RT, Miller JA. Epidemiology of pulmonary lesions in non-textile and cotton textile workers: a retrospective autopsy analysis. *Arch Environm Hlth* 1980;**35:(3)**:133–8.

34 Roach SA, Schilling RSF. A clinical and environmental study of byssinosis in the Lancashire cotton industry. *Br J Industr Med* 1960;**17**:1–9.

35 Rylander R, Haglind P, Lundholm M. Endotoxin in cotton dust and respiratory function decrement among cotton workers in an experimental card room. *Amer Rev Respir Dis* 1985;**131**:209–213.

36 Schachter EN, Brown S, Zuskin E, Beck GJ, Buck M, Kolack B, Bouhuys A. The effect of mediator modifying drugs in cotton bract-induced bronchospasm. *Chest* 1981;**79: 4(Suppl)**:73S–77S.

37 Schachter EN, Zuskin E, Buck MG, Witek TJ, Beck GJ, Tyler D. Airway reactivity and cotton bract-induced bronchial obstruction. *Chest* 1985;**87**:51–55.

38 Schilling RSF. Byssinosis in cotton and other textile workers. *Lancet* 1956;**ii**:261–5:319–24.

39 Taylor G, Massoud AAE, Lucas F. Studies on the aetiology of byssinosis. *Br J Industr Med* 1971;**28**:143–51.

40 Weill H. Problem solving in occupational airways disorders. *Chest* 1981;**79:4(Suppl)**: 1S–2S.

Chapter 15
Extrinsic Allergic Alveolitis

Extrinsic allergic alveolitis (hypersensitivity pneumonitis)

Extrinsic allergic alveolitis is caused by various organic materials including animal residues, moulds, spores, protozoa and chemical substances, some of which are classified under these headings in table 15.1. They have in common the property of existing as an aerosol of particles small enough to enter the alveoli (diameter < 1µm) and of generating in the host specific precipitating antibodies. The antigen–antibody reaction is associated with a brief influenza-like illness and with the development in the lung of multiple small granulomas. Evidence for the granulomas comes mainly from study of farmers' lung and bird handlers' lung. Their presence in related conditions can be inferred from the clinical features. Granulomas have not been demonstrated in humidifier fever and other diseases due to antigens spread in water droplets. The typical clinical episode of extrinsic allergic alveolitis develops a few hours after exposure, usually in the afternoon or evening. The exposure may be readily identifiable (e.g. to mouldy hay or to bird droppings) or be inconspicuous and the condition easily missed unless a comprehensive history is taken including occupational and leisure-time activities. Extrinsic allergic alveolitis should be suspected if the symptoms occur after a particular activity,

at a particular time during the week or on return to work after a weekend or holiday. Sometimes the characteristic acute symptoms are mild or absent; instead there is insidious development of mild or progressive diffuse interstitial fibrosis presenting at a later stage of the disease process with breathlessness on exertion. Examples of these two modes of presentation are given in table 15.2. The characteristic symptoms and physical signs can be reproduced by specific inhalation challenge. However, antibodies may not be detectable in some who respond to specific inhalation challenge, and may disappear in the chronic stage of the disease if exposure to the allergen has ceased. Antibodies also occur in exposed persons who are asymptomatic and apparently healthy. Thus, whilst the presence of antibodies is evidence for sensitization (2) it is not diagnostic and their role must be strongly influenced by constitutional and other factors (page 333).

Terminology

The occurrence of granulomata led Dickie & Rankin to describe this group of conditions as acute granulomatous pneumonitis, whilst the predominantly interstitial distribution suggested the name interstitial pneumonitis (Liebow). This distribution, together with

Table 15.1. Some causes of extrinsic allergic alveolitis

Antigen	Source or substrate	Condition	Reference
*Animal residues**			
Animal antigen (bovine, porcine, rodent etc.)	Danders, hair, serum, urine, pituitary snuff	Animal handlers' and furriers' lung, snuff takers' lung	73, 83, 86 81
Avian antigen (e.g. pigeon, budgerigar, turkey, etc.)	Bloom, droppings, feathers, serum	Bird fanciers' and handlers' lung	19, 22, 47
Coccus cactus	Carmine extraction	—	—
Sitophilus granaris	Grain and flour dust	Wheat weevil lung	84
Chemical substances			
Hydrochlorothiazide	Hypotensive therapy		68
Diisocyanates*	Adhesives and paints		74
Pyrethrum	Insecticide		72
Thermosetting resin*			77
Pauli's reagent (sodium diazobenzene sulphonate)			79
Moulds, other micro-organisms and spores			
Acanthamoeba	Humidifier sludge	Humidifier fever†	54
*Agaricus hortensis**	Mushroom spores	Mushroom workers' lung	92
Alternaria	Wood pulp	Pulp workers' disease	89
Aspergillus clavatus	Malt barley	Malt workers' lung	80
Aureobasidium pullulans (pullularia)	Redwood dust	Sequoiosis	75
	Sauna	Water droplet antigen disease	62
Bacillus subtilis	Humidifier aerosol	Humidifier fever	64
Cryptostroma corticale	Stored maple logs	Maple bark disease	78, 96
Flavobacteria endotoxin	Humidifier aerosol, etc.	Humidifier fever†	56, 63, 65
Gram negative bacteria	Sewage, sludge	Water droplet antigen disease	58
*Merulius lacrymans**	Dry rot spores		85
*Micropolyspora faeni**	Mouldy hay	Farmers' lung, etc.	41
Mucor liemalis	Wood chippings	Wood trimmers' disease	69
	Red pepper (paprika)	Paprika splitters' lung	93
Naegleria gruberi (amoeba)	Humidifier aerosol	Humidifier fever†	58, 59
Paecilomyces varotii	Wood chippings	Wood trimmers' disease	69
Penicillium casei and roqueforti	Cheese making	Cheese washer's disease	71
Penicillium chrysogenum and cyclopium	Wet linoleum, etc.		
Penicillium frequentans	Wet stacked cork	Suberosis	67, 87
Pleurotus florida	Mushroom spores	Mushroom workers' lung	90
Rhizopus rhizopodiformis	Wood chippings	Wood trimmers' disease	69
Thermoactinomyces-			
Candidus	Air conditioner aerosol	Humidifier fever	55, 60
Sporobolomyces†	Straw		—
Sacchari, Vulgaris	Sugar can fibre (bagasse)	Bagassosis	13, 14
Actinobifida dichotomica	Mushroom compost	Mushroom workers' lung	88, 13

* May also cause occupational asthma (page 361).
† A form of water droplet antigen disease.

Table 15.2.   Examples of the acute and chronic forms of extrinsic allergic alveolitis

	Acute	Chronic
Occupation	Pigeon fancier	Budgerigar fancier
Patient	Middle-aged man	Elderly lady
History	Acute episodes	Progressive breathlessness
Presentation	Early	Late
Insight	Good (reads the journals)	Nil
Diagnosis	Patient	Physician (if at all)
Disablement	Nil between episodes	Considerable
Response to treatment	Good	Poor

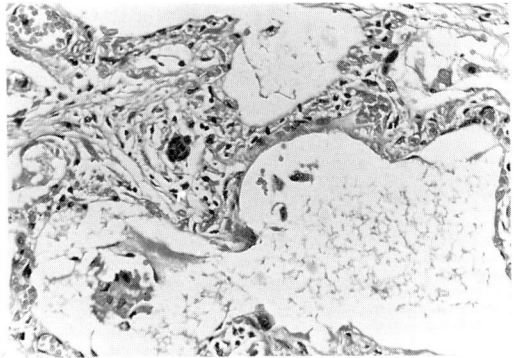

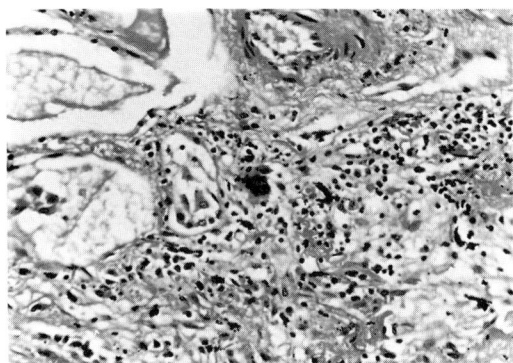

Fig. 15.1. Pulmonary granuloma from a patient with bird fanciers' lung showing multinucleated giant cells and interstitial fibrosis. In the upper view fibrinous exudate lines distal alveolar spaces, and in the lower one there is extensive lymphocytic infiltration (medium power views). (By courtesy of T. Ashcroft.)

dependence on a hypersensitivity reaction to inhaled antigens, was the basis for Pepys' term extrinsic allergic alveolitis and this was subsequently expanded by Seal to extrinsic allergic bronchiolo-alveolitis, and by Laitinen and colleagues to broncho-alveolitis (45) which more nearly described the anatomical distribution of the lesions. However, this terminology relates particularly to farmers' lung, bird fanciers' lung and other conditions in which the effective dose of antigen is relatively large, the pathological changes are known from lung biopsy and autopsy material and the condition is liable to progress beyond the acute stage. It is not necessarily appropriate for humidifier fever (ventilator pneumonitis) and related conditions (here called water droplet antigen disease) in which the effective dose is often small, the involvement of the lung may be trivial, the pathology is unknown and a chronic stage has only once been identified.

Acute phase

The primary lesion. The acute phase of extrinsic allergic alveolitis is accompanied by oedema of alveolar walls with infiltration by lymphocytes, plasma cells and occasional eosinophils; these changes constitute interstitial pneumonitis. There may be hyperplasia of alveolar type 2 cells, some of which convert to fibroblasts. Foam-laden macrophages occur in the interstitial tissue or in the lumen of small airways. Histiocytes, epithelioid cells and multinucleated giant cells of the Langhans type form noncaseating granulomata (fig. 15.1). The giant cells contain lamellated bodies. The granulomata may be separated by collagen fibres from the adjacent tissue and in some circumstances contain the causative vegetable material. They usually occur in interalveolar septa in the centres of lobules and in the walls of terminal and respiratory bronchioles where they may obstruct the lumen; the walls of small pulmonary arteries may be thickened by swelling of muscle fibres and by the presence of epithelioid cells; these changes predispose to pulmonary hypertension. Necrosis of the vessel walls has not been observed (28, 48, 49). Granulomata also

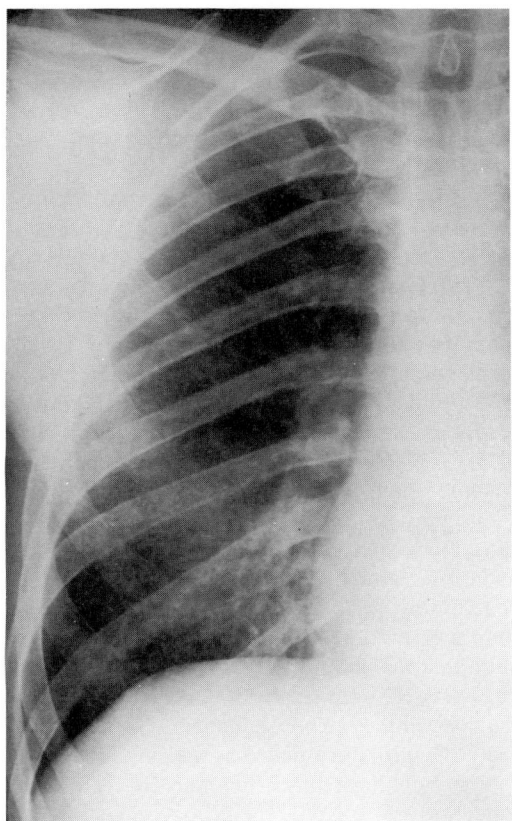 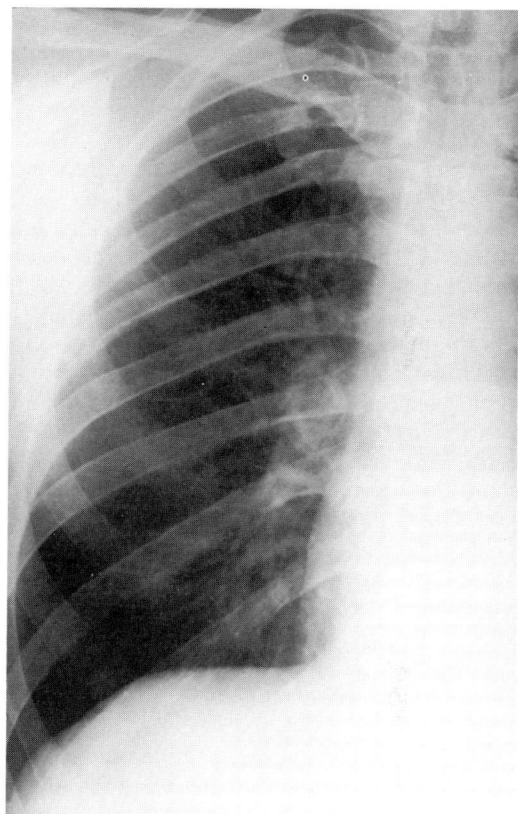

Fig. 15.2. Acute farmers' lung. Right chest radiographs of a farm worker aged 40 years who one morning in January experienced breathlessness and wheeze whilst giving hay to cows. Later that day he was febrile, had a productive cough, and went to bed 'feeling like death'. On examination, inspiratory crepitations were heard at the lung bases. The chest radiograph showed diffuse shadowing (left) and the forced vital capacity was reduced; there was no airflow obstruction (FEV$_1$/FVC 87%) No treatment was given and the patient subsequently lost weight. Six months later the chest radiograph had reverted to normal (right), but the patient complained of cough, phlegm and wheeze which was aggravated by exposure to hay. Assessment of lung function revealed airflow obstruction which responded to inhaled salbutamol, and reductions in total lung capacity and transfer factor; however, the radiographs suggested that the latter indices were probably improving at this time. Precipitins against *M. faeni* were present in the serum. The patient had had an acute episode of farmers' lung. He eventually made a full recovery but the picture was complicated by his developing asthma. This was only partially controlled by regular inhalations of salbutamol and becotide supplemented by intermittent courses of oral prednisolone.

occur in the nasal and bronchial mucosa and may be responsible for rhinitis and/or delayed airflow obstruction coming on 6h after acute exposure in some subjects (1). Desquamation of bronchial epithelium can occur and may predispose to bronchial hyperreactivity (45). The granulomatous lesions of the lung resemble those of sarcoidosis but the latter are larger and more clearly demarcated (7). In addition, in sarcoidosis, the granulomas are usually peripheral in the lobule, along the lymphatics, the bronchovascular sheath and in the hilar lymph nodes.

Clinical features. The acute phase of extrinsic allergic alveolitis (EAA) is an influenza-like illness which typically develops 6h after the onset of exposure (range 4–12h). The subject feels chilled, shivers, develops a fever and often has pain and tenderness in the muscles (myalgia). Cough, which is dry or productive of small amounts of sputum, is common; occasionally the sputum is blood stained. The appetite is lost and there may be headache, nausea, sometimes with vomiting, a sensation of tightness or restriction to expansion of the chest, and breathlessness on exertion in which the breathing is more shallow and rapid than usual. In one outbreak the volume flow of urine was conspicuously increased at the onset of the fever (54). Myocarditis has occasionally occurred as a complication. These features may be preceded by airflow obstruction in some atopic subjects (see chapter 16: Occupational Asthma).

On clinical examination the subject may be restless, apprehensive and cyanosed. The fever is accompanied by increased cardiac and respiratory frequencies. On auscultation of the lower half of the chest fine crackles (râles or crepitations) may be heard towards the end of inspiration. The symptoms and signs are of variable intensity from mild to severe and this influences their duration which may be from 12h to up to 2 or 3 weeks. Subsequently the subject may feel off colour for one or more days but complete symptomatic recovery is usual.

Re-exposure to the antigen can precipitate another acute episode, but if exposure is continuous or repetitive (for example, at weekends in the case of a pigeon fancier), the condition may progress through a subacute to a chronic phase described below. If the exposure is mild, or the patient's sensitivity is slight, the acute phase may go undetected and the patient presents with chronic disease (table 15.2).

Radiographic appearance. In the acute phase the chest radiograph can be normal or show the presence of multiple small opacities which are usually distributed centrally in the lung fields (fig. 15.2); in severe cases there may be larger diffuse or blotchy opacities resembling acute pulmonary oedema. The changes usually resolve completely but with repeated exposure may progress to irregular opacities which are a feature of the chronic condition (see below). Hilar enlargement and pleural effusion are rare and usually have some other cause.

Results of blood analysis. A differential blood white cell count may reveal mild polymorphonuclear leucocytosis and lymphopenia, the latter perhaps due to migration of T lymphocytes into the lung (see below). The erythrocyte sedimentation rate is often increased. The serum levels of immunoglobulin classes IgA, IgG or IgM are increased and there is usually evidence for increased consumption of complement with formation of C3b and C5a. The serum contains specific precipitins.

Lung function. Assessment of lung function is seldom carried out during the first acute episode: it is sometimes done in relation to a subsequent one or to inhalation challenge. There is then a reduction of total lung capacity and its subdivisions including the inspiratory and vital capacities; the forced expiratory volume (FEV_1) may be reduced in consequence. This restrictive type of ventilatory defect is accompanied by a low static lung compliance and by features of defective gas transfer including a low transfer factor and diffusing capacity of the alveolar capillary membrane; and exercise hyperventilation with hypoxaemia. There may also be shallow breathing in which the tidal volume is reduced more than would be expected from the reduction of vital capacity (page 47). Hyperventilation lowers the arterial CO_2 tension (hypocapnia) but in some patients this is masked by co-existing ventilation-perfusion ($\dot{V}_A/\dot{Q}$) inequality which may even cause hypercapnia at rest; the $\dot{V}_A/\dot{Q}$ inequality also accentuates the hypoxaemia. Narrowing of large airways is uncommon and mainly limited to a small pro-

Table 15.3. Illustrative case of farmer's lung

History. The patient and her husband, who was a quarry man, looked after three cows on a smallholding in mid-Wales. One summer, for the first time, they used a bailer for their hay which was subsequently found to be mouldy. The following spring the patient (age 51 years, height 1.57m) experienced an acute febrile illness with breathlessness and expectoration of some greenish, blood-flecked sputum.

Examination. Coarse inspiratory crepitations were heard at the lung bases. Blood pressure was 160/105mmHg, the chest x-ray showed some diffuse mottling of both lung fields and the ECG showed evidence of left ventricular hypertrophy.

Lung function. The compliance, total lung capacity and subdivisions were slightly reduced but the ventilatory capacity, FEV_1 and airflow resistance were normal. The transfer factor (Tl) and its membrane component (Dm) were reduced and the exercise ventilation was increased to a greater extent breathing air than oxygen.

Diagnosis. The diagnosis of disease of the lung parenchyma due to farmers' lung was supported by the finding of precipitating antibodies against *M. faeni*.

Subsequent course. The condition cleared up during the summer and the advice to change over to making silage was rejected. However, after an illness the following winter the patient agreed to use a fine dust respirator which was carefully chosen to fit her face. This prevented further episodes.

		Subacute	3 months later	Reference value
Forced expiratory volume	(FEV_1, l)	2.30	2.45	2.25
Forced vital capacity	(FVC, l)	2.73	3.05	3.2
FEV_1/FVC	(%)	84	80	75
Total lung capacity	(TLC, l)	4.46	4.94	4.9
Residual volume	(RV, l)	1.49	1.65	1.7
Transfer factor	(Tl)*	4.5 (13)	6.7 (20)	7.7
Diffusing capacity of alv.membr.	(Dm)*	6.7 (20)	14.4 (43)	15
Vol. of blood in alv. caps.	(Vc, ml)	43	43	56
Lung compliance	(Cstat, l kPa^{-1})	1.2	1.4	2.0
Airflow resistance	(l min^{-1} kPa^{-1})	0.11	0.11	1.2
Exercise ventilation	($\dot{V}_E$45, l min^{-1}) air	39	24	24
	O_2	30	24	24

* mmol min^{-1} kPa^{-1} (ml min^{-1} mmHg^{-1}).

portion of atopic subjects, but narrowing of small airways may occur as part of the disease process. Lung function in a patient with farmers' lung is summarized in table 15.3 (also 11, 15, 40 and 44).

Chronic phase

Morbid anatomy. The epithelioid granulomatous lesions which occur in the acute stage of extrinsic allergic alveolitis either resolve over a period of weeks or months and disappear, or persist as chronic inflammatory lesions with lymphocytes predominating (7). Many of the numerous type 2 cells become fibroblasts and lay down fibrous tissue which occupies the interalveolar spaces previously thickened by oedema and cellular infiltrates. In this way, what was a reversible thickening becomes permanent. The fibrous tissue progressively contracts and so further reduces both lung volume and the calibre of smaller airways. The fibrosis is usually present in the upper and mid-zones of the lung but is variable in both site and distribution. Commonly, areas of fibrosis engulf complete acini whilst others are stretched to form cystic spaces (fig. 15.3). Alternatively, the fibrosis may be extensive but inconspicuous, when the contraction causes centrilobular emphysema. The changes are accentuated by arteritis leading to occlusion of the lumen of small pulmonary arteries and the resulting loss of nutrient contributes to the disappearance of normal lung parenchyma. The end stage is diffuse fibrosis or cystic (honeycomb) lung which is indistinguishable from that following fibrosing alveolitis and other chronic fibrosing disorders. The accompanying pulmonary hypertension causes dilatation of the large pulmonary arteries, hypertrophy of the right ventricle and in

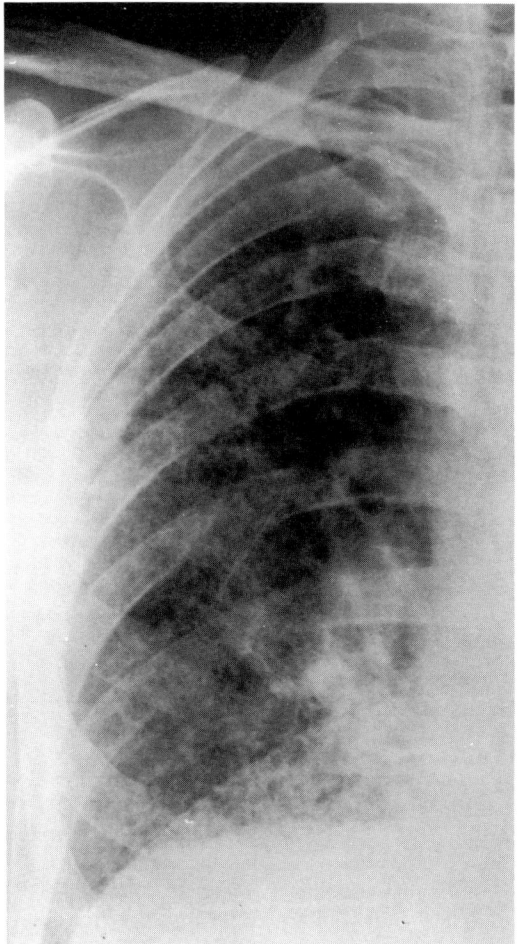
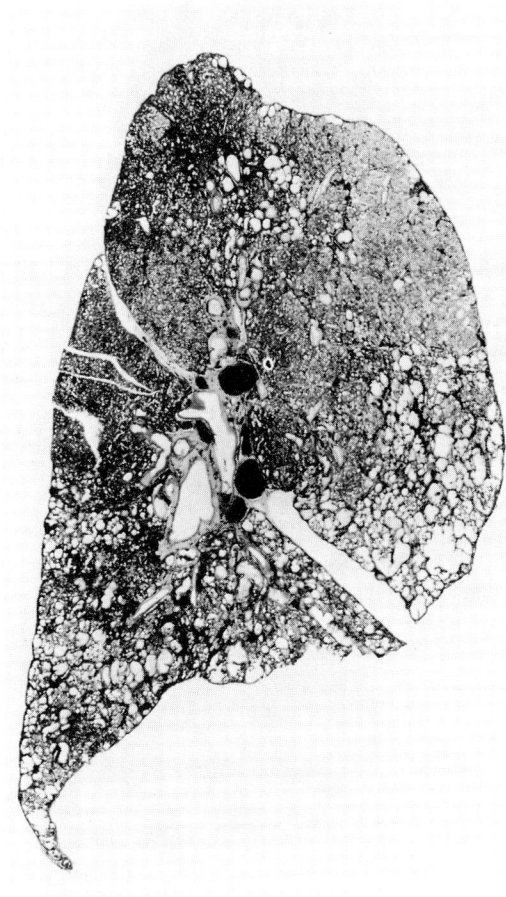

Fig. 15.3. Late stage extrinsic allergic alveolitis. This patient worked for 16 years as a collier, then for 15 years as a farm worker in Cumbria. Here at age 47 he presented with cough, breathlessness and weight loss; there was no history of acute episodes. The chest radiograph was reported as suggestive of acute on chronic farmers' lung; the precipitin test was strongly positive and there was a restrictive type of ventilatory defect. Over the next 7 years treatment with steroids did not prevent progression of the disease despite causing severe spinal osteoporosis. The patient developed finger clubbing and extensive pulmonary fibrosis (left): he became precipitin positive to *Aspergillus*, at the same time losing the reaction to *M. faeni* and died in gross respiratory failure with cor pulmonale. At post-mortem the lungs showed diffuse fibrosis with cystic changes. No coal dust foci were seen. (By courtesy of J. E. M. Hutchinson.)

severe cases, changes which are secondary to congestive cardiac failure, including congestion and cirrhosis of the liver.

Clinical features. Repeated episodes of acute extrinsic allergic alveolitis, or continuing mild exposure insufficient to cause symptoms, may lead to chronic changes which are mainly those of progressive diffuse interstitial fibrosis. The principal symptom is breathlessness on exertion which is seldom accompanied by wheeze except in the late stages. There may be a cough but characteristically this does not produce any sputum. Weight loss is common.

On clinical examination, clubbing of the fingers and fine inspiratory râles are sometimes observed but not so commonly as in cryptogenic fibrosing alveolitis and asbestosis. Cyanosis may or may not be detectable at rest but often becomes obvious during exercise. The chest is rather flat with diminished expansion and deviation of the trachea towards the more affected side. The breath sounds are usually loud and clear but there may be coarse added sounds or occasionally an inspiratory squawk described by Laennec as 'le cri d'un petit oiseau' (3).

With passage of time these typical features of diffuse interstitial pulmonary fibrosis become overlaid by others due to occurrence of complications. The patient often develops chronic bronchitis because of distortion of the airways by fibrous tissue (15, 44). Localized contraction of fibrous tissue in the upper and mid-zones causes compensatory emphysema at the lung bases; generalized contraction may lead to diffuse cystic changes which progress to honeycomb lung (49). Occasionally and atypically the chronic changes present as emphysema.

Disturbance of gas exchange causes hypoxaemia which in some patients is sufficiently intense to cause polycythaemia. The patient then exhibits cyanosis, has an enlarged red cell mass and often hypervolaemia; he or she is then vulnerable to episodes of vascular thrombosis, each with its attendant complications. The polycythaemia is sometimes accompanied by a raised serum erythropoietin concentration. The progressive pulmonary fibrosis reduces the pulmonary vascular bed by replacing lung tissue and distorting or narrowing small pulmonary arteries, and thus contributes to hypoxaemia

which itself causes pulmonary vasoconstriction; the resulting pulmonary hypertension leads to hypertrophy of the muscle of the right ventricle. The component of the hypertension which is attributable to hypoxic pulmonary vasoconstriction is usually small, except when the disease occurs in a person living at high altitude (30); it may be reversed by breathing oxygen, whereas the fixed component due to fibrous tissue does not change. The pulmonary heart disease may progress to congestive cardiac failure with swelling of the ankles and hepatic engorgement.

Chest radiography. In the chronic stage of extrinsic allergic alveolitis the chest radiograph usually exhibits small irregular opacities which characteristically affect mainly the upper and mid-zones (44). When acute episodes are superimposed on the chronic condition there may be evanescent rounded opacities as well. The profusion of irregular opacities usually increases with time and the opacities become larger, sometimes with intervening cystic spaces, which are then evidence of honeycomb lung (fig. 15.3). If the lesions are predominantly unilateral the trachea becomes drawn to the affected side. Increased transradiancy at the lung bases is evidence for compensatory emphysema; generalized emphysema may occasionally occur. Emphysema associated with chronic extrinsic allergic alveolitis is usually accompanied by small irregular opacities. However, the two conditions may occur independently. The coexistence of pulmonary hypertension is indicated on the chest radiograph by enlargement of the right ventricle and main pulmonary arteries.

Lung function. The changes in lung function (the tests are described in chapter 5) are typically those of restricted expansion of the lungs and defective gas transfer. There may be narrowing of small lung airways but the calibre of larger airways is typically normal or increased. Thus the total lung capacity and its subdivisions, and the exercise tidal volume, are usually reduced, but residual volume not invariably so. These changes are associated with a low static lung compliance and high recoil pressure. The low transfer factor may cause hypoxaemia and an increased ventilation during exercise. By contrast the airflow conductance and the forced

expiratory volume (FEV$_1$) are relatively normal
so the specific conductance and the FEV$_1$/FVC%
are normal or increased. This pattern of functional abnormalities is due to reduced distensibility of the lung and deranged function of the
lung parenchyma; their relative contributions to
the overall impairment may be assessed by
measurement of the compliance, recoil pressure,
transfer factor and physiological response to
exercise. The narrowing of small airways may be
suspected from the finding of a large residual
volume relative to total lung capacity, reduced
mixing index (VA'/VA) and decreased flow rate
at small lung volumes (MEF25%FVC). However,
any changes in these indices may also be due to
irreversible airflow obstruction secondary to
chronic bronchitis (15), or to emphysema (11).

Diagnosis of extrinsic allergic alveolitis

Acute phase. The features of acute extrinsic
allergic alveolitis resemble those of influenza
and the first episode is usually so diagnosed.
The correct diagnosis is made only after one or
more recurrences has led to recognition of the
characteristic features and identification of the
likely cause. Alternatively symptoms may
develop in members of a group sharing a common environment (e.g. home, or work place, cf.
page 294). Diagnosis requires careful assessment of the clinical and occupational history
and awareness of the differential diagnosis;
this includes infectious pneumonia due to
Legionella species (Legionnaires' disease), occupational asthma, which may coexist (chapter
16), acute bronchopulmonary aspergillosis,
ornithosis and silo-fillers' disease (chapter 13).
Other medical conditions which can be confused with EAA are acute bronchitis, atypical
pneumonia, miliary tuberculosis, acute fibrosing alveolitis and sarcoidosis. In sarcoidosis,
alveolitis is uncommon; there may be involvement of other organs and tissues of the body and
in approximately 75% of cases the Kveim test
will be positive. The diagnosis of extrinsic
allergic alveolitis may be made by observation
during a subsequent episode, especially if this
engenders the formation of antibodies; these can
be detected by immunodiffusion, or related
tests, which are more sensitive than estimation

of precipitating antibodies, and by a prick test.
The skin reaction is predominantly oedematous
in type, comes on approximately 6h after the
inoculation and lasts 24–36h (page 352). It may
be preceded by a transient immediate reaction
which is usually mediated by immunoglobulins
of the IgG type but may be mediated by IgE. But
neither the presence of antibodies nor a positive
Arthus-type skin reaction are diagnostic in the
absence of clinical signs, although they indicate
that some sensitization has occurred. The episode which initiated the index case usually
leads to more than one exposed person becoming sensitized so other members of the group,
even if asymptomatic, should be tested as well.
Broncho-alveolar lavage (BAL) can reveal an
increased number of activated T lymphocytes
and this may in future be the diagnostic method
of choice (35) but its specificity and sensitivity
are as yet unconfirmed. Lung biopsy may establish that granulomata are present. Fibre optic
bronchoscopy can be used though the success
rate is less than by open lung biopsy. The granulomata may not be found unless the disease is at
an early stage. They are evidence for extrinsic
allergic alveolitis but identify the cause only in
those rare cases in which the lesions contain
pieces of identifiable foreign material. The cause
may be confirmed by inhalation challenge
which simulates the natural exposure to the suspected antigen. The procedure is usually
regarded as safe. However, a positive result may
be associated with disagreeable symptoms and
the exposure carries a small risk of inducing
sensitization or progressive disease; it should be
carried out under controlled conditions in hospital and only when there is a need to confirm
sensitization to a hitherto unknown antigen, to
identify the active antigen in a mixture, or for
purposes of research. For the management of an
individual patient or factory incident there is
seldom any need for inhalation challenge;
instead the clinical information should be supplemented by observations during and after
exposure at work. The measurements should be
made on a day when other information suggests
that the exposure is likely to be relatively high.
The procedure is considered below.

Chronic phase. Diffuse interstitial pulmonary
fibrosis is the end result of many disease pro-

Table 15.4.   Responses to inhalation challenge. (By courtesy of G. Boyd.)

General:	Malaise, other symptoms, *pyrexia, *leucocytosis,
Functional:	Reductions in *lung volumes, transfer factor, arterial oxygen tension Increases in A-aDO$_2$, *exercise ventilation, *respiratory frequency
Serology:	Changes in specific antibodies, immune complexes, complement
Cellular:	Lymphocytes in lung washings (T cells) and *circulating blood
Other:	Changes in lung permeability, chemical compositon of lung washings, reactivity to antigen

* Recommended for use in assessment by Hendrick et al (6).

cesses, all of which may progress to honeycomb or cystic lung. They are sometimes complicated by chronic bronchitis or cor pulmonale. The condition can predispose to lung cancer (e.g. when due to scleroderma). In the absence of an acute phase a positive diagnosis of extrinsic allergic alveolitis may not be possible. Characteristic features include a history of exposure to a relevant antigen, radiographic changes which are predominantly in the upper two-thirds of the lung fields and infrequent finger clubbing or airflow obstruction; however, none of these features is invariable. One cannot rely on the presence of serum precipitating antibody because the titre falls when exposure ceases, and after about 3 years the test is usually negative (17, 23, 29, 40, 44). Even if it is positive the cause of the fibrosis may still be elsewhere. Similarly the characteristic epithelial granulomas disappear from the lung and are no longer detectable by lung biopsy. Inhalation challenge may still elicit a response but may also aggravate the condition. The diagnosis will depend on a balance of probabilities, both in favour of extrinsic allergic alveolitis and against other conditions which may have a similar effect upon the lung. The late stages of extrinsic allergic alveolitis are compared with those of cryptogenic fibrosing alveolitis, asbestosis and coal workers' cystic lung in table 15.5.

Testing for antibodies

The presence of precipitating antibodies against substances which may cause extrinsic allergic alveolitis is usually detected by the double diffusion technique of Ouchterlony. The method uses a Petri dish containing 1% agar in buffered solution in which are arranged a small central hole (well) and six equidistant peripheral wells; these are filled respectively with the sera under test, a source of antigen and reference sera. The proteins from the several wells diffuse outwards and if antibodies are present will participate in an antigen–antibody reaction; this is visible in the agar as an opaque line between the respective wells; if test and reference sera containing antibodies are placed in adjacent wells the lines between them will be continuous (fig. 15.4). If not they may either have a component of partial identity or will cross, depending on whether the sera had some antibodies in common or are dissimilar. The test is simple and useful but not specific for subclasses of antibody and only semi-quantitative. The serial dilutions also provide optimal conditions for a positive response which requires the presence of excess antigen. Greater specificity is achieved by first separating the serum proteins by electrophoresis along the length of a trough, then applying the immuno-diffusion technique transversely. Alternative techniques based on latex agglutination and haemagglutination, immuno-osmophoresis, enzyme-linked immunosorbent assay (ELISA) and immunofluorescence have also been described. More accurately quantitative results are obtained by radioimmunoassay (9) or ELISA (38); these techniques are specific for individual antigens, for example on the surface of spores of *Micropolyspora faeni*.

The radioimmunoassay method of Nielsen and colleagues has been used to detect antibodies against antigens in the capsule of *Micropolyspora faeni* spores and against pigeon 7S

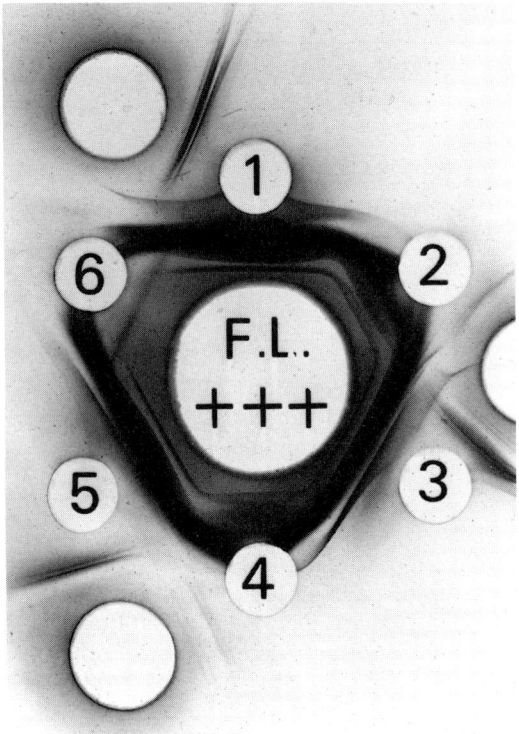

Fig. 15.4. Testing for precipitating antibodies. The central well of the agar plate contains serum from a case of farmers' lung. The wells 1–5 contain *M. faeni* antigen in the concentrations 20mg ml^{-1} (wells 1, 3 and 5) and 2mg ml^{-1} (wells 2 and 4). The outer wells (unlabelled) contain sheep antiserum to *M. faeni*. Antibodies from the patient's serum have combined with the antigens and precipitated within the gel forming precipitin lines. Each line corresponds to a different antigen combining with its appropriate antibody. The joining of lines from adjacent wells, best exemplified by the innermost continuous line, indicates an identical antigen in the *M. faeni* extracts 1–5. Well 6 contains *A. fumigatus* antigen in the concentration 20mg ml^{-1}. This has reacted with specific antibody in the patient's serum; the precipitin line crosses that of the reaction for *M. faeni* and is not continuous with it, indicating the presence of non-identical antigens. (By courtesy of J. H. Edwards.)

immunoglobulin which has been attached by an antigen–antibody reaction onto sheep red blood corpuscles (9). The test serum is treated with excess antigen to bind all the relevant antibodies and the resulting aggregates, after washing, are treated with excess antihuman globulin labelled with iodine-125. The aggregate so obtained is assayed using a scintillation counter. The result is reproducible to within 8%.

Inhalation challenge

The indications for inhalation challenge are considered under 'diagnosis'. To perform the challenge the subject inhales an appropriate aerosol in low concentration and the response over the subsequent 24h is monitored. The test material may be the natural antigen, for example from handling a pigeon or mouldy hay, a re-suspended aerosol, for example humidifier sludge, or a purified preparation which can be a filtered saline extract of one or more components of the antigen obtained by physical or chemical separation. The use of natural antigen ensures a normal presentation and response but the test is often difficult to set up and the dose is at best semi-quantitative. Processed antigen can be delivered in a known dose under controlled conditions but the presentation may be abnormal and the response may differ from that to the natural antigen. Thus the method to be used will depend on circumstances. An example of the preparation of antigen and the dose sequence is given later (page 355). The response should preferably comprise all that is experienced during the clinical episode (including both pulmonary and constitutional components) but the proportions appear to vary with the antigen. In the case of sensitization to *Micropolyspora faeni* (farmers' lung) and avian antigen (bird fanciers' lung) Hendrick and colleagues have suggested six criteria for a positive response (6): these and others are given in table 15.4. The induction of râles on auscultation of the chest and changes on the chest radiograph are evidence that the test dose which provoked them was too large. The topic merits more research.

A positive response to inhalation challenge is evidence that the substance, or one closely

Table 15.5. Comparison of the chronic forms of extrinsic allergic alveolitis (EAA), cryptogenic fibrosing alveolitis (CFA), asbestosis (A) and coalworkers' cystic lung (CCL).

	EAA	CFA	A	CCL
Aetiology	Environmental antigen	Unknown	Asbestos fibres	Not known (stellate nodules)
Clinical history	Characteristic exposure and onset	Non-specific	Asbestos exposure	Coalworker
Time course	6 weeks to 20 years	1–3 years	Usually slow	20–40 years
Clinical course	Variable; acute episodes	Progressive	Progressive	Progressive
Common symptoms	Breathlessness, cough, weight loss	Breathlessness	Breathlessness, cough	Breathlessness, wheeze
Finger clubbing	Uncommon	Common	Uncommon	Common
Fine râles	Uncommon	Common	Common	Common
Radiographic irregular opacities	Upper/mid zone	Not localized	Lower zones	Lower zones
other features	—	—	Pleural disease	p type opacities
Fibres or bodies in sputum/lavage	Rare	NPC	Common	NPC
Lung function				
Restrictive defect	Initially variable	(Yes)	Yes	No
Transfer defect	Initially variable	Yes	Yes	Yes
Airflow limitation	Late stage asthma may coexist	Late stage	Often	Late stage
Precipitating antibodies	Yes (up to 3 years)	NPC	NPC	NPC
Immunoglobins	Abnormal: not diagnostic	NPC		NPC
Skin sensitization	Variable	NPC	NPC	NPC
Response to inhalation challenge	Usual	NPC	NPC	NPC
Bronchoalveolar lavage	Cell type: not diagnostic (yet?)	No association		No information
Smoking prevalence	Below average	No association	Above average	Above average
Response to treatment	In early stages	In early stages	Symptomatic only	Symptomatic only
Pathology of DIPF	Preceded by granulomata	Discrete areas	Subpleural and basal	NPC
Honey combing	Common	Air cysts common	Inconspicuous	Yes
Pleural thickening	Variable	Uncommon	Commonly bilateral	No

NPC = not part of the condition. DIPF = diffuse interstitial pulmonary fibrosis.

related to it, is capable of causing the clinical episodes. A negative response may be a consequence of using too small a dose. Alternatively, the subject may not have been sensitive to the antigen. It is often difficult to decide whether to increase the dose or to try another antigen.

Prognosis

The prognosis in extrinsic allergic alveolitis depends on the antigen which is responsible, the susceptibility of the host and the intensity and duration of the exposure. It is also influenced by the stage of the illness when the condition is diagnosed; this is determined by the intensity of symptoms, the level of customary activity (which influences the stage of the disease at which breathlessness becomes obtrusive), the subjective attractiveness of the occupation causing the exposure, the patient's tolerance of discomfort and other aspects of personality. The prognosis is excellent when there have been only a few discrete episodes or when constitutional disturbance has outweighed the pulmonary effects. This is the case in most instances of water droplet antigen disease. Pulmonary fibrosis, however, is irreversible and when it has developed over many years, through insidious progression of the disease, improvement is unlikely. This is characteristically seen in committed farm workers and bird fanciers. There is every gradation in between. A long exposure and the presence of irregular opacities on the chest radiograph are of more adverse prognostic significance than the type of symptoms (episodic or persistent) and the findings on assessment of lung function. However, the intensity of exposure is also important as death has occurred from a single incident. The long-term prognosis is made worse if the patient is atopic, as this predisposes to airflow obstruction (e.g. figs. 15.2 and 15.6), and by smoking which predisposes to chronic bronchitis and emphysema. Paradoxically, before the acquisition of extrinsic allergic alveolitis, smoking exerts a protective influence by delaying the development of sensitization (see below). The prognosis is improved by avoidance or reduction of further exposure and by medical treatment. In the event of severe pulmonary hypertension it may also be improved by a sedentary lifestyle. The persist-

ence of precipitating antibodies is evidence of continuing exposure to the antigen so the reversal of a previously positive test is a favourable sign. However, despite the absence of precipitating antibodies there may still be increased consumption of autologous complement indicating the persistence of complement-consuming antibodies. Their presence is evidence for the continuing activity of the disease (20, 39). The persistence of raised serum levels of lysozyme and angiotensin converting enzyme has a similar connotation (52).

Treatment

The immediate treatment for the acute episode is withdrawal from exposure, rest and, in the event of material symptoms, the administration of oxygen and steroid drugs such as prednisolone, 40mg daily by mouth for 2–3 weeks with subsequent slow withdrawal. The use of steroids by inhalation is not effective and the use of sodium cromoglycate is contra-indicated (page 338). In the chronic phase of the disease withdrawal from exposure is still mandatory but there is no specific treatment. The patient will benefit from abandoning smoking and application of the symptomatic treatment and rehabilitation procedures described in chapter 19.

Following recovery from the acute episode or as part of the management of chronic disease, it is advisable to insist on a lifestyle which avoids further exposure. This often involves the affected person in a disagreeable decision about his or her employment, domicile, principal recreation or favourite pet, so the decision should be preceded by a full and sympathetic appraisal. Ways of reducing the exposure are discussed under 'prevention' below. Many of the procedures require a large measure of self-discipline and attention to detail and, while theoretically practicable, may not always be achievable. In these circumstances a more radical alternative such as a change of employment may be necessary and should then be pressed sympathetically. Inaction at this stage is not in the long-term interests of the patient.

Industrial injuries benefit. Extrinsic allergic alveolitis as a result of sensitization to an antigen arising from employment is a ground for industrial injuries benefit in the U.K. (page 8).

Predisposing factors

Some recorded causes of extrinsic allergic alveolitis are given in table 15.1 (page 321); the list is constantly being extended and additional substances will be identified in future. In some cases identification will come from clues provided by outbreaks of characteristic illness amongst persons sharing a common environment (e.g. an air-conditioned office). However, not all sensitizing agents are capable of producing disease. For example, the occurrence in New Guineans of precipitating antibodies against moulds growing in thatch roofs of houses is now well known (70, 66), yet no disease appears to have been reported from New Guinea despite intensive search. Precipitating antibodies were found by Pepys in coffee plantation workers and extrinsic allergic alveolitis was later diagnosed in one person employed in a factory processing coffee (95); however, the diagnosis was changed in the light of subsequent events (94). In view of these findings it is not surprising that amongst persons sensitized to active agents only a proportion acquire symptoms. Frequently, a number of potential antigens including moulds, bacteria and protozoa are present concurrently; this is the case during exposure to aerosol contaminated by constituents of humidifier sludge, sewage or moulding wood chippings. In different circumstances one or other of these agents is responsible for the incident but the cause of the variability is unclear. Where more than one person is affected the selective factors are at least partly environmental but personal habits and constitutional factors contribute to the acquisition of sensitivity and to clinical disease. One relevant habit is smoking; this reduces the extent of sensitization against *Micropolyspora faeni* in farmworkers and avian antigens in pigeon fanciers for a given level of environmental exposure (see below). The mechanism may be mechanical, smoking causing narrowing of airways and hence more complete clearance of airborne particles (chapter 4); alternatively or in addition it may be immunological, smoking attracting macrophages into the alveoli and stimulating their activity. Personal habits also help to determine the level of exposure; for example, amongst persons feeding cows some are more conscientious than others in separating out and shaking hay which has gone mouldy and inhale a larger dose of spores by so doing. The patient, whose case is described in table 15.3, falls into this category. Similar differences in exposure occur amongst pigeon fanciers.

Constitutional factors must contribute to susceptibility since some persons become sensitized more readily than others though, if the exposure is large enough, almost all do so eventually. It is not known if age influences the risk of sensitization. Atopic status appears not to influence susceptibility but it affects the subsequent course of the illness. A role for HLA antigens has been suggested and investigated in depth but so far with negative results (33, 42). In pigeon breeders a constitutional factor was suspected when P_1 antibodies were found to be more prevalent than amongst the general population. This turned out to be due to a P_1-like antigen present in pigeon blood and other antigenic material including house dust, but no association was found between P blood group phenotypes and sensitization to those antigens which cause bird fanciers' lung (18, 34). Stokes and colleagues found raised levels of immunoglobulin IgG3 in farmers with farmers' lung compared with other farmers (50). Both groups had increased amounts of total IgG and IgG1 relative to a non-farming population. The IgG3 excess is due to the possession of a particular Gm allotype and the observation suggests that these persons have above average susceptibility to farmers' lung. This finding has still to be confirmed. Persons who produce an above average amount of complement also appear to be at increased risk (20).

Mechanisms

Humoral pathway

Two separate mechanisms, one humoral and the other cellular, contribute to the formation of the granulomatous lesions and the subsequent pulmonary fibrosis of extrinsic allergic alveolitis. The humoral pathway entails the activation of complement to liberate the C3a, C5a and C3b fragments; the former fragments attract polymorphonuclear leucocytes, and the C3b fragment activates macrophages to liberate tissue enzymes which induce tissue necrosis, and to stimulate the laying down of fibrous tissue. The process of activation starts with a reaction involving antigen, antibody of the IgG or IgM type and complement to form a soluble immune complex. This initiates the process of degradation of complement components. The process is demonstrable in the skin of a sensitized person following the intradermal inoculation of antigen. An inflammatory reaction occurs some 6h later with aggregation of platelets, fibrin and leucocytes leading to tissue necrosis. This is the type III or Arthus reaction of Gell and Coombs and its time course resembles that of the 'delayed response' to inhaled antigen in persons with extrinsic allergic alveolitis. In such persons the occurrence of sensitization is associated with the development of precipitating antibodies able to activate complement; the antibodies are occasionally demonstrable in the pulmonary lesions. These characteristics led Pepys to suggest that extrinsic allergic alveolitis is a classical type III reaction involving the lung

parenchyma. However, in this event the pulmonary lesions should contain immune complexes but they are seldom demonstrable. In addition the lung lesion should be typical of the Arthus reaction but the latter is associated with inflammation and necrosis leading to fibrosis; by contrast extrinsic allergic alveolitis is characterized by granulomas and the lesion is not necrotic so an additional cellular mechanism must be responsible (see below). The activation of complement is a necessary stage in causation. Complement is involved in the disease process since in the acute and subacute stages its consumption is increased. However, this need not involve an antigen–antibody reaction. The antigens present in *Micropolyspora faeni*, and probably other substances, can activate complement directly by an alternative enzyme pathway. This may explain why some patients with extrinsic allergic alveolitis are precipitin negative. The presence of precipitating antibodies in the serum is evidence for sensitization; they appear not to be essential for manifestation of the disease which may occur without them (2).

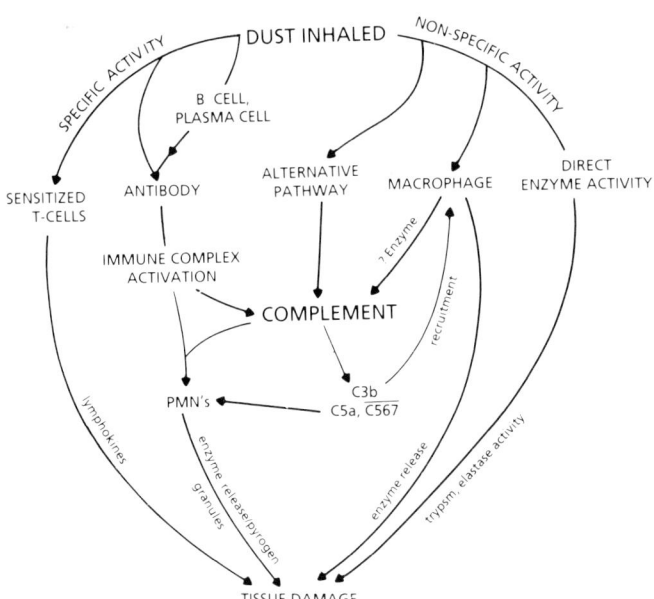

Fig. 15.5. Diagram illustrating the mechanisms of fibrogenesis in extrinsic allergic alveolitis. PMN is polymorphonuclear leucocyte. (By courtesy of J. H. Edwards.)

Cellular pathway

The agent causing extrinsic allergic alveolitis independent of circulating antibodies appears to arise from the cellular immune reaction of sensitized thymus-dependent T lymphocytes (T cells). These cells initiate the immune reaction to intradermal injection of tuberculin. The antigen combines with sensitized T cells which then release lymphokines; these substances attract and activate macrophages which are responsible for the granulomata appearing approximately 48h after the injection. In patients with extrinsic allergic alveolitis, challenge with appropriate antigen leads to activated T lymphocytes, which secrete lymphokines, appearing in the peripheral blood and in fluid obtained from the airways by bronchoalveolar lavage (16, 35). The cells in the airways migrate from the peripheral blood (10). These observations suggest that local cell-mediated hypersensitivity contributes to the pulmonary lesions of extrinsic allergic alveolitis through the release of lymphokines. How the sensitization of the T cells occurs is not known, but it may involve a direct effect of the antigen upon lung macrophages. Sensitization can also be induced by BCG or an intercurrent viral infection, as a result of their adjuvant properties.

In persons who readily develop IgG antibodies the tissue reaction is a specific response to the dust with delayed type hypersensitivity and immune complexes. The reaction can be triggered off by a tiny dose of antigen. Conversely, a large dose is needed to produce a reaction in previously unexposed subjects or those with minimal sensitization. The disease is then mediated via the alternative pathway, by enzymes from macrophages and by direct action of the dust. In subjects who have an intermediate level of sensitization, for example farmers with precipitins, both types of mechanism contribute; they are summarized in fig. 15.5.

Epidemiology

Accurate figures for the prevalence of sensitization, the incidence of acute episodes and the amount of chronic disease are difficult to obtain. This is partly because the antibody titre is an unreliable guide; it fluctuates with changes in exposure and returns to normal subsequent to withdrawal from exposure. In addition many acute episodes are not diagnosed at the time and cannot be confirmed retrospectively. Thus the reported figures probably underestimate the extent of the problem. Other confounding factors are the decline in smoking (which may protect), the otherwise good health of farm workers relative to other occupational groups and the present rapid changes in technology. Estimating the exposure by environmental monitoring is difficult since many of the relevant activities are performed on a small scale and individuals differ widely in the amount of dust to which they expose themselves; the exposure is usually reduced in response to symptoms (31). In addition, any dose–response relationship arising from the measurements will be different for sensitized and unsensitized individuals.

Prevalence. In studies of working populations precipitating antibodies have usually been found in 10–50% of those at risk, smokers being affected about half as often as non-smokers (21, 46). But table 15.6 shows that in some industries much higher prevalences, approaching 100%, have been reported. In most of these the working conditions have since been improved, and no longer resemble those which gave rise to these very high figures (e.g. 51). In large-scale operations, prevalences in excess of 1/1000 are now uncommon. In small-scale operations, family farms in areas of high rainfall and amongst amateur pigeon and budgerigar fanciers, the prevalences remain high. Thus amongst pigeon fanciers the prevalence of symptoms, whilst only 3.7% in those who were precipitin negative, rose to 78% in persons with a high titre (>30µg/ml, 31). The prevalence is often high in the early stages of use of any new substance which is capable of causing the disorder. This is a reason for vigilance and for investigating individual cases thoroughly.

Incidence rate. There have been few studies where the rate of development of sensitization has been investigated. Until recently amongst cork workers in Portugal the sensitization was usually acquired within the first 5 years after joining the industry and was not closely related to the environmental concentration (67). In

Table 15.6. Prevalence of extrinsic allergic alveolitis (EAA) and/or positive serology (Precip +)

		No. of subjects	EAA (%)	Precip + (%)	Ref.
1	Bagassosis; paper mill workers	140	49	—	12
2	Bird handlers' lung				
	Budgerigar fanciers	117	3.4	17.1	27
	Coeliac disease	61	4.9	35	5, 26
	Pigeon breeders	146	7.5	13	25
		339	—	38	36
		53	21	66	24
		256	—	30.4 (av)	21 (also 31)
	Poultry farmers	339	—	22.4	37
	Turkey growers	205	6.3	11	22
3	Cheese washers		12 (av)	—	71
4	Farmers' lung Devon	137	2.2–11.7*	27.0	46
	Wales	96	5.4–12.9	56.3	46
	Scotland, Orkney and Ayrshire	507	8.6	41	43
	East Lothian	148	2.3	—	43
5	Malt workers	701	5.2	—	80
6	Mushroom spawning shed workers	23	26	—	91
	Mushroom workers	100	2	—	76
7	Pig keepers	20	5	30	83
8	Suberosis	568	23	38	67
9	Water droplet antigen disease				
	Air conditioner	27	14.8	—	55
	Cooling water Heavily exposed	21	71	90	61
	Minimally exposed	350	2.6	23	61
	Humidifier Operating theatre	60	15	38	57
	Office staff	47	23	54†	54
	Tap water	539	19.4	—	63

(av) = average.
* Depending on criteria used.
† Estimated from subsample.

other circumstances sensitization is acquired within a shorter time span down to about six weeks.

Dose–response relationship. A clear association between crude estimates of exposure and the prevalence of clinical disease has been observed in all circumstances where it has been looked for. The circumstances include workers in different processes, for different durations and in environments which have changed either for better or worse following the introduction of hygiene measures or new methods or equipment. A dose–response relationship is also apparent in temporal changes which occur in some circumstances. Thus seasonal variations in disease activity due to variations in exposure have been observed for farmworkers where the peak incidence is at the end of the winter and in pigeon fanciers where the peak incidence is towards the end of the summer racing season (32). Incidents of humidifier fever have occurred on Mondays after weekends when the building was shut up but the heating left on (54). Most of these observations have been based on relatively simple indices of exposure as the antigen is often present in very low concentration which is difficult to measure accurately. There does not appear to have been any study in which the results of environmental or personal sampling have been related prospectively to the development of sensitization or of clinical disease. Such a study might arise from monitoring the effects of improved environmental control following an outbreak.

Prevention

Extrinsic allergic alveolitis is a consequence of sensitization to one or more of the antigens listed in table 15.1. The antigen is in the form of an aerosol of particle size 1μm or less which enters the body via the respiratory tract. It is able to do this because the cleansing mechanisms against small particles, although over 90% efficient (chapter 4), are not perfect, and the immunological defences are not effective against this class of material. Sensitization does not occur through intact skin but may occur following implantation or inoculation, as in attempted hyposensitization therapy for asthma (82). Sensitization appears not to occur via the gastrointestinal tract but the possibility of it doing so is one of several explanations for the sensitization to avian and other antigens which may occur in coeliac disease (see below).

Prevention of extrinsic allergic alveolitis is effected by (i) avoiding the formation of antigen, (ii) stopping it from becoming airborne, (iii) purifying contaminated air, (iv) enhancing the body's defence mechanisms.

Avoiding formation of antigen. Most of the antigens which cause alveolitis are derived from moulds, bacteria or protozoa, growing on a variety of substrates in the presence of heat and moisture. The antigens will not be formed if the growth of these organisms can be discouraged by physical or chemical means. For example, the moisture content of hay or grain can be reduced below the critical level (about 15%) by hot-air drying, or the temperature of humidifier systems can be raised to a level (above 70°C) at which growth is impossible. Air conditioning

and humidifying systems in which the air is recirculated are intrinsically more prone to biological contamination than open systems and there is the risk that adjacent structures (such as glass-fibre insulation) may harbour the antigenic organisms. These structures should be cleaned regularly but chemical anti-fungal agents (biocides) should be avoided because of the risk that they may enter the air-supply and be inhaled. Under other circumstances 1% propionic acid applied to the fresh material is effective and may be used for the prevention of bagassosis, suberosis, farmers' lung and the disease associated with wood pulp, maple bark, wood chippings and other materials. Similarly hypochlorite solution may be used for grain. At all times the accumulation of waste material, in which mould might grow, should be avoided and buildings, stores and warehouses should be sufficiently well maintained and ventilated to keep them dry. Alternatively the process can be abandoned. An example of this is the transition from the making of hay to the making of silage in areas of high rainfall.

Stopping antigen from becoming airborne. The prevention of moulding at source is an ideal which may not be practicable on account of the nature of the process, or for economic or other reasons. In these circumstances the best palliative is to prevent the formation of aerosol. This is done successfully for bagasse which can be maintained fully saturated with water from the time when the sugar is extracted, through the processes of storage, baling, transportation and during manufacture into board, paper and other products.

Reducing inhalation of antigen. Many processes require conditions which promote moulding including the cultivation of mushrooms, the germination of barley for manufacturing beer and spirits, the intensive rearing of birds and other livestock and an increasing number of industrial processes based on fermentation. Mushrooms also produce spores which are antigenic. In these circumstances the formation of aerosol is inevitable, though in the case of grain the amount of antigen may be reduced by measures to reduce contamination with moulds. It may be possible to contain the aerosol within a closed environment in which the process is performed automatically. If this is not possible the concentration of aerosol should be kept at a low level by general and local ventilation. Personal protection can be ensured by wearing an air-ventilated hood such as the airstream helmet, or a respirator, fitted with a high efficiency filter. The filter will remove the spores or other source of antigen and, provided the equipment is used correctly, will provide adequate protection in most circumstances (e.g. 4). Personal protective equipment is also of use for clinical management in the event of sensitization occurring (table 15.3).

Enhancing the body's defences. Prevention by enhancing the body's defences against inhaled antigens is theoretically attractive but so far has little to recommend it. The practice of smoking will delay the onset of sensitization but the disadvantages of smoking more than offset this advantage. The use of drugs to promote the

immune defences of the body is not yet feasible and the use of sodium cromoglycate or other agent which might prevent the allergic manifestations is contra-indicated by the possibility that this will only obscure and not retard the underlying process.

In general the prevention of extrinsic allergic alveolitis due to moulds, other micro-organisms and spores is much less difficult than preventing that due to animal residues and on this in particular there is need for more research. One development is the identification of classes of persons whose susceptibility is above or below the average (see predisposing factors above).

Additional information

Bagassosis. The stem of sugar cane after it has been crushed for the extraction of sugar syrup is called bagasse. It is a source of cellulose fibre for

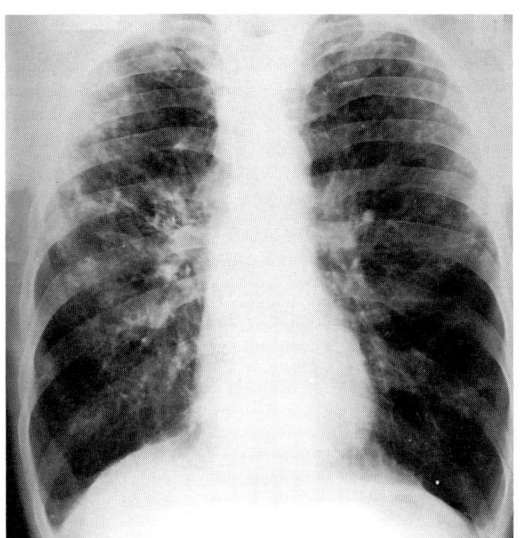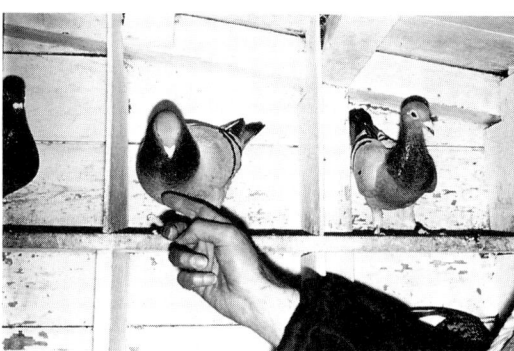

Fig. 15.6. Chest radiograph showing upper and mid-zone irregular opacities and increased basal translucency in a 40-year-old coal worker who reported keeping pigeons for 2 years from age 16. He was a non-smoker. Since early adulthood he had experienced regular nocturnal wheeze and breathlessness with episodes of bronchitis: these led to his losing progressively more and more time from work. The forced expiratory volume was reduced and was improving by inhaling salbutamol. Recently the patient was losing weight and had had a haemoptysis. This led to chest radiography and to a diagnosis of pneumoconiosis of coal workers. However, the patient had never worked on the coal face and the radiographic appearances were atypical. In addition, the static lung compliance and transfer factor were reduced (respectively 47% and 61% of the reference values) and the serum contained antibodies against pigeon residues. Enquiry revealed that he was still keeping and racing the birds. He had chronic pigeon fanciers' lung with asthma due to increased bronchial reactivity to pigeon antigen.

making paper and board, as fuel, and other applications, including as garden mulch. Bagasse also provides a culture medium for growth of micro-organisms including *Thermoactinomyces sacchari*; their spores give rise to sensitization and the clinical features of bagassosis. The risk is world-wide since sugar cane is grown in most sub-tropical countries and the bagasse is exported to many industrialized countries including the U.K., but the majority of cases of bagassosis have been reported from the U.S.A. The features of bagassosis resemble those of other forms of extrinsic allergic alveolitis. (For references, see page 341.)

Bird handlers' lung. Persons who rear chickens, turkeys and other birds risk developing bird handlers' lung of occupational origin, but the antigens differ in their potency. In practice the majority of cases arise from keeping pigeons as a hobby (fig. 15.6) or budgerigars (parakeets) as pets. Pigeon fanciers often become sensitized to the bloom, feathers, droppings or egg yolk of their birds (table 15.1); their serum antibody titre may then rise during the pigeon racing season and episodes of acute extrinsic allergic alveolitis may occur, particularly in the late summer. In atopic individuals the condition may present with rhinitis or asthma (fig. 15.6). Chronic disease may occur as a result of repeated exposures which often start in childhood; the risk of chronic disease is aggravated by awareness of the problem leading to fanciers taking sufficient precautions to prevent acute episodes but not to eliminate exposure altogether. Ventilation, good housekeeping and respirators (e.g. airstream helmet, chapter 3) are used for this purpose. The extent of disease is sometimes concealed but of its wide prevalence amongst the fraternity there is little doubt (31). Most derivatives of the birds are highly antigenic, both for extrinsic allergic alveolitis and other types of sensitization; thus pigeon blood contains an antigen resembling that present in the human blood group P_1. This leads to many pigeon fanciers having a raised P_1 antibody titre despite their not having come in contact with the P_1 blood groups (page 333). This antibody appears to be devoid of ill-effects. Antibodies against hen egg yolk and bird serum may also be

present in the serum of patients with coeliac disease (5, 23, 26). The association appears to reflect incomplete denaturation of ingested protein in this condition and is not a precursor of extrinsic allergic alveolitis. However, the two conditions may coexist. Diagnosis may be confirmed by identification of the specific antibody either using one of the immunoelectrophoretic methods described above or by inhalation challenge.

Budgerigar fanciers seldom develop acute attacks of extrinsic allergic alveolitis but may develop chronic disease from repeated sub-clinical exposure. The clinical features are summarized in table 15.2. Many persons are at risk in the U.K. where some 12% of households keep pet birds (27). Those who develop the condition are often elderly people living alone who have kept a bird for many years and enjoy its company; they are probably mostly non-smokers. Their pulmonary fibrosis is usually irreversible but may be liable to further aggravation.

The clinical features, diagnosis, epidemiology and prevention of bird handlers' lung resemble that of other forms of extrinsic allergic alveolitis. (For references, see page 342.)

Farmers' lung. In the west of Britain and in Iceland the association of breathlessness with bad hay has been known for many generations. The acute episodes were first described by Campbell in 1932, the condition was so called by Pickles in 1944 and the changes in lung function were first described in detail by Dickie & Rankin in 1958. The positive precipitin test against *Micropolyspora faeni* was first reported by Pepys and colleagues in 1961.

The condition is associated with the process of moulding in damp hay and cereals. Moulding begins when the moisture content exceeds about 20%; it is due initially to growth of *Aspergillus* and related fungi which through their metabolism raise the temperature in the hay and form water by oxidation. This raises the water content to above 35% and the temperature to about 50°C; the conditions are then right for growth of heat-tolerant *Thermoactinomyces vulgaris* and *Micropolyspora faeni* (also called *Faenia rectivirgula*) whose spores give rise to sensitization. The mycelium forms a white powder containing the spores which readily become airborne once the bales of hay have dried out.

Hay is made by cutting fresh grass which is dried in the sun on the ground or on poles or fences, collected, compressed into bales and stored in stacks. Moulding is likely to occur if the hay is baled prematurely or if wet weather prevents the completion of the drying process. Thus regions of high rainfall are at risk; dry areas are not. Hay which is stacked loose may continue to dry after collection and the introduction of balers by preventing further drying increases the risk of spoiling. This may be overcome by good farm practices supplemented if necessary by artificial drying. The use of 1% propionic acid will prevent moulding in the bales and in grain. With grass the problem may be circumvented by converting the grass into silage instead of hay. This practice is reducing the incidence of extrinsic allergic alveolitis amongst farmers in parts of the U.K. with a high rainfall. However, thermophilic organisms are also present in other vegetable matter, including chopped straw used as bedding for cattle kept in barns during the winter months. The extension of this method of intensive farming could lead to a resurgence of farmers' lung (Axford, personal communication).

Exposure to spores of *Micropolyspora faeni* occurs when the bales of mouldy hay are opened and fed to cattle; this takes place in the winter and early spring. Acute episodes of farmers' lung are likely to occur at that time of year and are accompanied by a rise in the serum titre of specific antibodies amongst the persons who are at risk (fig. 15.2 and table 15.3). There is also a rise in titre amongst the cattle; affected cows may cough and suffer an abortion or decline in milk production. Farmers' wives and their children were formerly at risk along with their menfolk but their exposure appears to be diminishing with changes in farm practices leading to milking herds being concentrated into relatively large units.

Compared with the acute effects the long-term effects of sensitization are less well documented. Persons who are sensitized but asymptomatic probably revert to normal on withdrawal from exposure. Those who have several acute episodes or are repeatedly exposed may progress to diffuse interstitial fibrosis (e.g. fig. 15.3). They may, however, develop nonspecific inflammation or bronchitis from regular exposure to inert dust (52), or become sensitized to allergens which give rise to allergic rhinitis, hay fever or occupational asthma. (For references, see page 342.)

Water droplet antigen diseases (including humidifier fever). Episodes of acute influenza-like illness with impairment of lung function may occur following sensitization to any of a number of antigens which are dispersed in water droplets. The antigens have been obtained from air conditioners, humidifiers, dehumidifiers, saunas, sewage and improperly purified domestic water supplies. A common feature of many of the episodes is the availability of a culture medium for growth of micro-organisms in or near a heat exchange system or similar structure. The resulting sludge contains many micro-organisms in symbiotic association, including thermoactinomyces, pullularia, bacterial toxins and amoebae (table 15.1). These organisms have all been associated with positive precipitin reactions, indicating sensitization, and have provoked typical acute episodes on inhalation challenge. Many buildings (offices, factories, laboratories, operating theatres) and many processes use equipment which might permit the growth of these organisms. The design of the heat exchange system and the extent to which it is maintained in a clean condition contribute to whether or not significant contamination will occur and, if so, which organism eventually becomes dominant. Very often it is the amoeba.

In some episodes of water droplet antigen disease the clinical, radiographic and physiological features are typical of extrinsic allergic alveolitis (e.g. 53); however, in the majority the constitutional effects are more conspicuous than the impairment of lung function. A reduction in vital capacity in association with narrowing of small airways appears to be a constant feature. In one such episode the provocation of symptoms by inhalation challenge did not lead to a reduction in transfer factor or to an increase in the consumption of complement (57, 59). Many episodes affect workers in modern air-conditioned buildings (page 294). Anecdotal evidence suggests that the episodes are seldom investigated and whilst long-term sequelae are believed to be rare, the possibility has not been explored systematically. There is no information on the morbid anatomy of the lung and the evidence for alveolitis is meagre; nevertheless, the illnesses have much in common with extrinsic allergic alveolitis including the clinical features, the presence of precipitating antibodies and the simulation by inhalation challenge. The differences may be due to the antigens being dispersed in droplets and droplet nuclei which are hygroscopic and readily cleared from the lung, rather than being carried on the surface of spores or in solid particles which are cleared less rapidly. Alternatively the constitutional disturbance may be due to bacterial endotoxins acting directly and not via an antigen–antibody reaction. However, neither of these hypotheses is supported by direct evidence and there is a clear need for more research. (For references, see page 343.)

Other conditions. Some of the many other forms of extrinsic allergic alveolitis are given in table 15.1 where they are classified in terms of the probable antigen. In all cases, with the partial exception of water droplet antigen disease which is discussed above, the presentation and clinical features conform to the descriptions given in this chapter. Some of the reports are of single cases or episodes, whilst others describe sensitization or clinical symptoms affecting large numbers of people. For the latter some epidemiological information on prevalence is summarized in table 15.6. Many of these outbreaks are due to a single antigen but, in some, more than one antigen may have contributed to the burden of ill-health; extrinsic allergic alveolitis of mushroom workers, poultry farmers using deep litter, wood trimmers and some water-workers fall into this category. For further details of the individual conditions the references which are cited should be consulted.

References

For additional references the relevant specialist journals should be consulted.

General aspects of extrinsic allergic alveolitis

1 Avila R. Some aspects of occupational asthma. *Clin Allergy* 1983;**13**:191–5.
2 Burrell R, Rylander R. A critical review of the role of precipitins in hypersensitivity pneumonitis. *Eur J Respir Dis* 1981;**62**:332–43.
3 Earis JE, Marsh K, Pearson MG, Ogilvie CM. The inspiratory 'squark' in extrinsic allergic alveolitis and other pulmonary fibroses. *Thorax* 1982;**37**:923–6.
4 Gourley CA, Braidwood GD. The use of dust respirators in the prevention of recurrence of farmer's lung. *Trans Soc Occup Med* 1971;**21**:93–5.
5 Hendrick DJ, Faux JA, Anand B, Piris J, Marshall R. Is bird fancier's lung associated with coeliac disease. *Thorax* 1978;**33**:425–8.
6 Hendrick DJ, Marshall R, Faux JA, Krall JM. Positive alveolar responses to antigen inhalation provocation tests: their validity and recognition. *Thorax* 1980;**35**:415–27.
7 Kawanami O, Basset F, Barrios R, Lacronique JG, Ferrans VJ, Crystal RG. Hypersensitivity pneumonitis in man. Light and electron-microscopic studies of 18 lung biopsies. *Am J Pathol* 1983;**110**:275–89.
8 Moore VL, Hensley GT, Fink JN. An animal mode of hypersensitivity pneumonitis in the rabbit. *J Clin Invest* 1975;**56**:937–44.
9 Nielsen KH, Parratt D, Boyd G, White RG. Use of radio-labelled antiglobulin for quantitation of antibody to soluble antigens rendered particulate: application to human sera from "pigeon fancier's lung syndrome". *Int Arch Allergy* 1974;**47**:339–50.
10 Turner-Warwick M. Immunological features of allergic alveolitis. Cited by Parkes RW. *Occupational Lung Disorders* 2nd edition. 1982: p 414.
11 Warren CPW, Tse KS, Cherniack RM. Mechanical properties of the lung in extrinsic allergic alveolitis. *Thorax* 1978;**33**:315–21.

Bagassosis

12 Hearn CED. Bagassosis: an epidemiological, environmental and clinical survey. *Br J Industr Med* 1968;**25**:267–282.
13 Lacey J. Thermoactinomyces sacchari sp. nov., a thermophilic actinomycete causing bagassosis. *J Gen Microbiol* 1971;**66**:327–38.
14 Salvaggio J, Arquembourg P, Seabury J, Buechner H. Bagassosis. *Am J Med* 1969;**46**: 538–44.

15 Weill H, Buechner HA, Gonzalez E, Herbert SJ, Aucoin E, Ziskind MM. Bagassosis: a study of pulmonary function in 20 cases. *Ann Int Med* 1966;**64**:737–47.

Bird handlers' lung

16 Allen DH, Basten A, Woolcock AJ. Studies of cell-mediated and humoral immunity in bird breeder's hypersensitivity pneumonitis. *Am Rev Respir Dis* 1977;**115**:45A (Supplement).

17 Allen DH, Williams GV, Woolcock AJ. Bird breeder's hypersensitivity pneumonitis: progress studies of lung function after cessation of exposure to the provoking antigen. *Am Rev Respir Dis* 1976;**114**:555–66.

18 Andersen P, Christensen KM, Jensen BE, Axel K, Laursen JCS, Geday H, Lundsgaard A, Anderson HK. Antibodies to pigeon antigens in pigeon breeders. *Eur J Resp Dis* 1982;**63**: 113–21.

19 Banham SW, McKenzie H, McSharry C, Lynch PP, Boyd G. Antibody against a pigeon bloom extract: a further antigen in pigeon fanciers' lung. *Clin Allergy* 1982;**12**:173–8.

20 Berrens L, Guckers CL, van Dijk A. The antigens in pigeon-breeders disease and their interaction with human complement. *Ann NY Acad Sci* 1974;**221**:153–62.

21 Boyd G, Madkour M, Middleton S, Lynch P. Effect of smoking on circulating antibody levels to avian protein in pigeon breeder's disease. *Thorax* 1977;**32**:651.

22 Boyer RS, Klock LE, Schmidt CD, Hyland L, Maxwell K, Gardner RM, Renzetti AD Jr. Hypersensitivity lung disease in the turkey raising industry. *Am Rev Respir Dis* 1974;**109**:630–5.

23 British Thoracic Society. A national survey of bird fancier's lung including its possible association with jejunal villous atropy. *Br J Dis Chest* 1984;**78**:75–87.

24 Christensen LT, Schmidt CD, Robbins L. Pigeon breeders' disease—a prevalence study and review. *Clin Allergy* 1975;**5**:417–30.

25 Elgefors B, Belin L, Hanson LA. Pigeon breeder's lung: clinical and immunological observations. *Scand J Respir Dis* 1971;**52**: 167–76.

26 Faux JA, Hendrick DJ, Anand BS. Precipitins to different avian serum antigens in bird fancier's lung and coeliac disease. *Clin Allergy* 1978;**8**:101–8.

27 Hendrick DJ, Faux JA, Marshall R. Budgerigar fancier's lung: the commonest variety of

allergic alveolitis in Britain. *Br Med J* 1978;**ii**:81–4.

28 Hensley GT, Garancis JC, Cherayil GD, Fink JN. Lung biopsies of pigeon breeders' disease. *Arch Path* 1969;**87**:572–9.

29 Lee TH, Wraith DG, Bennett CO, Bentley AP. Budgerigar fancier's lung: The persistence of budgerigar precipitins and the recovery of lung function after cessation of avian exposure. *Clin Allergy* 1983;**13**:197–202.

30 Lupi-Herrera E, Sandoval J, Bialostozky D, Seoane M, Martinez ML, Bonetti PF, Reyes P, Barrios R. Extrinsic allergic alveolitis caused by pigeon breeding at a high altitude (2240 metres). *Am Rev Respir Dis* 1981;**124**:602–7.

31 McSharry C, Banham SW, Lynch PP, Boyd G. Antibody measurement in extrinsic allergic alveolitis. *Eur J Respir Dis* 1984;**65**:259–65.

32 McSharry C, Lynch PP, Banham SW, Boyd G. Seasonal variation of antibody levels amongst pigeon fanciers. *Clin Allergy* 1983;**13**:293–9.

33 Muers MF, Faux JA, Ting A, Morris PJ. HLA-A, B, C and HLA-DR antigens in extrinsic allergic alveolitis (budgerigar fancier's lung disease). *Clin Allergy* 1982;**12**:47–53.

34 Munro AC, Inglis G, Lynch PP, Boyd G. A survey of P_1 antibodies in Scottish pigeon fanciers. *Clin Allergy* 1980;**10**:643–50.

35 Schuyler MR, Thigpen TP, Salvaggio JE. Local pulmonary immunity in pigeon breeder's disease. *Ann Intern Med* 1978;**88**:355–8.

36 Scribner GH, Barboriak JJ, Fink JN. Prevalence of precipitins in groups at risk of developing hypersensitivity pneumonitis. *Clin Allergy* 1980;**10**:91–5.

37 Wuthe H, Bergmann K-Ch, Vogel J. Frequency of lung function disturbances and immunological status of industrial poultry farmers. *Eur J Respir Dis* 1981;**62**(Suppl.113):38–9.

Farmers' lung

38 Bamdad S. Enzyme-linked immunosorbent assay (ELISA) for IgG antibodies in farmer's lung disease. *Clin Allergy* 1980;**10**:161–71.

39 Berrens L, Ridder G de, Boer F de. Longitudinal studies of immunological parameters in farmer's lung. *Scand J Respir Dis* 1977;**58**: 205–14.

40 Braun SR, doPico GA, Tsiatis A, Horvath E, Dickie HA, Rankin J. Farmer's lung disease: long-term clinical and physiologic outcome. *Am Rev Respir Dis* 1979;**119**:185–91.

41 Cross T, Maciver AM. The thermophilic actino-

mycetes in mouldy hay. *Micropolyspora faeni* sp. nov. *J Gen Microbiol* 1968;**50**:351–9.

42 Flaherty DK, Braun SR, Marx JJ, Blank JL, Emanuel DA, Rankin J. Serologically detectable HLA-A, B and C loci antigens in farmer's lung disease. *Am Rev Respir Dis* 1980;**122**:437–43.

43 Grant IWB, Blyth W, Wardrop VE, Gordon RM, Pearson JCG, Mair A. Prevalence of farmer's lung in Scotland: a pilot survey. *Br Med J* 1972;**i**:530–4.

44 Hapke EJ, Seal RME, Thomas GO, Hayes M, Meek JC. Farmer's lung: a clinical, radiographic, functional and serological correlation of acute and chronic stages. *Thorax* 1968;**23**:451–68.

45 Heino M, Monkare S, Haahtela T, Laitinen LA. An electron-microscopic study of the airways in patients with farmer's lung. *Eur J Respir Dis* 1982;**63**:52–61.

46 Morgan DC, Smyth JT, Lister RW, Pethybridge RJ, Gilson JC, Callaghan P, Thomas GO. Chest symptoms in farming communities with special reference to farmer's lung. *Br J Industr Med* 1975;**32**:228–34.

47 Reed CE, Sosman A, Barbee RA. Pigeon-breeders' lung. A newly observed interstitial pulmonary disease. *J Am Med Ass* 1965;**193**:261–5.

48 Reyes CN, Wenzel FJ, Lawton BR, Emanuel DA. The pulmonary pathology of farmer's lung disease. *Chest* 1982;**81**:142–6.

49 Seal RME, Hapke EJ, Thomas GO, Meek JC, Hayes M. The pathology of the acute and chronic stages of farmer's lung. *Thorax* 1968;**23**:469–89.

50 Stokes TC, Turton CWG, Turner-Warwick M. A study of immunoglobulin G subclasses in patients with farmer's lung. *Clin Allergy* 1981;**11**:201–7.

51 Terho EO, Heinonen OP, Lammi S. Incidence of farmer's lung leading to hospitalization and its relation to meteorological observations in Finland. *Acta Med Scand* 1983;**213**:295–8.

52 Turton CWG, Firth G, Grundy E, Rigden BG, Smyth JT, Turner-Warwick M. Raised enzyme markers of chronic inflammation in asymptomatic farmer's lung. *Thorax* 1981;**36**:122–5.

Water droplet antigen disease

53 Anderson K, McSharry CP, Boyd G. Radiographic changes in humidifier fever. *Thorax* 1985;**40**:312–3.

54 Ashton I, Axford AT, Bevan C, Cotes JE. Lung function of office workers exposed to humidifier fever antigen. *Br J Industr Med* 1981;**38**:34–7.

55 Banaszak EF, Thiede WH, Fink JN. Hypersensitivity pneumonitis due to contamination of an air conditioner. *N Engl J Med* 1970;**283**:271–6.

56 Belin L. Prevalence of symptoms and immuno-response in relation to exposure to infected humidifiers. *Eur J Respir Dis* 1980;**61** (Suppl.107):155–62.

57 Cockcroft A, Edwards J, Bevan C, Campbell I, Collins G, Houston K, Jenkins D, Latham S, Saunders M, Trotman D. An investigation of operating theatre staff exposed to humidifier fever antigens. *Br J Industr Med* 1981;**38**:144–51.

58 Edwards JH. Humidifier fever. MRC Symposium (1977). *Thorax* 1977;**32**:653–63.

59 Edwards JH, Cockcroft A. Inhalation challenge in humidifier fever. *Clin Allergy* 1981;**11**:227–35.

60 Fink JN, Banaszak EF, Baroriak JJ, Hensley GT, Kurup VP. *et al.* Interstitial lung disease due to contamination of forced air systems. *Ann Intern Med* 1976; **84**:406–13.

61 Friend JAR, Palmer KNV, Gaddie J, Pickering CAC, Pepys J. Extrinsic allergic alveolitis and contaminated cooling-water in a factory machine. *Lancet* 1977;**i**:297–300.

62 Metzger WJ, Patterson R, Fink JN, Semerdjian R, Roberts M. Sauna-takers' disease. *J Am Med Ass* 1976;**236**:2209–11.

63 Muittari A, Kuusisto P, Virtanen P, Sovijarvi A, Gronroos P, Harmoinen A, Antila P, Kellomaki L. An epidemic of extrinsic allergic alveolitis caused by tap water. *Clin Allergy* 1980;**10**:77–90.

64 Parrott WF, Blyth W. Another causal factor in the production of humidifier fever. *J Soc Occup Med* 1980;**30**:63–8.

65 Rylander R, Haglind P, Lundholm M, Mattsby I, Stenqvist K. Humidifier fever and endotoxin exposure. *Clin Allergy* 1978;**8**:511–16.

Other causes of extrinsic allergic alveolitis

66 Anderson HR. Respiratory abnormalities and ventilatory capacity in a Papua New Guinea Island Community. *Am Rev Respir Dis* 1976;**114**:537–48.

67 Avila R, Lacey J. The role of penicillium frequentans in suberosis. (Respiratory disease in workers in the cork industry.) *Clin Allergy* 1974;**4**:109–17.

68 Beaudry C, Laplante L. Severe allergic pneumonitis from hydrochlorothiazide. *Ann Intern Med* 1973;**78**:251–3.

69 Belin L. Clinical and immunological data on "wood trimmer's" disease in Sweden. *Eur J Respir Dis* 1980;**61**(Suppl.107):169–76.

70 Blackburn CRB, Green W. Precipitins against extracts of thatched roofs in the sera of New Guinea natives with chronic lung disease. *Lancet* 1966;**ii**:1396–7.

71 Campbell JA, Kryda MJ, Treuhaft MW. Cheese worker's hypersensitivity pneumonitis. *Am Rev Respir Dis* 1983;**127**:495–6.

72 Carlson JE, Villaveces JW. Hypersensitivity pneumonitis due to pyrethrum. *J Am Med Ass* 1977;**237**:1718–9.

73 Carroll KB, Pepys J, Longbottom JL, Hughes DTD, Benson HG. Extrinsic allergic alveolitis due to rat serum protein. *Clin Allergy* 1975;**5**:443–56.

74 Charles J, Bernstein A, Jones B, Jones DJ, Edwards JH, Seal RME, Seaton A. Hypersensitivity pneumonitis after exposure to isocyanates. *Thorax* 1976;**31**:127–36.

75 Cohen HI, Merigan TC, Kosek JC, Eldridge F. A granulomatous pneumonitis associated with red wood sawdust inhalation. *Am J Med* 1967;**43**:785–94.

76 Craig DB, Donevan RE. Mushroom worker's lung. *Can Med Ass J* 1970;**102**:1289–93.

77 doPico GA, Rankin J, Chosy LW, Reddan WG, Barbee RA, Gee B, Dickie HA. Respiratory tract disease from thermosetting resins. *Ann Intern Med* 1975;**83**:177–84.

78 Emanuel DA, Wenzel FJ, Lawton BR. Pneumonitis due to cryptostroma corticale (maple bark disease). *N Engl J Med* 1966;**274**:1413–8.

79 Evans WV, Seaton A. Hypersensitivity pneumonitis in a technician using Pauli's reagent. *Thorax* 1979;**34**:767–70.

80 Grant IWB, Blackadder ES, Greenberg M, Blyth W. Extrinsic allergic alveolitis in Scottish malt workers. *Br Med J* 1976;**i**:490–3.

81 Harper LO, Burrell RG, Lapp NL, Morgan WKC. Allergic alveolitis due to pituitary snuff. *Ann Intern Med* 1970;**73**:581–4.

82 Kaad PH, Ostergaard PAA. The hazard of mould hyposensitization in children with asthma. *Clin Allergy* 1982;**12**:317–20.

83 Katila ML, Mantyjarvi RA, Ojanen TH. Sensitisation against environmental antigens and respiratory symptoms in swine workers. *Br J Industr Med* 1981;**38**:334–8.

84 Lunn JA, Hughes DTD. Pulmonary hypersensitivity to the grain weevil. *Br J Industr Med* 1967;**24**:158–61.

85 O'Brien IM, Bull J, Creamer B, Sepulveda R, Harries M, Burge PS, Pepys J. Asthma and extrinsic allergic alveolitis due to Merulius lacrymans. *Clin Allergy* 1978;**8**:535–42.

86 Pimentel JC. Furrier's lung. *Thorax* 1970;**25**:387–98.

87 Pimentel JC, Avila R. Respiratory disease in cork workers (suberosis). *Thorax* 1973;**28**:409–23.

88 Sakula A. Mushroom worker's lung. *Br Med J* 1967;**iii**:708–10.

89 Schlueter DP, Fink JN, Hensley GT. Wood-pulp workers' disease: a hypersensitivity pneumonitis caused by Alternaria. *Ann Intern Med* 1972;**77**:907–14.

90 Schulz KH, Felten G, Hausen BM. Allergy to the spores of *Pleurotus florida*. *Lancet* 1974;**i**:29.

91 Stewart CJ. Mushroom worker's lung—two outbreaks. *Thorax* 1974;**29**:252–7.

92 Stewart CJ, Pickering CAC. Mushroom worker's lung. *Lancet* 1974;**i**:317. See also refs 76 and 91.

93 Uragoda CG. A comparative study of chilli grinders with paprika splitters. *J Soc Occup Med* 1983;**33**:145–7.

94 Van den Bosch JMM, Van Toorn DW, Wagenaar SS. Coffee worker's lung: Reconsideration of a case report. *Thorax* 1983;**38**:720.

95 Van Toorn DW. Coffee worker's lung: A new example of extrinsic allergic alveolitis. *Thorax* 1970;**25**:399–405.

96 Wenzel FJ, Emanuel DA. The epidemiology of maple bark disease. *Arch Environm Hlth* 1967;**14**:385–9.

Chapter 16
Occupational Asthma

A person who develops episodes of chest tightness, wheeze and breathlessness may have asthma. The usual definition is due to Scadding; asthma is a disease characterized by wide variations over short periods of time in resistance to flow in intrapulmonary airways. The common feature is airflow limitation which varies in intensity from hour to hour. It is due to increased release of chemical substances which cause the respiratory smooth muscle to contract; the provoking agent may be external to the subject or unknown, hence the subdivision of asthma into extrinsic or cryptogenic.

Extrinsic asthma is subdivided into those cases where the bronchoconstriction is mediated by immunoglobulins of the class IgE and those where other mechanisms are responsible. IgE mediated asthma occurs in persons who develop IgE antibodies in response to commonly encountered antigens. Some 20% of the population readily exhibit this characteristic which is recognized by an immediate reaction to allergy skin tests. The reactors are said to be atopic; they are at risk of developing extrinsic atopic asthma. Extrinsic non-atopic asthma also occurs. Both these types of extrinsic asthma may be provoked by substances encountered at work. For the condition to be occupational, the asthma should be associated with employment; the employment should entail exposure to a sensitizing agent and

other cases of occupational asthma should have occurred in the same or a similar job. A firm diagnosis requires objective confirmation. This is necessary because asthma is only one of several causes of variable airflow obstruction and only a minority of such cases, less than 15%, are occupational. The diagnosis of occupational asthma carries important implications for employment.

To make a diagnosis of occupational asthma the physician may need to visit the place of work and to initiate special investigations which are not required for the management of non-occupational asthma. The investigations include environmental monitoring, serial measurement of the peak expiratory flow rate, radioallergosorbent testing (RAST), non-specific bronchial provocation with histamine, methacholine or sulphur dioxide, and inhalation challenge. The clinical features and the techniques of investigation are described below. Whenever the diagnosis is made there are problems concerning treatment, return to work, and protection of other exposed persons. Furthermore, details of causation and the manner in which the agent provokes its response may shed light on immunological processes and bronchial pharmacology. Partly on this account the study of occupational asthma has attracted the interest of specialists in many related disciplines; experimentation, speculation and controversy are rife and have made occupational asthma one of the liveliest and fastest growing topics in respiratory medicine.

Conditions associated with atopic status.

Atopic persons readily develop IgE antibodies in response to commonly encountered antigens. They become sensitized by brief exposure to weak antigens in low concentration; others who are not atopic may nonetheless be sensitized by heavy exposure to a strong antigen and there is every gradation in between. A person's place on the continuum is determined by genetic factors so atopy runs in families. Atopy carries an increased risk of illness associated with antigen–antibody reactions mediated by immunoglobulins of the species IgE. The reactions are immediate and have been classified as type I by Gell & Coombs; the skin reaction is commonly used to make the diagnosis of atopy. For this purpose the test should be performed using extracts of grass pollen, house dust mite, cat fur and *Aspergillus fumigatus*. The procedure is described on page 351. The atopic individual may be allergic to some foods, for example shell fish, or to drugs, for example penicillin. In infancy there is an increased risk of developing infantile eczema. In childhood wheezy bronchitis, recurrent conjunctivitis, itchy skin, hay fever or perennial rhinitis, often manifested by sneezing, are relatively common and may presage the developing of classical extrinsic asthma in the second or third decades of life. Overall the atopic individual has a greater than 25% chance of developing one or other manifestation and of those with wheezy bronchitis, approximately 50% at some time experience symptoms typical of asthma. The antecedent bronchiolitis is now classified as asthma by some paediatricians. It can predispose to chronic bronchitis later in life (chapter 17). Atopic status also predisposes to bronchopulmonary aspergillosis (page 284) but the risk is very small. The serum IgE level normally rises with age into early adult life, when the risk of asthma is greatest, then gradually declines. The level is increased in the presence of any manifestation of sensitization.

Extrinsic atopic asthma

Most cases of asthma in an atopic subject have their onset in adolescence or early adult life. The patient often gives a history of 'wheezy bronchitis' during childhood or other manifestation of atopy. The asthma is seasonal when it is due to pollen from grass, rag weed or other vegetation. It may develop a few months after the introduction of a domestic pet into the household or may be due to sensitization to house dust mite (*Dermatophagoides pteronyssinus* or *farinae*); the condition will then disappear on moving to a mite-free environment, for example to live at moderate altitude. More often the aetiology is multifactorial with several allergens, cold air, exercise and irritants all causing wheezing. In addition to the common antigens numerous other sensitizing agents can cause asthma by the IgE mechanism which, therefore, operates mainly in atopic individuals but is by no means confined to them. The exposure to the antigen may arise during the course of employment.

In extrinsic atopic asthma the bronchoconstriction comes on within a few minutes of exposure, there is an immediate positive cutaneous reaction to the responsible antigen and the serum IgE concentration is increased. The number of eosinophils in blood and sputum is also usually increased. The bronchoconstriction is usually prevented by sodium cromoglycate or reversed by use of a bronchodilator aerosol; it is not much affected by corticosteroid drugs. According to the definition extrinsic atopic asthma does not occur in individuals who are not atopic. However, this is an over-simplification. Most non-atopic individuals (i.e. those who are negative on skin testing with common allergens) can develop IgE mediated asthma if the exposure is sufficient. Thus the term 'atopic asthma' is unsatisfactory.

Extrinsic non-atopic asthma

An external agent which is capable of causing asthma in any individual independent of his atopic status or serum IgE concentration gives rise to extrinsic non-atopic asthma. This definition implies that the condition is mediated by some mechanism other than IgE. Several such mechanisms have been identified, of which some are common to several antigens whilst others are unique to one. In these cases the asthma can usefully be designated by either or both the substance and the type of hypersensitivity reaction. However, chemicals of the isocyanate group can cause both atopic (IgE mediated) and non-atopic asthma so these two classes of extrinsic asthma are not mutually exclusive. The two classes also overlap in the time of the response. That of IgE mediated asthma is immediate whilst the response in non-atopic asthma is either immediate or delayed or both types of response may occur. They are described under occupational asthma below.

Cryptogenic asthma

Asthma which is not associated with sensitization to a specific antigen or a raised serum concentration of IgE may be said to be cryptogenic in that the cause is at present unknown. Within this category there is a subgroup of patients in whom the asthma usually develops in middle age (hence late onset asthma), is not seasonal in incidence and often persists despite bronchodilator therapy; eosinophilia is common and there is usually a good response to corticosteroid drugs. Some of these patients have other features suggestive of an immunological disorder including autoantibodies to smooth muscle, thyroid or gastric antibodies, antinuclear factor or prodromal polyarteritis nodosa. The patient may be homozygous for HLA W6. These associations provide some support for the designation of the conditions as intrinsic asthma but since the mechanisms are unknown the term is at present of limited usefulness. The practice of classifying as intrinsic any asthma that does not entail an antigen–antibody reaction is misleading and should be abandoned.

Features common to all types of asthma

The occurrence of variable or paroxysmal wheeze and breathlessness resulting from narrowing of lung airways is essential for the diagnosis of asthma. Cough and rhinitis or paroxysmal sneezing may also occur; the cough is sometimes prominent after exercise. The symptoms often develop first in the early hours of the morning and are frequently worst at this time. They may wake the patient or the spouse from sleep and can mimic the nocturnal dyspnoea of left ventricular failure. In a patient with chronic airflow obstruction the aggravation caused by recurrent infection may give rise to a similar picture. The physical signs and radiographic appearance of the chest are not specific for asthma. The diagnosis is usually made from the history, together with the finding of physiological evidence for airflow limitation which is partly or completely reversed by therapy. The lung function changes are described below. Between asthma attacks the airways usually have an increased tendency to constrict. This hyperreactivity may be demonstrated by non-specific provocation tests including inhalation challenge with cold damp air, histamine or methacholine and the performance of strenuous exercise. The procedures are described later. Unfortunately the tests of non-specific hyperreactivity are not diagnostic. Some asthmatics do not react so give false negative responses, while positive responses may be elicited following a virus infection or the inhalation of an irritant substance. The subject of asthma has been reviewed by Clark & Godfrey (2), and by others cited on page 368. Classified references are given subsequently.

Occupational asthma

Occupational asthma is caused by exposure at the place of work to a sensitizing bronchoconstrictor substance. The exposure has the special features that the times of the daily onset and termination are known or can be estimated, the exposure recurs usually for 5 days each week and the time interval between the exposure and the resulting bronchoconstriction can be ascertained. In the case of IgE mediated asthma, conjunctivitis and rhinitis may also occur, the time interval is short, usually a few minutes (hence immediate-onset asthma), and the association with the causative agent is often easily recognized. Asthma mediated by short-term sensitizing IgG (also called short-latency IgG), behaves similarly. Other sensitizing bronchocontrictor substances give rise to a delayed response which can occur after an interval of 4h or only after 12h or longer (hence delayed-onset asthma); the association with an exposure at the workplace is then less direct and if one is suspected the mechanism may not be obvious. The differential diagnosis then includes specific airway sensitization (occupational asthma), alveolitis with a cell-mediated response (extrinsic allergic alveolitis) or non-specific stimulation of bronchial irritant receptors by an irritant substance present in the workplace. The bronchoconstrictor response may have been potentiated by the responsible agent also causing inflammation, by a recent virus infection or by the subject also having non-occupational asthma or chronic bronchitis associated with smoking cigarettes. Irritant substances which can cause non-specific bronchoconstriction include chlorine, ozone, sulphur dioxide and any inert respirable dust. In addition some substances which can cause occupational asthma, for example colophony and isocyanates, also act as non-specific irritants; however, except when the airways are hyperreactive for some other reason the effective irritant concentration is higher than that which bronchoconstricts as a manifestation of sensitization.

Delayed onset extrinsic allergic asthma comes on after an interval which is usually about 5h but may be 1–12h; an intradermal skin test yields a response after a similar or slightly longer delay (page 351). The response is sometimes mediated by an immunoglobulin of the class IgG. The bronchoconstriction is sustained, involves small airways and is accompanied by hypersecretion of mucus and oedema of the bronchial mucosa. Sometimes there is cough, fever, malaise and myalgia. Some subjects show a dual response, i.e. both an immediate Type 1 response and a delayed response. The delayed response can be prevented by sodium cromoglycate or corticosteroid drugs but it is usually relieved only transiently by bronchodilator drugs. In this, delayed-onset asthma differs from IgE mediated asthma in which adrenergic bronchodilator drugs and sodium cromoglycate are highly effective but corticosteroid drugs typically are not (figs. 16.6 and 16.7, page 356). When exposure ceases, resolution of delayed-onset asthma is gradual, often taking more than 24h; there may be spontaneous recurrences, often during the night, or the condition may persist more or less continuously for weeks or months; it is then indistinguishable from late-onset intrinsic asthma. Subsequently the subject may be left with hyperreactive airways which constrict readily in response to challenge by histamine, methacholine, sulphur dioxide or exercise. The hyperreactivity may be temporary or last for a number of years, a further point of resemblance to intrinsic asthma. The diagnosis of occupational asthma is considered on page 358.

Lung function in asthma

The characteristic feature is airflow limitation developing in response to the sensitizing agent and relieved by treatment or cessation of exposure. During an isolated acute episode the flow limitation is mainly in the larger airways. It is readily measured as a reduction in forced expiratory volume or peak expiratory flow and this change reflects an increase in airflow resistance which can be demonstrated by whole body plethysmography. The increase in resistance is mainly due to a rise in bronchomotor tone and is reversed by inhalation of salbutamol or other β adrenergic drugs.

In the absence of treatment the subject obtains some relief from the increased resistance by subconsciously increasing the lung volume at end expiration (functional residual capacity). There is an accompanying increase in residual volume and a reduction in forced expiratory flow at small lung volumes. Following cessation of exposure the increased airflow resistance slowly reverts to normal, usually within an hour or two, as discussed above. The lung function is usually completely normal between attacks; routine assessment at such a time is of no help in diagnosis. However, the airways may readily constrict in response to exercise or other non-specific stimuli.

If the exposure is insufficient to cause acute attacks or if the subject's airways are hyperactive there may be persistent narrowing of small airways; the residual volume is increased and the forced expiratory flow (MEF25%FVC) is reduced (page 103). The larger airways may or may not be affected during the day but are likely to be narrowed in the early morning and late at night on account of exaggeration of the normal diurnal rhythm (fig. 16.1, below). This may be associated with an abnormal rise in plasma histamine.

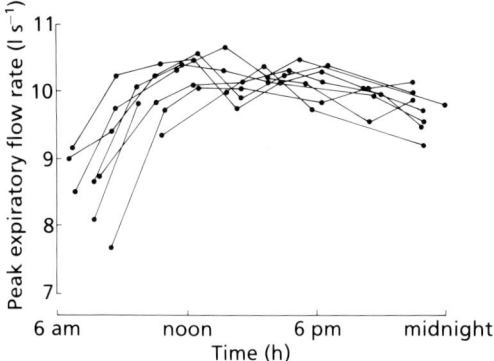

Fig. 16.1. Circadian measurements of peak expiratory flow rate in a pigeon fancier (precipitin positive) with exercise induced airflow limitation. There was a morning dip pattern which was reproducible from day to day. The pattern during 2 weeks without exposure was no different from that for other weeks, suggesting that the obstruction was not related to exposure.

Persistent asthmatic symptoms are accompanied by more marked airway narrowing and with correspondingly reduced forced expiratory flow rates, an increased residual volume, unequal distribution of inspired gas and hypoxaemia without much hypercapnia. Persistent cough with or without production of sputum may develop concurrently. The breathlessness on exertion and clinical plus radiographic features of air trapping may suggest a diagnosis of emphysema; however, unlike in emphysema, the transfer factor and K_{CO} are normal or increased, whilst lung compliance and recoil pressure are either normal or Cl is reduced and Pmax increased. Thus, while full assessment of lung function will exclude a diagnosis of emphysema, the diagnosis and management of occupational asthma usually requires no more than measurement of FEV, or PEFR. The use of periodic measurements of the peak flow

rate throughout the working day, at weekends and holidays, and the changes in FEV_1 in response to inhalation challenge are described subsequently.

Basic immunology

According to the model of Gell & Coombs allergic asthma is a Type 1 immunological reaction mediated by specific IgE immunoglobulins attached to cells in the bronchi, while alveolitis is a distinct clinical and immunological condition characterized by fever, dry cough, absence of bronchoconstriction, and mediated by circulating IgG precipitins (Type 3 reaction). In practice there is sometimes overlap of the clinical features of these two conditions. Exposure to bacillary enzymes and western red cedar, for example, commonly causes both early bronchoconstriction and, subsequently, fever accompanied by signs of alveolitis, while bronchoconstriction is sometimes a feature of farmers' lung. The clear distinction between Type 1 and Type 3, while still applying to the majority of cases, has thus become blurred and confused in a minority. Our present state of knowledge allows us to perceive only faintly how these two mechanisms interweave and interreact. Their relationship to other mechanisms for release of mediator substances such as by cotton dust (page 314) and grain dust (page 363) is also unknown.

The immediate Type 1 (or anaphylactic) reaction occurs in sensitized individuals and causes immediate-onset asthma following inhalation of antigen and a weal and flare reaction when the antigen is inoculated into the skin. It is due to antibody on the surface of mast cells or basophils combining with the corresponding antigen. The reaction leads to the release of pharmacologically active amines and other substances. Mast cells are secretory tissue cells with a granular cytoplasm which are found throughout the body. In the lung they occur mainly in the bronchial epithelium between the columnar cells and the basement membrane, in the blood they are carried as basophils which form a small proportion of the circulating leucocytes. The antibody is usually immunoglobulin E (IgE, also called reagin), but may be IgG. IgE (molecular

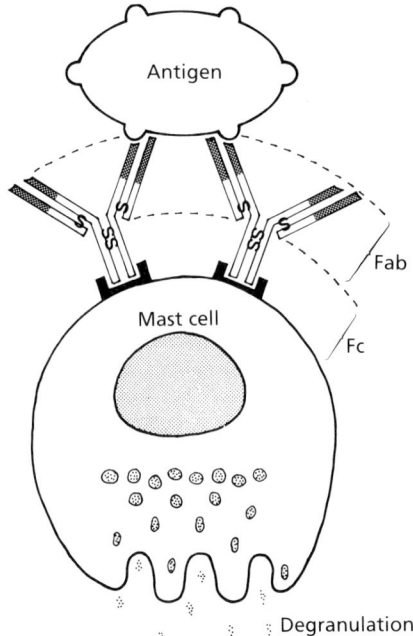

Fig. 16.2. Activation of a mast cell by IgE combining with its corresponding antigen. The terminal part of the Fab piece of IgE binds with its homologous antigenic determinant on the antigen; this causes an allosteric conformation change in the IgE molecule. The change is transmitted via the Fc piece to the mast cell receptor where it initiates the biochemical reactions which lead to degranulation. Two adjacent IgE molecules must bind the antigen for this to take place. Small molecules (e.g. toluene diisocyanate) initiate bridging by binding to larger carrier molecules; in this role they act as haptens. (By courtesy of J. H. Edwards.)

weight 200,000 Daltons) is produced mainly in lymphoid tissue of the upper respiratory tract. It is capable of binding both to receptors on the surface of mast cells or basophils and to the antigen. In the case of whole antigens (danders, pollen, mites, etc.) binding is onto the antigenic determinant of the material, but for antigenic substances of low molecular weight, binding is effected via a carrier protein. Such substances are called haptens (e.g. platinum salts, phthalic anhydride, toluene diisocyanate, etc.). The IgE molecule attaches to the antigen by its antibody binding fraction (Fab piece) and to the mast cell by its crystalline fraction (Fc piece, molecular

weight 55,000 Daltons). The fractions may be separated by splitting the IgE molecule with papain. Each Fab piece has two binding sites and each Fc piece has one (fig. 16.2). When two adjacent IgE molecules attach to the antigen this results in a change in shape which triggers the cell receptor via the Fc piece. There is then a local increase in concentration of cyclic adenosine monophosphate (C-AMP), via adenyl cyclase and methyl transferase, and release of arachidonic acid from the phospholipid of the cell membrane, via phospholipase. Granules within the cell which contain preformed active amines absorb water and by the action of cyto-skeletal proteins move towards the surface of the cell where they release the active material. The process consumes energy and requires the presence of calcium ions. The active agents include histamine which in the skin causes a weal and erythema. In the respiratory tract it gives rise to increased secretions of mucus and reflex bronchoconstriction which is mediated through the irritant receptors and vagi (page 47). In higher concentration histamine also acts directly on the airways and lung parenchyma. Other preformed mediators are heparin, enzymes and chemotactic factors for anaphylax-is, neutrophils and eosinophils (table 16.1). However, of greater importance is the new for-mation of active substances by metabolism of arachidonic acid. This is the precursor of prosta-glandins including PGD2 and PGF2a, which constrict bronchial smooth muscle, and of leuk-otrienes. Leukotriene B4 and related substances are chemotactic for eosinophils and other cells. Leukotrienes C4, D4 and E4 make up the slow reacting substance of anaphylaxis (SRS-A). These agents constrict peripheral airways, increase capillary permeability and stimulate production of mucus rich in glycoprotein which, therefore, has a high viscosity. The eosi-nophils attracted by the eosinophil chemotactic factor (ECF) contain a base protein which is cytotoxic; it aggravates the damage to tissues caused by the preformed enzymes from mast cells and by the newly formed SRS-A and other substances. Many of these substances contribute to delayed-onset asthma. Their formation in IgE mediated asthma is due to a high level of circu-lating antibody; they then give rise to the

Table 16.1. Mast cell mediators (for further information see text)

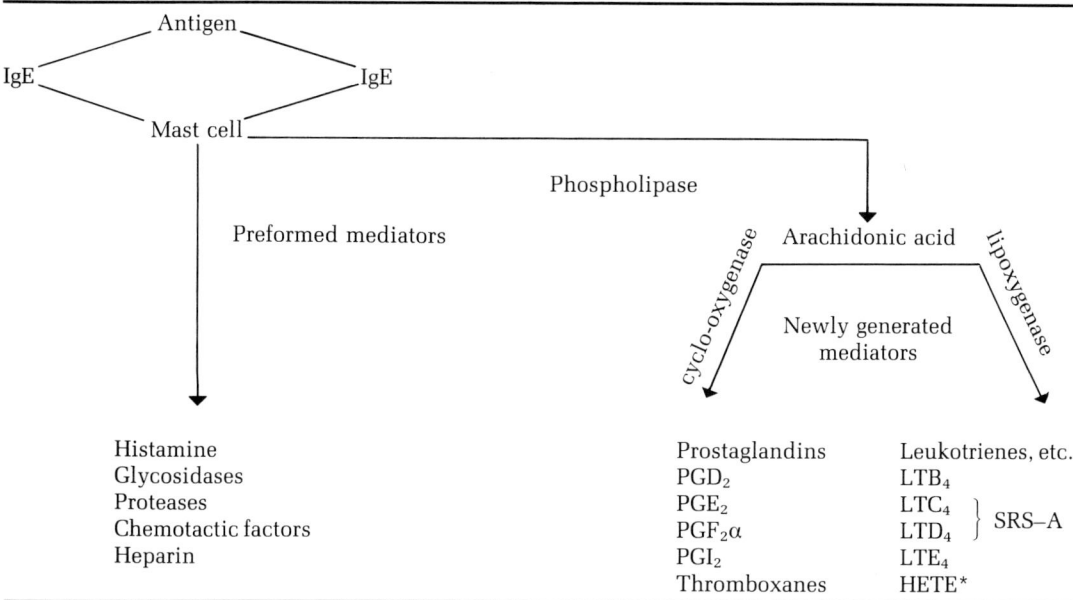

* Hydroxy-eicosa tetraenoic acid.

delayed part of the dual response which is, therefore, a feature of Type 1 asthma in highly atopic individuals or those exposed to a strong antigen.

The delayed or Type 3 reaction is associated with infiltration of the skin or bronchial epithelium by inflammatory cells; these are attracted by the neutrophil chemotactic factor (NCF) from sensitized mast cells. The neutrophils reinforce the action of the prostaglandins and leukotrienes described above. The reaction is usually mediated by specific IgG but is often sluggish in the absence of specific IgE antibodies; these appear to potentiate the response. The delayed cutaneous reaction described below can also be induced by IgE alone. On this account, amongst persons with bird fanciers' lung or farmers' lung those who are atopic are at increased risk of also having asthma (chapter 15). Most cases of occupational asthma are due to the formation of specific IgE against the inhaled antigen: examples are given in table 16.3 below. Some are due to IgG or IgM whilst in other instances the mechanism has still to be unravelled: examples are given in table 16.2.

Skin testing

An immediate response to a skin prick test is evidence for sensitization which is usually but not invariably mediated by the skin-sensitizing antibody IgE. The test is normally performed on the anterior surface of the forearm by pricking the skin through a drop of antigen. A fine hypodermic needle is inserted obliquely into the dermis just far enough to lift it gently, but not far enough to draw blood. Any bleeding is evidence that the insertion has been made too deeply. Because of the risk of generalized anaphylaxis reaction intradermal injection is best avoided. However, it is sometimes used in delayed onset asthma to indicate the presence of specific IgG. The associated delayed skin reaction is described below.

A positive immediate response comprises an itchy urticarial weal of diameter 2–15mm surrounded by an evanescent erythema of diameter 10–40mm. The weal diameter at 15min is commonly used as an index. Usually about half a dozen antigens of common substances known to cause Type 1 asthma are tested together with an

Table 16.2. Hypothetical explanations for production of asthma in absence of specific IgE

	Non-specific irritation	Histamine release	Other causes
Toluene diisocyanate	+	—	May block β adrenergic receptor sites
Tartrazine	—	—	Specific IgD against phenyl sulphonic moiety
Plicatic acid	+	+	May activate complement
Avian residues	—	—	Specific IgG in atopic subjects
Cladosporium, penicillins, etc.	—	—	Specific IgG precipitating antibodies
Ethanol	—		May produce bronchoconstrictor substance
Colophony	+	—	Specific IgM
Furfuryl alcohol	+	—	Not known
Formaldehyde	+	+	

inactive control solution. The latter is used to eliminate the risk of a 'false positive' reaction, which is mainly limited to subjects with dermatographia. A positive reaction to two or more antigens is evidence for atopic status. In addition the suspected occupational allergen may be used; a method for its preparation is described below. A positive reaction is evidence for the production of a specific IgE against the extract being tested. Where contact with the material is solely occupational this is evidence of a reaction to such exposure; an example is sensitization to rat urinary protein which is seldom acquired in other ways. In the case of substances which are potent sensitizers the positive prick test may also be evidence of disease; this is usually the case with platinum salts. In other circumstances the majority of reactors are usually asymptomatic. The allergens from locust tissue cross-react with antibodies against house-dust mites so in this circumstance a positive reaction may be no more than confirmation of atopic status. However, despite these difficulties in interpretation, the prick test is a valuable tool, especially when the diameter of the weal is used semi-quantitatively to assess the response to an alteration in exposure or to look for a change in susceptibility to disease. A negative result does not exclude an occupational cause for the asthma because reactions in the skin and in the bronchi are not always identical. A delayed reaction to the prick test usually occurs

at approximately 8h (range 4–24h) and comprises a red indurated papule with surrounding oedema. This is called an Arthus reaction. The diameter of the papule is usually recorded at 4h, 8h and then daily for up to 3 days. Histologically there is often necrosis and phagocytic cells are present which, with suitable immunofluorescent staining, can be shown to contain IgG antibody. On this account the Arthus reaction is of great theoretical importance. In practice a delayed reaction to prick test is very uncommon and the majority of patients with a dual or delayed bronchoconstriction do not show it.

Radioallergosorbent test (RAST)

This test is used for detecting the presence in serum of IgE antibody which is specific for a particular antigen, and thus helps to identify which of a number of antigens may be the cause of the patient's symptoms. The information which it provides overlaps with that from the skin prick test but RAST can be used for a number of substances for which no skin test is available. RAST is also more reproducible and often more convenient but it is more expensive so should only be performed on patients whose serum IgE is abnormally high (>350µg/ml). Some of the IgE antibodies which can be detected by this method are given in table 16.3. The presence of a positive RAST is not evidence that the sensitizing antigen has caused the

Table 16.3.   Some substances which give rise to asthma associated with specific IgE and a positive radioallergosorbent test (RAST) (The list is being added to almost daily, but not all are commercially available for RAS testing.)

B. subtilis proteinase	Papain
Castor wax	Platinum salts‡
Cockroach and other insects	Quillaja bark (saponin)
Coffee beans (green)	Reactive dyes‡
Gum acacia	Rodent serum and urine
Gum tragacanth	Tetrachlorophthalic anhydride‡
Ipecacuanha	Trimellitic anhydride‡
Isocyanates*†‡	Western red cedar

* Positive in only some individuals (see text).
† False positives can occur.
‡ Conjugated with human serum albumin.

patient's symptoms, nor does a negative RAST indicate that a previous episode was not due to the antigen.

The test is performed by incubating the subject's serum with a suspected antigen which is attached to a paper disc, wall of a test tube or other convenient surface. If there are specific antibodies in the serum they bind firmly with the antigen and are not dislodged during subsequent washing. The attached antigen––antibody complexes are then incubated with purified antibody to human IgE which is labelled with radioisotope. This leads to the radioisotope becoming attached to the antigen–antibody complexes in amounts which relate directly to the quantity of specific IgE present in the serum. Once a specific IgE has been identified it can be used in a RAST inhibition assay which is an analogous procedure for detecting the presence of a specific antigen. RAST may also be used for detecting specific IgG.

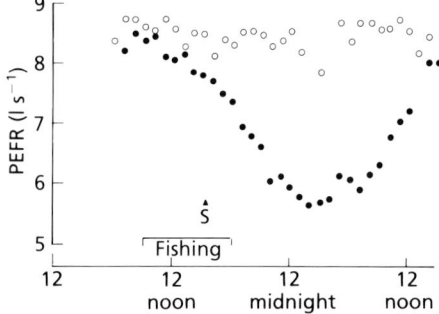

Fig. 16.3. Circadian measurements of peak expiratory flow rate demonstrating delayed onset asthma in a patient sensitized to *Calliphora* (blue bottle) maggots used as fish bait. Except for a few results in the middle of the night each point is the mean of five daily recordings. Symptoms (indicated by S) were associated with the presence of a circulating IgG antibody. (By courtesy of Stockley *et al* (32).)

Inhalation challenge testing

At work

Occupational asthma arises from exposure to an antigen or hapten which is inhaled during the course of or in connection with employment. The resulting airflow limitation can be monitored by serial measurement of lung function, usually the forced expiratory volume (FEV_1) or peak expiratory flow (PEF). The peak expiratory flow is measured with a portable peak-flow meter (e.g. Wright); this should preferably be fitted with an encoder which conceals the results from the subject and provides a check on the accuracy of transcription (page 92). The subject makes his own measurements every 2h from waking to bed time daily for a suitable period. Five days can be sufficient to establish a consistent pattern (e.g. fig. 16.3) but a longer period is usually required. The period should include weekends and preferably 2 consecutive weeks away from the suspected exposure: these may be during a holiday, during a change of work or during a period of protection provided by wearing a respirator (page 58). If the employment has been contributing to the airflow limitation, it will be found that the peak-flow rate is significantly lower while the subject is working normally than when he is not exposed. This test may reveal a deterioration soon after entering the workplace or after being at work for a few hours, a progressive deterioration throughout the week or a persistently low value which rises after a holiday (figs. 16.4 and 16.5). The test is

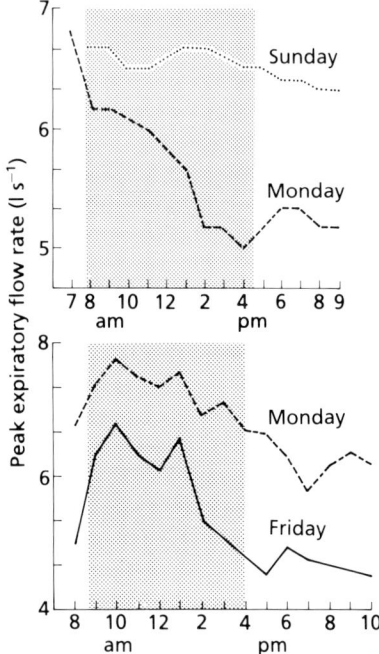

Fig. 16.4. Circadian measurements of peak expiratory flow rate (PEFR) in two electrical workers with occupational asthma resulting from exposure to colophony (indicated by stippling). The upper record (subject A) showed an initial followed by a delayed reaction on a Monday following a symptom-free weekend. The result for Friday (not included) showed a morning dip which masked the initial fall in PEFR. The lower record (subject B) showed a morning dip. The delayed reaction was progressively more pronounced and occurred from a lower level of PEFR as the week advanced. The result for Sunday (not illustrated) was similar to that for Friday. Recovery only occurred the following Monday (fig. 16.5). (By courtesy of Burge *et al* (90).)

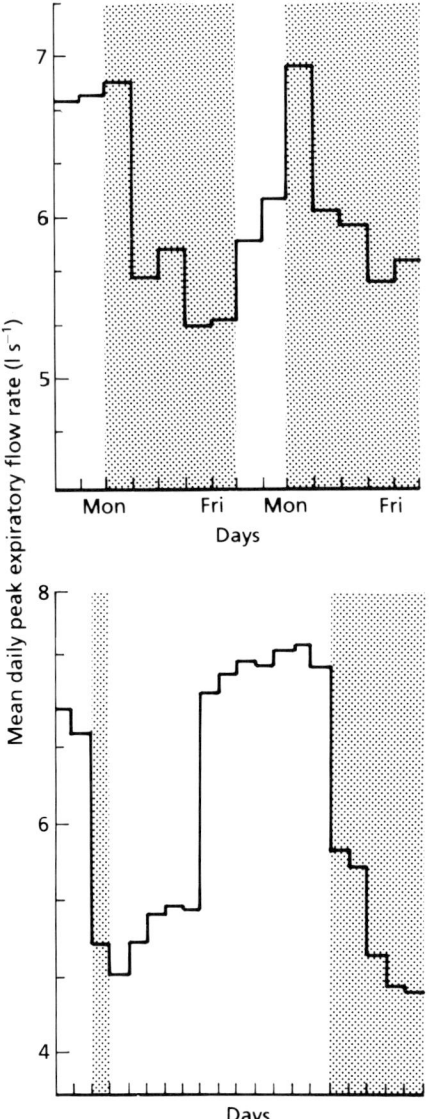

Fig. 16.5. Mean daily levels of peak expiratory flow rate (PEFR) in two electrical workers with occupational asthma resulting from exposure to colophony (indicated by stippling). In the upper record (subject B) the PEFR fell on Mondays (fig. 16.4) and remained relatively low for the rest of the working week. Recovery took 3 days. The lower record (subject C) began when the patient returned to work after 3 weeks' absence. One day's work exposure resulted in asthma lasting 6 days. (By courtesy of Burge *et al* (91).)

simple and the result is informative if the subject is both reasonably competent and well-motivated. As an alternative or for preliminary investigation of a suspected occupational allergen the investigator may measure the subject's peak flow or FEV_1 at the start and towards the end of one or more working days. Measurements should be begun as soon as occupational asthma is suspected and whilst the subject is still working normally, otherwise he may be moved to another section or the process changed before the diagnosis is established.

In the hospital laboratory

Bronchial challenge provides information on a subject's responsiveness to the allergen, information which may be necessary for treatment and for advice on future employment; the test carries a small risk of precipitating severe airways obstruction, alveolitis (page 330) or even death so it should be undertaken with circumspection. However, if the choice is between properly supervised challenge and return to an unregulated environment at work which is believed to have caused severe asthma, the former is the more acceptable. In practice this choice should not have to be made. Positive indications for challenge testing are to investigate a hitherto unsuspected antigen and to identify a specific antigen amongst several to which the subject may be exposed; the information is often of unique value towards planning for the future. Challenge should not be undertaken for medico-legal purposes (page 361) and in occupations where occupational asthma is a recognized hazard, monitoring at work should be used instead.

Challenge should be undertaken only when the patient is in a stable state with no material airflow obstruction (e.g. $FEV_1 > 80\%$ predicted when off drugs) and not within a week of previous exposure to the suspected antigen or to histamine. It should preferably be carried out in a manner which mimics exposure at work such as painting, welding, soldering or sifting (table 16.4). The manoeuvre should be performed in a booth or small chamber ventilated to outside air within the hospital complex. Full safety precautions should be available, including nebulized and intravenous bronchodilator drugs, intravenous hydrocortisone, oxygen and facilities for respiratory and cardiac resuscitation (79). The inhaled concentration of test substance should not exceed the hygiene standard and should be less than that experienced at work. Challenge can also be undertaken using a nebulized aerosol of an aqueous extract of the material in question. This should be prepared as a 10% weight-for-volume suspension in phosphate buffered saline. The suspension is agitated for 24h at 4°C, filtered, dialysed against phosphate buffered saline, freeze-dried, resuspended at an appropriate concentration (which might be in the range 0.01–10mg/ml) and sterilized using a multipore filter. The concentration should initially be less than that which causes a positive prick test. The subject should

Table 16.4.   Examples of types of inhalation challenge (see also 9)

Painting or spraying	Polyurethane paint, formaldehyde, shellac, trimellitic anhydride, ethylene diamine, dimethyl ethanolamine
Soldering	Colophony, stainless steel welding
Nebulized aqueous extract or solution	Plicatic acid, flour protein, rat urine, *M. lacrymans*, *B. subtilis* proteinase
Sifting dust	Western red cedar, quillaja bark
Sifting anhydrous lactate with substance added	Platinum salts, penicillin, reactive dyes, cephalexin, piperazine dihydrochloride
Mixing sand with substance added	Furfuryl alcohol and resin

not be taking bronchoactive drugs at the time. When an immediate response is expected the FEV_1 or peak expiratory flow rate should be monitored. A delayed response can also reduce the FEV_1 but this is not invariable. It may only affect the flow rate in small airways in which case the MEF25%FVC obtained from the expiratory flow volume curve (page 98) is the index of choice. The procedure should normally start at 9.00 a.m. so that measurements of lung function can be made throughout the day, initially at 5min intervals and subsequently every hour. On day 1 the subject is instructed in the procedure and control measurements are made. On day 2 and if necessary subsequent days, graded exposures are given and later these are repeated using a refined extract or after administration of sodium cromoglycate or other protective agent. Thus in a study of the effects of colophony (pine resin) Burge, Pepys and colleagues initially had their subjects inhale one natural breath of soldering fume, followed by three and six breaths at 15min intervals if no reaction had occurred by then. On 4 subsequent days if no reaction had occurred the subjects breathed fumes on three occasions for 1 and 2min, 5min, 20min and 60min, with the subject re-applying the heated

iron to the solder every 30s throughout the exposure (90). Other examples are given in table 16.4. In the case of an uncomplicated immediate response the measurements may be discontinued or checked infrequently after the flow rate has returned to the initial value but if a delayed response is suspected they should be continued into the following day. The results of the challenge test are analysed graphically (figs. 16.6 and 16.7) or used to construct a dose–response relationship; an immediate response is related to the logarithm of the dose but a late response may not be quantifiable and in this circumstance is reported as present or absent or in terms of the mean FEV_1 for the 12h following challenge.

Testing for non-specific bronchial hyperreactivity

Airway calibre reflects the tone of bronchial smooth muscle; the calibre is usually increased by atropine and β sympathetic stimulating drugs and in asthmatics is reduced by β blockade with propanolol. The calibre is also reduced by histamine, analogues of acetyl choline (e.g. methacholine) and other agents acting through the

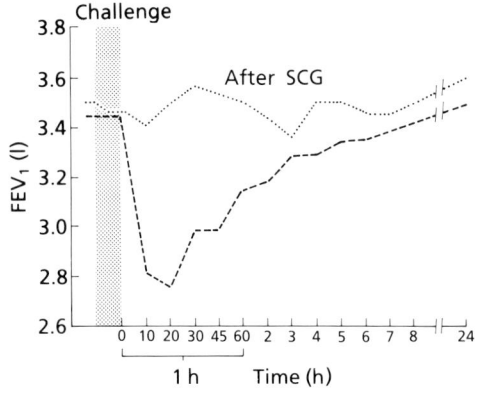

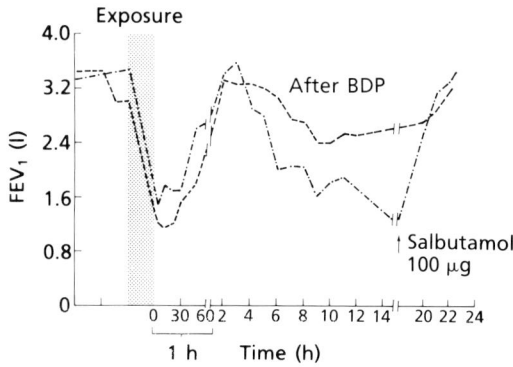

Fig. 16.6. Immediate response of forced expiratory volume (FEV_1) to challenge with ammonium hexachlorplatinate in a platinum refinery worker. The immediate onset asthma was prevented by pretreatment with sodium cromoglycate (SCG) but not by placebo treatment (not shown). (By courtesy of Pepys *et al* (74).)

Fig. 16.7. Dual response of forced expiratory volume (FEV_1) to challenge with rye flour in a baker. The delayed but not the immediate asthmatic reaction was largely prevented by pretreatment with beclomethasone dipropionate (BDP) but not by placebo treatment (not shown). (By courtesy of Hendrick *et al* (45).)

parasympathetic nervous system. The sensitivity to non-specific bronchoconstrictor agents is increased in healthy people after viral infections of the respiratory tract, in asthmatics, in persons with hay fever and in those recovering from occupational asthma, particularly of the delayed-onset type (for example, that associated with sensitization to isocyanate). The reactivity can also be increased by inhalation challenge or ingestion of the sensitizing substance in dosage too small to cause bronchoconstriction. The presence of non-specific bronchial hyperreactivity is usually assessed in terms of the dose of histamine or methacholine which reduces the forced expiratory volume by 20% (designated provocation concentration 20% or PC20) or the specific airway conductance by 35% (PC35 sGaw). The PC20 FEV_1 is the more reproducible index and the test is more widely available but the end-point appears to reflect a greater degree of bronchoconstriction. Recommendations for standardizing the challenge procedure have

been made by several organizations (3, 12) but a number of technical points have still to be resolved. Hyperreactivity may also be assessed by the occurrence of airflow limitation in response to exercise or breathing cold air. The subject should preferably be asymptomatic, have no material airflow obstruction and not be taking any medication at the time of testing.

The histamine provocation test is performed by alternating measurements of forced expiratory volume with inhalations of dilute solutions of histamine, either for 2min from a Wright nebulizer, or five vital capacity breaths from a demand nebulizer (e.g. De Vilbiss) or five tidal breaths from a dosimeter. The FEV_1 is measured 90s after the inhalation is completed. Using a Wright nebulizer with a gas flow rate of 8 l min^{-1} and solution volume of 5ml the initial histamine concentration is 0.3mg ml^{-1}; the dose is doubled for each subsequent inhalation up to a maximum concentration of 32mg ml^{-1}. If there has been any airflow limitation it is reversed with

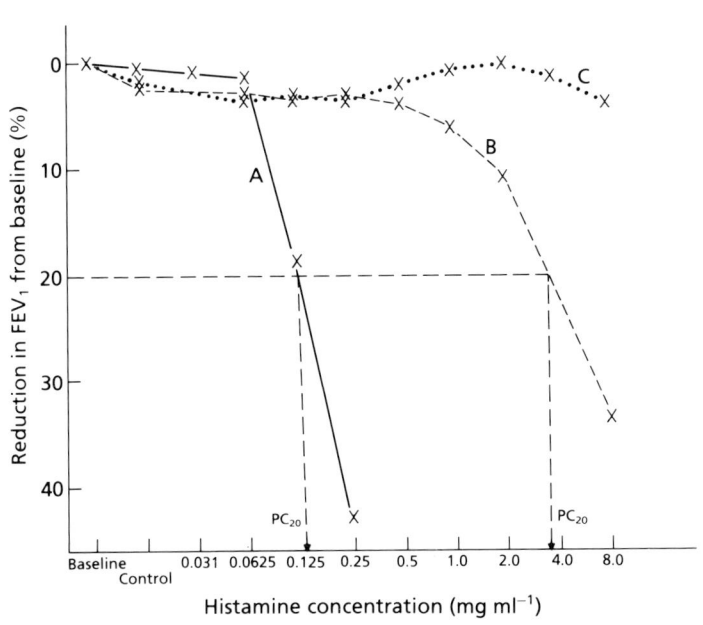

Fig. 16.8. Testing for bronchial hyperreactivity. The subjects complained of episodic breathlessness which was thought to be due to asthma: the FEV_1 was normal between attacks. Subjects inhaled saline and then graded doses of histamine solution from a Wright nebulizer for 2min with 3min intervals between. During these times measurements of forced expiratory volume were made every 0.5min. Subject A showed marked hyperreactivity; subject B was moderately reactive; subject C did not react to histamine in the dosage used. The small reduction in FEV_1 occurring after the control inhalation of saline was probably physiological; a larger reduction would have been an indication for postponing the histamine challenge as the result could not have been interpreted satisfactorily. (By courtesy of N. P. Keaney and B. King.)

salbutamol or other β stimulant drug. The PC20 is obtained by interpolation of the semi-log plot of FEV_1 on histamine concentration (fig. 16.8). Alternatively the cumulative dose of histamine may be so plotted when the index is designated PD20. The methacholine test is performed similarly using doses in the range 0.01–25mg ml^{-1}; it is equally effective and yields a quantitatively similar, though not identical, result but the ensuing airflow limitation is sometimes less easily reversed than is the case with histamine.

Exercise-induced airflow limitation (EIA) is assessed by measurement of FEV_1 before and 6min after moderately heavy exercise. Either running, cycling or stepping exercise of duration 6min may be used; swimming is unsuitable as it provides a less powerful constrictor stimulus than other forms of exercise. A reduction in FEV_1 in excess of 10% which is reversed by subsequent inhalation of salbutamol aerosol is positive evidence for EIA. The bronchoconstriction is due to constrictor stimuli acting on airways which are both unduly responsive and have a raised bronchomotor tone prior to stimulation. The bronchomotor tone is further increased if the exercise entails breathing cold air as this initiates reflex bronchoconstriction via receptors in the large airways supplied by branches of the vagi. The test is suitable for children and for physically active adults but is often inappropriate in the elderly. For these subjects in particular a cold air provocation test may be performed at rest. The patient hyperventilates through the mouth a mixture of CO_2 in air which has been cooled to $-10°C$ via a cooling coil in a refrigerator or bucket of ice and salt. The asthmatic response to exercise or to cold air is blocked by the prior administration of cromoglycate. When it occurs the response is followed by a refractory period of duration, approximately 4h.

Diagnosis of occupational asthma

A history of attacks of asthma developing for the first time during a period of employment which entailed exposure to a known allergen, with abatement of symptoms on withdrawal from exposure and recurrence on re-exposure, is strong evidence for occupational asthma. More often the picture is less clear-cut; the patient gives a history of chronic ill-health with wheeze, cough and phlegm or breathlessness developing at night or coming on during the day, but without acute episodes or clear association with exposure. The chronic illness may have been preceded by a single acute illness from which there was apparently complete recovery. In childhood there may have been episodic wheeze, cough or breathlessness characteristic of childhood asthma but with a symptom-free interval prior to the recurrence in question. There may have been a history of atopic illness or of asthma or hay fever amongst first-degree relatives. To assess the possible role of occupation, the employment history, the family background, the mode of onset and subsequent course of the illness, the relationship to exposure to known allergens and the atopic status should be established. The occupational history should identify all the known allergens in the plant including raw materials, primary products, additives, contaminants and breakdown products (see table 16.7). For processes entailing the use of resins, paints, glues, varnishes or chemicals, the identification can be difficult (table 16.5), especially as the active substances

Table 16.5. Examples of occupations which may entail exposure to isocyanates or epoxy compounds

Manufacture of adhesives, aircraft, boats, insecticides, motor vehicles, paints, ships, wire
Process workers with paint, plastics, polyurethanes, resins, rubber, textiles
Tradesmen including electricians, insulation engineers, laminators, meat processors, painters, shipyard burners, upholsterers, wood workers
Chemists (including organic chemists), farmers, firemen, salvage and scrap dealers

might have become airborne in any of a number of ways. The movement of personnel and the ventilation currents of air within the plant should be considered. If the patient is working, a peak flow chart should be obtained, as discussed above. If there is a commercial test solution available a skin prick test should be performed;

alternatively, a measurement of serum concentration of IgE and a RAS test (page 352) may be carried out. If none of these investigations gives a helpful result the possibility that non-specific bronchial hyperreactivity is present may be assessed using exercise, cold air, histamine or methacholine (page 356). Each stage in the enquiry will bring the investigator nearer to the correct diagnosis; however, this always rests on a balance of probabilities. The association of exposure to a known antigen, subsequent appropriate symptoms and peak flow chart, skin sensitization and a positive RAST make a positive diagnosis highly probable, especially if there have been previous cases of asthma at the works. However, where some feature is atypical or antedates the first exposure, the occurrence of a positive skin test or RAST is not proof that the asthma, if any, is occupational. Conversely, a negative RAST does not exclude if there had been an interval of one or more years since last exposure. In these circumstances inhalation challenge testing is sometimes regarded as a final arbiter. This is correct for a patient giving a history of typical acute episodes which are reproduced by the inhalation. In these circumstances the diagnosis was probably never in doubt. Similarly, in a patient with a history of asthma since childhood, a positive response to challenge is merely evidence of multiple sensitization, not of a primary occupational disorder. A false positive result may be obtained by challenge with an irritant substance; this possibility can be investigated by repeating the challenge on a volunteer control patient with extrinsic atopic asthma. A false negative result may be obtained if too low a dose of antigen is employed or if too long a time has elapsed since last exposure. In these circumstances repeated challenge may reactivate the disease; indeed in some instances even a single challenge has been followed by persistent asthma or bronchial hyperreactivity. Thus the question of occupational asthma should be decided before the challenge is undertaken. The procedure is then used to identify the specific cause in those patients where the advantage of possessing the information more than offsets the disadvantages. The principal advantage is guidance in planning a future career; the disadvantages are the con-

siderable cost in time and resources, and the small risk that the condition may be aggravated by undergoing the test.

Prevalence of occupational asthma

The prevalence of occupational asthma at a workplace can be established by undertaking an occupational survey. The survey commonly arises from discovering a single case in a previously unremarkable factory or other unit of employment. Factors contributing to the presentation of the first case include exceptionally heavy exposure, a constitutional reactivity to the allergen and a personality which is very perceptive of airflow limitation. Experience shows that the index case seldom occurs on its own. Other cases usually coexist but are misdiagnosed or apparently less severe or concealed out of ignorance, low expectations of good health or fear of being put out of employment. Very often the exposed workers are few in number and this makes the task of surveying them appear easy. On other occasions it is laborious because the allergen has not been identified, exposure is affected by circulation patterns within the plant and the identification of new cases is difficult for the reasons given above.

The study should preferably include the whole plant. The diagnostic criteria should include symptoms from the upper or lower respiratory tract, airflow limitation before and after administration of a sympathomimetic aerosol, a raised serum IgE and a positive skin prick test or RAST. Initially the survey is likely to be undertaken without regard to the time of day but observation at the beginning and end of a shift are almost always more informative. A test of bronchial hyperreactivity is sometimes included in the survey and contributes to description of the respiratory morbidity; however, a positive result is not specific for asthma (see above).

Occupational asthma usually affects about 5% of persons who are exposed to the sensitizing agent; this is, for example, the prevalence in workers exposed to toluene diisocyanates or to wood dust from western red cedar. It rises to approximately 30% in persons exposed to insect, mammal or bird residues of moderate antigenicity (page 361) and to 50–100% with exposure to highly antigenic material such as complex salts of platinum. The prevalence reflects the intensity and duration of exposure, the antigenicity of the material, the incidence of smoking and the host susceptibility.

Management of occupational asthma

The management of occupational asthma should, where possible, be firmly based on a clear identification of the cause, assessment of the general and local environment in the workplace and consideration of risk factors particular to the affected person.

The aim of management is to prevent the patient having any contact with the allergen, even within the hygiene standard. There should also be no risk of exposure arising from unintended spillage. Sometimes this can be done by changing the process but usually it means a change of work for the patient, perhaps a transfer to another department or to another factory. Sometimes the installation of local exhaust ventilation may allow the patient to return to his former work but any such return should be carefully supervised, with daily measurements of peak flow or FEV_1. Recurrence of symptoms is most frequent in those whose bronchi remain hyperreactive.

Medical treatment (page 407) is sometimes used to enable the patient to continue to work. Ideally it should not be necessary and the use of systemic corticosteroid drugs for this purpose is highly undesirable. The question of treatment more often arises for asthma which is mild and readily controlled by inhalation therapy with a β-adrenergic drug, possibly supplemented by beclomethasone diproprionate or sodium cromoglycate. The treatment can allow the patient to return to his former work for a few months while awaiting a transfer to other work or improvements in his working environment. But it is not a long-term solution.

Prognosis

Clinical experience suggests that the prognosis for occupational asthma is excellent in those persons who are diagnosed soon after the onset of symptoms, in whom the underlying lung function is normal, where there is normal bronchial reactivity to non-specific stimulation and when the antigen or hapten is both unique to the employment and does not overlap with common antigens, for example house dust mite. Prognosis might be expected to be below average in persons sensitized to antigens which are widely distributed in the environment (for example, isocyanates); in addition the risk is different for those who form IgE antibodies very readily (i.e. atopic individuals) compared with others, but whether or not this leads to their having a poor prognosis is unknown. Information on prognosis in occupations where there is a risk of occupational asthma is meagre and there is urgent need for longitudinal studies of whole populations including ex-employees. In the case of individuals the prognosis is poor where he or she has struggled to continue to work, often with inadequate medication, where there is superimposed irreversible airflow limitation and when the non-specific bronchial reactivity is increased. Many of these patients become sensitized to other antigens or develop a condition which resembles intrinsic asthma. These considerations provide a strong indication for early diagnosis and for measures to prevent the occurrence of occupational asthma (16).

Prevention

The occurrence of a single case of occupational asthma should lead to a detailed scrutiny of the workplace (chapter 3) which should conform to the hygiene standard (table 1.7, page 16). The health of other employees and recent ex-employees should be looked into. In addition the episode should instigate a review of the medical criteria for entry to the job. In most instances atopy should not be a contra-indication (page 80) but subjects with pre-existing chest disease, particularly when accompanied by bronchial hyperreactivity, probably should be excluded.

Industrial injuries benefit

In the U.K. occupational asthma following exposure to certain specified materials is a prescribed

Table 16.6. Causes of occupational asthma which are accepted for Industrial Injuries Benefit in the U.K. (Additional causes will be accepted in future.)

Platinum salts	Antibiotics
Isocyanates	Cimetidine
Epoxy resin curing agents	Wood dusts
	Ispaghula
Colophony fumes	Castor bean dust
Proteolytic enzymes	Ipecacuanha
Animals and insects in laboratories	Azodicarbonamide
Dust from grain or flour	

Table 16.7. Working classification of substances which cause occupational asthma

Mammalian and bird residues	Table 16.8
Arthropods and molluscs	Table 16.9
Tree dust, bark or sap	Table 16.10
Vegetable products including grain	Table 16.11
Micro-organisms and spores	Table 16.12
Enzymes	See text
Drugs (including antibiotics)	Table 16.13
Dyes	See text
Metal salts	Table 16.14
Other chemical substances:	
Isocyanates	Table 16.15
Colophony (pine resin)	Table 16.14
Epoxy compounds	Table 16.14
Furfuryl alcohol	Table 16.14
Formaldehyde	Table 16.14

disease under the National Insurance (Industrial Injuries) Act, so that affected persons are eligible for industrial injuries benefit. The materials to which the regulations at present apply are given in table 16.6. More substances will be specified in due course. For the purpose of assessing a claim the diagnosis is based on a balance of probabilities and does not include procedures which are invasive. Instead since identical symptoms can arise from pre-existing asthma or from coincident non-occupational asthma (or even from chronic bronchitis) the applicant is usually given the benefit of any doubt that is present. The subject is considered in more detail on page 8.

Examples of occupational asthma

Classification of substances which may cause occupational asthma is difficult for a number of reasons. There is a very wide range of sensitizing substances, some of which are common to different classes of allergen. There are also wide gaps in our knowledge of mechanisms and frequently a subject is exposed to several possible causative agents. A farmer handling grain may be sensitized to grain, pollen, mites, fungal spores, animal residues or chemicals used for treating crops. Similarly, a poultry vendor has recently been described who was sensitized not to bird residues or litter but to colophony (pine resin) which he used for stripping the feathers. In these circumstances a simple classification is possibly less likely to mislead than a sophisticated one based on our present incomplete knowledge. In the investigation of patients the classification should never be used as a substi-

tute for a comprehensive history. Some classes of substances which may cause occupational asthma are listed in table 16.7; they are commented on below. Classified references describing the individual occupational asthmas begin on page 369.

Mammalian and avian residues

Sensitizing agents which have been shown to cause asthma include the serum, pelts and urines of rats and mice and the danders and wool of other animals. Animal laboratory workers are particularly at risk and may develop an immediate-onset asthma which is mediated

Table 16.8. Some mammalian and avian residues which cause occupational asthma of the immediate or delayed type

Avian residues* (delayed/dual)	Danders† (immediate)	Rodent (immediate)
Budgerigars	Cat	Saliva
		Serum
Chickens	Cow	Urine
Pigeons	Dog	(Fur)
Turkeys	Pig	(Pelt)

* Also cause extrinsic alveolitis (as does mammalian pituitary snuff).
† Also wool, pelt, gastric and pancreatic enzymes.

by specific IgE. Delayed or dual responses are uncommon. The asthma is usually preceded or accompanied by rhinitis and sometimes by skin rashes or urticaria. Atopic individuals are more likely to develop symptoms compared with persons who are not atopic, but the risk is not confined to them and is apparently not increased by the coexistence of hay fever, though this may lead to aggravation of symptoms at times of high pollen counts. In addition atopic subjects who have contracted extrinsic allergic alveolitis (EAA) from mammalian or animal residues can also develop delayed-onset asthma; the responsible agents include feathers, faeces, urine and serum of pigeons, budgerigars and poultry, and pituitary snuff (table 16.8).

Arthropods and molluscs

Ramazzini in 1713 observed that 'small fragments of dead silkworms as well as locust larvae and caterpillars possess some sort of noxious and corrosive acrimony injurious to the lungs'. Many species of crustacea, insects and mites cause immediate, delayed or dual onset asthma in sensitized persons. Conjunctivitis and rhinitis also occur and are often the most commonly reported allergic symptoms. In these instances the asthma is of the immediate-onset type and is associated with a raised serum level of specific IgE. Asthma of the delayed-onset type is usually IgG mediated (fig. 16.3, page 353). The species include locusts, cockroaches, grasshoppers and crickets which appear to have antigens in common with the house dust mite; thus atopic individuals who are already sensitized to the house

dust mite are at increased risk if they work with these species and vice versa. Breeding or processing shrimps, prawns, oysters and crabs, can cause occupational asthma, as can preparing marine sponge. People exposed to silkworms are also at risk: the antigens cross-react with those for some butterflies and moths and so persons breeding these insects may be vulnerable. Storage mites infest grain, straw, flour and related foodstuffs, on the cob, in barns, mills, warehouses and other places. Sensitization to the mites is a cause of rhinitis and asthma in persons handling grain products; those at risk include farmers, millers, bakers, food handlers and even housewives (table 16.9).

Tree dust, bark or sap

Bark and sawdust from many trees may cause asthma of immediate or delayed onset (table 16.10). The best documented is that due to western red cedar which gives rise to delayed onset or persistent asthma in a small proportion (approximately 5%) of exposed persons; such persons may also experience increased bronchial reactivity and may develop chronic bronchitis. The active agent appears to be plicatic acid which is known to activate complement and by this means may induce inflammation in the airways. The cause of the asthma is not known because, whilst specific IgE antibodies have been demonstrated in some subjects, they are not present in others who are affected. In this the condition differs from asthma due to quillaja bark which is the source of saponin. Individuals sensitized to the pulverized bark develop an

Table 16.9. Some arthropod and mollusc residues which cause occupational asthma (references page 369)

	Insects	Crustacea	Mites	Spiders
Beetles	Housefly maggots	Crabs	House dust†	
Butterflies	Locusts‡	Prawns	Cheese	
Caterpillars	Moths	Shrimps	Flour	
Cockroaches	Silkworms	Molluscs	Grain	
Crickets	Sewer flies	Oysters	Straw	
Grasshoppers	Weevils*	Squids		

* Including bean weevil and grain weevil (*Sitophilus granarius*).
† *Dermatophagoides pteronyssinus* and *farinae*.
‡ e.g. *Locusta migratoria migratoroides*, also *Schistocerca gregaria*.

Table 16.10   Trees of which the dust, bark or sap can cause occupational asthma (references, page 369)

Species	Reaction
Abiruana (*Pouteria*)	Dual
African maple (*Triplochiton scleroxylon*)	Specific IgE
African zebra wood (*Microberlinia*)	Specific IgE
Boxwood	Dual
California red wood (*Sequoia semper virens*)	Dual
Cedar of Lebanon (*Cedrus libani*)	Delayed
Cocabolla (*Dalbergia retusa*)	Immediate
Iroko (*Chlorophora excelsa*)	Dual
Kejaat (*Pterocarpus angolensis*)	Dual
Mahogony	Dual
Oak	Immediate
Obeche (as for African maple)	
Paw paw tree (*Carica papaya*)	Dual
Ramin (*Gonystytus bancanus*)	Delayed (EAA)
Samba (as for African maple)	
Soap bark (*Quillaja saponaria*)*	Specific IgE
Tanganyika aningre	Immediate (RAST neg.)
Western red cedar (*Thuja plicata*)*	Dual

EAA = Extrinsic allergic alveolitis.
* Active agent listed in table 16.11.

immediate-onset asthma with rhinitis and erythema associated with the formation of specific IgE antibodies. The sensitizing agent is quillaic acid; it is chemically related to gum acacia which is a cause of printers' asthma and to gum tragacanth (mentioned below). These substances share common antigens. Bark and wood dust from many other trees may also cause asthma of the immediate or dual onset types including oak, iroko, mahogany and African zebra wood; the mechanisms are in most instances not yet understood.

Vegetable products (including grain)

Many vegetable products are direct causes of occupational asthma (table 16.11); in other instances they act as non-specific irritants or provide the vehicle for other allergens including mites, spores and chemical substances. Allergic asthma which is associated with specific IgE is reported following exposure to gum acacia used in printing (see above), gum tragacanth used in confectionery and sweets, green coffee beans, castor beans and bean products. Sensitization arises from the dust of castor beans (*Ricinus communis*), which are transported in porous

Table 16.11.   Some vegetable products which can cause occupational asthma (references page 369); see also Table 16.10.

Bromelin (pineapple protease)	Papain*
	Paprika (plant)
Castor beans and wax	Pine oil‡
Citrus fruit peel‡	Plicatic acid*
Coffee beans (green)	Quillaic acid*
Flour proteins†	Saponin*
Freesia (plant)	Sunflower pollen
Grain pollen	Tamarind seeds
Gum acacia (hence printer's ink)	
	Tea dust
Gum tragacanth	Terpentine‡
Hops‡	Tobacco dust
Ipecacuanha (dust)	
Ispaghula§ (husks)	

* From trees listed in table 16.10.
† Wheat, triticale, rye, barley, oats, rice, maize.
‡ Contain β myrcene, α pinene or related terpene.
§ Also called plantago ovata or psyllium.

hessian sacks, and from pomace which is the residue after the oil has been extracted. Wax made from the pomace is antigenic; the oil itself is not. The pomace contain ricin and other antigens. It is used as an agricultural fertilizer and can cause occupational asthma in oil mill operatives, transport workers and farmers. The wax has a high viscosity and a high resistance to heat, cold and pressure so has a host of applications in medicine, toiletry and industry; these provide numerous opportunities for the development of sensitization. Grain farmers and handlers may develop asthma from grain pollen, flour protein (fig. 16.7, page 356, also table 16.11) and grain dust. The latter is also a nonspecific irritant which can cause a material reduction in vital capacity and other changes in lung function. McCarthy and her colleagues have suggested that this response is mediated via release of leukotrienes (49). In some instances the asthma results from sensitivity to mites or spores present in the grain and not the grain itself, for example, the grain weevil *Sitophilus granarius*, the mite *Glycyphagus destructor* and the mould *Cladosporium*. Dust from tea, tobacco, hops and other plants also gives rise to asthma. In the case of hops the volatile oil β myrcene is the probable sensitizer. It also occurs in citrus fruit peel and pine oil but the mechanism is not established.

Spores

Fungi grow on plant products of all sorts and produce an abundance of spores, many of which give rise to occupational asthma (table 16.12); others cause extrinsic allergic alveolitis while some spores may cause both, but seldom in the same subject; *Micropolyspora faeni*, which is the cause of farmers' lung, and *Merulius lacrymans*, which causes dry rot in timber, fall into this category. Farmers and others are also exposed to mouldy hay, grain or compost supporting a growth of *Cladosporium*, *Alternaria* or other species which can cause immediate-onset asthma; in this event precipitating antibodies may be present in the serum. Mushroom spores may similarly give rise to an immediate asthma with rhinorrhoea and positive skin prick test. However, there is no eosinophilia, the serum level of IgE is within normal limits, precipitating antibodies are not demonstrable in the serum and the mechanism of this asthma remains unexplained. Mushroom growers and personnel manufacturing dried mushroom soup are at risk.

Enzymes

Digestive enzymes are obtained from the mammalian gastrointestinal tract, bacteria and plants and many of these substances can give rise to occupational asthma of the immediate or dual onset type which is identified by specific IgE antibodies. They include trypsin and other pancreatic enzymes, *Bacillus subtilis* proteinase which is used in the manufacture of detergent washing powders and papain from the latex of the paw paw tree which grows in many subtropical countries. Papain in particular has many applications including that of meat tenderizer, a cleanser for beer and textiles, and use in the production of many cosmetics, foods and drugs.

Drugs

Antibiotics and other drugs can give rise to asthma which is usually of the delayed-onset type. Some drugs which occasionally act in this way are listed in table 16.13. The risk is greatest amongst those engaged in manufacture but some pharmacists and a few persons who ingest the products as patients or as consumers of meat from treated animals have also been affected. Asthma sometimes occurs after exposure to ethanol; the mechanism is unknown (table 16.2, page 352). Aspirin, which inhibits the activity of prostaglandin synthetase, occasionally causes asthma but has sometimes been found to relieve it. These actions have been attributed to different consequences of reduced synthesis of pro-

Table 16.12. Some micro-organisms which cause occupational asthma: they also cause extrinsic allergic alveolitis (Table 15.1, page 321)

Alternaria	*Merulius lacrymans*
Aspergillus niger	*Micropolyspora faeni*
Cladosporium	Mushroom (various species)
Humidifier sludge	*Paecilomyces*
	Verticillium

Antigen may be present in spores, culture fluid or breakdown products.

Table 16.13. Some antibiotics and other drugs which cause occupational asthma (references, page 370)

Ampicillin	Hexachlorophene
Aspirin	Methyldopa
6 Aminopenicillanic	Piperazine
acid	dihydrochloride
Benzyl penicillin	Salbutamol
Cephalosporin	intermediaries
Chloramine T	Spiramycin*
Cimetidine	Sulphathiazole
Ethanol	Sulphonechloramides
Halazone	Tetracycline

* Also adipic acid (additive).

staglandins in the lung. However, some aspirin sensitive subjects also react to tartrazine, for which a specific IgD antibody has been demonstrated (68), so the mechanism of aspirin asthma cannot yet be regarded as established.

Dyes

During both manufacture and commercial use some reactive dyes act as sensitizing agents, causing an immediate-onset asthma with rhinitis and a raised titre of specific IgE. Delayed-onset asthma occurs with some diazonium salts including diazonium chloride which is used in photoreproduction as a coupling agent. The food dye tartrazine also causes asthma: a possible mechanism is given above.

Metal salts

Salts of a number of metals which have been reported as causes of asthma include sodium aurothiomalate, aluminium fluoride and sulphate (page 265), nickel sulphate and carbonyl, sodium and potassium dichromate and complex salts of platinum especially ammonium tetra- or hexa-chlorplatinate (fig. 16.6, page 356). Asthma due to chromium and nickel salts has occurred during their production, and during the use of these substances in the welding of stainless steel (pages 248, 250 and 298). Asthma due to platinum salts is of immediate and dual onset, mediated by specific IgE and often associated

with rhinitis, urticaria and contact dermatitis; these features in conjunction with asthma have been called platinosis but the term implies a pneumoconiosis. The condition is an allergy to reactive platinum halide compounds. It has been reviewed by Pepys (9). Exposure to the reactive compounds can occur during refining or using platinum, for example, in electroplating jewellery and as a catalyst in the chemical and oil refining, and motor industries. Allergic reactions develop in a high proportion of exposed persons, with those who are atopic being at increased risk (71). An antibody response is also readily produced in hooded Lister rats.

Other chemical substances

A host of chemical substances can cause occupational asthma amongst producers, users and those exposed to debris or waste products (table 16.14). In many instances the active ingredient is known, but in complex mixtures more than one sensitizing agent may be present and unravelling the cause of the asthma may not be easy.

Isocyanates. Flexible and rigid foams for upholstery, packing and padding, surface sealing compounds, paints, plastics and many other products are made from polyurethanes so large numbers of workers are exposed to these compounds (table 16.5). Some of the workers are also exposed to other sensitizing agents including ethylene-diamine (page 368). The polyurethanes are complex long chain esters; they are produced by reaction of a polyalcohol (polyol) with one of a number of isocyanates, usually toluene diisocyanate (TDI) but also diphenyl methane diisocyanate (MDI), hexamethylene diisocyanate (HDI, an ingredient of paint for motor car bodies), and other compounds (table 16.15). N-Methyl morpholine and other amines are used in the process as catalysts and cross-linking agents, and hardeners are used to achieve the desired consistency. The isocyanates form vapours by evaporation, heating or combustion and they readily react with protein. They are the commonest cause of occupational asthma and also act as non-specific irritants to the eyes, skin and lungs (table 13.14, page 293). The asthma may be of immediate or dual onset and often persists for days or weeks after with-

Table 16.14.   Some chemical substances which cause occupational asthma (with references, see also 9)

Abietic acid; see colophony		Fluorocarbon (heated)	
Acrylic resin	106	Formaldehyde	102–104
Adipic acid; see table 16.3		Furfuryl alcohol	101
Amino-ethyl-ethanolamine	107	Hexachlorophene	
Aluminium salts; see page 265		Hexamethylene diisocyanate†	
Ammonium tetrachlorplatinate; see platinum		Isocyanates	75–87
		N-Methyl morpholine	77
Azodicarbonamide	108	Naphthalene diisocyanate†	
Chloramine		Nickel salts	9, 73
Chromate salts	73	Perspex (plexiglas) powder	98, 106
Cobalt sulphate; see page 273		Persulphate salts; see page 368	
Colophony	88–93	Phthalic acid*	
Diazonium chloride; see dyes		Platinum salts	9, 71, 74
Dichromates of sodium and potassium	72	Polyols (polyalcohols)	77, 84
Diphenyl methane diisocyanate†		Tetrachlorophthalic anhydride*	
Dyes	69–70	Toluene diisocyanate†	
Epoxy curing agents	94–100	Triethylene tetramine *	
Ethanolamine derivatives	107, 109	Trimellitic acid*	
Ethylene-diamine	105		

* See epoxy curing agents.
† See isocyanates.

drawal from exposure, or after inhalation challenge. Some exposed persons also develop bronchial hyperreactivity to histamine and a few develop extrinsic allergic alveolitis (page 83, 86). Amongst persons exposed regularly to isocyanates probably less than 5% become sensitized, but these individuals develop severe asthma at concentrations well below the threshold limit value of 0.02ppm (85). A positive skin reaction to prick testing with TDI–human serum albumen complex (TDI, HSA) may occur but is not invariable and atopy is not a predisposing factor. The mode of action of isocyanates is the subject of much recent research. In lymphocytes treated with isoprenaline, TDI reduces the rise in cyclic 3′5 adenosine monophosphate (cAMP) which would otherwise occur; this suggests that isocyanates act by blocking β adrenergic receptor sites (81). However, the effect is present using lymphocytes from normal as well as from sensitized donors so there must be an additional mechanism. This is independent of non-specific bronchial hyperreactivity since not all patients with TDI asthma have an increased response to histamine. The asthma is possibly IgE mediated in those patients who have an increased plasma level of specific IgE (assessed as a positive RAST, 87). Serum from patients exposed only to TDI can react both to this substance and to MDI or HDI. However, in a patient RAST positive to MDI and P-TMI the antibodies were specific and did not cross-react (82).

Amongst exposed persons the proportion of RAST positives ranges from 18% to 80% depending on the intensity of the exposure and the sensitivity of the patient to isocyanate, but

Table 16.15.   Some isocyanate compounds (see also pulmonary oedema, page 292)

2,4-Toluene diisocyanate	$CH_3C_6H_4(NCO)_2$	TDI
Diphenylmethane-4,4-diisocyanate	$CH_2(C_6H_4NCO)_2$	MDI
Hexamethylene diisocyanate	$(CH_2)_6(NCO)_2$	HDI
1,5,-Naphthylene diisocyanate	$C_{10}H_6(NCO)_2$	NDI
p-Tolyl isocyanate	$CH_3C_6H_5NCO$	p-TMI

the majority of cases of isocyanate asthma are RAST negative so are not IgE mediated. In addition some asymptomatic workers are RAST positive (80). These findings suggested to Butcher and colleagues that the positive RAST might be detecting antibody acting against human serum albumen which had been altered by contact with isocyanate and not against a specific isocyanate hapten. In patients exhibiting a delayed or late reaction to MDI and HDI specific IgG antibodies have been demonstrated so the asthma can be produced by more than one immunological mechanism. Development of sensitization to the amine catalysts referred to above might contribute to asthma in some process workers (77). The amines can increase the bronchial reactivity to histamine. However, the catalyst is not used in TDI production so asthma amongst producers of TDI must have some other explanation. The topic is the subject of much current research.

Colophony (pine resin). Pine resin is used as flux in soldering where it contributes to the melting and spreading of the solder and prevents oxidation of the heated material; it is used as an adhesive for labels and sticking plaster, as a reodorant and in other ways. The sensitizing agents appear to be abietic acid and its derivatives; they cause rhinitis, contact dermatitis and asthma of the immediate and delayed onset types in association with a raised serum concentration of IgM (figs. 16.4 and 16.5, pages 354 and 355). Extrinsic allergic alveolitis can also occur. Burge has observed that the average latency between first exposure and onset of symptoms is 4 years (range 1 month to 23 years). The incidence of asthma reflects the atmospheric concentration of colophony which itself varies with the temperature at which the soldering is undertaken. Very high concentrations, as may occur during a fire, cause acute irritation of the upper respiratory tract. This irritant reaction is accompanied by bronchial hyperreactivity to histamine. It usually improves following withdrawal from exposure, unlike the asthma which may persist. Other causes of asthma in solderers are toluene diisocyanate (a constituent of polyurethane) or trimellitic anhydride (a constituent of epoxy resin) if the wire which is being soldered is coated with either of these substances.

Epoxy compounds. Epoxy compounds are so called on account of having an oxygen atom attached to two adjacent carbon atoms. This group reacts with any of a number of others to yield relatively stable substances. The compounds are used as plasticizers in vinyl chloride polymerization, as curing agents in the manufacture of epoxy resins and for paints, dyes, lacquers and other products. Epoxy resins are tough and durable and have a high electrical resistance. On account of these properties they are used for adhesives, mouldings, surface coatings and in reinforced plastics. The curing agents include phthalic acid anhydride ($C_8H_4O_3$, PAA) and trimellitic acid anhydride ($HOCOC_6H_3(CO)_2O$, TMA), which are most active when heated, and triethylene tetramine (TTA) which is used at ambient temperature. Vapour from the curing agents in high concentration causes irritation of the respiratory tract. In lower concentration the vapour causes sensitization in a small proportion of persons who are exposed; the symptoms include conjunctivitis, rhinitis, immediate and delayed onset asthma, malaise and other features of alveolitis. Anaemia can occur in persons who are highly sensitized. The uncured resin may cause dermatitis but does not appear to affect the lung. Sensitization is due to the curing agent acting as a hapten by combining with protein in the airways and serum to produce autogenous antigen; this stimulates a specific IgE mediated antibody response which contributes to the immediate onset asthma. A RAS test is then usually positive. The delayed reaction and the anaemia have been associated with a specific IgG against TMA–protein complex. Sensitization to the curing agents may occur in any of a number of occupations (table 16.5); they include meat packers whose asthma is an uncommon but interesting example. In packaging the meat, fumes are generated during cutting the polyvinyl chloride (PVC) wrapping material with a hot wire, during sealing the ends on a heated pad and during heating the label to activate the epoxy resin adhesive. The fumes are irritant and can cause sensitization. The asthma is usually due to PAA present in the adhesive but sensitization may also occur to epoxidized soya bean oil which is used as a plasticizer. In addition the respiratory tract may be irritated by hydro-chloric acid which is liberated when PVC is heated. Thus in this as in many other situations there are a number of possible causes for the asthma. Diagnosis is usually based on a detailed occupational history and the result of the RAS test, but these procedures may need to be supplemented by others (page 358).

Furfuryl alcohol. Furan-based resins are used extensively in foundries for making casting moulds which do not need preliminary baking. The resin contains furfuryl alcohol whilst phosphoric and sulphuric acids are used as a catalyst. The material causes a late onset asthma and increased bronchial reactivity. The acids also irritate the eyes and may burn the skin.

Formaldehyde (formalin). Formaldehyde is the starting point for innumerable chemical processes including manufacture of the resins phenol- melamine- and para-formaldehyde and urea formaldehyde which is used in glue and as plastic foam for wall insulation and other applications. Formalin is liberated when these substances are heated or treated with acid; it is also used as a disinfectant, fungicide and hardening agent in biological and medical work and in the tanning, textile, rubber and plastics industries.

Formaldehyde acts as an irritant of the eyes, nose and respiratory tract and occasionally causes asthma which may be of the immediate or delayed-onset types; in the latter event it is associated with the presence of precipitating antibodies in the serum. Derivatives of formaldehyde may also cause release of histamine from lung tissue. Other possible actions of formaldehyde are considered on page 259.

Other chemicals. Immediate and delayed onset asthma have been observed as a result of sensitization to many substances including polymerized acrylic resin (perspex or plexiglas), amino-ethyl-ethanolamine which is a constituent of flux used in aluminium solder and dimethyl ethanolamine which is a hardening agent for spray paint. Delayed onset asthma may occur with azodicarbonamide which is used as a blowing agent in the production of expanded foam plastics, ethylene-diamine which is widely used in manufacture of vinyl chloride and other plastics, as a solvent for shellac in lacquer, as an accelerator in TDI foam, in foundry moulding, and in the rubber industry, sodium or potassium persulphate which is a bleaching agent used in tinting hair (page 305) and many other substances. In most cases there is increased bronchial reactivity to histamine which persists for a time after withdrawal from exposure.

References

Articles on occupational asthma appear in numerous journals, including *Clinical Allergy, Journal of Allergy and Clinical Immunology* and journals of thoracic and occupational medicine. The following are a selection.

General

1 Barnes P, Fitzgerald G, Brown M, Dollery C. Nocturnal asthma and changes in circulatory epinephrine, histamine and cortisol. *N Engl J Med* 1980;**303**:263–7.

2 Clark TJH, Godfrey S (Eds). *Asthma*, 2nd edn. London: Chapman and Hall, 1983.

3 Eiser NM, Kerrebijn KF, Quanjer PH (Eds). Guidelines for standardization of bronchial challenges with (nonspecific) bronchoconstricting agents. *Bull Europ Physiopathol Respir* 1983;**19**:495–514. *See also* Hendrick DJ *et al*, *Am Rev Resp Dis* 1986;**133**:600–4.

4 Gwynn CM, Ingram J, Almousawi T, Stanworth DR. Bronchial provocation tests in atopic patients with allergen-specific IgG$_4$ antibodies. *Lancet* 1982;**i**:254–6.

5 Hariparsad D, Wilson N, Dixon C, Silverman M. Oral tartrazine challenge in childhood asthma: effect on bronchial reactivity. *Clin Allergy* 1984;**14**:81–5.

6 Harries MG, Burge PS, O'Brien IM. Occupational type bronchial provocation tests: testing with soluble antigens by inhalation. *Br J Industr Med* 1980;**37**:248–52.

7 Higgs CMB, Laszlo G. Coded peak flow measurement and the perception of asthma. *Thorax* 1982;**37**:780.

8 Martin AJ, Landau LI, Phelan PD. Asthma from childhood at age 21: the patient and his disease. *Br Med J* 1982;**284**:380–2.

9 Pepys J. Occupational respiratory allergy. *Clinics in Immunology and Allergy* 1984;**4(i)**: 1–196.

10 Platts-Mills TAE, Tovey ER, Mitchell EB, Moszora H, Nock P., Wilkins SR. Reduction of bronchial hyperreactivity during prolonged allergen avoidance. *Lancet* 1982;**ii**:675–7.

11 Pullan CR, Hey EN. Wheezing, asthma and pulmonary dysfunction 10 years after infection with respiratory syncytial virus in infancy. *Br Med J* 1982;**284**:1665–9.

12 Ryan G, Dolovich MB, Roberts RS, Frith PA, Juniper EF, Hargreave FE, Newhouse MT. Standardization of inhalation provocation tests: two techniques of aerosol generation and inhalation compared. *Am Rev Respir Dis* 1981;**123**:195–9.

13 Salvaggio JE. Occupational asthma: overview and mechanisms. *J Allergy Clin Immunol* 1979;**64**:646–9.

14 Weill H, Turner-Warwick M (Eds). Occupational lung diseases. In: *Lung Biology in Health and Disease*. Volume 18. New York: Marcel Dekker. 1981.

15 Weill H. Epidemiologic and medical-legal aspects of occupational asthma. *J Allergy Clin Immunol* 1979;**64**:662–4.

16 Yeung M, Grzybowski S. Prognosis in occupational asthma. *Thorax* 1985;**40**:241–3.

Animal and bird residues (see also chapter 15, Extrinsic Allergic Alveolitis, page 341)

17 Cockcroft A, Edwards J, McCarthy P. Role of pre-employment allergy screening in animal workers. *Eur J Respir Dis* 1981;**62**:Suppl 113:42–3.

18 Cockcroft A, McCarthy P, Edwards J, Andersson N. Allergy in laboratory animal workers. *Lancet* 1981;**i**:827–30.

19 Edwards JH, McConnochie K, Trotman DM, Collins G, Saunders MJ, Latham SM. Allergy to inhaled egg material. *Clin Allergy* 1983;**13(5)**: 427–32.

20 Harries MG, Cromwell O. Occupational asthma caused by allergy to pigs' urine. *Br Med J* 1982;**284**:867.

21 Newman Taylor A, Longbottom JL, Pepys J. Respiratory allergy to urine proteins of rats and mice. *Lancet* 1977;**ii**:847–9.

22 Walls AF, Longbottom JL. Comparison of rat fur, urine, saliva and other rat allergen extracts by skin testing: RAST and RAST inhibition. *J Allergy Clin Immunol* 1985;**75**:242–51.

Arthropods

23 Baldo BA, Krilis S, Taylor KM. IgE-mediated acute asthma following inhalation of a powdered marine sponge. *Clin Allergy* 1982;**12**: 179–86.

24 Burge PS, Edge G, O'Brien IM, Harries MG, Hawkins R, Pepys J. Occupational asthma in a research centre breeding locusts. *Clin Allergy* 1980;**10**:355–63.

25 Cartier A, Malo JL, Forest F, Lafrance M, Pineau L, St.-Aubin J-J, Dubois J-Y. Occupational asthma in snow crab processing workers. *J Allergy Clin Immunol* 1984;**74**:261–9.

26 Cuthbert OD, Jeffrey IG, McNeill HB, Wood J, Topping MD. Barn allergy among Scottish farmers. *Clin Allergy* 1984;**14**:197–206.

27 Davies RJ, Green M, Schofield NMcC. Recurrent nocturnal asthma after exposure to grain dust. *Am Rev Respir Dis* 1976;**114**:1011–9.

28 Gaddie J, Legge JS, Friend JAR, Reid TMS. Pulmonary hypersensitivity in prawn workers. *Lancet* 1980;**ii**:1350–2.

29 Ingram CG, Jeffrey IG, Symington IS, Cuthbert OD. Bronchial provocation studies in farmers allergic to storage mites. *Lancet* 1979;**ii**:1330–2.

30 Kang B, Vellody D, Homburger H, Yunginger JW. Cockroach cause of allergic asthma. *J Allergy Clin Immunol* 1979;**63**:80–6.

31 Kino T, Oshima S. Allergy to insects in Japan: II. The reaginic sensitivity to silkworm moth in patients with bronchial asthma. *J Allergy Clin Immunol* 1979;**64**:131–8.

32 Stockley RA, Hill SL, Drew R. Asthma associated with a circulating IgG antibody to *Calliphora* maggots. *Clin Allergy* 1982;**12**:151–5.

Wood

33 Chan-Yeung M, Giclas PC, Henson PM. Activation of complement by plicatic acid, the chemical compound responsible for asthma due to western red cedar *(Thuja plicata)*. *J Allergy Clin Immunol* 1980;**65**:333–7.

34 Chan-Yeung M, Vedal S, Kus J, Maclean L, Enarson D, Tse KS. Symptoms, pulmonary function and bronchial hyperreactivity in Western red cedar workers compared with those of office workers. *Am Rev Respir Dis* 1984;**130**:1038–41.

35 Hinojosa M, Moneo I, Dominguez J, Delgado E, Losada E, Alcover R. Asthma caused by African maple *(Triplochiton scleroxylon)* wood dust. *J Allergy Clin Immunol* 1984;**74**:782–6.

36 Lam S, Tan F, Chan H, Chan-Yeung M. Relationship between types of asthmatic reaction, nonspecific bronchial reactivity, and specific IgE antibodies in patients with red cedar asthma. *J Allergy Clin Immunol* 1983;**72**:134–9.

37 Raghuprasad PK, Brooks SM, Litwin A, Edwards JJ, Bernstein IL, Gallagher J. Quillaja bark (soap-bark)-induced asthma. *J Allergy Clin Immunol* 1980;**65**:285–7.

Vegetable products including grain (see also Arthropods above)

38 Baur X, Fruhmann G. Allergic reactions,

including asthma, to the pineapple protease bromelain following occupational exposure. *Clin Allergy* 1979;**9**:443–50.

39 Block G, Tse KS, Kijek K, Chan H, Chan-Yeung M. Baker's asthma. Studies of the cross-antigenicity between different cereal grains. *Clin Allergy* 1984;**14**:177–85.

40 Davison AG, Britton MG, Forrester JA, Davies RJ, Hughes DTD. Asthma in merchant seamen and laboratory workers caused by allergy to castor beans: analysis of allergens. *Clin Allergy* 1983;**13**:553–61.

41 Dosman JA, Cotton DJ, Graham BL, Li KYR, Froh F, Barnett GD. Chronic bronchitis and decreased forced expiratory flow rates in lifetime non-smoking grain workers. *Am Rev Respir Dis* 1980;**121**:11–16.

42 Enarson DA, Vedal S, Chan-Yeung M. Rapid decline in FEV_1 in grain handlers. *Am Rev Respir Dis* 1985;**132**:814–7.

43 Gauss WF, Alavie JP, Karol MH. Workplace allergenicity of a psyllium containing bulk laxative. *Allergy* 1985;**40**:73–6.

43 Gleich GJ, Welsh PW, Yunginger JW, Hyatt RE, Catlett JB. Allergy to tobacco: an occupational hazard. *New Engl J Med* 1980;**302**:617–19.

45 Hendrick DJ, Davies RJ, Pepys J. Bakers' Asthma. *Clin Allergy* 1976;**6**:241–50.

46 Jones RN, Hughes JM, Lehrer SB, Butcher BT, Glindmeyer HW, Diem JE, Hammad YY, Salvaggio J, Weill H. Lung function consequences of exposure and hypersensitivity in workers who process green coffee beans. *Am Rev Respir Dis* 1982;**125**:199–202.

47 Lehrer SB, Karr RM, Muller DJG, Salvaggio JE. Detection of castor allergens in castor wax. *Clin Allergy* 1980;**10**:33–41.

48 Luczynska CM, Marshall PE, Scarisbrick DA, Topping MD. Occupational allergy due to inhalation of ipecacuanha dust. *Clin Allergy* 1984;**14**:169–75.

49 McCarthy PE, Cockcroft AE, McDermott M. Lung function after exposure to barley dust. *Br J Industr Med* 1985;**42**:106–10.

50 Machado L, Olsson G, Stålenhelm G, Zetterström O. Dust exposure challenge test as a measure of potential allergenicity and occupational disease risk in handling of ispaghula products. *Allergy* 1983;**38**:141–4. See also McConnochie K *et al.* *Thorax* 1985;**40**:702(Abstract).

51 Newmark FM. Hops allergy and terpene sensitivity: an occupational disease. *Ann Allergy* 1978;**41**:311–2.

52 Yach D, Myers J, Bradshaw D, Benatar SR. A respiratory epidemiologic survey of grain mill workers in Cape Town, South Africa. *Am Rev Respir Dis* 1985;**131**:505–10.

53 Zuskin E, Valic F, Kanceljak B. Immunological and respiratory changes in coffee workers. *Thorax* 1981;**36**:9–13.

Micro-organisms and spores

54 Burge PS, Finnegan M, Horsfield N, Emery D, Austwick P, Davies PS, Pickering CAC. Occupational asthma in a factory with a contaminated humidifier. *Thorax* 1985;**40**:248–54.

55 Darke CS, Knoweldon J, Lacey J, Milford Ward A. Respiratory disease of workers harvesting grain. *Thorax* 1976;**31**:294–302.

56 Dijkman JH, Borghans JGA, Savelberg PJ, Arkenbout PM. Allergic bronchial reactions to inhalation of enzymes of bacillus subtilis. *Am Rev Respir Dis* 1973;**107**:387–94.

57 O'Brien IM, Bull J, Creamer B, Sepulveda R, Harries M, Burge PS, Pepys J. Asthma and extrinsic allergic alveolitis due to *Merulius lacrymans*. *Clin Allergy* 1978;**8**:535–42.

58 Symington IS, Kerr JW, McLean DA. Type 1 allergy in mushroom soup processors. *Clin Allergy* 1981;**11**:43–7.

59 Topping MD, Scarisbrick DA, Luczynska CM, Clarke EC, Seaton A. Clinical and immunological reactions to *Aspergillus niger* among workers in a biotechnology plant. *Br J Industr Med* 1985;**42**:312–8.

Enzymes

60 Novey HS, Keenan WJ, Fairshter RD, Wells ID, Wilson AF, Culver BD. Pulmonary disease in workers exposed to papain: clinico-physiological and immunological studies. *Clin Allergy* 1980;**10**:721–31.

61 Pepys J, Hargreave FE, Longbottom JL, Faux J. Allergic reactions of the lungs to enzymes of bacillus subtilis. *Lancet* 1969;**i**:1181–4.

Drugs

62 Ayres J, Ancic P, Clark TJH. Airways responses to oral ethanol in normal subjects and in patients with asthma. *J Roy Soc Med* 1982;**75**:699–704.

63 Coutts II, Lozewicz S, Dally MB, Newman-Taylor AJ, Burge PS, Flind AC, Rogers DJH. Respiratory symptoms related to work in a factory manufacturing cimetidine tablets. *Br Med J* 1984;**288**:1418.

64 Coutts II, Dally MB, Newman Taylor AJ, Pickering CAC, Horsfield N. Asthma in workers manufacturing cephalosporins. *Br Med J* 1981;**283**:950.

65 Geppert EF, Boushey HA. An investigation of the mechanism of ethanol-induced broncho-constriction. *Am Rev Respir Dis* 1978;**118**: 135–9.

66 Hagmar L, Bellander T, Bergöö B, Simonsson BG. Piperazine-induced occupational asthma. *J Occup Med* 1982;**24**:193–7.

67 Szczeklik A, Gryglewski RJ, Czerniawska-Mysik G. Relationship of inhibition of prostaglandin biosynthesis by analgesics to asthma attacks in aspirin-sensitive patients. *Br Med J* 1975;**i**:67–9.

68 Weliky N, Heiner DC. Hypersensitivity to chemicals. Correlation of tartrazine hypersensitivity with characteristic serum IgD and IgE immune response patterns. *Clin Allergy* 1980;**10**:375–94.

Dyes

69 Alanko K, Keskinen H, Björksten F, Ojanen S. Immediate-type hypersensitivity to reactive dyes. *Clin Allergy* 1978;**8**:25–31.

70 Graham V, Coe MJS, Davies RJ. Occupational asthma after exposure to a diazonium salt. *Thorax* 1981;**36**:950–1.

Metal salts (see also page 303)

71 Dally MB, Hunter JV, Hughes BG, Stewart M, Newman Taylor AJ. Hypersensitivity to platinum salts: a population study. *Am Rev Respir Dis* 1980;**121(Suppl)**:230.

72 Keskinen H, Kalliomäki P-L, Alanko K. Occupational asthma due to stainless steel welding fumes. *Clin Allergy* 1980;**10**:151–9.

73 Novey HS, Habib M, Wells ID. Asthma and IgE antibodies induced by chromium and nickel salts. *J Allergy Clin Immunol* 1983;**72**:407–12.

74 Pepys J, Pickering CAC, Hughes EG. Asthma due to inhaled chemical agents—complex salts of platinum. *Clin Allergy* 1972;**2**:391–6.

Isocyanates

75 Bascom R, Kennedy TP, Levitz D, Zeiss CR. Specific bronchoalveolar lavage IgG antibody in hypersensitivity pneumonitis from diphenylmethane diisocyanate. *Am Rev Respir Dis* 1985;**131**:463–5.

76 Baur X. Immunologic cross-reactivity between different albumin-bound isocyanates. *J Allergy Clin Immunol* 1983;**71**:197–205.

77 Belin L, Wass U, Audunsson G, Mathiasson L. Amines: possible causative agents in the development of bronchial hyperreactivity in workers manufacturing polyurethanes from isocyanates. *Br J Industr Med* 1983;**40**:251–7.

78 Burge PS, O'Brien IM, Harries MG. Peak flow rate records in the diagnosis of occupational asthma due to isocyanates. *Thorax* 1979;**34**: 317–23.

79 Butcher BT. Inhalation challenge testing with toluene di-isocyanate. *J Allergy Clin Immunol* 1979;**64**:655–7.

80 Butcher BT, O'Neil CE, Reed MA, Salvaggio JE. Radioallergosorbent testing with p-tolyl mono-isocyanate in toluene diisocyanate workers. *Clin Allergy* 1983;**13**:31–4.

81 Butcher BT, Salvaggio JE, O'Neil CE, Weill H, Garg O. Toluene diisocyanate pulmonary disease: immunopharmacologic and mecholyl challenge studies. *J Allergy Clin Immunol* 1977;**59**:223–7.

82 Chang KC, Karol MH. Diphenylmethane diisocyanate (MDI)-induced asthma: evaluation of the immunologic responses and application of an animal model of isocyanate sensitivity. *Clin Allergy* 1984;**14**:329–39.

83 Charles J, Bernstein A, Jones B, Jones DJ, Edwards JH, Seal RME, Seaton A. Hypersensitivity pneumonitis after exposure to isocyanates. *Thorax* 1976;**31**:127–36.

84 Danks JM, Cromwell O, Buckingham JA, Newman Taylor AJ, Davies RJ. Toluene diisocyanate induced asthma: evaluation of antibodies in the serum of affected workers against tolyl mono-isocyanate protein conjugate. *Clin Allergy* 1981;**11**:161–8.

85 Diem JE, Jones RN, Hendrick DJ, Glindmeyer HW, Dharmarajan V, Butcher BT, Salvaggio JE, Weill H. Five-year longitudinal study of workers employed in a new toluene diisocyanate manufacturing plant. *Am Rev Respir Dis* 1982;**126**:420–8.

86 Malo JL, Ouimet G, Cartier A, Levitz D, Zeiss R. Combined alveolitis and asthma due to hexamethylene diisocyanate (HDI), with demonstration of crossed respiratory and immunologic reactivities to diphenylmethane diisocyanate (MDI). *J Clin Immunol* 1983; **72**:413–19.

87 Pezzini A, Riviera A, Paggiaro P, Spiazzi A, Gerosa F, Filieri M, Toma G, Tridente G. Specific IgE antibodies in twenty-eight workers with diisocyanate-induced bronchial asthma. *Clin Allergy* 1984;**14**:453–61.

Colophony

88 Burge PS. Occupational asthma in electronics

workers caused by colophony fumes: follow-up of affected workers. *Thorax* 1982;**37**:348–53.

89 Burge PS, Edge G, Hawkins R, White V, Newman Taylor AJ. Occupational asthma in a factory making flux-cored solder containing colophony. *Thorax* 1981;**36**:828–34.

90 Burge PS, Harries MG, O'Brien I, Pepys J. Bronchial provocation studies in workers exposed to the fumes of electronic soldering fluxes. *Clin Allergy* 1980;**10**:137–49.

91 Burge PS, O'Brien IM, Harries MG. Peak flow rate records in the diagnosis of occupational asthma due to colophony. *Thorax* 1979;**34**:308–16.

92 Hendy MS, Beattie BE, Burge PS. Occupational asthma due to an emulsified oil mist. *Br J Industr Med* 1985;**42**:51–4.

93 So SY, Lam WK, Ya D. Colophony-induced asthma in a poultry vendor. *Clin Allergy* 1981;**11**:395–9.

Epoxy resin curing agents

94 Bardana EJ (Jr), Andrach RH. Occupational asthma secondary to low molecular weight agents used in the plastic and resin industries. *Eur J Respir Dis* 1983;**64**:241–51.

95 Bernstein DI, Zeiss CR, Wolkonsky P, Levitz D, Roberts M, Patterson R. The relationship of total serum IgE and blocking antibody in trimellitic anhydride-induced occupational asthma. *J Allergy Clin Immunol* 1983;**72**:714–19.

96 Fawcett IW, Newman Taylor AJ, Pepys J. Asthma due to inhaled chemical agents—epoxy resin systems containing phthalic acid anhydride trimellitic acid anhydride and triethylene tetramine. *Clin Allergy* 1977;**7**:1–14.

97 Howe W, Venables KM, Topping MD, Dally MB, Hawkins R, Law JS, Newman Taylor AJ. Tetrachlorophthalic anhydride asthma: evidence for specific IgE antibody. *J Allergy Clin Immunol* 1983;**71**:5–11.

98 Kennes B, Garcia-Herreros P, Dierckx P. Asthma from plexiglass powders. *Clin Allergy* 1981;**11**:49–54.

99 Patterson R, Addington W, Banner AS, Byron GE, Franco M, Herbert FA, Nicotra MB, Pruzansky JJ, Rivera M, Roberts M, Yawn D, Zeiss CR. Antihapten antibodies in workers exposed to trimellitic anhydride fumes: a potential immunopathogenetic mechanism for the trimellitic anhydride pulmonary disease-anemia syndrome. *Am Rev Respir Dis* 1979;**120**:1259–67.

100 Pauli G, Bessot JC, Kopferschmitt MC, Lingot G, Wendling R, Ducos P, Limasset JC. Meat wrappers' asthma: identification of the causal agent. *Clin Allergy* 1980;**10**:263–9.

Furfuryl alcohol

101 Cockcroft DW, Cartier A, Jones G, Tarlo SM, Dolovich J, Hargreave FE. Asthma caused by occupational exposure to a furan-based binder system. *J Allergy Clin Immunol* 1980;**66**:458–63.

Formaldehyde

102 Burge PS, Harries MG, Lam WK, O'Brien IM, Patchett PA. Occupational asthma due to formaldehyde. *Thorax* 1985;**40**:255–60.

103 Hendrick DJ, Lane DJ. Occupational formalin asthma. *Br J Industr Med* 1977;**34**:11–18.

104 Nordman H, Keskinen H, Tuppurainen M. Formaldehyde asthma—rare or overlooked? *J Allergy Clin Immunol* 1985;**75**:91–9.

Other chemicals

105 Lam S, Chan-Yeung M. Ethylenediamine-induced asthma. *Am Rev Respir Dis* 1980;**121**:151–5.

106 Lozewicz S, Davison AG, Hopkirk A, Burge PS, Boldy DAR, Riordan JF, McGivern DV, Platts BW, Davies D, Newman Taylor AJ. Occupational asthma due to methyl methacrylate and cyanoacrylates. *Thorax* 1985;**40**:836–9.

107 Pepys J, Pickering CAC. Asthma due to inhaled chemical fumes—amino-ethyl ethanolamine in aluminium soldering flux. *Clin Allergy* 1972;**2**:197–204.

108 Slovak AJM. Occupational asthma caused by a plastics blowing agent, azodicarbonamide. *Thorax* 1981;**36**:906–9.

109 Vallieres M, Cockcroft DW, Taylor DM, Dolovich J, Hargreave FE. Dimethyl ethanolamine-induced asthma. *Am Rev Respir Dis* 1977;**115**:867–71.

Chapter 17
Chronic Bronchitis and Emphysema: Roles of Smoking, Occupation and Air Pollution

Chronic bronchitis
Chronic airflow limitation
Smoking as a cause of chronic lung disease
*Causes of chronic bronchitis (environmental and
    social, medical, occupational)*
Emphysema
Management
Industrial Injuries Benefit

Amongst working men in the U.K. chronic bronchitis and emphysema are the commonest cause of respiratory impairment and disablement and of loss of time from work. The principal aetiological factor is fume from cigarette smoke but occupational dusts and vapours can cause chronic bronchitis, both in isolation and by aggravating the effects of the cigarettes. Chronic bronchitis also occurs as a complication of progressive massive fibrosis, extrinsic allergic alveolitis, asbestosis and occupational asthma due to colophony or isocyanates. The view is taken that chronic bronchitis arising in the course of an occupation does not differ from that due to other causes; by contrast emphysema in coal workers can be specifically associated with simple pneumoconiosis (chapter 9).

Chronic bronchitis

Chronic bronchitis is defined as the occurrence of productive cough, with phlegm on most days for as much as 3 months in the year, for at least 2 successive years (33). The diagnosis is made on the basis of answers to standard questions; these are contained in the MRC Questionnaire on Respiratory Symptoms and other questionnaires based on it (page 81). Phlegm comes from the mucous glands in the walls of bronchi and goblet cells throughout the respiratory tract (page 71). Secretion is stimulated by inhaled particles and vapours. In chronic bronchitis the glands hypertrophy and thereby thicken the subepithe-

lium of the bronchial walls; the thickening is often visible at bronchoscopy. At post-mortem (fig. 17.1) it may be measured using the Reid index, which is the ratio of the gland thickness to the thickness of the airway wall internal to the cartilage. The measurement is made in the right main bronchus. In healthy persons the gland/wall ratio is in the range 0.14–0.36. Patients with established chronic bronchitis have an increased Reid index (43). The bronchial epithelium also contains an increased number of goblet cells and some malfunctioning columnar cells whose cilia beat in a contra-flow direction; this action obstructs the movement of secretions towards the pharynx.

Chronic bronchitis is often complicated by episodes of acute chest illness when the phlegm is increased in quantity and can be purulent. The illnesses are a cause of sickness absence from work but in adult life are seldom serious, except when the patient also has airflow limitation or emphysema. At one time these conditions were considered to be inevitable sequels to chronic hypersecretion. However, Fletcher and others have shown that chronic bronchitis is compatible with normal lung function and a normal life expectation; thus serious complications are not inevitable (18, 19). Their occurrence is usually due to the separate but overlapping effects of inhaled fumes on the secretory cells to cause hypersecretion, on the airway walls to limit airflow and on the lung parenchyma to cause emphysema. Any one complication can occur without the others so each should be specified. Similarly the underlying chronic bronchitis, if present, should be referred to as such and not incorporated in chronic obstructive bronchitis, or chronic bronchitis and emphysema (19). Industrial bronchitis has been used to describe the condition occurring in a dusty occupation or more specifically by Morgan to describe hypersecretion associated with an occupational exposure but not accompanied by airflow limitation (35). Some occupations where chronic bronchitis can be a problem are given in table 17.1 but in the

absence of a dose–response relationship or evidence that the bronchitis is distinguishable from that due to other causes, its description as industrial is not helpful. The aetiology is almost certainly multifactorial (page 378). Obstructive bronchiolitis occurs in airways of diameter less than 3mm; it is usually asymptomatic and hence difficult to diagnose. The condition can follow exposure to fume or dust, for example grain dust, a viral infection of the respiratory tract or a connective tissue disorder such as rheumatoid arthritis; the aetiology may then be included in the name, for example viral obstructive bron-

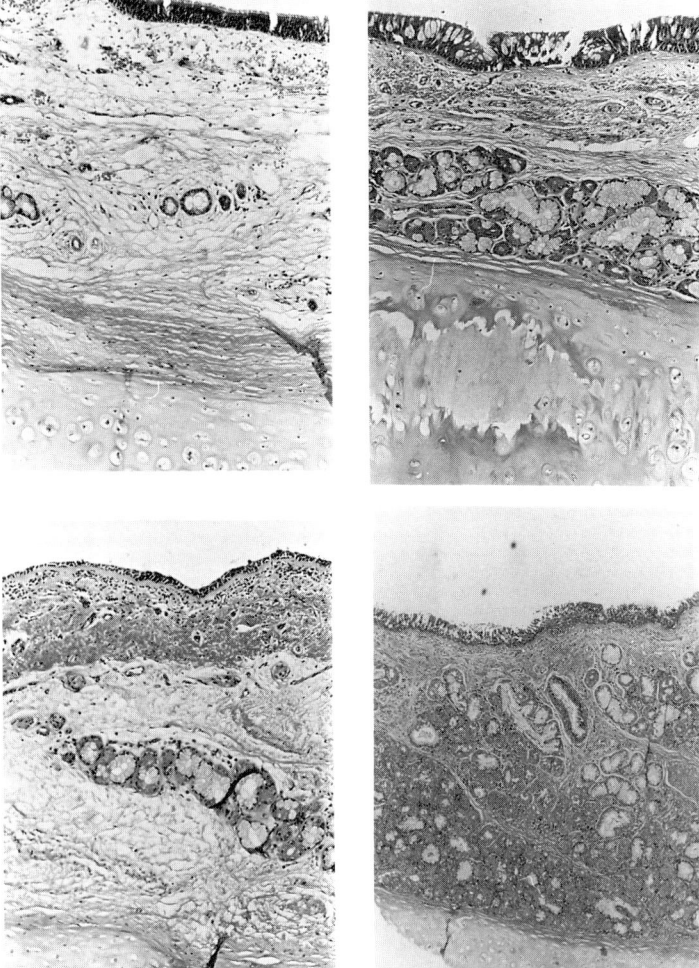

Fig. 17.1. Histological low power views of epithelium from the right main bronchus showing normal and hypertrophic submucosal glands. For the four specimens the Reid index (gland thickness ÷ wall thickness internal to the cartilage) was respectively approximately 0.1, 0.25, 0.55 and 0.9. The latter two subjects had chronic bronchitis. (By courtesy of T. Ashcroft.)

Table 17.1. Occupational dusts and fumes which increase the prevalence of chronic bronchitis

Source of substance	Comment
Asbestos mining	Smoking a more important factor (29)
Coal mining	Dose–response relationship (42, 44)
Coolant-lubricant aerosols	Dose–response relationship (3, also page 274)
Coke	Oven workers especially (55)
Cotton and flax	No dose relationship of symptoms (chapter 14)
Fire fighting	Many substances, exposure variable (53, also page 276)
Foundry	Effect additive with smoking (12)
Grain handling	Can cause asthma (chapter 16) (15)
Man-made mineral fibres	No dose relationship of symptoms (56)
Mining siliceous ore	May interact with smoking (21, 47, 55)
Slate quarrying and dressing	(22)
Sulphur dioxide	Also constituent of urban air pollution
Welding	Relationship to exposure (2, 10, 38)
Wood (western red wood, cedar, etc.)	Can cause asthma (chapter 16)

chiolitis. Chronic bronchitis is often present concurrently.

The cough and expectoration which result from hypersecretion can interrupt the performance of physical work but chronic bronchitis is not a cause of breathlessness unless respiratory impairment coexists. The impairment usually takes the form of airflow limitation.

Airflow limitation

Obstruction in large airways (diameter >3mm)

In chronic bronchitis the mucus may temporarily obstruct the bronchi until cleared by coughing. Persistent obstruction is caused by enlarged mucous glands and by thickening of the subepithelium due to local inflammation with oedema. These processes summate to progressively narrow the airways; however, flow limitation is not invariable. When it occurs it is commonly accentuated by an increase in tone of the bronchial smooth muscle; this is contributed to by tobacco smoke, environmental or occupational irritants, atopic status (page 346), nonatopic bronchial hyperreactivity and genetic predisposition (Pi type MZ). The non-specific bronchoconstrictor response to inhaled aerosol is mainly reflex from stimulation of irritant receptors (page 67) but in high dosage a direct local response also occurs.

Flow limitation in large airways causes an obstructive type of ventilatory defect with reductions in peak expiratory flow rate and forced expiratory volume, prolongation of expiration and a rise in airways resistance; the changes are progressive and accentuate the normal deterioration of lung function which occurs from age 25 years onwards (page 103). The average decline in forced expiratory volume in asymptomatic non-smokers, the effects of exposure to a respirable aerosol and the additional

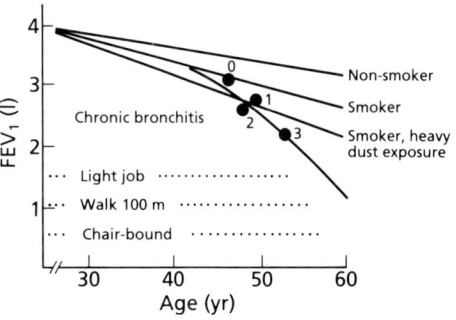

Fig. 17.2. Diagram illustrating the relationship of forced expiratory volume to age in coal miners for smokers, men with heavy dust exposure and those with bronchitis (graded 0–3) compared with non-smokers. The horizontal lines indicate the approximate exercise ability of men with reduced levels of FEV_1. The figure is based on the model of Fletcher *et al* (18) and the cross-sectional survey findings of Rogan *et al* (44); it has been published previously (9).

deterioration associated with respiratory symptoms, are illustrated in fig. 17.2. The effects are readily detectable by longitudinal study of groups of subjects or, if the deterioration is sufficient to cause breathlessness on exertion, by study of individuals. The respiratory impairment is often not apparent from measurements made at one point in time because the only standard of comparison is then the reference value which has wide-range confidence limits (coefficient of variation 15%). A deviation from the reference value in excess of 1.64 standard deviations is usually an indication of abnormality. However, whilst large airway narrowing is a cause of breathlessness, it probably does not shorten life unless, as is usually the case, the smaller airways are affected as well.

Obstruction in small airways

Narrowing of small airways of diameter less than 3mm may result from infection, non-infective inflammation, interstitial oedema or the cellular response to accumulated dust. It may be functional due to bronchiolar constriction, or dynamic from a diminution in lung surfactant or loss of elastic and collagen fibres in the lung parenchyma; these normally exert a retractive force which tends to hold the airways open. Causes of narrowing include infection, smoking, diffuse emphysema, diffuse fibrosis associated with asbestosis or extrinsic allergic alveolitis and a raised left atrial pressure. However, except with heavy exposure to dust or when the patient is in left heart failure, narrowing confined to small airways seldom causes much breathlessness. The condition can be diagnosed from a reduced forced expiratory flow rate at small lung volumes (MEF25%FVC). The forced expiratory volume is usually moderately reduced, the closing volume is increased and, except in extrinsic allergic alveolitis, the residual volume is often large relative to the elastic recoil pressure. The single breath nitrogen test and similar single breath indices of uneven lung function show evidence of abnormality. The airflow limitation reduces the oxygen tension in affected alveoli; this causes local reflex vasoconstriction of small pulmonary arteries. When many such arteries are affected the pulmonary arterial pressure rises relative to cardiac output. Initially this occurs on exercise; subsequently it is present at rest and leads to diversion of pulmonary blood flow from the bases to the upper zones of the lungs. Right ventricular hypertrophy ensues and there is a risk of congestive cardiac failure, especially during episodes of chest infection. The clinical syndrome is usually accompanied by chronic bronchitis. Emphysema may coexist but is not the main feature. Dornhorst described the patient in the late stages of bronchiolitis as being blue and bloated, contrasting his state with that of the emphysematous patient who was typically pink and puffing, hence blue bloater (or type B) and pink puffer (type A, page 381). The type B patient is typically of stocky physique, has hypoxaemia which is of comparable intensity at rest and on exercise, and hypercapnia which is accentuated by exercise. Before the onset of congestive cardiac failure a tendency to hypoventilation may be detected by a rise in blood carbon dioxide tension and buffering capacity. The treatment of the condition is considered in chapter 19. It should be noted that the forced expiratory volume is affected by narrowing of both large and small airways and reflects the grade of breathlessness (page 399): it is, therefore, an appropriate index of respiratory impairment in persons with chronic lung disease.

Smoking as a cause of chronic lung disease

Tobacco smoke is an aerosol of tar, nicotine and other substances suspended in a mixture of gases including carbon monoxide and other products of incomplete combustion. The carcinogenic substance, 3,4-benz(a)pyrene, is present in the tar which contains many irritant substances. These stimulate production of mucus from mucous glands, activate lung irritant receptors to initiate reflex bronchoconstriction, cause degranulation and local release of histamine from mast cells and interfere with the function of cilia. The bronchoconstriction increases the proportion of inhaled particles which impact at bifurcations of large airways; as a result fewer deposit by sedimentation in the periphery of the lung (page 69). In small conducting airways tobacco smoke causes bronchiolitis (8); this obstructs the flow of gas and leads to premature airway closure during expiration. In second order respiratory bronchioles tobacco smoke causes emphysema which is, therefore, centrilobular in distribution (fig. 17.3).

The serum levels of IgA, IgG and IgM are reduced by smoking and the levels of IgE and blood eosinophils are increased (23, 39, 52). The reductions in immunoglobulins may increase the susceptibility to respiratory infections of smokers and their young children (7). The increase in IgE may alter the subject's response to inhaled antigens in the direction of bronchoconstriction rather than an alveolar reaction (chapter 16); it may also contribute to an increased bronchoconstrictor response to inhaled histamine in some smokers (19).

Not all subjects are affected by tobacco smoke but when compared with non-smokers the smokers have approximately 3 times the prevalence of chronic bronchitis and the average decline with age of forced expiratory volume is materially greater: this is illustrated in fig. 17.2. A similarly enhanced deterioration with age is apparent in other indices which reflect airway patency; thus as evidence of narrowing of small airways the closing volume is increased and forced expiratory flow rate at small lung volumes is reduced. The development of emphysema is indicated by a decline in transfer factor and K_{CO}, although part of this loss is attributable to changes in the perfusion of the lung which are reversed by abstaining from smoking.

Variability in the response to tobacco aerosol

Individuals differ in their response to tobacco smoke; some of the variation is intrinsic but most is a result of differences in exposure. This is due to the interplay of many factors.

(a) *Consumption of tobacco.* Cigarette smokers consume between one and 100 cigarettes per day; the consumption is weakly negatively correlated with the nicotine content of the tobacco.

(b) *Inhalation.* The amount of aerosol inhaled is affected by the smoking pattern including the rate of airflow, the duration of each 'drag' and the extent to which it is deliberately drawn into the lung. Compared with cigarettes made from Virginian tobacco the inhalation is usually less for cigar tobacco and those cigarettes which have an alkali fume (e.g. Gauloises); this is due to the higher pH facilitating the absorption of nicotine from the buccal mucosa. However, cigar smokers who formerly smoked Virginian tobacco usually continue to inhale (31). Smokers who leave long stubs or allow the cigarette to burn spontaneously inhale less than others who do not.

(c) *Composition of the aerosol.* Cigarettes contain nicotine and tar and in the process of combustion liberate carbon monoxide; the average amount of nicotine per cigarette is approximately 1.3mg. The nicotine contributes to addiction to smoking but is not a direct cause of ill-health. The tar content ranges from 30mg per cigarette (high tar) to 10mg per cigarette (low tar). Tar is a cause of respiratory symptoms and lung cancer and fitting filters to the cigarettes confers some protection. The tar appears not to influence the development of airflow limitation (48). The concentration of carbon monoxide in tobacco smoke is determined by conditions at the site of combustion. A low concentration is achieved by having the tobacco loosely packed, using filters with ventilation holes and leaving a long unsmoked butt; however, these practices are not popular. Carbon monoxide in cigarette smoke reduces the exercise capacity and contributes to ischaemic heart disease. It has still to be shown that the measures to produce safer cigarettes have a beneficial effect.

(d) *Other air pollution.* This can exert an additive effect or it can interact. The interaction is positive for some occupational fumes discussed below but smoking lowers the incidence of extrinsic allergic alveolitis (chapter 15).

(e) *Individual susceptibility.* Individual susceptibility often becomes apparent at the onset of smoking and leads to the sensitive person not acquiring the habit. Self-selection has the effect that in some studies young smokers have been found to have superior lung function compared with the current non-smokers; the latter include the majority of asthmatics, persons with increased bronchial reactivity to histamine and those who experienced wheezy bronchitis during childhood (51). However, even in adolescence, smoking reduces the lung function and increases the prevalence of respiratory symptoms (1, 49).

The dose of aerosol may be estimated by asking the questions on smoking from the MRC Questionnaire of Respiratory Symptoms (1976) (page 81), supplemented by retrospective information on previous brands. Salivary or urinary continine may be used as a marker of exposure (25). An indication of smoking habits can be obtained by measuring the blood concentration of carboxyhaemoglobin or the alveolar concentration of carbon monoxide. The latter is usually in the range 0–5 ppm in non-smokers and 10–50 ppm in smokers. The level is correlated positively with the number of cigarettes smoked per day and negatively with the time since the last cigarette. The half-time for disappearance of carbon monoxide from the blood is approximately 4h at rest and less on exercise (page 271). As well as smokers, non-smokers may also be exposed to tobacco fumes, especially those who travel in early morning buses, have workmates or spouses who smoke, or who regularly attend public houses or working-mens' clubs. The resulting passive smoking is associated with a higher incidence of lung cancer (13) and a reduced ventilatory capacity compared with non-exposed persons (27).

Discontinuing smoking

The abandonment of smoking usually leads to a reduction or disappearance of daily cough and phlegm; there are often improvements in forced expiratory volume and transfer factor, particularly in young smokers. The permeability of the alveolar epithelium, which is high amongst smokers, is significantly reduced (26). In older subjects the decline in lung function with age usually reverts to the rate for non-smokers (18). The mortality from chronic bronchitis, emphysema and pulmonary heart disease also improves. Over about 7 years the rates fall to a quarter of those for current smokers (14). The capacity for exercise increases due to reductions in the blood concentrations of carbon monoxide and nicotine and an improvement in transfer factor; however, in some subjects the effect is masked by a rapid gain in weight. This is due to an increased appetite and a tendency to nibble,

chew or suck between meals. In most instances the beneficial effects predominate; the subject experiences better health and there is reduced mortality from chest illness, lung cancer and other smoking-related diseases, including myocardial infarction.

In some countries the number of smokers is increasing (50) and even in the U.K., despite considerable publicity, over 40% of men and 35% of women continue to smoke (45), but the majority of adults are now non-smokers. In 1981 in England and Wales, smoking was responsible for some 63,000 respiratory deaths, almost all of which could have been prevented by not smoking. The excess mortality is predominantly in areas of heavy industry which were formerly polluted and where there is additional exposure to occupational dusts and vapours. However, the ill-effects of smoking are greatly in excess of those due to occupation (16) or to air pollution (37).

Environmental and social causes of bronchitis

Babies born to parents who smoke have more chest illnesses in early life than those born to non-smokers. Children who grow up in areas of high environmental pollution have more respiratory symptoms and lower ventilatory function relative to stature than those in less polluted areas. Families who cook their meals using coal gas have more respiratory abnormality than those who cook by electricity. Users of open fires which burn solid fuel are more at risk of symptoms than those who do not; they include the families of coal miners who selectively fall into this category because of their entitlement to free coal. These effects are small and in some instances relate only to children but there is increasing evidence that they contribute to the burden of adult chronic bronchitis in the population as a whole. The prevalence of bronchitis is proportionally greater amongst men than women by a factor of 5 or 10 to 1 depending on which index is used. The sex ratio is fairly constant between social classes but there is a 5-fold increase in prevalence from social class 1 where it is low to social class 5 where it is high. An important factor contributing to the social class gradient is smoking, which is practised by over 50% of men in social class 5 compared with 25% in social class 1, but the gradient persists after smoking is allowed for. This is also the case for the difference between men and women which appears to be at least partly genetically determined. There may also be an ethnic factor with persons of African origin being less susceptible than Caucasians.

Medical causes of bronchitis

As well as general predisposing factors there are specific medical conditions which seem to be forerunners of chronic bronchitis in adult life. They include respiratory syncitial virus infection in infancy, broncho-pneumonia secondary to whooping cough in children who have not been fully immunized, and childhood asthma which does not go into complete remission. Atopic status by itself does not appear to contribute to chronic bronchitis, nor does chronic sinusitis. Conditions which specifically damage or distort the lung predispose to bronchitis; they include bronchiectasis, kyphoscoliosis, cystic fibrosis and diffuse or localized pulmonary fibrosis. On this account chronic bronchitis is a common complication of progressive massive fibrosis, asbestosis and extrinsic allergic alveolitis of occupational origin.

Occupational causes of bronchitis

Prevalence

Any occupational factor contributing to bronchitis is superimposed on all the other predisposing factors listed in the last three sections, including smoking, environmental, social and medical factors. The occupational factor seldom operates in isolation and the resulting bronchitis is rarely of the large airway type described by Morgan (page 374). Usually there is evidence for narrowing of small airways as well, for example a reduction in flow rates at small lung volumes or an increase in closing volume or residual volume. In coal miners an increased residual volume (RV) may also be due to focal emphysema associated with simple pneumoconiosis but, in its absence, when the forced expiratory volume is reduced, the RV is usually increased (36). Overall the bronchitis which develops in persons exposed to occupational dusts and fumes is not detectably different from that due to other causes; occupational bronchitis is not a distinct clinical entity. Some occupations carry an increased risk of bronchitis (table 17.1) but because the cases cannot be identified individually the risk can only be expressed in numerical terms. From a review of many traditionally dusty occupations, including coal mining, foundry work, gold mining and work with cotton and flax, Gilson found that compared with persons not exposed to dust the prevalence of bronchitis was on average in the ratio 2:1 with a range of from 1:1 to 3:1 (21). The ratio in grain handlers was also of this order (15). Amongst workers in many of these occupations the average ventilatory capacity was lower, reflecting narrowing of the airways (54); examples are given in table 17.2 and fig. 17.2. The latter shows the average decline in forced expiratory volume with age in coal miners with chronic bronchitis,

Table 17.2. Percentage of smokers and of men with respiratory symptoms amongst shipyard workers (Data of Cotes, Feinmann, Rennie and Chinn)

	Age group			
	16–19	20–29	30–44	45–70
Cigarette smokers	37	46	52	57
Other smokers	—	1	1	3
Ex-smokers	4	14	24	29
Non-smokers	59	39	23	11
Cough and phlegm >3 months in year	2.1	15.8	25.9	37.4
Breathless, grade 3 or above	0	1.3	9.6	19.9
Wheeze most days or nights	2.4	9.7	16.9	24.5
FEV_1 > 2 SD below expected	NA	NA	7.3	17.5

superimposed on the declines associated with smoking and with exposure to coal dust. The average reduction in FEV_1 attributable to persistent cough and phlegm in working miners who were not noticeably breathless was 0.08 l; in those who were also breathless on exertion the average reduction was 0.43 l. Similarly, amongst shipyard workers (10) the average reduction in FEV_1 associated with chronic bronchitis was 0.15 l. The reduction was greater at 0.36 l in those men who also experienced wheeze on most days or nights. These average changes are very small; they are of practical significance because they are superimposed on those due to age and other factors and because some individuals are more affected than others. On this account the average change does not give a true picture of the extent of abnormality and there is need for a better way of presentating such findings (19).

Interaction with smoking

Oldham working with Lloyd Davies found that the effect on the prevalence of bronchitis of a life-time of foundry work was equivalent to smoking 250 cigarettes per day; the two effects were independent and additive (12). In other studies there was interaction between smoking and dust exposure, including positive interaction in the case of gold miners (47) and in some studies of cotton and asbestos workers (55). In these instances the dust-exposed smokers had a greater amount of respiratory ill-health than would have been expected from adding together the effects of dust exposure in non-smokers and of smoking in persons not exposed to dust. A similar positive interaction has been reported for men exposed to fumes from welding or caulker-burning. Smokers exposed to these fumes may exhibit increased loss of time from work (30). In one study the interaction was strongest for ex-smokers, suggesting that welders with chronic bronchitis abandoned smoking in order to continue in their occupation (10). At the anecdotal level a number of men commented to this effect and a similar observation has been made of grain elevator operators by Dosman (15).

Negative interaction between smoking and an occupational hazard has been observed in some studies including those by Bouhuys, McDonald and their associates (4, 29). Negative interaction between smoking and some causes of extrinsic allergic alveolitis has also been observed (page 333). Negative interaction implies that the occupationally-exposed smoker has a smaller chance of developing respiratory symptoms or that these are of lesser intensity than is the case for his non-smoking colleague. Its occurrence could be evidence for a protective effect. Alternatively the distribution of susceptibility within the population might have been altered by pre-employment examination excluding susceptible individuals or by those who developed symptoms moving to other work and not being available for study; in this event a real positive interaction might be missed. Intuitively the combination of tobacco fumes and an occupational irritant might be expected to conform to the additive model. In practice the interactive model is frequently observed; persons exposed to such an irritant have a strong reason for abandoning smoking.

Relationship to exposure

Occupational dusts and vapours contribute to bronchitis by direct action and not by sensitization, so the exposure should give rise to a positive dose–response relationship; the presence of such a relationship is strong evidence for the association being causal. Thus in the coal-mining industry Rae and his colleagues found a significant association between the measured dust exposure and the prevalence of symptoms in men up to the age of 45 years (42). No similar association was observed in the older subjects, possibly because by this age the effect of other causes of bronchitis obscured the pattern. Similar relationships between prevalence and exposure have now been obtained in many occupations (e.g. 3, 10, 38). Such studies clearly demonstrate that occupation contributes to the burden of chronic bronchitis; exposure to diesel fumes does not appear to do so (page 275). However, much of the information is retrospective and relates to conditions in the past; present-day conditions are usually considered to be better but this is conjectural in the absence of evidence. The evidence is obtained by prospective longitudinal studies. Such studies should be undertaken in industries at risk so that the occupational component of chronic bronchitis can finally be eliminated. The methodology is considered in chapter 6.

Relationship to acute effects

Acute irritation of the respiratory tract occurs with exposure to many substances used in industry: in some instances the substances are also sensitizing agents and may cause occupational asthma rather than bronchitis (table 17.3). Toluene diisocyanate, formaldehyde, colophony and epoxy resin are examples. Other irritants including chlorine gas, vanadium pentoxide and some fumes to which fire fighters are exposed may occasionally give rise to chronic bronchitis, but dose is important and the evidence is not conclusive (28, 53). These and other lung irritants are considered in chapter 13.

Table 17.3. Some substances which may acutely irritate the respiratory tract without causing chronic bronchitis (see also table 13.14, page 293)

Acetaldehyde	Nitrogen dioxide*†
Ammonia	Phenol
Beryllium salts	Selenium dioxide and anhydride
Chlorine	Tetrachlorphthalic anhydride‡
Colophony (pine resin)‡†	Trimellitic anhydride‡
Formaldehyde‡†	Toluene diisocyanate‡†
Hydrochloric acid	Vanadium pentoxide

* May cause bronchial hyperreactivity without asthma.
† Progression to chronic bronchitis may occur.
‡ Is cause of occupational asthma (Chapter 16).

Emphysema

Emphysema is characterized by expansion of distal air spaces with destruction of their walls (5). The change usually affects the alveoli of second order respiratory bronchioles and is called centrilobular or centriacinar emphysema. It occurs particularly in the upper lobes and apices of the lower lobes. These parts of the lung

are the principal sites of deposition of irritant gases including tobacco smoke (40); they are also subject to mechanical stress caused by gravity acting on the pyramidal shape of the lung. The amount of centrilobular emphysema increases with age and smoking. Emphysema may also occur diffusely throughout the acinus, a condition known as panacinar emphysema. This condition is either distributed widely throughout the lung or present mainly in the lung bases. It is then usually due to a reduced blood concentration of α_1 antitrypsin (see aetiology below). The gross anatomy of the two types is illustrated in fig. 17.3. Other types described by Reid (43), include compensatory emphysema which follows shrinkage of lung tissue, (for example, that due to progressive massive fibrosis (chapter 9)), scar emphysema in which the shrinkage and the associated emphysema are both localized round an area of fibrosis, and cystic or honeycomb lung when the walls of some enlarged air spaces are thickened by fibrous tissue. However, these names are descriptive and do not indicate the mechanisms.

Clinical features

Centrilobular emphysema is a common finding at post-mortem in male smokers, but such symptoms as occur are often due to coincident chronic bronchitis. Emphysema presents with breathlessness which occurs initially during strenuous exercise but subsequently on mild exertion and later at rest. It may be accompanied by cyanosis on exertion but not by hypercapnia or polycythaemia and the resting arterial blood oxygen tension is usually in excess of 9kPa (70mmHg) until a late stage in the disease; the favourable blood picture is maintained by relative hyperventilation at rest which may be apparent on clinical examination. These features are the basis for Dornhorst's description of the patient being pink and puffing (hence pink puffer or type A as distinct from blue bloater, page 376). The patient is usually lean and often of above average height. He may show pursed-lip breathing. Finger clubbing is not a feature of emphysema. The chest is often enlarged in its anteroposterior diameter and its expansion limited. The percussion note is typically hyper-

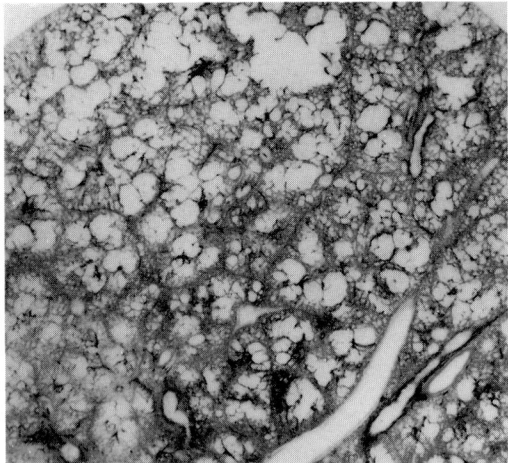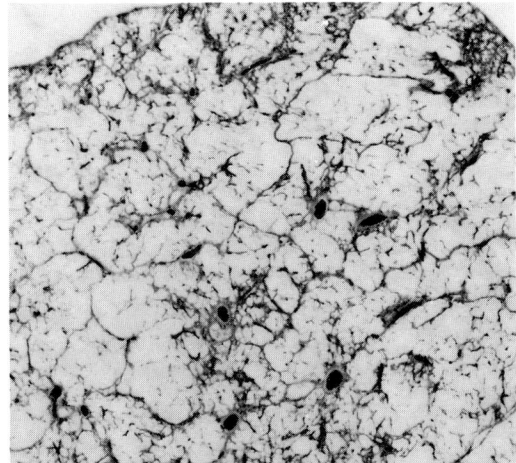

Fig. 17.3. Large lung sections showing emphysema. *Left*: Partially confluent centrilobular emphysema with normal lung tissue in the periphery of the lobules. The clinical features were of a pink puffer (type A). *Right*: Gross panlobular emphysema with almost no normal lung. Atypically the clinical features were of a blue bloater (type B).

resonant and the breath sounds faint with no added sounds. The electrocardiogram is normal until a late stage in the disease when it shows evidence of right ventricular hypertrophy. The condition may then progress to congestive cardiac failure but this is more often a late consequence of chronic airflow limitation without emphysema. Chest radiography reveals an increased anteroposterior diameter, a low, flat diaphragm and increased transradiancy with attenuated vascular markings, particularly at the periphery of the lung. The transradiancy can be assessed quantitatively by computer-assisted tomography (CAT scan) which can now be used as a screening test (17).

Lung function

The destruction of lung tissue which occurs in emphysema has two important consequences which together give rise to breathlessness. First, the area of alveolar capillary membrane available for gas exchange is reduced; this reduces the transfer factor and KCO, and thus causes hypoxaemia and increased ventilation on exercise. The latter may be further augmented by an increase in the volume of gas which is wasted in

ventilating an increased physiological deadspace. Second, the loss of tissue reduces the elastic recoil of the lung. This is the prime cause of the clinical features of emphysema. The effects are apparent at all phases of respiration. During sustained expiration the reduced elastic recoil allows the airways to collapse prematurely, thus trapping air in the lung and increasing the residual volume and the closing volume and capacity. Tidal breathing then takes place at an increased lung volume; the chest becomes over-inflated and the efficiency of respiratory muscles is reduced. During forced expiration the tendency for airways to collapse is accentuated and this dynamic compression contributes to reductions in forced expiratory volume and other indices of forced expiratory flow. The reduced elastic recoil is also associated with an increase in static lung compliance; the total lung capacity is usually increased in consequence. The emphysema and the associated increase in lung distensibility are not distributed uniformly throughout the lung so the distribution of inspired gas is uneven. These changes increase the physiological deadspace and impair indices of lung gas distribution. The tests are described in chapter 5.

Aetiology

Emphysema is due to loss of tissue from the interlacing mesh of fibres which give the lung its elasticity. The loss represents a shift in the balance between the processes of tissue breakdown and resynthesis, both of which occur continuously throughout life; resynthesis becomes less efficient with increasing age. Breakdown is accelerated by proteolytic enzymes acting on the amorphous component of elastic tissue and by oxidizing agents which may inactivate the antiproteases present in blood plasma (6). Both classes of agent can enter the respiratory bronchioles via the airways or reach the alveolar capillaries via the blood stream. Examples of airborne entry are papain or B. subtilis protease aerosol in persons handling these substances and gaseous ozone or nitrogen dioxide (pages 290 and 285); the latter are present in tobacco smoke and in fumes liberated by many industrial processes. Proteases and oxidants are also present in polymorphonuclear leucocytes (polymorphs) which are attracted into the lung by smoking, and in alveolar macrophages which are attracted by most inhaled substances. Some substances, including cadmium oxide present in cigarette smoke, stimulate the macrophages to have large lysosomes; these contain an increased amount of enzyme and so have an enhanced potential for proteolysis. Leakage of enzymes from macrophages occurs during ingestion of particles and also during their subsequent digestion if the phagocytic vacuoles do not close properly (24). The leakage contributes to the centrilobular emphysema associated with smoking and possibly also to that associated with haematite mining and with simple pneumoconiosis of coal workers. It does not occur to a notable extent with silicosis, possibly because silica dust, being more toxic, kills the macrophages and causes fibrosis instead.

Protection against proteases is conferred by antiproteases and macroglobulins present in blood plasma (46). The best documented is alpha-1 antitrypsin (α1AT) which is a polymorphic protein identified by specific protease inhibitor (Pi) typing; it is inherited on two autosomal co-dominant genetic alleles. Approximately 0.02% of persons inherit the homozygous phenotype PiZZ; they have a reduced plasma level of α1AT and often develop emphysema in middle life, smokers earlier than non-smokers. The heterozygous phenotype PiMZ does not carry an increased risk of emphysema: the possibility that it may contribute to the common types of chronic airflow obstruction is discussed by Madison and colleagues (32). The emphysema associated with alpha-1 antitrypsin deficiency is panacinar and predominantly basal because the trypsin, now without its coating of inhibitor, reaches the lung in the mixed venous blood and is then distributed mainly to the lung bases. The aggravating effect of smoking is probably due to tobacco smoke both inactivating other plasma antipro-

Table 17.4. Occupational pollutants which may contribute to emphysema

Substance	Experimental evidence	Source	Occurrence in man
Aluminium fume	No	Smelting	Secondary to fibrosis (page 265)
B. subtilis protease	Yes	Enzyme detergents	With heavy exposure (34)
Cadmium	Equivocal	Smelting, etc.	With heavy exposure, otherwise coincidental (11)
Coal and other dusts	No	Mining and handling	Centriacinar (pages 171, 280) Compensatory in PMF
Cotton	No	Processing cotton	Probably coincidental (chapter 14)
Nitrogen dioxide	Yes (57)	Silos, explosives, welding	Not confirmed (page 285)
Ozone	Equivocal	Welding, electrical discharge	No evidence (page 290)
Papain	Yes (41)	Carica papaya	Not reported

teases (20) and attracting protease-rich cells into the acinus.

Occupational causes of emphysema

Occupational pollutants may impinge on any part of the complex system just described and on the lung tissue itself. Some substances which have been suspected of causing emphysema in these ways are listed in table 17.4. In most instances the positive evidence comes from animal experiments whilst the information in man is often anecdotal. This is not surprising since early emphysema has only recently become detectable during life, the exposures are often intermittent and poorly documented, the adverse effects are enhanced by smoking, and susceptibility is influenced by constitutional factors. Occupational emphysema has been demonstrated following heavy exposure to cadmium fumes and to *B. subtills* protease. It occurs as a complication of simple pneumoconiosis in coalminers and haematite miners. Emphysema also occurs when there is advanced progressive massive fibrosis; the distribution is then usually peripheral and the mechanism is probably shrinkage of the PMF leading to expansion of pre-existing subclinical emphysema. However, the subject of occupational emphysema is ill-understood. It is likely to advance now that a means of early diagnosis has become available.

Management

The management of suspected occupational bronchitis should be tackled at several levels. Where possible an occupational survey should be undertaken with a view to establishing prevalence, severity and the relationship to exposure. The exposure should then be reduced by appropriate environmental hygiene measures supplemented, if appropriate, by the issue and fitting of respirators (chapter 3). Medical treatment (chapter 19) should include the strong advice to abandon smoking. The possibility of changing to a light job in a non-dusty situation should be considered and, if appropriate, undertaken early in the course of the illness, but not before the abandonment of smoking.

Industrial injuries benefit

In the U.K. at the time of writing neither occupational bronchitis nor emphysema alone or together are recognized as conferring entitlement to industrial injuries or disablement benefit (though the possibility of emphysema following exposure to cadmium is under consideration), but limited benefit is available if these conditions aggravate disablement associated with pneumoconiosis (chapter 9). Chronic bronchitis occurs with modestly increased frequency in many occupations but there is, at present, no way of identifying, in an individual, whether his bronchitis is due to his work or not. It is such a common complication of smoking that the award of benefit to all who might apply would be impractical as well as unfair to the non-smoking majority of the adult population. The position would change if investigation of dose–response relationships (with allowance made for the effects of smoking) identified some occupations in which the occurrence of occupational bronchitis was both frequent and irrefutable. In such an occupation the development of chronic bronchitis by a lifetime non-smoker would be strong grounds for benefit.

References

1 Adams L, Lonsdale D, Robinson M, Rawbone R, Guz A. Respiratory impairment induced by smoking in children in secondary schools. *Br Med J* 1984;**288**:891–85.

2 Antti-Poika M, Hassi J, Pyy L. Respiratory diseases in arc welders. *Int Arch Occup Environm Hlth* 1977;**40**:225–30.

3 Bake B, Larsson S, Mossberg B, (Eds). Chronic bronchitis in non-smokers. *Eur J Respir Dis* 1982;**63**:Suppl 118.

4 Bouhuys A, Zuskin E. Chronic respiratory disease in hemp workers. A follow-up study 1967–1974. *Ann Intern Med* 1976;**84**:398–405.

5 CIBA Symposium. Terminology, definitions and classification of chronic pulmonary emphysema and related conditions. *Thorax* 1959;**14**:286–99.

6 Cohen AB, James HL. Reduction of the elastase inhibitory capacity of alpha-antitrypsin by peroxides in cigarette smoke. *Am Rev Respir Dis* 1982;**126**:25–30.

7 Colley JRT, Holland WW, Corkhill RT. Influence of passive smoking and parental phlegm on pneumonia and bronchitis in early childhood. *Lancet* 1974;**ii**:1031–4.

8 Cosio MG, Hale KA, Niewoehner DE. Morphologic and morphometric effects of prolonged cigarette smoking on the small airways. *Am Rev Respir Dis* 1980;**122**:265–71.

9 Cotes JE. Respiratory Disablement: Problems and opportunities. *J Soc Occup Med* 1983;**33**: 5–12.

10 Cotes JE, Feinmann EL, Male VJ, Rennie FS. Respiratory health of shipyard workers. *Thorax* 1984;**39**:691.

11 Davison AG, Fayers PM, Newman Taylor AJ, Venables KM, Darbyshire JH, Pickering CAC, Holden H, Smith NJ, Mason H, Scott M. Cadmium inhalation and emphysema. *Thorax* 1986;**41**:714(Abstract). *See also* Editorial Cadmium and the lung. *Lancet* 1973;**ii**:1134–5.

12 Davies TAL. *Respiratory disease in foundrymen: report on a survey.* London: HMSO. 1971.

13 Doll R. Prospects for prevention. *Br Med J* 1983;**286**:445–53.

14 Doll R, Peto R. Mortality in relation to smoking: 20 years' observations on male British doctors. *Br Med J* 1976;**ii**:1525–36.

15 Dosman JA, Cotton DJ. *Occupational Pulmonary Disease: focus on grain dust and health.* New York: Academic Press. 1980.

16 Elmes PC. Relative importance of cigarette smoking in occupational lung disease. *Br J Industr Med* 1981;**38**:1–13.

17 Flenley DC, White KF. Topics in chronic bronchitis and emphysema. In: Flenley DC, Petty TL (eds). *Recent Advances in Respiratory Medicine 4.* Edinburgh: Churchill Livingstone. 1986.

18 Fletcher C, Peto R, Tinker C, Speizer FE. *The Natural History of Chronic Bronchitis and Emphysema.* Oxford: Oxford University Press: 1976.

19 Fletcher CM, Pride NB. Definitions of emphysema, chronic bronchitis, asthma and airflow obstruction: 25 years on from the Ciba symposium. *Thorax* 1984;**39**:81–5.

20 Gadek JE, Fells GA, Crystal RG. Cigarette smoking induces functional anti-protease deficiency in the lower·respiratory tract of humans. *Science* 1979;**206**:1315–6.

21 Gilson JC. Occupational Bronchitis? *Proc R Soc Med* 1970;**63**:857–64.

22 Glover JR, Bevan C, Cotes JE, Elwood PC, Hodges NG, Kell RL, Lowe CR, McDermott M, Oldham PD. Effects of exposure to slate dust in North Wales. *Br J Industr Med* 1980;**37**:152–62.

23 Gulsvik A, Fagerhol MK. Smoking and immunoglobulin levels. *Lancet* 1979;**i**:449.

24 Hutchison DCS. Enzymes, inhibitors and emphysema. *Bull Eur Physiopathol Respir* 1978;**14**:1–10.

25 Jarvis MJ, Russell MAH, Feyerabend C, Eiser JR, Morgan M, Gammage P, Gray EM. Passive exposure to tobacco smoke: saliva cotinine concentrations in a representative population sample of non-smoking schoolchildren. *Br Med J* 1985;**291**:927–9.

26 Jones JG, Lawler P, Crawley JCW, Minty BD, Hulands G, Veall N. Increased alveolar epithelial permeability in cigarette smokers. *Lancet* 1980;**i**:66–8.

27 Kauffmann F, Tessier JF, Oriol P. Adult passive smoking in the home environment: a risk factor for chronic airflow limitation. *Am J Epidemiol* 1983;**117**:269–80. *See also* Brunekreef B, *et al.* *Int J Epidemiol* 1985;**14**:227–230.

28 Lees REM. Changes in lung function after exposure to vanadium compounds in fuel oil ash. *Br J Industr Med* 1980;**37**:253–6.

29 McDonald JC, Becklake MR, Fournier-Massey G, Rossiter CE. Respiratory symptoms in chrysotile asbestos mine and mill workers in Quebec. *Arch Environm Hlth* 1972;**24**: 358–63.

30 McMillan GHG. The health of welders in naval dockyards: Welding, tobacco smoking and absence attributed to respiratory disease. *J Soc Occup Med* 1981;**31**:112–8.

31 McNicol MW, Turner JAMcM. Nicotine, carbon monoxide and heart disease. *Lancet* 1982;**i**:40.

32 Madison R, Mittman C, Afifi AA, Zelman R. Risk factors for obstructive lung disease. *Am Rev Respir Dis* 1981;**124**:149–53.

33 Medical Research Council. Definition and classification of chronic bronchitis for clinical and epidemiological purposes. *Lancet* 1965;**i**: 775–9.

34 Mitchell C, Gandrevia B. Loss of pulmonary elastic recoil due to heavy occupational exposure to proteolytic enzymes used in the detergent industry. *Proc IVth ILO International Pneumoconiosis Conference, Apimondia, Burcharest.* 1971.

35 Morgan WKC. Industrial bronchitis. *Br J Industr Med* 1978;**35**:285–91.

36 Morgan WKC, Burgess DB, Lapp NL, Seaton A, Reger RB. Hyperinflation of the lungs in coal miners. *Thorax* 1971;**26**:585–590.

37 Morris SC, Shapiro MA, Waller JH. Adult mor-

tality in two communities with widely different air pollution levels. *Arch Environm Hlth* 1976;**31**:248–54.

38 Oxhoj H, Bake B, Wedel H, Wilhelmsen L. Effects of electric arc welding on ventilatory lung function. *Arch Environm Hyg* 1979;**34**:211–7.

39 Pantin CFA, Merrett TG. Smoking and IgE levels. *Br Med J* 1982;**284**:744.

40 Pearson MG, Vinitski S, Chamberlain MJ, Morgan WKC. Regional deposition of particles in the lung during cigarette smoking. *Thorax* 1984;**39**:716–7.

41 Pushpakom R, Hogg JC, Woolcock AJ, Angus AE, Macklem PT, Thurlbeck WM. Experimental papain-induced emphysema in dogs. *Am Rev Respir Dis* 1970;**102**:778–89.

42 Rae S, Walker DD, Attfield MD. Chronic bronchitis and dust exposure in British coalminers. In: Walton WH (ed): *Inhaled Particles III*: Old Woking. Surrey: Unwin. 1971. Vol.II:883–96.

43 Reid L. *The Pathology of Emphysema*. Chicago: Yearbook Medical Publishers. 1967.

44 Rogan JM, Attfield MD, Jacobsen M, Rae S, Walker DD, Walton WH. Role of dust in the working environment in development of chronic bronchitis in British coal miners. *Br J Industr Med* 1973;**30**:217–26.

45 Royal College of Physicians. *Health or Smoking? A follow-up report*. London: Pitman Medical. 1983.

46 Stockley RA. Proteolytic enzymes, their inhibitors and lung diseases. *Clin Sci* 1983;**64**:119–26.

47 Sluis-Cremer GK, Walters LG, Sichel HS. Chronic bronchitis in miners and non-miners: an epidemiological survey of a community in the gold-mining area in the Transvaal. *Br J Industr Med* 1967;**24**:1–12.

48 Sparrow D, Stefos T, Bossé R, Weiss ST. The relationship of tar content to decline in pulmonary function in cigarette smokers. *Am Rev Respir Dis* 1983;**127**:56–8.

49 Tager IB, Muñoz A, Rosner B, Weiss ST, Carey V, Speizer FE. Effect of cigarette smoking on the pulmonary function of children and adolescents. *Am Rev Respir Dis* 1985;**131**:752–9.

50 Taha A, Ball K. Smoking and Africa: the coming epidemic. *Br Med J* 1980;**280**:991–3.

51 Tashkin DP, Clark VA, Coulson AH, Bourque LB, Simmons M, Reems C, Detels R, Rokaw S. Comparison of lung function in young nonsmokers and smokers before and after initiation of the smoking habit. *Am Rev Respir Dis* 1983;**128**:12–16.

52 Taylor RG, Gross E, Joyce H, Holland F, Pride NB. Smoking, allergy and rate of decline in FEV_1. *Thorax* 1984;**39**:695.

53 Unger KM, Snow RM, Mestas JM, Miller WC. Smoke inhalation in firemen. *Thorax* 1980;**35**:838–42.

54 Valentin H. *Forschungsbericht Chronische Bronchitis und Staubbelastung Am Arbeitsplatz*. Tel 2. H. Valentin, Boppard. 1981.

55 Weill H, Diem J. Relationships between cigarette smoking and occupational pulmonary disease. In: Dosman JA, Cotton DJ (Eds), *Occupational Pulmonary Disease*. New York: Academic Press: 1980:65–75.

56 Weill H, *et al*. In: *WHO: Biological effects of man-made mineral fibres. Euro reports and studies 81*. Copenhagen: WHO: 1984:385.

57 World Health Organization. Oxides of nitrogen. Environm Health Criteria, 4. Geneva: WHO. 1977.

Chapter 18
Exercise Tests and Respiratory Disablement

Maximal exercise
Submaximal tests of physical fitness
Physiological response to submaximal exercise
Respiratory disablement (definitions, types of impairment,
  methods for assessing ability to take exercise)

Heavy physical exertion is either an explosive effort of brief duration or it is sustained. Explosive effort is expended during lifting, wrenching and other movements which require physical strength. The energy comes from within specialized muscle fibres which differ in structure and function from those which support sustained activity. The distinctive features of the two systems are summarized in table 18.1. Physical strength is measured using dynamometers and these have a place in sports medicine, orthopaedic surgery and rehabilitation; they can be used in occupational medicine. Respiratory muscle strength is measured in terms of the maximal pressure which can be developed against a closed shutter. It has contributed to understanding of the changes in vital capacity associated with diving (chapter 7) but the measurement is not made routinely.

Sustained physical work entails expenditure of energy which normally comes from oxidation of glycogen and other substances; the additional oxygen is obtained by increased ventilation and perfusion of the lungs and increased blood flow to the active muscles. Breathlessness develops as the oxygen supply system approaches its capacity. The capacity is increased by physical training. It is reduced by inactivity, disease of the lungs or cardiovascular system, or a reduced ability of the blood to transport oxygen.

An exercise test is used to assess a person's capacity for exercise or physical fitness; it provides insight into the causes of exertional dyspnoea, contributes to the evaluation of disablement, and is essential for the supervision of training. Oximetry during exercise and measurement of the ventilatory response to submaximal

exercise also contribute to the assessment of lung function. The exercise test may be used to obtain the ventilatory and circulatory responses to submaximal exercise or it may be continued through to the symptom-limited maximal exercise capacity. If the latter is not measured directly it can be estimated from the submaximal results (table 18.2). It can also be estimated from body mass, age and other variables (table 18.5).

The maximal oxygen uptake of a group of healthy persons of the same age and sex has a wide range (±20%) but the variation within one individual in different states of training is relatively narrow (±5%). The large variation between subjects is mainly genetically determined. It has the effect that the exercise capacity of an individual is relatively independent of his state of training so can be assessed approximately by a single measurement. The fitness status of a group of subjects can also be assessed at one point in time, but that of an individual requires serial measurements or special tests.

Maximal exercise

The capacity for exercise can be expressed as a power output in watts. It is usually reported as the maximal oxygen uptake; this is also called the aerobic capacity which can be attained during exercise of increasing intensity ($\dot{n}O_2$ max). The aerobic capacity expressed per kg body mass reflects the ability to transport oxygen from the air to the active muscles and in part measures what is loosely called physical fitness. As an index it is unsatisfactory (table 6.7, page 119) but it is convenient. The determinants of

Table 18.1. Features of two types of effort

	Explosive effort	Sustained effort
Activity	Turn, lift, throw	Climb, swim, build
Determinants	Muscle strength, skill	High oxidative capacity of muscle
Muscle fibres		
Fibre type	2 (A and B), fast twitch	1 and 2, slow twitch
Enzyme site	Cytoplasm	Mitochondria
Enzyme types	Lactate dehydrogenase	MyosinATPase
	Myokinase	Succinate dehydrogenase
Oxidative capacity	Low	High
Recovery	Slow	Rapid if aerobic throughout

Metabolic pathway

Carbohydrate + NAD

Initial

$$\boxed{\begin{array}{c} CP + ADP \\ \downarrow \\ C + ATP^* \end{array}} \qquad \begin{array}{c} \downarrow \\ Pyruvate + NAD_2H + ATP^* \\ | \end{array}$$

Final

$$\begin{array}{c} Lactate\ dehydrogenase \\ \downarrow \\ Lactate + NAD \end{array} \qquad \begin{array}{c} Krebs\ cycle + substrate \\ cytochrome\ chain + O_2 \\ \downarrow \\ CO_2 + H_2O + NAD + ATP^* \end{array}$$

Respiratory component

Small; oxygen debt afterwards | Depends on lung function and muscle blood flow

CP = phosphocreatine; C = creatine; NAD = nicotinamide-adenine-dinucleotide; ADP = adenosine diphosphate; ATP = adenosine triphosphate.
* ($\rightarrow$ADP + muscle contraction).

the aerobic capacity are indicated in fig. 18.1. A high aerobic capacity is a condition of employment as a member of a mine rescue team (31) and for some types of deep sea diving (15, and chapter 7); it is important for membership of a fire brigade (5) and other occupations entailing strenuous work. Persons with respiratory impairment or ischaemic heart disease develop symptoms which prevent their attaining the aerobic capacity; the end-point is then the symptom limited maximal oxygen uptake. This quantity and the associated maximal exercise ventilation and cardiac frequency provide useful guides to disablement, the response to treatment and the future career prospects.

Maximal exercise testing is safe when performed with proper precautions. The test should be preceded by a medical examination and car-ried out on a treadmill or other ergometer under the supervision of trained personnel; the electrocardiogram should be monitored continuously. For this purpose the ECG leads should be over the sternum and at the cardiac apex (3). A medical practitioner should be within close call. Full resuscitation facilities should be available and the laboratory staff trained in their use. The blood pressure should be recorded at intervals during the exercise.

In patients with respiratory impairment the recovery after maximal exercise is rapid and the test is usually well tolerated. However, when, as in most healthy persons, exercise is limited by the capacity of the cardiovascular system recovery afterwards is slow due to the energy demands being met in part anaerobically. Metabolism of the accumulated lactic acid takes

DETERMINANTS OF CAPACITY FOR PHYSICAL WORK

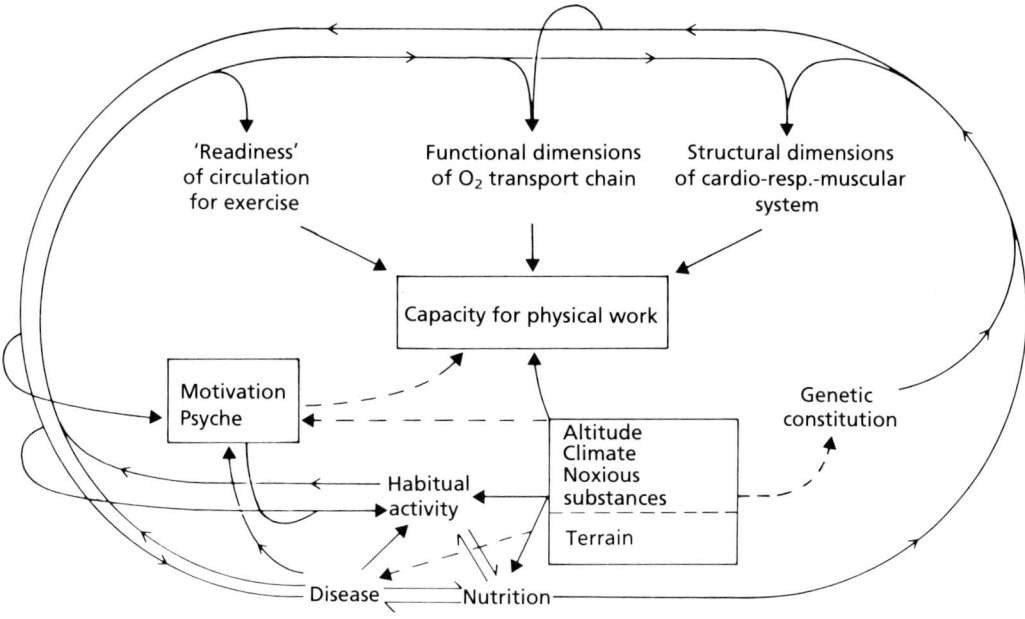

Fig. 18.1. Determinants of capacity for physical work. (Source: Cotes *et al* (20).)

approximately 1h (half time, 10min), the depleted muscle glycogen stores may take up to 48h to refill and repair of minor trauma may take several days. Thus for sedentary subjects maximal exercise is disagreeable and an alternative is needed. This may be a field test of exercise performance or a test of submaximal exercise.

Laboratory tests of maximal exercise

Assessment of the physiological response to exercise has been greatly improved by the recent development of autonomic equipment which provides an on-line display of oxygen uptake and related variables. This can be used to modify the work protocol whilst the test is in progress. On a cycle ergometer the work rate is increased progressively by increasing the loading on the flywheel; the increments of work per min are 10–25W and the rate of pedalling is kept constant (usually at 60 per min). To increase the load during treadmill walking both the belt

speed and the incline are increased, the former in the range 7–270m min^{-1} (1/4-10mph) and the latter between horizontal and an incline of 15°. The Bruce treadmill protocol (6) is widely used but an alternative which takes less time and does not entail concurrent speed and incline changes is more convenient. Using a treadmill both healthy persons and patients can achieve their maximum starting from rest but on a cycle ergometer healthy persons should do this in two stages starting with a submaximal test. The test of maximal performance then starts at a work load just below that at which the respiratory exchange ratio (ratio of carbon dioxide output to oxygen uptake) is unity ($R=1.0$), or at which the cardiac frequency is 70% of the predicted maximum (table 18.2). Examples of work protocols are given in table 18.3. The end-point of the maximal exercise test is when the subject develops symptoms, when the electrocardiogram or blood pressure become abnormal or when the subject attains the physiological

Table 18.2. Linear regression equations which describe aspects of the physiological response to exercise of men and women in an erect posture. (See also table 18.5, page 393.)

Aspects of function	Relationship	SD	Reference
(a) *Healthy subjects*			
Ventilation on oxygen uptake	$\dot{V}_E$(l min^{-1})† $= 0.5 \, \dot{n}O_2$ (mmol min^{-1})* $+ 2$	5.4	(13)
Tidal volume on vital capacity	Vt_{30} (l) $= 0.13$ VC (l) $+ 0.87$	0.22	(13)
Oxygen uptake during cycling	$\dot{n}O_2$ (mmol min^{-1}) $= 0.53$ W (watts) $+ 0.31$ BM(kg) -4.1	4.0	(13)
Cardiac frequency on oxygen uptake and fat free mass	$f_C = 34 + 1590 \, \text{FFM}^{-1}$ (kg) $+ 58 \, \text{FFM}^{-1} \, \dot{n}O_2$ (mmol min^{-1})*	12%	(16)
Maximal cardiac frequency	f_C (min^{-1}) $= 210 - 0.65$ age (yr)	19	(2)
Cardiac frequency at 80% maximal workrate	f_C (min^{-1}) $\simeq 160 - 0.52$ age (yr)	16	
Respiratory exchange ratio at $\dot{n}O_2 = 45$ mmol min^{-1} on age	$RER_{45} = 9.75 \times 10^{-4}$ age (yr) $+ 0.79$	0.08	(36)
Maximal O_2 uptake on $\dot{n}O_2$ at RER $= 1.0$	See Table 18.5 (reference values) Table 18.8		
(b) *Subjects with respiratory impairment*			
Indirect maximal breathing capacity from FEV$_1$	I MBC (l min^{-1}) $= 37 \, \text{FEV}_1$ (l) $- 2.8$	8%	(13)
Maximal exercise ventilation on FEV$_1$	$\dot{V}_{Emax,ex}$, (l min^{-1}) $= 33.1 \, (\text{FEV}_1)^{0.73}$ (Fig. 18.10)	0.19	(19)
Maximal O_2 uptake on FEV$_1$ and $\dot{V}_{E45}$	$\log_e \dot{n}O_2max$ (mmol min^{-1}) $= 4.45 + 0.55 \log_e \text{FEV}_1$ (l) $- 0.022 \, \dot{V}_{E45} + 0.2$ if working	0.205	(19)

* When uptake of oxygen is measured in l min^{-1} the coefficient for $\dot{n}O_2$ should be multiplied by $(10^3 \div 22.4)$.
† For female subjects the ventilation is about 10% higher.
FFM = fat free mass; BM = body mass.

maximal oxygen uptake (defined below). The symptoms which limit exercise include breathlessness, ischaemic pain (angina or intermittent claudication), cough, expectoration, giddiness and fatigue (33). Immediately exercise is discontinued the subject should say why he stopped; this ensures that the symptoms are recorded correctly and enables the observer to assess the subject's breathlessness. The assessment is helped by handing the subject the request in writing and asking him to read it aloud before he makes his reply. The subject is then asked to rate the effort which he put into the test by completing the Borg scale of perceived exertion (table 18.6). Cardiovascular indications for terminat-

ing the exercise include a run of three or more ventricular ectopic beats or five such beats in 1min, progressive ST depression (>2mm), ventricular tachycardia, a fall of systolic blood pressure or a rise above the range 225–275mmHg. In the absence of these abnormalities the exercise is terminated when the oxygen transport system has reached capacity: this is indicated by the uptake of oxygen reaching a virtual plateau (to within 4 mmol min^{-1}) despite a further rise in the rate of work. Accompanying features include the attainment of a maximal cardiac frequency (table 18.2), a greatly increased blood lactic acid concentration which may be as high as 10mmol l^{-1}, and a respiratory exchange ratio

Table 18.3. Work protocols for assessing maximal oxygen uptake

	Cycle ergometer			Treadmill			
	Healthy person		Patient	Healthy person		Patient	
Test	Submax.	Max.	Combined	Combined		Combined	
Starting point	Rest	W at $R=1.0$ $-20W$	Rest	3kph	Incline 4°	1.5 kph	Incline 4°
Increment per min	15W	20W	10W	1kph	1°	0.5kph	1°
End point	$R=1.0$	$\dot{n}O_2$max	$\dot{n}O_2$max (SL)†	$R=1.0^*$	$\dot{n}O_2$max	3kph*	$\dot{n}O_2$max (SL)†

W = Watts; kph = kilometres per hour; SL = Symptom-Limited.
* Treadmill is inclined to 4° at this point and exercise continued.
† Exercise may also be terminated at $\dot{n}O_2 = 45$ mmol min^{-1}.

in excess of 1.1. In subjects who exercise to the point of incapacitating breathlessness the ventilation minute volume approximates to the predicted maximal breathing capacity (table 18.2, also fig. 18.10, below). The result is reported as maximal work rate on the ergometer or maximal oxygen uptake. The latter is preferable, especially for treadmill exercise where the relationship of oxygen uptake on treadmill setting and body mass is variable even when using a fixed protocol. For the average healthy man the maximal oxygen uptake on the treadmill is approximately 130mmol min^{-1} (SD 18) (2.9 l min^{-1} (SD

Table 18.4. Maximal oxygen uptake (cycle ergometer) for men in different occupations ($n \simeq 30$)

	Fire brigade (5)	Mine rescue (31)	Heavy industry (36)	Divers (15)
Age	29.5	31.2	25.0	34.8
Body mass (kg)	79.4	75.2	71.4	81.3
Body fat (%)	20.4*	17.3	14.7	18.9
fCmax (min^{-1})	186	184	190	183
$\dot{n}O_2$max (mmol/min)	132*	150†	152	144†
$\dot{n}O_2$max/kg	1.68*	2.04†	2.12	1.8†

* Different from mine rescue ($P<0.05$).
† 90% of treadmill results.

0.4)); that on the cycle ergometer is approximately 10% lower. The equivalent per kg body mass is 1.8mmol kg^{-1} min^{-1} (40ml kg^{-1} min^{-1}) with a range for unfit to very athletic subjects of ±20% (2, 33). Average values for some occupational groups are given in table 18.4 and reference values in table 18.5.

Field tests. The exercise performance of most subjects may be assessed by measuring the time taken to undertake a specified task, for example, ascending twelve flights of stairs, running 3km or completing a round of circuit training. Performance may also be assessed in terms of the maximal amount of work done in a specified time, for example the distance walked in 12min. This test is of proven value for patients with respiratory disease; a 6min test is equally useful (7, 25). The walk is often on a level corridor but a treadmill may be used instead. In both healthy and disabled subjects the result is influenced by the mental attitude to illness and mood of the patient (26, 34) and is improved by physical training (e.g. 9, fig. 19.2, page 411). At the end of the test the intensity of the perceived exertion should be assessed using the scale of Borg (table 18.6).

Submaximal tests of physical fitness

A maximal exercise test is only performed satisfactorily by a minority of unselected subjects. Some refuse or do not try hard enough whilst others, especially in older age groups, develop ECG abnormalities; in one study 40% dropped out on this account (15), though several of these completed a subsequent test. Many more people will complete a submaximal test of physical fitness. Such tests entail the measurement and interpretation of cardiac frequency during or after exercise. Alternatively the frequency or other variable is used to estimate the maximal oxygen uptake which is then compared with the reference value. The relationship of cardiac frequency to oxygen uptake during exercise is illustrated in fig. 18.2: the frequency relative to the fat-free mass is increased in persons who take little exercise. The recovery of cardiac frequency after exercise is illustrated in fig. 18.3. Recovery is slow in persons who are not fit. The recovery pulse frequency is measured during the Harvard pack test (24). To perform the test the subject steps 30 times per min for 5min on

and off a platform usually of height 40.6cm (16in) carrying a load of 22kg or one-third of body weight, whichever is greater. The subject uses both arms and legs, the former via hand grips above the step (fig. 18.4). The test is very strenuous and requires close observation; this is both to ensure that the subject lifts his centre of gravity through the full height of the step in time with the metronome, and to monitor the electrocardiogram. Neglect of this precaution has been associated with death. The Harvard pack test is best replaced by a less strenuous one in which the cardiac frequency is measured during the exercise. The frequency at a standard rate of work on a cycle ergometer, treadmill or step can be used as an index of fitness (table 18.7). The results are intercorrelated and provide a less strenuous alternative to the Harvard pack test

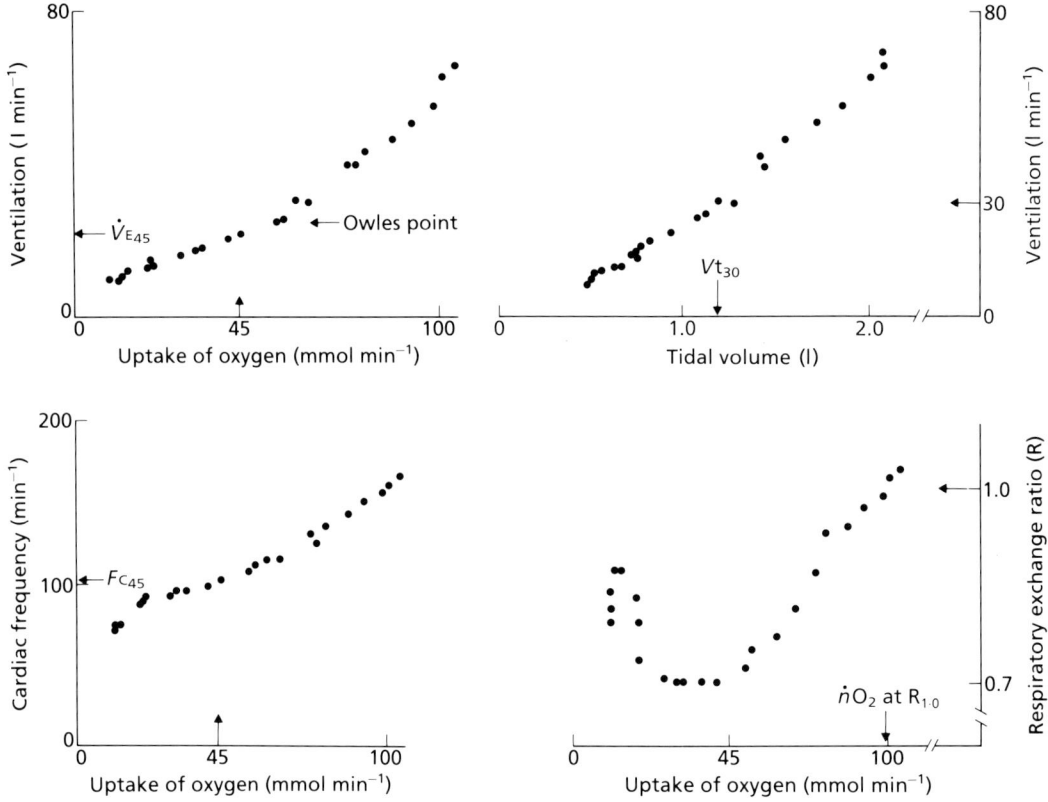

Fig. 18.2. Intermediate results of a submaximal progressive exercise test in a healthy subject showing the derivation of the indices f_{C45}, $\dot{V}_{E45}$, Vt_{30} and $\dot{n}O_2$ at $R = 1.0$. For details see text.

(17, 31). However, none of the tests accurately predict the maximal oxygen uptake. Traditionally this is estimated by extrapolating the regression of submaximal exercise cardiac frequency on oxygen uptake (fig. 18.2) up to the maximal frequency predicted for the subject's age (table 18.2). Unfortunately the method is inaccurate because the relationship is not linear and the maximal frequency is not known precisely. Greater accuracy is achieved by basing the prediction on the oxygen uptake at a respiratory exchange ratio of unity ($R_{1.0}$) and other variables (table 18.8).

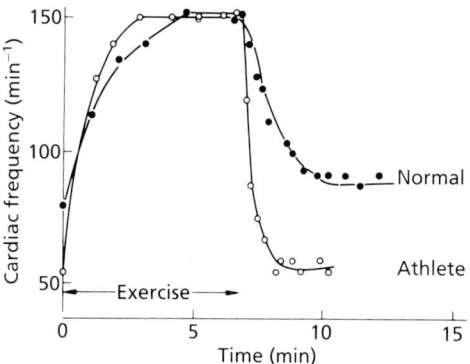

Fig. 18.3. Cardiac frequency during exercise showing the rise at the start and the recovery afterwards taking place more slowly in an unfit subject compared with an athlete in training. This difference is the basis for the Harvard pack index. (Source: Cotes (13), p. 310.)

Table 18.5. Reference equations for maximal oxygen uptake in healthy men using a cycle ergometer (mmol min⁻¹: for l min⁻¹ divide by 44.6)

Source	(23)	(36)
Coefficient terms		
Age (yr)	−1.03	−0.95
Stature (cm)	1.11	—
Body mass (kg)	0.84	—
Fat free mass (kg)	—	1.43
Activity score (1–4)	6.7	6.3
Smoking (yes/no)	—	−8.1
Constant term	−103	70
Mean $\dot{n}O_2$max*	129	128
Standard error	18.5	17.3

* Age 35 yr, st. 1.73 m, wt. 70 kg,
FFM 56 kg, activity score 2.5, ½ smoker.

These tests are suitable for reasonably healthy subjects; they underestimate the exercise tolerance of persons who are very anxious or who over-ventilate. The procedures over-estimate the exercise tolerance of respiratory patients in whom the limiting factor is breathlessness secondary to respiratory impairment; in these circumstances the symptom-limited maximal oxygen uptake can be estimated from forced expiratory volume and ventilation during submaximal exercise (page 402). The procedures described in this section also over-estimate the exercise tolerance of patients who are limited by other incapacitating symptoms for example, angina pectoris, intermittent claudication or muscular or skeletal pain.

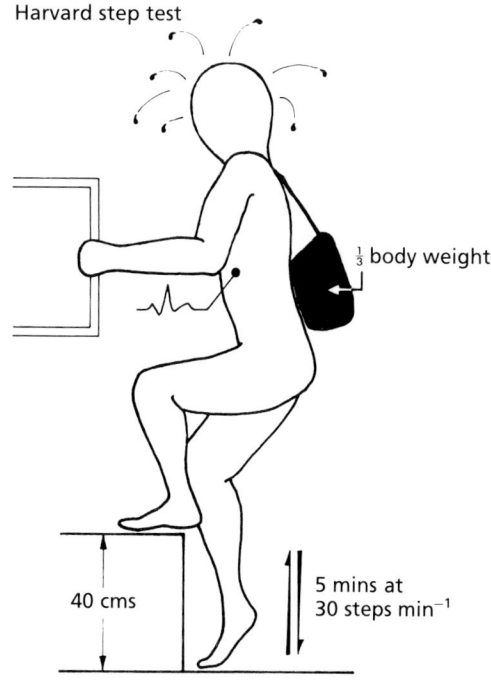

Fig. 18.4. Harvard pack test.

The physiological response to submaximal exercise

Aspects of measurement. For exercise of all but very short duration energy is generated in the active muscles by oxidation of carbohydrate and fat. The additional consumption of oxygen entails increases in ventilation and cardiac output by means of increases in tidal volume, respiratory frequency, cardiac frequency and stroke volume. The carbon dioxide output also increases. The non-invasive measurement of these and related variables during exercise of progressively increasing intensity provides invaluable information on the physiological response to exercise. The measurement of stroke volume is seldom necessary but the other variables should be recorded during routine testing. Because of the many factors involved the rate of external work done is not equivalent to the oxygen uptake. Other indices including those of lung mechanics, arterial blood gases and transfer factor may also be obtained during exercise; the mechanics indices are mainly of research interest; the others are considered under gas exchange below. Examples of protocols for progressive exercise on a cycle ergometer and treadmill are given in table 18.3. A step test can also be modified for the same purpose (28). The saddle of the cycle should be adjusted so that the leg is straight at the end of the thrust; the cycling frequency should be 60 per min. Using a treadmill the means of slowing or stopping should be explained to the subject and a safety harness or padded board used to prevent injury in the event of a fall. A period of

practice exercise should precede the test which should be carried out in a relaxed atmosphere; time should be allowed for digestion after a meal.

Ventilation minute volume (and/or tidal volume) are measured with a dry gas meter, or respiratory anemometer, or pneumotachograph and integrator. The equipment should have a resistance to flow of not more than 0.1kPa (1cmH$_2$O) at a flow rate of 100 l min^{-1} and volumetric calibration should be carried out at several rates of gas flow using a gas syringe or pump (fig. 5, 6, page 95). Respiratory frequency should be recorded. The concentrations of oxygen and carbon dioxide in the mixed expired gas are obtained by gas analysers sampling distal to a gas mixing chamber (fig. 18.5). Oxygen uptake ($\dot{n}O_2$), carbon dioxide output ($\dot{n}CO_2$) and respiratory exchange ratio ($\dot{n}CO_2/\dot{n}O_2$) are obtained from these measurements. Cardiac frequency obtained electronically from the R waves of the electrocardiograph (ECG), is displayed each minute; the ECG is displayed on a visual monitor. The interrelationships between the variables are illustrated in fig. 18.2 and the four quadrants of this graph should be available for inspection during or at the end of the test (10): the display is provided by a microprocessor or computer linked to the transducers (e.g. P.K. Morgan Scientific Instruments). The reported result should include the ventilation, cardiac frequency and respiratory exchange ratio at an oxygen uptake of 45mmol min^{-1}, the tidal volume at a minute volume of 30 l min^{-1} and the values for these indices in the last half minute of the test. The oxygen uptake at $R=1.0$ and the highest attained oxygen uptake should also be reported together with the reason why the test was discontinued (see exercise limitation below).

Ventilation minute volume. The relationship of ventilation to consumption of oxygen (fig. 18.2) is linear at low and intermediate intensities of work and may be described by a linear regression equation (table 18.2). The relationship is independent of body mass and in most able-bodied persons is independent of age, though ventilation is increased in smokers (18), the elderly (29) and persons who breathe with a small tidal volume (36). Very fit subjects have low values whilst women have rather higher

Table 18.6. Rating score for perceived exertion of Borg (4)

Score	Approximate description
7	Very, very light
9	Very light
11	Fairly light
13	Somewhat hard
15	Hard
17	Very hard
19	Very, very hard (the limit)
20	Beyond endurance

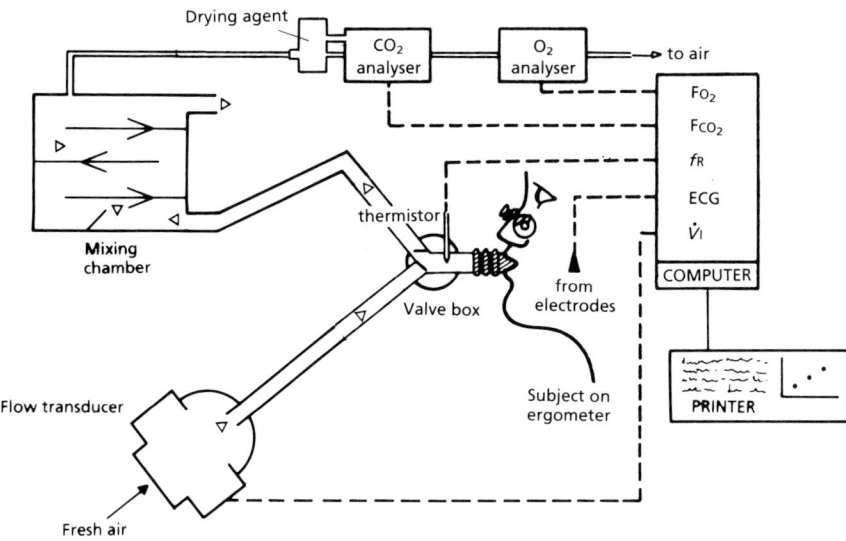

Fig. 18.5. Basic equipment necessary for exercise testing. (Source: Cotes (13), p. 306.)

values than men, but the difference is small. The ventilation at any designated uptake of oxygen may be used as an index, for example 45mmol min⁻¹ (1.0 l min⁻¹) when the mean ventilation of the average man is 24 (SD 5.4) l min⁻¹ (i.e. $\dot{V}_{E45}$ = 24 l min⁻¹) and the corresponding respiratory exchange ratio (R_{45}) is 0.83. The ventilatory cost of exercise ($\dot{V}_{E45}$) is increased as part of the syndrome of defective gas transfer in diseases of the lung parenchyma, including emphysema, extrinsic allergic alveolitis and asbestosis; in the latter condition $\dot{V}_{E45}$ has been found to be a more sensitive guide to abnormality than vital capacity or transfer factor (18). Exercise ventilation is also increased slightly in the presence of uneven lung function when it is due to enlargement of the physiological deadspace. Other causes of an increase in exercise ventilation include previous pleurisy, mitral stenosis and cyanotic congenital heart disease. In addition the lung disease may reduce the maximal ventilation and hence the work capacity.

At rates of work approaching the maximum the ventilation is increased relative to the consumption of oxygen (fig. 18.2). The increase is due to insufficient delivery of oxygen to the active muscles leading to the production of lactic acid. The acidaemia and reduced tissue pH stimulate breathing and the curve steepens. The

place on the curve where the rise occurs is called Owles' point or anaerobic threshold. It may be identified by inspecting the curve or defined mathematically or considered in terms of an increase in respiratory exchange ratio (R), from the resting value of approximately 0.8, to 1.0 or more. In subjects with healthy lungs the consumption of oxygen at this point provides a good guide to the capacity for exercise (35). Owles' point occurs at a relatively low consumption of oxygen in unfit subjects and those whose body dimensions do not permit a high capacity for exercise. It occurs at a high level in subjects who are athletic or have undergone physical training.

The relationship of ventilation to tidal volume (Hey plot) is linear up to a tidal volume of approximately half the vital capacity; at higher levels of ventilation the tidal volume is relatively constant or diminishes (fig. 18.2). Any further increase in ventilation minute volume is secured by an increase in respiratory frequency. The relationship may be described in terms of the tidal volume at a minute volume of 30 l min⁻¹ (Vt_{30}). The mean result for an average man is 1.4 (SD 0.22) l. Vt_{30} varies with vital capacity (table 18.2). It is reduced when there is stimulation of juxtacapillary receptors (J receptors) in the lung parenchyma, as occurs in left heart failure and sometimes in beryllium disease (chapter 11); the respiratory frequency is then disproportionately increased (tachypnoea). Exercise tidal volume may also be reduced and respiratory frequency and minute ventilation increased by unfamiliarity with the test procedure, by apprehension and by voluntary rapid breathing; these changes may occur in and invalidate an assessment of disablement (q.v.). In some circumstances tachypnoea is an indication that the subject will benefit from physical training.

Cardiac frequency. The relationship of cardiac frequency to uptake of oxygen is usually linear (fig. 18.2): its extrapolated lower limit at zero uptake of oxygen is in the range 40–80min and its upper limit is maximal cardiac frequency (fC_{max}). Reference values for fC_{max} are given in table 18.2. As in the case of ventilation the relationship may be represented by the cardiac frequency at any designated consumption of oxygen, for example, at 45mmol min^{-1} (1.0 l min^{-1}) when the mean cardiac frequency of the average man is 105 min^{-1} (SD 18) (i.e. fC_{45}=105 min^{-1}). The accuracy of prediction may be improved by taking into account the quantity of body muscle since this partially determines the size of the heart and hence the stroke volume (SV) to which the frequency (fC) is reciprocally related (i.e. $fC=Qt/SV$, where Qt is cardiac output). The muscle may be estimated as fat free mass which is obtained from body mass and measurements of skinfold thickness (chapter 5). The relationship of cardiac frequency to fat free mass is given in table 18.2. Cardiac frequency relative to oxygen uptake (e.g. fC_{45}) declines slightly with increasing age. A low cardiac frequency relative to oxygen uptake, fat free mass and age is usually evidence for a high level of habitual activity, and vice versa. Normal subjects with a relatively high cardiac frequency are likely to benefit from exercise training, but it must be remembered that a rapid pulse on exertion is a feature of heart disease, and of anaemia.

Gas exchange. Gas exchange may be investigated non-invasively during progressive exercise by measuring the transfer factor and the arterial oxygen saturation. The transfer factor (chapter 5) on average increases by approximately 20% between rest and an oxygen uptake of 45mmol min^{-1} but fails to do so when the pulmonary vascular bed is restricted, as in some cases of diffuse interstitial fibrosis (8). The arterial oxygen saturation falls during exercise in subjects in whom there is defective gas transfer, such as patients with asbestosis (fig. 18.6). The desaturation is partially corrected by a consequent increase in ventilation which raises the oxygen tension in alveolar gas; desaturation is most conspicuous in patients with a below average ventilatory response. The saturation may be measured by an ear oximeter. Direct measurement of gas tensions by sampling and analysis of arterial blood reduces the acceptability of the procedure and is seldom justifiable.

Exercise limitation (see also Respiratory Disablement below). Unpleasant symptoms may cause the subject to stop exercising or the operator may terminate the test because of abnormal signs (described under maximal exercise above) or because the rate of work or other index has reached a predetermined target. An appropriate end-point for the test is the attainment of 80% of $\dot{n}O_2$max estimated from heart rate as this is adequate for revealing latent ischaemic heart disease by electrocardiography. Progression towards this work rate can be monitored by observing the cardiac frequency as it approaches the reference value (table 18.2). Alternative end-points are a cardiac frequency of 150min^{-1}, an oxygen uptake of 22, 45 or 67mmol min^{-1} (0.5–1.5 l min^{-1}), a respiratory exchange ratio of unity ($R=1.0$) or, during cycle ergometry, a specified work rate, for example, 100W. The subsequent report should describe clearly what symptoms were experienced and why the exercise was discontinued. If appropriate a segment of the electrocardiogram should be included. Scores for breathlessness (considered below) and for perceived exertion (table 18.6, page 392) should also be reported.

Respiratory disablement

Definitions

These definitions are based on recommendations of WHO (37) in preference to other schemes, of which some are reviewed elsewhere (1, 14).

Respiratory impairment. Inhaled dusts and vapours and pathological conditions of the lung impair its function; the attributes which may be affected include production and clearance of secretions, airways calibre, gas exchange, respiratory control and musculo-skeletal function. Any such abnormalities constitute respiratory impairment. They can be assessed in terms of specific symptoms such as cough, production of sputum and wheeze or as changes in lung function; the techniques for assessment are described in chapter 5. The impairment is a cause of 'loss of faculty' under the U.K. Social Security Act of 1975 (chapter 1).

Respiratory disablement. During activity a person with respiratory impairment experiences breathlessness on exertion or has a reduced exercise performance as a result of persistent cough or related symptom. The loss of performance constitutes respiratory disablement. It is assessed in terms of exercise capacity. The rating of disablement and methods for its assessment are considered below.

Respiratory handicap. Respiratory disablement may be a social disadvantage with respect to (1) social intercourse, which may be affected by productive cough or wheeze, (2) recreation, which may be affected by breathlessness, or (3) employment, which may be affected by these or other factors. The social disadvantage consti-

tutes a respiratory handicap. However it should be noted that handicap may occur without disability. For example, a radiographic abnormality, such as progressive massive fibrosis in coal miners, may indicate that a change of work is advisable even in the absence of symptoms. Conversely disablement may occur without handicap in the case of a person of sedentary inclination whose maximal exercise performance is reduced by respiratory impairment without this encroaching on his normal activities. For a given level of impairment the handicap varies directly with age and with the physical requirements of employment, the journey to work or leisure pursuits; it usually varies inversely with educational attainment and financial status (11).

Disablement due to impaired lung function

Respiratory impairment is considered in chapter 5 (page 101). The impairments which contribute most to respiratory disablement are a reduced ventilatory capacity, usually recorded as the forced expiratory volume (FEV_1, page 93), and an increased ventilatory cost of exercise, represented by the ventilation at an oxygen uptake of 45mmol min^{-1} ($\dot{V}_{E45}$). The FEV_1 is reduced by airflow obstruction; this has a greater effect

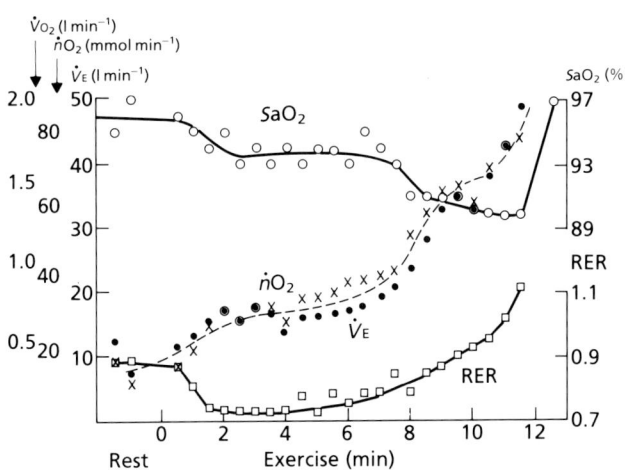

Fig. 18.6. Ergometry. Ventilation minute volume ($\dot{V}_E$, ●), oxygen consumption ($\dot{n}O_2$, ×), oxygen saturation (SaO_2, ○) and respiratory exchange ratio (RER, □) during progressive exercise in a 53-year-old lagger with mild asbestosis. His transfer factor was 75% of expected and he had moderately severe airflow obstruction. Onset of desaturation coincided with a material increase in oxygen consumption. The desaturation would have been greater but for a consequent increase in ventilation and hence in respiratory exchange ratio. The saturation returned to normal within 1min of the end of exercise.

upon exercise capacity than the same loss of FEV_1 as a consequence of reduced lung expansion. Obstruction which is largely confined to expiration, as occurs in emphysema, is usually less disabling than the same loss of ventilatory capacity, due to chronic bronchitis, in which the airway narrowing reduces the flow rates during inspiration as well. Conversely the $\dot{V}_{E45}$ is usually increased relatively more by defective gas transfer leading to hypoxaemia which is confined to exercise than by ventilation perfusion inequality, in which the hypoxaemia is also present at rest. Voluntary overbreathing and voluntary shallow rapid breathing may simulate these abnormalities, but can be detected by the methods considered below. The extent of respiratory disablement is assessed by measuring the symptom-limited maximal oxygen uptake. This should be appropriate to the subject's respiratory impairment. The appropriateness may be gauged by using the prediction equation for maximal oxygen uptake in terms of FEV_1 and $\dot{V}_{E45}$ given in table 18.2. Despite expectations to the contrary (1) respiratory disablement cannot be assessed accurately from FEV_1 and transfer factor.

The disablement associated with a given loss of lung function increases with age. This increase has two components. Firstly, lung function declines with age so when performing a standard task (for example, walking at 5km h^{-1}) the older person has less reserve capacity than a younger one. Secondly, the internal work done in performing a given task, and hence its oxygen cost, increases with age. As a result the ventilation needed for the performance of the task increases with age. The way these two processes combine to the detriment of the older person is illustrated in fig. 18.7.

Capacity for exercise is influenced not only by impairment of lung function but also by the state

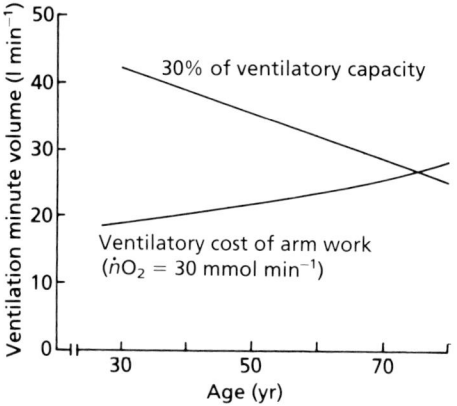

Fig. 18.7. Ventilatory capacity and ventilatory cost of exercise as a function of age in healthy men. The displayed ventilatory capacity is 30% of maximal breathing capacity calculated from FEV_1 and the ventilatory cost of exercise is for arm work requiring an uptake of oxygen of 30mmol min^{-1}. With increasing age, the ventilatory capacity decreases but the ventilatory cost of exercise rises. The changes lead to age-related breathlessness with consequent loss of exercise capacity despite the lung function and ventilatory response to exercise remaining 'normal' throughout. (Source: Cotes (11).)

Table 18.8. Equation for estimating $\dot{n}O_2$max (mmol min^{-1}) in healthy men from the results of submaximal cycle ergometry (for l min^{-1} divide by 44.6). (Source: Weller et al, 36.)

$$\dot{n}O_2\text{max} = 70.1 + 0.63\dot{n}O_2 \text{ at } R_{1.0} \text{ (mmol min}^{-1})$$
$$+ 0.78 \text{ fat free mass (kg)}$$
$$- 0.29\ f_{C45}(\text{min}^{-1})$$
$$- 0.86\% \text{ fat}$$

Standard error of estimate 12.0mmol min^{-1}
Coefficient of variation 9.0%

Table 18.7. Submaximal tests of physical fitness (31)

Ergometer	Setting	Duration	Index
Treadmill	80m per min	6min	f_C in 6th min
Step	Height 32cm	6min	f_C in 6th min
Cycle	100W, 125W, 150W	2min × 3	Work rate at f_C=150 per min

f_C=cardiac frequency.

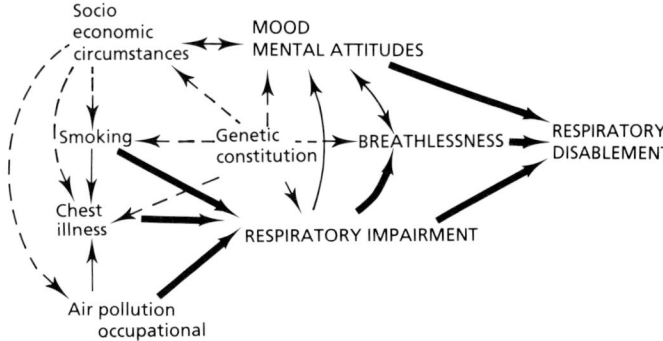

DETERMINANTS OF RESPIRATORY DISABLEMENT

Fig. 18.8. Diagram indicating the many intrinsic and environmental factors which can contribute to respiratory disablement. Some of the factors are discussed in Chapter 17.

of physical training, by the proportion of body mass which is fat rather than muscle and by some other variables. Thus, after allowing for FEV_1 and $\dot{V}_{E45}$ the maximal oxygen uptake of patients with chronic lung disease shows a significant positive correlation with fat free mass and a negative correlation with cardiac frequency during moderate exercise (fC_{45}) (19). Partly for this reason the correlation between loss of ventilatory ability (e.g. FEV_1) and the extent of breathlessness is weak. Some contributory factors are indicated in table 18.9. An important one not shown in the table is the mental attitude of the subject to his illness, his health generally and the treatment which he is receiving. For a given level of respiratory impairment a hopeful attitude is associated with a higher exercise capacity than a pessimistic one (26, 34). The mental attitude is the outcome of interaction between the personality and personal experience of ill-health (fig. 18.8). As with other factors which contribute to breathlessness the mental attitudes exhibit large differences between subjects. For this reason, unless fully allowed for, they contribute to the scatter in

cross-sectional analyses. Their effect is less in longitudinal studies in which changes within individuals are examined. Thus, when a change in breathlessness occurred in a group of coal miners it was usually highly correlated with a change in body fat, vital capacity, and some indices derived from an exercise test (table 18.10).

Methods of assessing ability to take exercise

Questionnaire. Questions about habitual activity may be added to the questionnaire on respiratory symptoms. They should include both the activities associated with work (e.g. getting to work) and leisure-time activities; intensity of effort and duration or number of episodes per week should be recorded. The information may be rated on a 4-point scale reflecting minimal active, below and above average active and a high level of activity such as is associated with participation in competitive sport. In a recent study, after allowing for physical dimensions and body composition, the

Table 18.9. Indices which describe clinical grade of breathlessness of 601 shipyard workers

Clinical grade = $0.55 + 0.02$ age $+ 3 \times 10^{-4}$ age^2 $- 0.53$ FEV_1
The grade was increased if the subject had angina ($+ 1.07$), chronic bronchitis ($+ 0.73$)
or a history of previous pneumonia ($+ 0.22$).
On average there was also an increase associated with exposure to welding fumes.

Data of Cotes, Feinmann, Male, Rennie and El Gamal.

Table 18.10.   Variables from multiple regression analysis which describe the change in grade of breathlessness over 9 years of 111 coal-miners.
(Arrows indicate direction of change associated with an increase in grade of breathlessness.)

(a) Full assessment		(b) Simple assessment	
maximal O_2 consumption	↓	body mass	↑
K_{CO}	↓	forced vital capacity	↓
tidal volume on maximal exercise	↑	bronchitis score	↑
forced vital capacity	↓		
body mass	↑		
Variance accounted for: 85%		Variance accounted for: 73%	

Source: Musk *et al* (27).

activity score contributed significantly to description of maximal oxygen uptake (table 18.8).

Visual analogue scale. The simplest visual analogue scale is a 10cm line representing the range of variation of the quantity which is being considered, in this case exercise capacity or breathlessness. The ends of the line represent the lower and upper limits, for example, 'confined to bed' to 'can run mile in 4min', or 'not breathless' to 'extremely breathless'. The subject indicates the point on the line which describes his own circumstances. The procedure can be carried out at interview or, in the case of breathlessness, at the end of exercise. It can also be done each minute during exercise by means of a visual display controlled from the ergometer. The method may be made more specific by adding a descriptive scale as in fig. 18.9.

Descriptive rating scales. A descriptive rating scale lists a series of alternatives in order of progressively increasing abnormality or normality. The former constitutes a disability scale of which the best known is the clinical grades of breathlessness of Fletcher; these form part of the MRC Questionnaire of Respiratory Symptoms (chapter 5). The subject is asked to compare his or her ability to take exercise with that of a healthy person of the same age. The continuity of the scale breaks down when there is notable disablement. The alternative is an ability scale which describes what the subject can do rather than what he cannot. In practice the two approaches may be combined as is done in table 18.11. The ability scale may be amplified in many ways; an example is given below.

The score for ability or disability is usually obtained by the subject replying to questions.

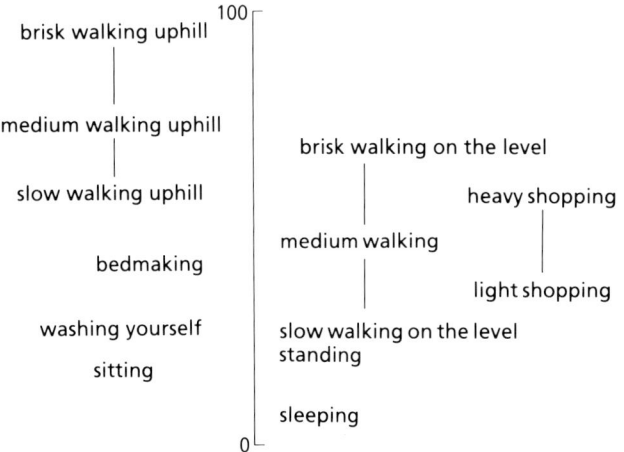

Fig. 18.9. Diagram for rating the ability to take exercise. The subject marks the central vertical line at what he considers to be the appropriate point; the ability score is the distance in cm from the origin (0). (By courtesy of McGavin *et al* (25).)

Table 18.11. Clinical grade of breathlessness, ability score and average FEV_1 of men with chronic lung disease (11)

Description	Clinical grade	Ability score	FEV_1
Is living: needs help with feeding	—	8	0.3
With help can dress and sit out of bed	—	7	0.5
Can converse, walk 10m, bath with help	—	6	0.7
Can walk 100m, sing, climb eight stairs	—	5	1.1
Can walk 400m	4	4	1.6
Can walk unlimited distance at slow pace	3	3	2.1
Can walk at normal pace on level ground without becoming breathless	2	2	2.6
Can hurry on level ground and walk uphill without undue breathlessness	1	1	3.1

There is wide individual variation reflecting motivation, age and other factors (table 18.9 and fig. 18.11).

Alternatively it may be based on direct observations of the person at home or in other circumstances, for example getting to or from the place of assessment. This can provide a lower limit for the estimated ability. The respiratory component of the score can also be predicted from the lung function either alone (table 18.12) or in combination with other variables (table 18.2). The validity to this approach has been discussed above; it is obviously invalid if cardiovascular disease, anaemia, arthritis or muscular weakness contribute to the total disability.

Ergometry. The direct measurement of exercise ability by ergometry is technically straightforward. In practice the measurement presents few difficulties for the person with respiratory impairment whose exercise is limited by breathlessness and who is prepared to do his best. The end point is incapacitating breathlessness which may be confirmed by observing and conversing with the subject, by a visual analogue scale and by comparing the maximal exercise ventilation ($\dot{V}_E$max ex) with the maximal breathing capacity (MBC); the latter may be estimated from FEV_1 (table 18.2). The ratio $\dot{V}_E$max/MBC is the dyspnoeic index which, at the breaking point, should approach or, in the case of patients with a very low FEV_1, slightly exceed 100%. Alternatively a reference value for $\dot{V}_E$max may be obtained from FEV_1 or from FEV_1 and peak respiratory flow rate (21). This is done in fig. 18.10 where the confidence limits indicate the range of values in persons who were breathless at the point of discontinuing exercise. Lower levels of $\dot{V}_E$max are almost always evidence for exercise being limited by some factor other than breathlessness; however, the possibility that in some persons the limitation reflects an increased responsiveness to all potentially noxious stimuli merits fuller investigation (32).

Table 18.12. Criteria for severe respiratory impairment* (Source: Epler *et al* (22) *see also* table 5.11, page 103)

	Index	%predicted	Av. value†
Chronic airflow obstruction	FEV	<40%	1.25l
Interstitial lung disease	FVC and Tl_{CO}	<50% <40%	2.0l 3.6mmol min^{-1} kPa^{-1} 11ml min^{-1} mmHg^{-1}

* Severe breathlessness during walking 216m in 4min.
† Man age 55 years, height 1.72m.

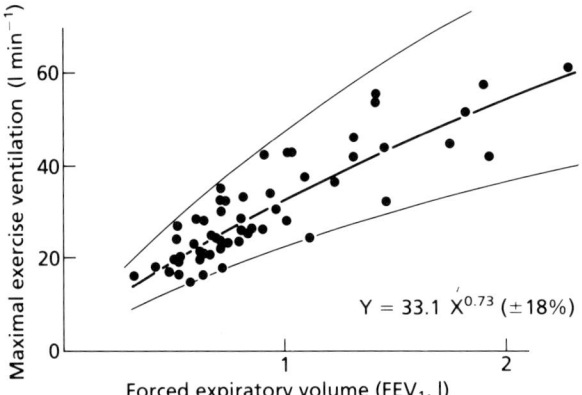

Fig. 18.10. Relationship of maximal exercise ventilation to forced expiratory volume for well-motivated patients with chronic lung disease. In patients not limited by breathlessness or in whom motivation is suspect the ventilation is often below the lower confidence limit. (Source: Cotes *et al* (19).)

Recovery from breathlessness due to respiratory impairment occurs within 5min, so the procedure is usually quite acceptable to the respiratory patient. It may be combined with measuring the physiological response to submaximal exercise which provides potentially useful additional information. Difficulty is experienced if the subject coughs or expectorates during the test, reports breathlessness prematurely, complains that he cannot get air into the chest, or alters the rate and depth of breathing by voluntary action; an inappropriate pattern of breathing may be detected by using the relationship of ventilation to tidal volume (Hey plot) which is illustrated in fig. 18.2 and the relationship of tidal volume at a ventilation of 30 l min^{-1} to vital capacity which is given in table 18.2. Voluntary hyperventilation may be detected from the relationship of ventilation to oxygen uptake (fig. 18.2); a high initial ventilation which subsequently reverts towards normal is diagnostic. In addition the respiratory exchange ratio is increased compared with the reference value (table 18.2). If the ratio rises steeply during exercise this may be due to voluntary overbreathing or to hypoxaemia secondary to defective gas transfer; the latter may be recognized by use of an ear oximeter to measure the arterial oxygen saturation and by repeating the test during breathing oxygen. Where the disturbance to breathing is confined to the last few minutes of exercise the maximal oxygen uptake may be estimated from the ventilation during submaximal exercise

($\dot{V}_{E45}$) and the forced expiratory volume (table 18.2).

In contrast to persons with respiratory impairment, who are limited by respiratory factors, most other subjects are limited by the capabilities of the cardiovascular system. The exercise capacity is obtained as maximal oxygen uptake ($\dot{n}O_2$max); this is either determined by direct measurement or estimated using a submaximal test of physical fitness (page 393). The directly measured value should meet the criteria given on page 390; where it does not the limitation is usually associated with symptoms, for example fatigue, dizziness, palpitations or those given above. The validity of the result should be assessed in the light of these and other features of the case. Interpretation of the result is more difficult when the $\dot{n}O_2$max is estimated from other variables since their measurement provides further stages at which error may be introduced (see below).

Disablement ratings. Disablement may be rated as 100% if the subject is unable to double his resting oxygen uptake. It is zero if the subject is normally asymptomatic or is able to attain his or her predicted maximal oxygen uptake. Grading for intermediate levels of exercise ability may be expressed on a disability scale as a percentage of the reference value (table 18.5). For subjects limited by respiratory symptoms the numerator is symptom-limited $\dot{n}O_2$max; otherwise it is the value calculated from FEV_1 and $\dot{V}_{E45}$ (table 18.2). The percent disablement is of limited usefulness (e.g. fig. 18.7). It is not closely related to the lung function or to the rating for respiratory impairment (table 5.11, page 103). Alternatively the oxygen uptake may be scored on an ability scale and related to the oxygen cost of the activities which the subject might wish to undertake; some costs are illustrated in fig. 18.11. Over an 8h shift a normal person, in whom exercise is circulation limited, is able to sustain 40% of the observed maximal oxygen uptake (2). This percentage appears not to apply to subjects with respiratory limitation; it is probably higher and also related to the level of respiratory impairment. The topic merits further research.

Relation to compensation

The assessment of disablement is of great value when considering fitness for employment, a change of job, re-employment or rehabilitation. It is also widely used as a basis for industrial injuries benefit. For this application the disablement is only one component of the assessment which is likely to include the extent of respiratory impairment, the respiratory handicap and an assessment of prognosis. The prognosis is mainly determined by the underlying disease process, but is also related to the extent of the loss of function and the level of pulmonary arterial pressure. The indices of lung function

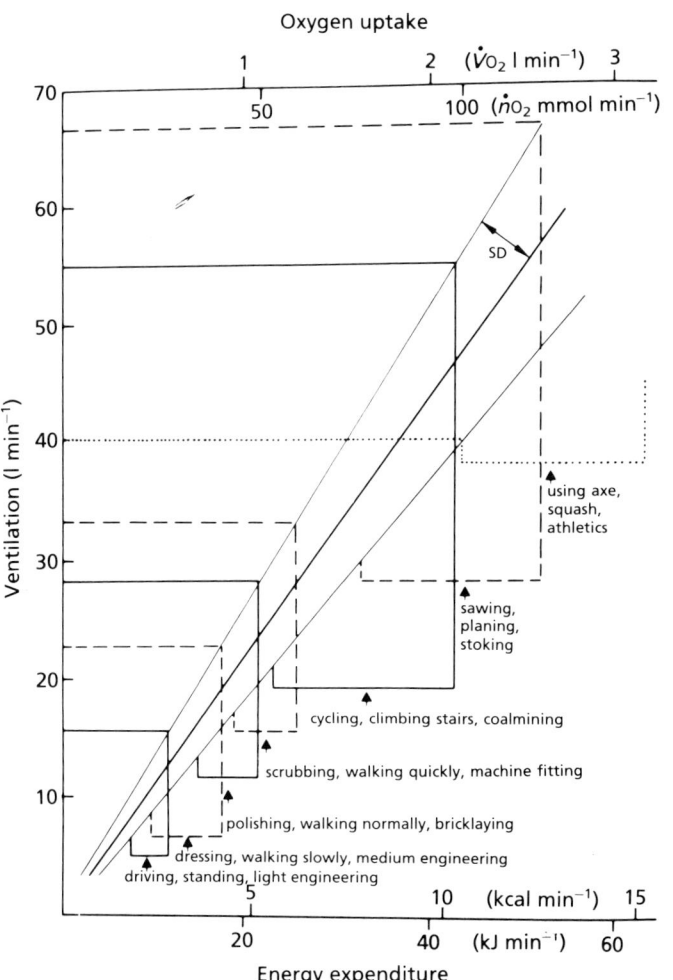

Fig. 18.11. Average energy and ventilatory costs of activities for healthy men. In women the ventilatory costs are similar but the energy costs are approximately 10% lower. Ventilation is increased by age, smoking, respiratory symptoms and other factors; it is below average in persons who are physically fit. (Source: Cotes (12).)

which are informative are those affected by the disease and by airflow obstruction or other change due to secondary involvement of lung airways. In the early and intermediate stages the prognosis is related to grade of breathlessness whilst in the later stages this role is taken on by the capacity for exercise, arterial oxygen tension, pulmonary arterial blood pressure and presence of hypercapnia during exercise breathing oxygen (13).

All persons coming to the laboratory for the first time are more or less anxious or apprehensive and this can influence their performance of lung function and exercise tests. Claimants for compensation are, perhaps, more prone to anxiety than others. Much depends on their presenting an adequate account of their condition and so they tend to brood on their symptoms and any associated grievance. The resultant anxiety can cause a genuine deterioration of their initial illness, especially of the intensity of dyspnoea. It can also lead to a conscious or unconscious lack of co-operation in the performance of function tests and this affects the results. It is, therefore, important that the technician who supervises the tests should gain the trust of the subject and should administer the tests with a subtle blend of sympathy and authority. It is equally important that the doctor who interprets the results should be aware of the effects of imperfect co-operation. He should suspect faulty co-operation when the results of one test are inconsistent with those of another. When tests are correctly performed the vital capacity manoeuvres undertaken in the course of measurement of the ventilatory capacity, lung volumes, transfer factor and lung compliance should bear a sensible relationship to each other and to the tidal volume during exercise (table 18.2). There should be reasonable consistency in the minute by minute results which make up the four index tests during exercise (fig. 18.2). The maximal exercise ventilation should be appropriate for the level of FEV_1 (fig. 18.9) and the respiratory exchange ratio should not be unduly high, but it should not be forgotten that these last two are affected by heart disease, anaemia and a transfer defect. Moreover the symptoms, clinical signs, function tests and performance of exercise should be consistent with one another (e.g. fig. 18.12). Inconsistency is the basis for the clinical impression of 'functional overlay', so well known to the astute physician. These considerations suggest that the physiological assessment should form part of a medical consultation and not take place at a tribunal. At a consultation it is possible to discuss with the patient how the findings of his assessment can be used to promote his health or to select suitable employment. It is very desirable to do this, and thus to build up the patient's confidence and obtain his full co-operation. Some of the steps which may be taken to help the patient are described in the next chapter.

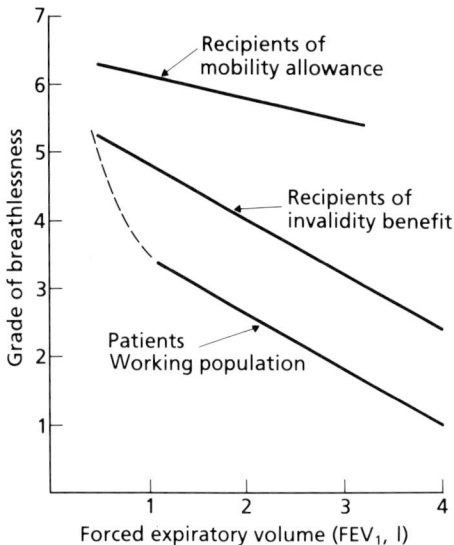

Fig. 18.12. Relationship of grade of breathlessness to forced expiratory volume for men receiving allowances on account of chronic bronchitis and/or emphysema, compared with coal miners attending hospital as patients and with men assessed during a survey of shipyard workers. Many of the claimants had disproportionate breathlessness. (Data of Pearce *et al* (30) and unpublished.)

References

1 American Thoracic Society. Evaluation of impairment/disability secondary to respiratory disorders. *Am Rev Resp Dis* 1986;**133**:1205–9.
2 Åstrand PO, Rodahl K. *Textbook of Work Physiology*, 2nd edition. London: McGraw-Hill: 1977.

3 Blackburn H, Taylor HL, Okamoto N, Rautaharj
   P, Mitchell PL, Kirkhof AC. Standardisation of
   the exercise electrocardiogram. A systematic
   comparison of chest lead configurations
   employed for monitoring during exercise. In:
   Physical activity and the heart: proceedings.
   Karvonen MJ, Barry AJ (Eds), Springfield, Ill:
   Thomas. 1967:101–33.

4 Borg G. Psychological aspects of physical
   activities. In: *Fitness, Health and Work Capacity*. Larson LA (Ed). New York: Macmillan:
   1974:141.

5 Brown A, Cotes JE, Mortimore IL, Reed JW. An
   exercise training programme for firemen. *Ergonomics* 1982;**25**:793–800.

6 Bruce RA, Kusumi F, Hosmer D. Maximal oxygen intake and nomographic assessment of
   functional aerobic impairment in cardiovascular disease. *Am Heart J* 1973;**85**:546–62.

7 Butland RJA, Pang J, Gross ER, Woodcock AA,
   Geddes DM. Two-, six-, and 12-minute walking
   tests in respiratory disease. *Br Med J* 1982;
   284:1607–8.

8 Chu SS, Cotes JE. Lung transfer factor and Kco
   at cardiac frequency 100 beats/min as a guide to
   impaired function of lung parenchyma. *Thorax*
   1984;**39**:524–8.

9 Cockcroft AE, Saunders MJ, Berry G. Ran-
   domised controlled trial of rehabilitation in
   chronic respiratory disability. *Thorax* 1981;**36**:
   200–3.

10 Cotes JE. Response to progressive exercise: a
   three-index test. *Br J Dis Chest* 1972;**66**:169–84.

11 Cotes JE. Assessment of disablement due to
   impaired respiratory function. *Bull Eur Physiopath Resp* 1975;**11**:210P–17P.

12 Cotes JE. The ventilatory cost of activity. *Br J
   Industr Med* 1975;**32**:220–3.

13 Cotes JE. *Lung Function*, 4th edn. Oxford:
   Blackwell Scientific Publications, 1979.

14 Cotes JE. Respiratory disablement: problems
   and opportunities. *J Soc Occup Med* 1983;**33**:
   5–12.

15 Cotes JE. Exercise fitness of divers. *Proceedings
   of Symposium on Fitness to Dive*, Institute of
   Environmental and Offshore Medicine, University of Aberdeen: 1984.

16 Cotes JE, Berry G, Burkinshaw L, Davies CTM,
   Hall AM, Jones PRM, Knibbs AV. Cardiac frequency during submaximal exercise in young
   adults: relation to lean body mass, total body
   potassium and amount of leg muscle. *Quart J
   Exp Physiol* 1973;**58**:239–50.

17 Cotes JE, Dicken C, Evans DL, Johnson GR,
   Kalinowska EB, MacIntyre IM, Saunders MJ.
   Prediction of Harvard pack index from the
   result of an 11 min progressive exercise test and
   anthropometric measurements in coalminers.
   Ergonomics 1979;**22**:1353–61.

18 Cotes JE, Feinmann EL, Male VJ, Rennie F.
   Respiratory health of shipyard workers. *Thorax*
   1984;**39**:691(Abstract).

19 Cotes JE, Posner V, Reed JW. Estimation of
   maximal exercise ventilation and oxygen
   uptake in patients with chronic lung disease.
   Bull Europ Physiopathol Respir 1982;**18**(Suppl
   4):221–8.

20 Cotes JE, Reed JW, Mortimore IL. Determinants
   of capacity for physical work. In: *Energy and
   Effort*. Harrison GA (ed). London: Taylor and
   Francis: 1982;**22**:39–64.

21 Dillard TA, Piantadosi S, Rajagopal KR. Prediction of ventilation at maximal exercise in chronic air-flow obstruction. *Am Rev Respir Dis*
   1985;**132**:230–5.

22 Epler GR, Saber FA, Gaensler EA. Determination of severe impairment (disability) in
   interstitial lung disease. *Am Rev Resp Dis*
   1980;**121**:647–59.

23 Jones NL, Makrides L, Hitchcock C, Chypchar
   T, McCartney N. Normal standards for an
   incremental progressive cycle ergometer test.
   Am Rev Respir Dis 1985;**131**:700–8.

24 Keen EN, Sloan AW. Observations on the Harvard step test. *J Appl Physiol* 1958;**13**:241–3.

25 McGavin CR, Artvinli M, Naoe H, McHardy
   GJR. Dyspnoea, disability and distance walked:
   comparison of estimates of exercise performance in respiratory disease. *Br Med J*
   1978;**ii**:241–3.

26 Morgan AD, Peck DF, Buchanan DR, McHardy
   GJR. Effects of attitudes and beliefs on exercise
   tolerance in chronic bronchitis. *Br Med J*
   1983;**286**:171–3.

27 Musk AW, Bevan C, Campbell MJ, Cotes JE.
   Factors contributing to the clinical grade of
   breathlessness in coalworkers with pneumoconiosis. *Bull Eur Physiopathol Respir* 1979;**15**:
   343–55.

28 Nagle FJ, Balke B, Naughton JP. Gradational
   step tests for assessing work capacity. *J Appl
   Physiol* 1965;**20**:745–8.

29 Patrick JM, Bassey EJ, Fentem PH. The rising ventilatory cost of bicycle exercise in the seventh decade: a longitudinal study of nine healthy men. *Clin Sci* 1983;**65**:521–6.

30 Pearce SJ, Posner V, Robinson AJ, Barton JR, Cotes JE. "Invalidity" due to chronic bronchitis and emphysema: how real is it? *Thorax* 1985;**40**:828–31.

31 Robertshaw SA, Reed JW, Mortimore IL, Cotes JE Afacan AS, Grogan JB. Submaximal alternatives to the Harvard Pack index as guides to maximal oxygen uptake (physical fitness). *Ergonomics* 1984;**27**:177–85.

32 Rosser R, Guz A. Psychological approaches to breathlessness and its treatment. *J Psychosom Res* 1981;**25**:439–47.

33 Shephard RJ. *Human Physiological Work Capacity (IBP 15).* Cambridge: University Press: 1978.

34 Sprake CM, Cotes JE, Reed JW. Correlates of 6 min walking distance and maximal oxygen uptake in chronic lung disease. *Clin Sci* 1984;**66**:57P.

35 Wasserman K, Whipp BJ, Koyal SN, Beaver WL. Anaerobic threshold and respiratory gas exchange during exercise. *J Appl Physiol* 1973;**35**:236–43.

36 Weller JJ, El-Gamal FM, Parker L, Reed JW, Bridges NG, Chinn DJ, Cotes JE. Estimating the capacity for exercise of shipyard workers. *Clin Sci* 1985;**68**:(Suppl 11):45P. (Abstract).

37 World Health Organisation. *International Classification of Impairments, Disabilities and Handicaps.* Geneva: WHO: 1980.

Chapter 19
Management of Respiratory Impairment

Early diagnosis
Medical treatment
Aids to increased activity
Re-employment

Early diagnosis

Both occupational lung diseases and chronic bronchitis usually develop insidiously and they may occur together. Unfortunately both conditions are commonly regarded as being untreatable except perhaps by changing jobs or abandoning smoking and this advice is often unwelcome; thus the request for medical help is frequently deferred. This pessimistic attitude to occupational lung disease should be abandoned because much can be done to help. For example, early diagnosis often permits arrest or reversal of respiratory impairment and, if a change of job is essential, early diagnosis enables the change to be made without duress and at a convenient time.

Medical treatment

Occupational lung disease may be identified by a regular surveillance programme; this will probably include chest radiography or serial measurement of forced expiratory volume. A condition diagnosed in this way is usually asymptomatic. Alternatively, occupational disease may be suspected from the development of respiratory symptoms (for example, breathlessness on exertion) or from chest illness leading to loss of time from work. The illness is likely to be managed by the general practitioner but its occurrence should lead the works medical department to investigate the circumstances. The medical condition may be due directly to the occupational exposure, to a known complication (for example, lung cancer in a person previously exposed to asbestos), or to chronic bronchitis, emphysema or asthma. Chronic bronchitis is usually a consequence of smoking but may be aggravated by the occupational exposure or form part of occupational lung disease (chapter 17). Emphysema is seldom of occupational origin except in coalworkers with pneumoconiosis, whilst asthma may be occupational or not, depending on circumstances. The diagnosis, including the likely aetiology, will be made by clinical examination supplemented by chest radiography, assessment of lung function, environmental monitoring or inhalation challenge; the methods are described in preceding chapters.

Early diagnosis is of the greatest importance and a major responsibility of the occupational physician. The diagnosis should lead to action under one or more of the headings which are listed below. In addition, specific treatment should be administered where appropriate such as for extrinsic allergic alveolitis, beryllium disease or occupational asthma. These aspects are discussed in the chapters describing the conditions. The present chapter reviews the general management of chronic chest illness, whether occupationally related or not. It is based on a report of a working party of the Royal College of Physicians (2); this should be consulted for further details and references.

Clean air. The first principle of treatment is to ensure that the patient is not exposed to air containing contaminants which can readily be removed or avoided. At the work place this is achieved by controlling occupational air pollution, providing a no smoking zone and, if the patient is a smoker, persuading him to abandon the habit. In many circumstances, if this advice is followed, the medical condition will improve considerably, even in the absence of other measures. Outside working hours the patient should avoid contaminated atmospheres, including tobacco smoke in public rooms or single-decker buses where smoking is permitted, fumes from a poorly controlled domestic fire or stove or irritant gases from hot ash.

Bronchodilation. Obstruction to airflow is the principle cause of breathlessness in most patients with occupational lung disease. Much of it is irreversible but there is usually a reversible component, especially in patients who also have chronic cough and expectoration or regular wheeze. The identification and relief of this reversible airflow obstruction is an essential component of treatment. Reversibility should be assessed using a selective β-adrenergic stimulant drug given by inhalation. An improvement in FEV_1 or related index of 10% after 10–60min is an indication for continued therapy. Further improvement in ventilatory function or exercise performance may occur over several weeks of regular medication. This may take the form of salbutamol, terbutaline or other similar preparation given as an aerosol every 4h. An inadequate response to beta-agonists should lead to a similar trial of a corticosteroid drug, usually prednisolone 40mg daily for 1–3 weeks with subsequent withdrawal (fig. 19.1). If the trial is successful it should be followed by a trial of steroids by inhalation–beclomethasone dipropionate as four inhalations each of 50µg twice daily or betamethasone valerate in twice this dose. Subsequent dosage should be adjusted to secure clinical benefit without complications.

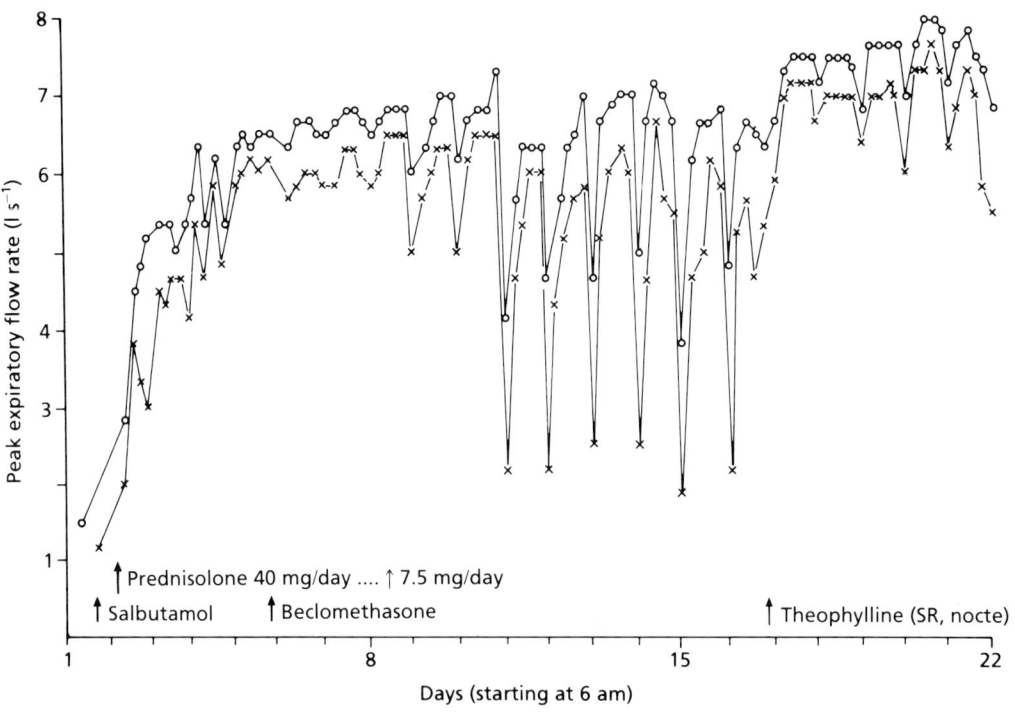

Fig. 19.1. Serial measurements of peak expiratory flow rate over 3 weeks, showing stages in the establishment of a suitable bronchodilator regimen in a patient with severe airflow limitation. Salbutamol by inhalation only had a small effect (indicated by distance between the two lines). The condition responded to oral prednisolone in high dosage. Changing to maintenance dose plus inhaled beclomethasone resulted in loss of control, which was re-established when an evening dose of slow release theophylline was added to the regimen. (By courtesy of S. J. Pearce.)

Ipratropium bromide is an atropine analogue drug which is locally active after inhalation and, in the dosage 20μg every 4h, is often of value for patients with chronic obstructive bronchitis, either in preference or in addition to a β stimulant. A slow release theophylline preparation such as aminophylline in the dosage 10–15mg per kg per day is sometimes also useful. Sodium cromoglycate may be of use for subjects with variable airways obstruction, especially exercise-induced asthma. The dosage may then be 20mg by inhalation up to six times daily. The use of this drug in patients with occupational asthma is considered on page 360.

The drugs are normally administered as aerosols or small particles from a suitable dispenser and adequate instruction should be given in its use. This should usually include a practical demonstration with a dummy dispenser. The operator breathes out to residual volume, inserts the nozzle between the lips, activates the mechanism and takes a full inspiration to total lung capacity. The breath is then held for a few seconds. Neglect of this technique, which is usually due to inadequate demonstration, is a very common cause of treatment failure. Alternative methods and appliances for ensuring efficient inhalation are available for the subject who cannot or will not use an aerosol properly. The old and disabled have particular problems in this respect.

Control of infection. Acute exacerbations of chest illness occur during the course of chronic lung disease but their cause is often obscure and not associated with obvious bacterial infections. Chemotherapy is needed in only that minority of episodes which are characterized by fever, leucocytosis, radiographic consolidation and mucopurulent sputum containing drug-sensitive organisms. Patients with recurrent episodes should be supplied with a reserve course of antibiotics, to take at the onset of infection, before they have made contact with their general practitioners. In addition there is sometimes a case for low dose prophylactic anti-bacterial chemotherapy to be taken at the start of a common cold with a view to preventing secondary bacterial infection. Continuous prophylactic chemotherapy is seldom effective; it should be replaced by reserve course chemotherapy,

except possibly for the few patients who under supervision benefit from early treatment but left to their own devices fail to start the tablets in time. Immunoprophylaxis by vaccination provides some protection against influenza. It should be administered in the form of killed flu vaccine to patients with seriously impaired lung function in order to prevent acute exacerbation. Immunization against other organisms is not yet satisfactory.

Clearing secretions. Patients who produce much sputum or who have difficulty with expectoration may be helped by one of several forms of physiotherapy which, after instruction, may be carried out at home. Probably the most useful is controlled coughing in which the subject performs a series of controlled coughs (huffs) starting from full inspiration. The huffs may be augmented by external chest compression and interspersed with relaxed breathing. The procedure may be combined with postural drainage and should be performed under conditions of full bronchodilation. Very breathless patients are often helped by breathing oxygen via nasal cannulae during the manoeuvres.

Other procedures which some patients find help them to clear secretions are intermittent positive pressure breathing and use of mucolytic drugs, but their use does not benefit the majority.

Oxygen therapy

Acute exacerbation. An acute chest illness may be accompanied by material hypoxaemia: this has a number of adverse consequences including raising the pulmonary vascular resistance, interfering with the conducting system of the heart and affecting gastro-intestinal, renal and central nervous function. On this account an arterial oxygen tension of 6.5kPa (50mmHg) or less is an indication for administering oxygen in low dosage, e.g. 2 l min^{-1} by nasal prongs or Edinburgh mask, or with a 24% or 28% Ventimask. All such patients should be admitted to hospital because a watch should be kept for hypoventilation, preferably by repeated blood gas analysis. If severe respiratory acidosis develops (e.g. arterial pH below 7.25, or [H$^+$] above 56nmol l^{-1}), there is a small place for respiratory stimulant drugs (e.g. doxapram), or intermittent positive pressure ventilation to supplement the primary treatment. However, particularly when the primary condition is pulmonary fibrosis and/or emphysema, the patient's life may be nearly unbearable between exacerbations, in which case he should not be ventilated.

Control of pulmonary hypertension. Pulmonary hypertension occurring in the course of pulmonary fibrosis is usually irreversible and not amenable to treatment. Hypertension may also be due to hypoxaemia secondary to uneven lung function. The hypoxaemia causes persistent pulmonary hypertension by inducing muscular hypertrophy in the walls of small pulmonary arteries. It also gives rise to polycythaemia which aggravates the hypertension and increases the risk of intravascular thrombosis. Sudden death may occur from interference with the conducting system of the heart. These complications of hypoxaemia may be ameliorated by long-term oxygen therapy. The patient takes the oxygen at night and sometimes is able to continue to work during the day. The dosage is 2 or 3 l min^{-1} via nasal cannulae for 15h per 24h day: the treatment is usually best given from an oxygen concentrator (e.g. Rimer-Birlec) as this is an economical source of domiciliary oxygen. Such concentrators are now available through the National Health Service. Specialist assessment is advised before they are prescribed.

Diuretics. Oedema associated with chronic chest disease is usually an indication of cor pulmonale. Frusemide or thiazide diuretics are useful and oxygen may have a synergistic effect in severe hypoxia. Spironolactone given along with a thiazide diuretic is sometimes helpful in resistant cases. Between acute episodes the oedema should be controlled by low dose maintenance therapy.

Aids to increased activity

Weight reduction. The onset of notable breathlessness on exertion often coincides with an increase in body weight which affects directly the energy costs and ventilatory costs of activity. In the absence of heart failure the additional weight is mainly fat and can be removed by dieting, not forgetting control of intake of alcohol and confectionery. All who are overweight should be encouraged to diet and their progress should be monitored by weekly weighing. This may be supplemented by measurement of body fat (chapter 5). Weight reduction in the obese can be guaranteed to produce a significant improvement in exercise tolerance.

Exercise training. The patient with chronic respiratory disability often leads a physically inactive life and becomes unfit in consequence. He then has a lower anaerobic threshold and high ventilatory cost of activity (chapter 18). His physical condition may be improved by exercise training such as walking, cycling, swimming or gymnastics. The exercise should be undertaken for at least 20min per day, 3 days per week for 6 weeks. Thereafter it should be continued in order that the improvement be maintained. Favourable responses include a sense of wellbeing, an increase of approximately 20% in the distance which can be walked in 12min (fig. 19.2) and a lengthening of the stride. There is no material improvement in lung function. Exercise training should preferably be supervised by a physiotherapist or respiratory health worker or be started at a rehabilitation centre, but at present these mainly supervise surgical cases.

Training the respiratory muscles. Recent work suggests that endurance training of the respiratory muscles raises the capacity for exercise by increasing the level of ventilation which can be sustained. The training is performed by breathing against an inspiratory resistance or by voluntary hyperventilation; progress is assessed by measuring the maximal ventilatory capacity over 4min, with carbon dioxide added to the respired gas to avoid hypocapnia. However, further studies are needed to confirm the benefit and to exclude harmful side-effects.

Breathing control. Slow breathing with emphasis on outward displacement of the abdominal wall and lower ribs during inspiration appears to reduce the breathlessness of some patients. However, objective evidence on the effectiveness of this breathing pattern is meagre and contradictory.

Portable oxygen. Oxygen during exercise reduces breathlessness and increases the capacity for exercise of most patients with gross ventilatory impairment (FEV_1 <1.0 l) as well as those whose exercise ventilation is increased by defective gas transfer. Non-smokers are helped to a greater extent than smokers. For use at home the oxygen may be piped from a large cylinder or oxygen concentrator; outside the home use may be made of a portable cylinder or liquid oxygen dispenser which is carried or mounted on a trolley. The flow rate is in the range 2–8 l min^{-1} depending on circumstances, which include whether or not the oxygen which flows during expiration is stored in a reservoir bag for use during the succeeding inspiration. The treatment presents practical difficulties as the equipment is expensive and not all patients benefit; those who do may be identified by a double blind trial of the effect of oxygen upon maximal walking distance. The trial should be carried out before treatment is recommended.

Walking aids. A trolley fitted with three large wheels and arm troughs is a convenient way of transporting oxygen equipment and of taking some weight off the legs. This device materially increases the distance which can be walked on level ground by patients who benefit from breathing oxygen. It may be made by modifying a conventional walking aid.

Re-employment

The onset of chest disease affects employment, particularly if the job is physically demanding, if there is exposure to irritant fumes or gases, or many stairs have to be climbed, or if the journey to work entails exposure to cigarette smoke. Initially the disability may be concealed, as other workers often protect a disabled colleague from the more arduous tasks. When it is obvious that he can no longer do his job the disabled person will have to find lighter work. A large firm can often transfer him to suitable work but small firms can absorb only a very limited number of disabled workers so may have to dismiss him. He may try job after job, frequently taking unsuitable work in an attempt to continue as breadwinner of his family. Sooner or later he may have to accept long-term invalidity benefit by which time it is too late to secure effective rehabilitation. This should be undertaken at the time of the first loss of a job with a view to returning to long-term employment. To this end, advice based on skilled assessment is available in the U.K. from any of the twenty-seven Employment Rehabilitation Centres (ERCs) of the Manpower Services Commission (MSC). The assessment comprises a 6-week course which is directed to improving physical capacity, restoring confidence, and producing a considered and practical recommendation about the type of work likely to lead to permanent resettlement. Approximately 27% of persons who attend on account of respiratory disability secure permanent work whilst some 16% fail to complete the course. Failure is mainly due to prolonged sickness absence resulting from referral being too late in the course of the disease, but inability to acquire new skills is also contributory.

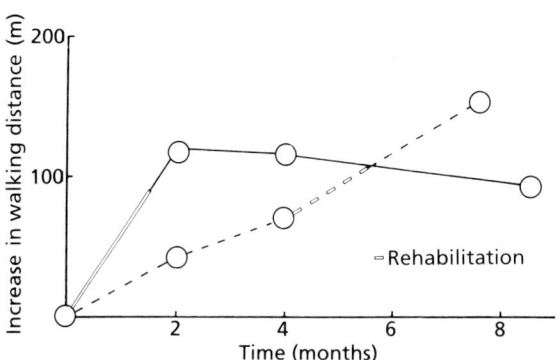

Fig. 19.2. Mean increase in distance walked in 12min by patients in a randomized trial of rehabilitation for chronic respiratory disability. Treatment significantly increased the walking distance and the maximal oxygen uptake, despite patients whose treatment was delayed (interrupted line) voluntarily increasing their level of activity from the time of entering the trial. The mean initial walking distance was 543m. (By courtesy of A. E. Cockcroft and colleagues (1).)

Access to ERCs is through one of the MSC's 50 Disablement Resettlement Officers (DROs) or the Employment Medical Advisor at the ERC. Referrals from all sources are welcomed. About 70% of applicants take up a place. The DROs have a responsibility for finding employment afterwards and ways of increasing their success-rate are now being considered. The Manpower Services Commission also supports sheltered workshops for disabled persons (e.g. Remploy Ltd) and sheltered industrial groups within industrial and commercial firms. It lends specific tools, makes grants for adapting premises, assists with excess fares to work and provides money to help persons registered with the DRO as disabled to set up in business on their own account. There is a job introduction scheme which effectively provides part of a wage for 6 weeks so that the disabled person and the prospective employer can undertake a trial of suitability for long-term employment. Some 60% of those so engaged are still in employment 6 months after the end of their introductory period. Financial support is also provided for full-time residential training at a Skill Centre, College of Further Education or Residential Training College for the Disabled.

The facilities for re-training and re-employment are offered with less enthusiasm to those with respiratory handicap than to other disabled persons. The reasons may include late referral, limited basic education, difficulty in adjusting to work with others who have a more conspicuous handicap, unpredictable attendance and the high concentrations of tobacco smoke encountered on many commercial and industrial premises as well as on public transport. These difficulties can often be overcome, though a suitable environment is not to be found at every workplace (fig. 19.3). It is an advantage if the building is of easy access, within easy travelling distance of home, and has a clean atmosphere. Ideally the work should be capable of being performed by the employee at his own pace. Night-shift work is usually well tolerated, as are jobs which entail light activity. Such jobs often have the additional advantage of better long-term prospects than employment which is entirely sedentary. Prospects such as these in a firm willing to employ a quota of genuinely disabled persons should provide a second career for those who really want one. This is a good solution to a situation which is distressingly common but which should never have arisen in the first place.

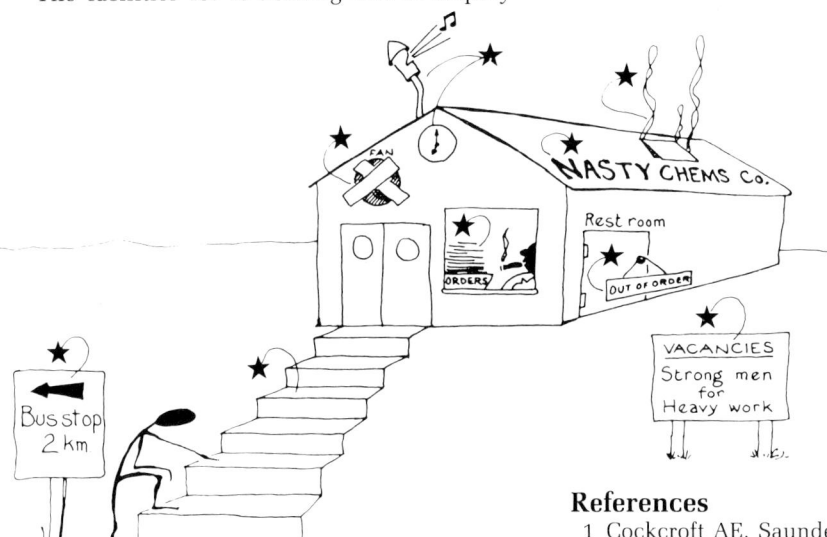

Fig. 19.3. 'A suitable environment is not to be found in every work place.' Adverse features are indicated by stars.

References

1 Cockcroft AE, Saunders MJ, Berry B. See page 405, ref. 9.
2 Royal College of Physicians. Report by the College Committee on Thoracic Medicine. Disabling chest disease: prevention and care. *J Roy Coll Physcn Lond* 1981;**15**:69–87.

Author Index

Page numbers in *italic* give locations of
the full reference citation.

Subject Index

Page numbers in *italics* give locations of references
which provide additional information.
Where entries are not in numerical order,
the principal entry is given first.